ISBN 978-0-483-39857-3
PIBN 10726891

4

THE

AMERICAN JOURNAL

OF THE MEDICAL SCIENCES

FOR OCTOBER 1856.

CONTRIBUTORS TO THIS VOLUME.

WM. J. ALEXANDER, M. D., *of Salem, Va.*

CHARLES E. BELLAMY, M. D., *of Columbus, Georgia.*

GEORGE C. BLACKMAN, M. D., *Professor of Surgery in the Medical College of Ohio.*

JOHN H. BRINTON, M. D., *of Philadelphia.*

CHARLES E. BUCKINGHAM, M. D., *of Boston.*

W. H. BYFORD, M. D., *of Evansville, Indiana.*

D. F. CONDIE, M. D., *of Philadelphia.*

JNO. C DALTON, JR., M. D., *Professor of Physiology in the College of Physicians and Surgeons of the City of New York.*

PLINY EARLE, M. D., *of New York.*

THOMAS ADDIS EMMET, M. D., *late Visiting Physician to the New York State Emigrant Hospital, Wards' Island.*

AUSTIN FLINT, M. D., *Professor of Clinical Medicine and Pathology in the University of Buffalo.*

CHARLES FRICK, M. D., *of Baltimore.*

WILLIAM A. HAMMOND, M. D., *Assistant Surgeon U. S. A.*

EDWARD HARTSHORNE, M. D., *one of the Surgeons to Wills Hospital.*

ISAAC HAYS, M. D., *of Philadelphia.*

F. HINKLE, M. D., *of Marietta, Lancaster Co., Pa.*

G. B. HOTCHKIN, M. D., *of Media, Pennsylvania.*

H. G. JAMESON, M. D., *late of Baltimore.*

JOSEPH JONES, M. D., *of Georgia.*

EDWIN C. LEEDOM, M. D., *of Plymouth, Montgomery Co., Pa.*

G. B. LINDERMAN, M. D., *of Mauch Chunk, Pennsylvania.*

H. C. MATTHEWS, *of St. Louis, Missouri.*

RICHARD McSHERRY, M. D., *of Baltimore.*

J. C. NOTT, M. D., *of Mobile, Alabama.*

ISAAC G. PORTER, M. D., *of New London, Connecticut.*

JOHN B. PORTER, M. D., *Surgeon U. S. A.*

W. RICHARDSON, M. D., *late Assistant Physician in the Hospital Blackwell's Island.*

B. ROEMER, M. D.

ALFRED STILLÉ, M. D., *Professor of Theory and Practice of Medicine in Pennsylvania College, Philadelphia.*

HORATIO R. STORER, M. D., *one of the Physicians to the Boston Lying-in Hospital.*

J. C. TABER, M. D., *of Charleston, S. C.*

R. P. THOMAS, M. D., *Professor of Materia Medica in the Philadelphia College of Pharmacy.*

JAMES D. TRASK, M. D., *of White Plains, New York.*

DAVID R. WALTON, M. D.

JAMES J. WARING, M. D., *of Washington, D. C.*

CHARLES W. WRIGHT, M. D., *Professor of Chemistry in the Kentucky School of Medicine.*

THE
AMERICAN JOURNAL
OF THE
MEDICAL SCIENCES.

EDITED BY

ISAAC HAYS, M.D.,

FELLOW OF THE PHILADELPHIA COLLEGE OF PHYSICIANS; MEMBER OF THE AMERICAN MEDICAL ASSOCIATION; OF THE AMERICAN PHILOSOPHICAL SOCIETY; OF THE ACADEMY OF NATURAL SCIENCES OF PHILADELPHIA, &c. &c. &c.

NEW SERIES.

VOL. XXXII.

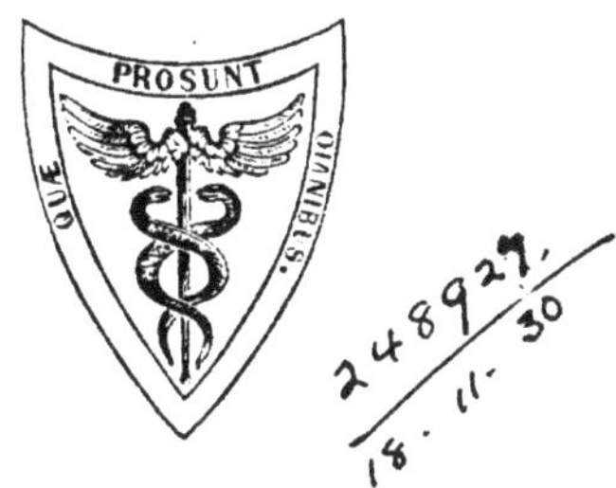

PHILADELPHIA:
BLANCHARD & LEA.

1856.

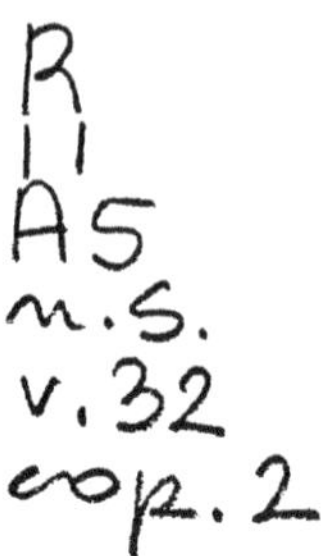

PHILADELPHIA:

T. K. AND P. G. COLLINS, PRINTERS.

TO READERS AND CORRESPONDENTS.

The following works have been received:—

Memoir on the Cholera at Oxford in the year 1854, with Considerations Suggested by the Epidemic. By Henry Wentworth Acland, M. D., F. R. S., F. R. G. S., etc., F. R. C. P., Physician to the Radcliffe Infirmary, etc. London: John Churchill and J. H. & J. Parker. Oxford: 1851. (From the Author.)

Digestion and its Derangements: The Principles of Rational Medicine Applied to Disorders of the Alimentary Canal. By Thomas K. Chambers, M. D., F. C. P., etc. London: John Churchill, 1856. (From the Author.)

Cours Théorique et Clinique de Pathologie Interne et de Thérapie Médicale. Par E. Gintrac, Professeur de Clinique Interne et Directeur de l'Ecole de Médecine de Bordeaux, &c. &c. &c. Tom. I, II, III. Paris: Germer Bailliere, 1853. (From the Author.)

On the Nature, Treatment, and Prevention of Pulmonary Consumption, and incidentally of Scrofula, with a Demonstration of the Cause of the Disease. By Henry McCormac, M. D. London: 1855. (From the Author.)

Deux Mémoires sur la Physiologie de la Moelle Epinière lus a l'Academie des Sciences le 27 Août et le 24 Sept. 1855. Par le Docteur E. Brown-Séquard, Lauréat de l'Académie des Sciences, etc. (From the Author.)

Recherches Expérimentales sur la Transmission Croisée des Impressions Sensitives dans la Moelle Epinière. Par le Docteur E. Brown-Séquard, Lauréat de l'Académie des Sciences. Paris, 1855. (From the Author.)

Propriétés et Fonctions de la Moelle Epinière: Rapport sur quelques Experiences de M. Brown-Séquard, lu a la Société de Biologie le 21 Juillet, 1855. Par M. Paul Broca, Professeur Agrégé à la Faculté de Médecine, etc. Paris, 1855. (From Dr. Brown-Séquard.)

Recherches Expérimentales sur la Production d'une Affection Convulsive Epileptiforme à la Suite de Lesions de la Moelle Epinière. Par le Docteur E. Brown-Séquard, Lauréat de l'Académie des Sciences, etc. Mémoire lu à l'Académie des Sciences, le 21 Jan. 1856. (From the Author.)

Thèse pour le Doctorat en Médecine. Presentée et contenue à la Faculté de Médecine de Paris. Par George Henry Brandt, né a Ponta-Delgada (São-Miguel-Iles Açores), Docteur en Médecine, Honore d'une Medaille pour le Cholera en 1849. Paris, 1855. (From Dr. E. Brown-Séquard.)

Human Physiology. By Robley Dunglison, M. D., LL. D., Professor of the Institutes of Medicine in Jefferson Medical College, Philadelphia. With five hundred and thirty-two Illustrations. Eighth edition, revised, modified, and enlarged; in two volumes. Philadelphia: Blanchard & Lea, 1856. (From the Publishers.)

New Remedies, with Formulæ for their Preparation and Administration. By Robley Dunglison, M. D., &c. Seventh edition, with numerous additions. Philadelphia: Blanchard & Lea, 1856. (From the Publishers.)

The Principles of Surgery. By James Miller, F. R. S. E., F. R. C. S. E., Author of a Treatise on the Practice of Surgery, Surgeon in Ordinary to the Queen for Scotland, etc. Fourth American, from the third and revised London edition. Illustrated by two hundred and forty engravings on wood. Philadelphia: Blanchard & Lea, 1856. (From the Publishers.)

The Dissector's Manual of Practical and Surgical Anatomy. By Erasmus Wilson, F. R. S., Author of a "System of Human Anatomy." The third American from the last revised London edition. Illustrated with one hundred and fifty-four wood engravings. Edited by William Hunt, M. D., Demonstrator of Anatomy in the University of Pennsylvania. Philadelphia: Blanchard & Lea, 1856. (From the Publishers.)

The Microscope aud its Revelations. By William B. Carpenter, M. D., F. R. S., F. G. S., Examiner in Physiology and Comparative Anatomy in the University of London, Professor of Medical Jurisprudence in University College, etc. With an Appendix, containing the Applications of the Microscope to Clinical Medicine, etc., by Francis Gurney Smith, M. D., Professor of the

Institutes of Medicine in the Medical Department of Pennsylvania College, etc. Illustrated by four hundred and thirty-four engravings on wood. Philadelphia: Blanchard & Lea, 1856. (From the Publishers.)

Atlas of Cutaneous Diseases. By J. Moore Neligan, M. D., Edin., M. R. I. A., Honorary Doctor of Medicine, Trinity College, Dublin, Fellow of the King and Queen's College of Physicians in Ireland, etc. etc. Philadelphia: Blanchard & Lea, 1856. (From the Publishers.)

A Practical Handbook of Medical Chemistry. By John E. Bowman, F. C. S., Professor of Practical Chemistry, King's College, London. Second American from the third and revised London edition, with Illustrations. Philadelphia: Blanchard & Lea, 1856. (From the Publishers.)

The Principles and Practice of Ophthalmic Medicine and Surgery. By T. Wharton Jones, F. R. S., Professor of Ophthalmic Medicine and Surgery in University College, London, Ophthalmic Surgeon to the Hospital, etc. With one hundred and ten Illustrations. Second American edition, with additions, from the second and revised London edition. Philadelphia: Blanchard & Lea, 1856. (From the Publishers.)

An Analytical Compendium of the Various Branches of Medical Science for the use and examination of Students. By John Neill, M. D., Surgeon to the Pennsylvania Hospital, Fellow of the College of Physicians, etc., and Francis Gurney Smith, M. D., Physician to St. Joseph's Hospital, Fellow of the College of Physicians, etc. A new edition, revised and improved, with three hundred and seventy-four Illustrations. Philadelphia: Blanchard & Lea, 1856. (From the Publishers.)

On Some Diseases of Women admitting of Surgical Treatment. By Isaac Baker Brown, F. R. C. S. (By Exam.), Surgeon Accoucheur to St. Mary's Hospital, Vice-President of the Medical Society of London, etc. etc. Illustrated by twenty-four wood engravings. Philadelphia: Blanchard & Lea, 1856. (From the Publishers.)

A Practical Treatise on Diseases of the Testis, and of the Spermatic Cord and Scrotum. With numerous wood engravings. By T. B. Curling, F. R. S., Surgeon to the London Hospital, Lecturer on Surgery at the London Hospital Medical College, etc. Second American from the second revised and enlarged English edition. Philadelphia, Blanchard & Lea, 1856. (From the Publishers.)

Medical Jurisprudence. By Alfred Taylor, M. D., F. R. S., F. R. C. P., and Lecturer on Medical Jurisprudence and Chemistry in Guy's Hospital. Fourth American from the fifth and improved London edition. Edited, with additions, by Edward Hartshorne, M. D., one of the Surgeons to Wills' Hospital, etc. Philadelphia: Blanchard & Lea, 1856. (From the Publishers.)

Headaches, their Causes and their Cure. By Henry G. Wright, M. D., M. R. C. S. L., L. S. A., Fellow of Royal Medico-Chirurgical Society, Physician to the St. Pancras Royal Dispensary. New York: S. S. and W. Wood, 1856. (From the Publishers.) London: John Churchill. (From the Author.)

Cases in Midwifery, with Remarks, by Thomas F. Cock, M. D., Physician to the New York Hospital. New York: S. S. & W. Wood, 1856.

The Medical Profession in Ancient Times. An Anniversary Discourse delivered before the New York Academy of Medicine, November 7, 1855. By John Watson, M. D., Surgeon to the New York Hospital. (Published by order of the Academy.) New York, 1856. (From the Author.)

Eulogy on the Life and Character of Theodoric Romeyn Beck, M. D., LL.D. Delivered before the Medical Society of the State of New York. By Frank H. Hamilton, M. D. Published by order of the Senate. Albany, 1856. (From the Author.)

The Causes and Curative Treatment of Sterility, with a preliminary Statement of the Physiology of Generation. By Augustus K. Gardner, A. M., M. D., Permanent Member of the American Medical Association, Fellow of the New York Academy of Medicine, Member of the Massachusetts Medical Society, etc. New York: De Witt & Davenport, 1856.

Remarks on Vesico-Vaginal Fistule, with an Account of a New Mode of Suture, and Seven Successful Operations. By N. Bozeman, M. D., of Montgomery, Ala. Louisville, 1856. (From the Author.)

Essay on Cholera Infantum, for which the prize of the New York Academy of Medicine was awarded, March 5, 1856. By James STEWART, M. D., Author of a "Practical Treatise on the Diseases of Children." New York, 1856. (From the Author.)

Transactions of the State Medical Society, transmitted to the Legislature February 8, 1856. Albany, 1856.

Proceedings of the Convention and of the Medical Society of the State of California, held in Sacramento, March, 1856. Sacramento, Cal., 1856.

Transactions of the South Carolina Medical Association at the extra meeting in Greenwood, July 18, 1855, and at the annual meeting in Charleston, February 6, 1856. Charleston, 1856.

Third Annual Report relating to the Registry and Returns of Births, Marriages, and Deaths in the State of Kentucky from January 1, 1854 to December 31, 1854. Frankfort, Ky., 1856.

Annual Report of the Officers of the Insane Asylum of the State of California for the year 1855. James Allen, State Printer.

Thirteenth Annual Report of the Managers of the State Lunatic Asylum at Utica. Albany, 1856.

City Registrar's Report on the Births, Marriages, and Deaths in the City of Providence during the year ending December 31, 1855. With an Appendix, showing the Mortality of Providence during fifteen years, from 1840 to 1854, inclusive. Providence, 1856.

Thirty-Ninth Annual Report on the State of the Asylum for the Relief of Persons Deprived of the use of their Reason. Published by direction of the Contributors. Third month, 1856. Philadelphia, 1856.

Report of the Joint Special Committee on the Census of Boston, May, 1855; including the Report of the Censors, with Analytical and Sanitary Observations. By JOSHUA CURTIS, M.D. Boston, 1856. (From the Author.)

The following Journals have been received in exchange:—

Gazette Médicale de Paris. February, March, April, and May, 1856.

Revue de Thérapeutique Médico-Chirurgicale. Par A. MARTIN-LAUZER. February, March, April, and May, 1856.

Journal de Médecine de Bordeaux. Redacteur en chef, M. COSTES. January and February, 1856.

Moniteur des Hôpitaux. March, April, and May, 1856.

Archives D'Ophthalmologie. Par M. A. JAMAIN. Nov. and Dec., 1855.

Annales Médico-Psychologiques. Par MM. les Docteurs BAILLARGER CARISE et MOREAU. April, 1856.

El Porvenir Médico. Periodico Oficial de la Academia Quirurgica Matritense. February, 1856.

Medical Times and Gazette. March, April, and May, 1856.

Edinburgh Medical Journal. March, April, and May, 1856.

Association Medical Journal. Edited by ANDREW WYNTER, M. D. February, March, and April, 1856.

Dublin Medical Press. March, April, and May, 1856.

The Glasgow Medical Journal. April, 1856.

Journal of Public Health and Sanitary Review. Edited by B. W. RICHARDSON, M. D. April, 1856.

The Journal of Psychological Medicine and Mental Pathology. Edited by FORBES WINSLOW, D. C. L. April, 1856.

The British and Foreign Medico-Chirurgical Review. April, 1856.

The Dublin Hospital Gazette. April, May, and June, 1856.

The Medical Chronicle, or Montreal Monthly Journal of Medicine and Surgery. Edited by W. WRIGHT, M. D., and D. C. MACCALLUM, M. D. April, May, and June, 1856.

The Boston Medical and Surgical Journal. Edited by Drs. SMITH, MORLAND, and MINOT. April, May, and June, 1856.

St. Louis Medical and Surgical Journal. Edited by Drs. LINTON and McPHEETERS. March and May, 1856.

The American Medical Gazette. Edited by D. M. Reese, M. D. April and June, 1856.

New Orleans Medical News and Hospital Gazette. Edited by Drs. Choppin, Beard, and Brickell. March, April, and June, 1856.

Atlanta Medical and Surgical Journal. Edited by Drs. Logan and Westmoreland. April and May, 1856.

The Medical Examiner. Edited by Samuel L. Hollingsworth, M. D. April, May, and June, 1856.

The North-Western Medical and Surgical Journal. Edited by N. S. Davis, M. D., and H. A. Johnson, M. D. March, April, May, and June, 1856.

The Cincinnati Medical Observer. Edited by Drs. Mendenhall, Murphy, and Stevens. April, May, and June, 1856.

New York Medical Times. Edited by H. D. Bulkley, M. D. April, May, and June, 1856.

The American Journal of Insanity. Edited by the Officers of the New York State Lunatic Asylum. April, 1856.

Southern Medical and Surgical Journal. Edited by Drs. Dugas and Rossignol. April, May, and June, 1856.

The American Medical Monthly. Edited by Edward H. Parker, M. D. April, May, and June, 1856.

Nashville Journal of Medicine and Surgery. Edited by W. K. Bowling, M. D., and Paul F. Eve, M. D. April and May, 1856.

The Peninsular Journal of Medicine and the Collateral Sciences. Edited by Z. Pitcher, M. D., and A. B. Palmer, M. D. April and May, 1856.

The Virginia Medical Journal. Edited by Drs. McCaw and Otis. April and June, 1856.

The Western Lancet. Edited by T. Wood, M. D. April, May, and June, 1856.

The American Journal of Dental Science. Edited by Chapin A. Harris, M. D., D. D. S., and A. Snowden Piggot, M. D. April, 1856.

The Medical and Surgical Reporter. Edited by S. W. Butler, M. D. April, May, and June, 1856.

The Medical Counsellor. Edited by R. Hills, M. D. April, May, and June, 1856.

The New Hampshire Journal of Medicine. Edited by Geo. H. Hubbard, M. D. April, May, and June, 1856.

The Monthly Stethoscope and Medical Reporter. Edited by G. A. Wilson, M. D., and R. A. Lewis, M. D. April, May, and June, 1856.

Buffalo Medical Journal. Edited by Sanford B. Hunt, M. D. April, May, and June, 1856.

The New York Journal of Medicine. Edited by S. S. Purple, M. D., and S. Smith, M. D. May, 1856.

The American Journal of Science and Arts. Edited by Profs. B. Silliman, B. Silliman, Jr., and D. Dana. May, 1856.

The Medical Independent. Edited by Henry Goadby, M. D., E. Kane, M. D., and L. G. Robinson, M. D. May and June, 1856.

American Journal of Pharmacy. Edited by William Procter, Jr. May, 1856.

Charleston Medical Journal and Review. Edited by C. Happoldt, M. D. May, 1856.

The Louisville Review. Edited by S. D. Gross, M. D., and T. G. Richardson, M. D. May, 1856.

The Ohio Medical and Surgical Journal. Edited by John Dawson, M. D., and R. Gundry, M. D. May, 1856.

Memphis Medical Recorder. Edited by A. P. Merrill, M. D. May, 1856.

Iowa Medical Journal. Edited by Drs. M. Gugin and Allen. March and April, 1856.

The Southern Journal of the Medical and Physical Sciences. Edited by Drs. Currey, Jones, Atchison, King, and Ramsey. May, 1856.

Quarterly Summary of the Transactions of the College of Physicians of Philadelphia, from November 7, 1855, to February 6, 1856, inclusive.

CONTENTS

OF THE

AMERICAN JOURNAL

OF THE

MEDICAL SCIENCES.

NO. LXIII. NEW SERIES.

JULY, 1856.

ORIGINAL COMMUNICATIONS.

MEMOIRS AND CASES.

REVIEWS.

BIBLIOGRAPHICAL NOTICES.

QUARTERLY SUMMARY

OF THE

IMPROVEMENTS AND DISCOVERIES IN THE MEDICAL SCIENCES.

FOREIGN INTELLIGENCE.

Anatomy and Physiology.

Materia Medica and Pharmacy.

Medical Pathology and Therapeutics, and Practical Medicine.

Surgical Pathology and Therapeutics, and Operative Surgery.

Ophthalmology.

Midwifery.

Medical Jurisprudence and Toxicology.

AMERICAN INTELLIGENCE.

Original Communications.

Domestic Summary.

Communications intended for publication, and Books for Review, should be sent, *free of expense*, directed to ISAAC HAYS, M. D., Editor of the American Journal of the Medical Sciences, care of Messrs. Blanchard & Lea, Philadelphia. Parcels directed as above, and (carriage paid) under cover, to John Miller, Henrietta Street, Covent Garden, *London;* or M. Hector Bossange, Lib. quai Voltaire, No. 11, *Paris*, will reach us safely and without delay. We particularly request the attention of our foreign correspondents to the above, as we are often subjected to unnecessary expense for postage and carriage.

ALL REMITTANCES OF MONEY, and letters on the *business* of the Journal, should be addressed *exclusively* to the publishers, Messrs. Blanchard & Lea.

☞ The advertisement-sheet belongs to the business department of the Journal, and all communications for it should be made to the publishers.

THE

AMERICAN JOURNAL

OF THE MEDICAL SCIENCES

FOR JULY 1856.

ART. I.—*Physical, Chemical, and Physiological Investigations upon the Vital Phenomena, Structure, and Offices of the Solids and Fluids of Animals.* By JOS. JONES, M. D., of Georgia. (An Inaugural Dissertation for the Degree of M. D., in the University of Pennsylvania.)

Preliminary Remarks.—These investigations were carried on during two summer vacations, in Liberty County, Georgia, where the author had access to the Fishes, Reptiles, Birds, and Mammalia inhabiting the sea, salt water rivers, marshes, and inland forests, swamps, and rice fields. Some of the difficulties which attended them will be evident from the following extract from Dr. Holbrook's admirable work upon North American Herpetology:—[1]

"The science which treats of the form, organization, habits, and history of Reptiles, has been more neglected than all other branches of Zoology; for the study of Reptiles offers difficulties more numerous and insurmountable than those presented by any other class of vertebrate animals. Inhabiting, for the most part, deep and extensive swamps, infected with malaria, and abounding with diseases during the summer months, when reptiles are most numerous, time is wanting to observe their modes of life with any prospect of success. Regarded, moreover, by most persons as objects of detestation, represented as venomous, and possessed of the most noxious properties, few have been hardy enough to study their character and habits."

Added to these difficulties which beset the way of the naturalist, the organic chemist and physiologist must often spend many fatiguing hours in fruitless attempts to secure alive the shy and wary Ophidians, Saurians, and Chelonians. After wading through the swamps and marshes for half a day, if a living subject should be secured, it must be carried home, and its blood and organs examined without delay. The difficulties of careful organic ana-

[1] North American Herpetology, by J. E. Holbrook, M. D., Vol. i. page 10, Philadelphia, 1836.

lysis, and physiological investigations, are greatly increased by the previous fatigues and exposures. We hope that those who are disposed to criticise the extent and character of these investigations, will remember the difficulties with which we had to contend.

My investigations extended over the four great classes of vertebrate animals, and did not embrace the invertebrate kingdom. It was necessary, also, to consider carefully the laws which govern the structure and development of invertebrate animals. The chapter upon their solids and fluids, contains a condensed summary of those facts and principles, mentioned by various modern and ancient Comparative Anatomists, which have an immediate bearing upon our investigations. The sections upon the structure and development of the circulatory and respiratory systems contain not only a condensed view of the important facts mentioned by the various writers, but also original observations made from numerous dissections, and accurate weights of the hearts and organs.

I cannot enter upon these investigations without first acknowledging the numerous and lasting obligations which I owe to my revered teacher and friend, Dr. Samuel Jackson, Professor of the Institutes of Medicine in the University of Pennsylvania. The greatest pleasure of this truly noble and generous philosopher, is to inspire the minds of his students with his own ardent love for the truth. If these investigations possess any value, it is due as much to his brilliant instruction, kind advice, and generous assistance, as to my own exertions. I would also return my hearty thanks to Dr. Edward Hallowell, of this city, for numerous opportunities of examining the viscera of rare reptiles.[1]

[1] To those who may wish to pursue the study of comparative anatomy, physiology, and chemistry, I would respectfully recommend the following works, which are readily accessible to American students.

It would be, perhaps, useless, to give a list of the numeous articles scattered throughout the different Journals, as it would be of service to those only who live in cities, and have access to large scientific libraries, and are without doubt well acquainted with these subjects.

Anatomy of the Invertebrata. By Siebold; translated by W. J. Burnett, M. D. Boston, 1854.

Anatomy of the Invertebrata. By Richard Owen. London, 1855.

Dana on Zoophytes. Philadelphia, 1846.

General Outline of the Organization of the Animal Kingdom. By Thomas Rymer Jones, F. R. S. London, 1855.

Wagner's Comparative Anatomy of the Vertebrate Animals. Translated by Alfred Tulk. New York, 1845.

Outlines of Comparative Physiology. By Louis Agassiz and A. A. Gould. Boston, 1848; republished in Bohu's Scientific Library. London, 1851.

Carpenter's Principles of Comparative Physiology. London, 1854, and Philadelphia, 1854.

Müller on the Glands. Translated by S. Solly. London, 1839.

Griffith's Cuvier's Animal Kingdom, 16 vols. London, 1832.

Vital Force.—In studying the progressive development of the blood, and the organs and apparatuses of the invertebrate and vertebrate kingdoms, we are met with difficulties at every step of our progress. Errors of observation, arising from imperfections of our senses and instruments, and errors arising from mental preconceptions and prejudices, obscure the light of truth. Another source of difficulty and error, arises from the complex nature of all the phenomena, and the limited extent of our knowledge. Oftentimes, those who have had the best opportunities for observing the secret operations of nature, have devoted their undivided time and attention simply to the description of the habits, exterior forms, and colours, of plants and animals. These observations are all useful, and aid profound researches by affording classifications, and determining the geographical distribution of living animals. They may give us a general insight into a few of the obvious phenomena of life, but they can never unfold the laws which regulate the development of the animal and vegetable kingdoms. A knowledge of these can only be ac-

North American Herpetology. By J. E. Holbrook, M. D., Professor of Anatomy in Medical College of the State of South Carolina. 5 vols. Philadelphia, 1842.

Human Anatomy. By J. Quain, M. D., and W. Sharpey, M. D. Philad., 1849.

Kölliker's Microscopical Anatomy. Translated under the direction of the Sydenham Society. Philadelphia, 1854.

Müller's Physiology. Translated by W. Baly, M. D. London, 1840.

The Chemistry of Animal and Vegetable Physiology. By G. J. Mulder. Translated by J. T. W. Johnson. London, 1849.

Simon's Animal Chemistry, with reference to the Physiology and Pathology of Man. Translated by G. E. Day. Philadelphia, 1846.

Traité de Chimie, Anatomique et Physiologique, &c. Par C. Robin and F. Verdeil. Paris, 1853.

Bernard and Robin on the Blood. Translated by Atlee. Philadelphia, 1854.

Memoirs on Respiration. By Lazarus Spallanzani. London, 1805.

Digestion. By Lazarus Spallanzani. London, 1800.

Lectures on the Physical Phenomena of Living Beings. By C. Matteucci. Translated by J. Pereira, M. D. Philadelphia, 1848.

Manual of Physiology. By W. S. Kirkes, M. D., and J. Paget. Philad., 1849.

Carpenter's Principles of Human Physiology. Philadelphia, 1856.

Carpenter's Principles of General Physiology, including Organic Chemistry and Histology. Philadelphia, 1854.

Longet—Treatise on Physiology. Translated by F. G. Smith, M. D. Philad., 1856.

Lehmann's Physiological Chemistry. Translated by G. E. Day, M. D., and edited by Prof. R. E. Rogers. Philadelphia, 1855.

Lehmann's Manual of Chemical Physiology. Translated by J. C. Morris, with an Essay on Vital Force, by Dr. Samuel Jackson. Philadelphia, 1856.

Manuals of Blood and Urine. By Griffith, Reese, and Markwick. Philad., 1848.

Golding Bird on Urinary Deposits. Philadelphia, 1854.

Bowman's Practical Chemistry. Philadelphia, 1849.

A Practical Handbook of Medical Chemistry. By J. E. Bowman. Philad., 1856.

Kidneys and Urine. By Berzelius. Philadelphia, 1843.

Prout on Urinary Diseases. Philadelphia, 1826.

quired by studying carefully all the chemical, physical, and vital phenomena, and by examining the development, structure, and function of all the organs, apparatuses, and systems, commencing with the simplest, and ascending to the most complex organism.

Although this science may be said to be but in its infancy, still we have facts sufficient to show, that there is a grand uniformity in the plan of the development of all the component parts of the animal kingdom. By this we do not mean, that the organs and apparatuses of every higher animal pass through in their development, successively, all the forms of those placed below in the scale of creation. Neither is it possible to arrange all animals in one straight line, commencing with the simple cell animalcule, and ending with the complicated organism of man. While the vital force which presides over the development of all organized beings has certain common properties, and fashions after certain common methods, inorganic and organic materials, still each species, genus, order, and class of animals has its own peculiar properties of the vital force, which acts according to fixed and immutable laws, established by the Creator, and which can be altered by him alone. We have a demonstration of this in the fact, that different species, genera, and classes of animals, have retained their identity from generation to generation, from the foundation of the world. All the facts of geology prove that the laws which regulate the development of animals, are fixed and immutable. Varieties may arise, but one species has never been transmuted into another by either physical or chemical influences. If this were not so, where would the foundation of the science of Natural History, in its most extended sense, be laid? The creation of a force, by whose modifications the physical and vital constitution of every living being on earth, in air or water, is precisely adapted to fulfil certain definite ends, necessarily presupposes a Creator, who constructed, comprehended, and controlled all the physical, chemical, and vital laws which regulate the universe. Whether the human mind will ever be able to grasp in one view all the modifications, phenomena, and laws of life, remains for future researches to show. The comprehension of the phenomena of life in the higher animals, necessarily requires not only a perfect knowledge of all the chemical and physical laws which govern all matter, but also of that subtle force, which, like the mind, has escaped the view of all observers.

Before proceeding to the physical, chemical, anatomical, and physiological investigations of the blood and organs of different animals, it is necessary that we should give sufficient proof of the existence of a vital force, distinct from the nervous, chemical, and physical forces.

Certain physiologists have denied the existence of a vital force. Others, admitting its existence, affirm that it is identical with nervous force; and nervous force they prove to be identical with electricity. According to this doctrine, the vital and nervous forces are purely physical phenomena.

Those who deny the existence of any peculiar vital or organizing force, must admit that suitable matter, placed under the requisite conditions for the production of living beings, will be capable of generating animals by simple physical and chemical means. Careful experiments have been performed by Dr. Joseph Leidy[1] and others,[2] by placing the elements of organic structures under all the requisite conditions for the commencement and maintenance of life action; and never have they discovered a single instance where a living being, animal or vegetable, even of the simplest structure, has been produced by these physical agents alone. Place a germ under these conditions of heat, moisture, and a supply of oxygen, and immediately it begins to develop an organized being. It is a universal law of nature, that every living being has descended from a germ, which was derived from a parent, and the first parent was the creation of the Deity. Through these microscopical points of matter have been transmitted from generation to generation, unchanged, all the peculiarities of each species, genus, and class. What a concentration of forces! Wherein does a germ differ from any other form of organized matter? The ultimate chemical elements are the same with a piece of muscle, and yet, when placed under precisely the same conditions, the one putrefies, whilst the other develops a living being. Have we here no proof of a special force?

Again: take two germs—they are alike in appearance, and ultimate chemical constitution, and require precisely the same conditions for their development, and yet one will form a cold-blooded animal, whose circulation is sluggish, nervous system imperfectly developed, the chemical and physical changes in its blood slow, and all the phenomena of life correspondingly feeble; whilst from the other will be developed a bird, whose circulation is rapid, nervous system highly developed, the changes in the elements of its tissues and blood incessant, and its temperature correspondingly high. Whence this difference? Does not this show that each species in the animal economy is endowed with its own special vital force? That this difference is due to this and this alone, is demonstrated by a fundamental law, that like causes produce like effects. If there be no vital force, organic matter placed in certain circumstances, and acted upon by definite chemical and physical laws, must always yield the same results. Organic matter placed in the situation of these germs, is invariably decomposed into simpler forms, and finally resolved into its ultimate chemical elements. Under the same circumstances, and acted upon by the same agents, the action of the germ is directly opposite, being that of construction, building up, instead of decomposition and destruction.

The chemical and physical forces always act in a direction directly oppo-

[1] Flora and Fauna within Living Animals, by Joseph Leidy. Smithsonian Contributions to Knowledge, vol. v. art. 2, 1853, p. 11.

[2] By F. Schulze, Berlin. Edinburgh New Philos. Journal, vol. xxiii. p. 165, 1837.

site to that of the vital force. The former are constant and invariable in their intensity and direction under like circumstances, whilst the latter varies in direction and intensity. When, therefore, they act simultaneously upon matter, the living being the resultant of these actions will be imperfectly or highly developed, according as the vital force is feeble or powerful.

The great distinction, then, between animals of different species and classes, depends originally upon the vital force, which presides over the development of every molecule of organized matter, and guides and controls all its physical and chemical actions. According to the perfection of this organic or vital force will be the development of the organic system, and centralization of the forces.

The lowest plants and animals consist of simple cells without any special organs or apparatuses. In these simple forms, the germ force is distributed equally through every molecule of matter. Trembley[1] performed a series of careful experiments upon reproduction by artificial sections in the Hydra. One hydra was cut in half, and each became a perfect animal; another was divided into three portions, and a head produced a tail, the middle portion a head and a tail, and the tail a head. New tentacles replaced those cut off, and a longitudinal cut in the body was soon united. Different individuals were engrafted upon each other, as is frequently done in trees. The heads and tails of two polyps were mutually changed, and they united perfectly, or what is still more curious, the tail of one may be substituted for the head of another; and if the tail of one be placed in the head of another, they unite heads and tails. A single hydra was divided into forty parts, and as many distinct animals were formed.

No such results have ever been obtained with the higher animals. According as the nervous system is developed, the index of the vital force, will be the centralization and perfection of all the forces. Hence, for the formation of the germ in the higher animals, we have special apparatuses. If the original germ cells of any organ or highly developed tissue be destroyed, they can never be replaced. The wound in the skin or muscles is never united by true skin or muscular fibres, but by the simplest form of tissue, the fibrous, which is analogous to that which composes the whole mass of the lower animals.

The next question which demands our attention is, whether or not the vital and nervous forces are distinct?

In nature there exist two great kingdoms. They both arise from one common origin—the organic cell. In the twilight of animal existence, the simple cell-animalcule can hardly be distinguished from the sporules of vegetables. The simplest forms of animals have been often confounded with

[1] A. Trembley, on Freshwater Polyps, 1 vol. 4to. Leyden, 1744; and Phil. Trans., vol. viii. of Abridgment, 1742. See also Baker's Natural History of the Polype, 8vo. London, 1743. Rare and Remarkable Animals of Scotland, by J. G. Dalyell, vol. i. p. 28. Prof. F. Forbes' British Star-Fishes, p. 199.

plants, by the best observers, and the character of many of these individuals is still involved in obscurity. Every day the distinctions between the two kingdoms are disappearing. Most of the important organic products which were thought to distinguish the vegetable from the animal, have been found in both kingdoms. Cellulose has been discovered in the brain,[1] spleen,[2] and liver; and sugar[3] is the constant product of the action of the liver from both nitrogenized and non-nitrogenized organic matters. Motion no longer separates the animal from the vegetable world. This property of matter appears to be most incessantly exercised in the minutest organisms. The motion of the minute ciliæ of vegetables is known to every one. The contraction of the leaves of the sensitive plant is a familiar example. The only distinction between the lowest orders of the two kingdoms, the Protozoa and Algæ, is that the former possess, to a certain extent, voluntary mótion.

In the vegetable kingdom, from the simple cell to the most complex and highly developed tree, we discover not the first rudiment of a nervous apparatus, or a cell-generating nervous force. Here we have the evidences of the existence of a force requiring the same conditions for its existence and operations—heat, moisture, oxygen, and a germ—which are necessary for the production of an animal organism entirely independent of any nervous system. Does not this fact demonstrate conclusively, that nervous force is entirely distinct from the vital?

The conclusion is sustained also by facts drawn from the animal kingdom. In the lowest forms of animals, not even the rudiment of a nerve-cell can be discovered, and yet these beings possess the attributes of vitality, and even nervous force. They carry on all the acts of digestion, secretion, nutrition, and growth; possess voluntary motions, and are capable of receiving impressions from without. Dana,[4] in his work upon Zoophytes, states that, upon pressing the tip of a branch of a large Alcyonium, in the Fejees, there was an immediate contraction of every polyp throughout the whole zoophyte, although extending to a breadth of four feet, and composed of many thousands of individuals. The existence of any special nervous system in these animals is denied by the best comparative anatomists of the present day, and yet they possess the sensation of higher animals, manifested in the

[1] By Rudolph Virchow (Virchow's "Arch," B. vi. h. 1, p. 135). Also, by G. Busk, F.R.S. Journal of Microscopical Science, No. vi. p. 101.

[2] By R. Virchow, Comptes Rendus, No. 23, December 2, 1853. Monthly Journal of Medical Science, January, 1854.

[3] By M. Claude Bernard, "Nouvelle Fonction du Foie," Paris, 1853, chap. 11. See also, Secretion of Sugar by the Liver, and its modification by disease, by M. Vernois. Monthly Journal Med. Sci., Nov. 1853, from Archiv. Gén., 1853. Dr. Gilb, on the Relation that Fat bears to the Presence of Sugar in the Livers of the Mammalia and Birds. Paper read before the Physiological Section of the Medical Society of London (April 10, 1854). See Abstract in American Journal Med. Sci., July, 1854, p. 211.

[4] Structure and classification of Zoophytes, by J. D. Dana, p. 14. Philadelphia, 1846.

selection of food, and the reception of impressions from light and foreign bodies.

Again—has any one ever discovered nerves or nerve-cells in a germ? The primary nerve-cells are not formed until after the commencement of change, and the formation of the germ material into cells. The apparatus for the generation of the nervous force is the product of the vital force.

It is a remarkable fact, and one which gives confirmation to these views, that the cells—the active agents in the formation of all the secretions, and separation of all the excretions—are always separated from the bloodvessels and nerves, and in no case do they come in contact. The cell of the most complicated structure differs, as far as its acts are concerned, in no essential degree from that of a vegetable or simple cell-animalcule. Every cell in the whole animal and vegetable economy is capable of carrying on the offices of nutrition, secretion, and growth, whether they be supplied with nervous force, or deprived of it. Every individual animal or vegetable, simple or complex, is composed of organic cells; therefore, the conclusion is inevitable, that development, nutrition, secretion, and excretion, are directed by the vital force, which is incorporated with, and presides over, every molecule of organized matter, directing and controlling all its physical and chemical laws, so that amidst innumerable and unceasing changes, the individuality of every organ, apparatus, and animal is preserved. According to the development of this force will be the perfection of the organism which it constructs.

I. *Solids and Fluids of Invertebrate Animals.*—Before commencing the consideration of the blood and organs of cold-blooded animals, it will aid us, in the study of the progressive development of the fluids and solids of organized beings, to review briefly the fluids, organs, and apparatuses of the invertebrate kingdom. The classification is that adopted by Siebold.[1]

This science is by no means perfect, and every system of classification must be more or less imperfect. It is impossible to represent upon paper the relation existing between different classes, and their mode of connection with each other. The lowest members of a class which stands high in the system of classification are often as low, or lower, in the development of the nervous system and all the organs, than classes which stand far below. Notwithstanding that the lowest members of each class resemble each other in the simplicity of their structure and the absence of special organs, still the study of the invertebrate kingdom as a unit reveals general lines or systems of development branching up from the simple cell-animalcule to the highly organized Cephalopod. Therefore, in studying accurately the progressive development of the fluids and solids of these animals, we must commence with the lowest members of each class, and proceed to the highest. In the present article, however, we

[1] Comparative Anatomy of the Invertebrata, by Siebold. Translated from the German by W. J. Burnett, M. D. Boston, 1854.

can do no more than present those anatomical and physiological details and principles which have an immediate bearing upon our researches upon the vertebrata.

In the lowest forms of the Protozoa, which are simple cells provided with vibratile ciliæ, and resembling closely the sporules of vegetables, we find neither organs nor a circulatory system. Careful microscopical researches have failed to detect a nervous system; and yet these animals appear, by their voluntary motions, to possess sensation. If a nervous system exists, it must be reduced to its molecular condition.

In the highest members of this group we discover the first rudiments of a circulatory system, and an attempt at the interchange of the fluids from different parts of the body.

All the Stomatoda have contractile pulsatory cavities situated in the denser and outer layers of the parenchyma of the body, varying in form, number, and arrangement in different species. During their expansion, these cavities become filled with a clear, transparent, colourless liquid, which disappears entirely during the contraction. These movements succeed each other, ofttimes, at regular intervals. In some cases, however, regularity between the diastole and systole cannot be determined, owing to the number of these pulsatory cavities. No bloodvessels communicate with these cavities, and no special walls have been discovered surrounding them; and the fluid which they contain, although analogous to blood, contains no corpuscles. By these simple means, corresponding to the structure of these animals, the fluids of the body are prevented from stagnation, and a free interchange of the nutritive elements promoted.

In the Polypi—inarticulate fleshy bodies, having a simple visceral cavity, with a single opening at the centre above, without intestines, without glands separate from the walls of the visceral cavity, with no distinction of sex, and an imperfectly developed nervous system in the highest and none whatever in the lowest—the circulatory system is rudimentary, and the fluid which it distributes nothing but the digested matters of the visceral cavity. This circulatory fluid contains a few spherical corpuscles, apparently albuminous, and a few oil-globules. According to Dr. T. Williams,[1] a few of these corpuscles appear to be nucleated, others appear to contain secondary cells, and others, again, are charged with minute granules. The fluid is incapable of coagulation, and contains albumen in very small amount. In the tubular axis of colonial Polyps, which communicates with the visceral cavities of all the individuals composing the colony, something analogous to the circulation of the blood was discovered, by Cavolini,[2] in 1785. His observations have been con-

[1] Memoir on the Blood-proper, and Chylaqueous Fluid of Invertebrate Animals, by Dr. T. Williams. Philos. Transact., 1852. Brit. and For. Med.-Chir. Review, vol. xii. p. 484.

[2] "Memorie per Servire alla Storia de' Polipi Marini." Naples, 1785.

firmed by Dana, Lister, and other observers. From the article of J. J. Lister,[1] published in the *Philosophical Transactions*, we quote the following interesting observations upon the vibratory motion of the contents of the tubular axis of colonial Polyps:—

"The current flowed in one channel, alternately backwards and forwards, through the main stem and lateral branches of a plume, and through the root as far as the opacity admitted of its being traced; sometimes it was seen to continue into the cells. The stream was throughout in one direction at one time; it might be compared to the running of sand in an hour-glass, and was sometimes so rapid in midtide that the particles were hardly distinguishable; but it became much slower when near the change. Sometimes it returned almost without a pause; but at other times it was quiet for a while, or the particles took a confused whirling motion for a few seconds; the current afterwards appearing to set the stronger for the suspension. Five ebbs and five flows occupied fifteen minutes and a half; the same average time being spent in the ebb as in the flow."

Professor Dana, in his work upon Zoophytes,[2] states that, in his observations upon one of the Sertularidæ, the vibrating contents of the tubular axis had a greenish tint, and appeared to be derived in part from the digested food of the stomach. This circulation of the products of digestion, without any elaboration by special organs, reminds us strongly of the formation of the fluid contents of cells in the vegetable kingdom.

The nervous system of the highest species of the Acalephæ is more developed than that of the Polyps, and the blood and circulatory system appear to be correspondingly highly developed. The nervous system, however, is in too imperfect a condition to call for the production of any special organs. In these transparent gelatinous animals a circulatory system has been described by Will.[3] Their entire bodies are traversed by canals, which receive water from the stomach, or directly from without, and, being lined by ciliæ, a constant renewal of the water is effected. These aquiferous canals, which should be regarded as a respiratory system, are accompanied and surrounded by vessels having exceedingly thin walls. These sanguiferous vessels are without ciliated epithelium, and have neither longitudinal nor circular fibres. In some species they contain a greenish fluid, with spheroidal and slightly elongated red corpuscles with large nuclei.[4] In others the corpuscles are brown; and in others, again, they are of a greenish colour. There is no regular circulation, the blood being shifted hither and thither by the irregular contractions of the body. According to Agassiz, the circulatory system opens directly by large tubes into the alimentary canal. The fluid, therefore, which they circulate is the direct product of digestion. The blood of the Acalephæ should be regarded as of a higher type than that of the Polyps, because its corpuscles are

[1] Philosophical Transactions, 1834, p. 369.

[2] P. 21.

[3] Horæ tergest, p. 34.

[4] These observations of Will are not sustained by those of Dana and Agassiz. See Contributions to the Nat. Hist. of the Acalephæ, by Agassiz. Boston, 1850, p. 260.

larger, contain more granules and oil-globules, and their cell-membranes are more distinct.

Much confusion and imperfection exists in the descriptions of the vascular sanguineous system of the Echinodermata, arising from the fact that the respiratory system has been often confounded with the circulatory. All the researches, however, show that the higher members of this order have a distinct circulatory system separated from the alimentary canal, composed of arterial and venous trunks, between which, in some species, there is an organ analogous to a heart. In some species, as the Holothurinæ, there is no distinct heart, but the vascular system is well defined. It consists of a ring around the œsophagus, which sends off a trunk, which may be compared to the aorta. This ramifies upon the intestines and genital organs. By a reunion of these ramifications a second trunk is formed, analogous to the vena cava. This divides into two vessels, which ramify upon the branchiæ. From the branchiæ arise two veins, which return to the aorta. The Echinodermata is the only class amongst the Radiata in which a proper circulation of the nutritive fluid takes place, and this is attended with a corresponding development of the nervous and muscular systems, and the organs of secretion. It is in this class that we first find the liver, in its rudimentary state, however, consisting of simple cæca opening into the digestive cavity. It is remarkable that the circulatory fluid does not exhibit corresponding marks of higher elaboration. It appears to differ from the contents of the digestive cavity only in a greater degree of concentration. This fact, connected with another asserted by Dr. Williams, that the movement of the circulatory fluid is mainly carried on by ciliary motion, renders it probable that more careful and extended researches will discover some communication between the digestive cavity and the circulatory system. According to Dr. T. Williams, the corpuscles resemble spherules, composed of hard and very minute granules of coagulated albumen, without any detectable nucleus or cell-wall, or oily particles, and are readily broken up into their individual molecules. In the Spiunculida, the highest order of this class, the corpuscles are more highly developed, being flat and irregularly oblong, having small, bright, highly refractive nuclei.

As each class in the invertebrate kingdom passes through very much the same stages of development, and, moreover, as the object of these observations is to develop principles which will guide us in our future researches, and not to enter into a minute description of all the anatomical details of the structure of the solids and fluids of these animals, which may be readily obtained elsewhere, we will pass directly to the consideration of the comparative anatomy and physiology of the Mollusca.

In the lowest families of the class Acephala, the nervous system consists of a simple ganglionic mass, the intestinal canal is a simple cavity, and the liver composed of small single or ramified glandular follicles, thickly set together, and covering a large part of the alimentary canal. The circulatory system and fluids are correspondingly feebly developed. In the lowest species the heart is simple, whilst in the higher it is composed of both auricles and ventricles. In Salpa the heart is simple, and forces the blood alternately backwards and forwards in different directions. In the Lamellibranchia the nervous system is distinct, and composed of a central ganglionic and a peripheric system. The senses and the muscular and organic systems are correspondingly highly developed. The liver is voluminous, distinct from the intestine, and consists of brown lobular masses. An excretory organ also makes its appearance, formerly called the gland of Bojanus. The circulatory system corresponds in perfection with the advance in the structure of the solids of the body. The heart is divided into three chambers, and surrounded with a large pericardium. Two lateral, triangular, thick-walled auricles receive the blood from the branchiæ, and send it into a single muscular ventricle. By the contraction of this ventricle, the blood is sent into the body by a posterior and anterior aorta; its return into the two auricles being prevented by valves. Here we have, for the first time, the type of heart which exists in vertebrate animals. The blood is colourless, and contains many pale granular globules, often indistinctly nucleated. According to Siebold, the blood-corpuscles of the Naiades have an irregular form, and run together when placed upon a watch-glass. This may be due to the coagulation of the fibrin. When treated with acetic acid, they separate, become clear and almost imperceptible, and a hitherto invisible nucleus is brought into view. In this reaction they resemble closely the blood-corpuscles of the vertebrata.

In the lowest members of the class Cephalophora a heart and circulatory system are absent, or exist in a rudimentary condition; the biliary organs consist of numerous small follicles surrounding the intestines; no traces of kidneys or salivary glands are present, and the nervous system is correspondingly rudimentary in its structure and arrangement. In the highest order of this class, the nervous system is more perfect, and the organs of vision and hearing present. The digestive apparatus is complicated, and in those individuals nourished by solid food we find highly developed salivary glands. The liver is isolated, and often divided into lobes of a brownish-green colour. The biliary canals arising from the hepatic lobules form two or more secretory ducts, which empty the bile into the stomach or intestines. The heart is always present, consisting of a thin-walled auricle, generally single and rarely double, and a single muscular ventricle. The heart is surrounded by a distinct pericardium. The circulation is analogous to that of higher animals. The arterial blood passes from the respiratory organs into the auricle, then into the ventricle, and is forced, through a very short aorta, over the body. The heart is generally situated in the bottom of the pulmonary cavity, or at the base of the branchiæ, its position depending generally upon that of the respiratory system. The two chambers of the heart are separated by a valve. The development of the respiratory system corresponds with the perfection of the nervous system and organs. In the lowest orders it is absent. The blood is colourless, except in Planorbis, in which it is red. It is often opalescent, and always poor in corpuscles. The corpuscles are colourless, smooth cells, with a granular, indistinct nucleus, which is rendered very distinct by the action of acetic acid. According to Leydig, the blood of Paludina contains two forms of corpuscles, one round, which becomes granular nucleated cells after the action of acetic acid, and the other provided at one side with processes which disappear under the action of acetic acid. The blood of the Cephalophora generally contains a small quantity of fibrin, which, when coagulated, forms a web uniting the globules in masses and rows.

We pass now to the last division of the Mollusca, the Cephalopoda, which may be considered as belonging to the former class, only more highly organized. They have the rudiments of an internal skeleton, and a well-developed muscular system. The nervous system is more highly developed than that of any class which we have thus far studied, having a central portion resembling the brain of the vertebrata, in the extraordinary increase of its ganglionic substance, and in being contained in a cartilaginous cranium. All the organs, except the spleen, which are found in the vertebrata, exist in this class. They have organs of sense corresponding in perfection with the development of the nervous system; digestive apparatus complicated in structure; salivary glands highly developed; a pancreas present in some species; the liver present in all, and consists of a compact glandular mass, with distinct excretory ducts; kidneys also present. The circulatory system does not appear to be more highly developed than that of the other mollusca, the principal characteristics of which have been already described. The blood shows an elaboration corresponding to the perfection of the organs and apparatuses of the Cephalopoda. It coagulates spontaneously upon standing, and the number of corpuscles is greatly increased. They inclose numerous granules, thus resembling the colourless corpuscles of the vertebrata. The majority of the blood-corpuscles are colourless; some few, scattered here and there, have a violet hue.

II. *Fluids and Solids of Vertebrate Animals.*—1. Circulatory and Respiratory Systems. A minute investigation of all the varieties of the circulatory system of vertebrate animals would occupy more than a lifetime, and complete descriptions would fill large volumes. In this paper, we can do nothing more than give those general outlines of the development of the circulatory and respiratory systems, which are absolutely necessary to enable us properly to understand the physical, chemical, and physiological phenomena of the different classes of animals. Commencing with the lowest of all vertebrate animals, the connecting link with the invertebrata, we will ascend rapidly to the highly organized Mammalia.

The circulatory system of the Amphioxus, or Branchiostoma (Lancelet), resembles closely that of some of the Annelida, as the Eunice, in its division and the distribution of numerous pulsatile dilatations upon the different vascular trunks. Müller enumerates as belonging to the circulatory system of this singular animal, the following parts:—

1. The Arterial Heart, a thick vessel of uniform calibre, situated in the median line, immediately beneath the branchial chamber, between the arches forming the framework of that cavity. Posteriorly, it is continuous with the heart of the vena cava. From its sides are given off the bulbs of the branchial arteries, varying in number with that of the branchial arches, from twenty-five to fifty on each side. These bulbs are situated at the commencement of the branchial arteries, and by their contractions propel the blood into the capillary network surrounding the branchial arches.

2. The Aortic Heart, which discharges the function of a systemic heart.

3. The Heart of the Vena Portæ, a long contractile vessel which runs along the under surface of the intestine as far as the hepatic organ.

4. The Heart of the Vena Cava, which is opposite to the heart of the vena portæ, and lies superiorly to the hepatic cæca. The contraction of these hearts succeed each other at regular intervals. Each in turn becomes filled with the colourless blood, whilst the others successively contract. The blood does not appear to be more highly elaborated than that of the Cephalopods, and contains none of the coloured corpuscles of higher vertebrate animals.

The respiratory system is formed upon an equally degraded type. The branchial apparatus is placed in the same cavity in which are lodged the liver, kidneys, generative apparatus, and greater portion of the intestinal tube. A similar arrangement is seen in the respiratory system of many of the invertebrata. The nervous and organic systems are correspondingly simple in their structure. The canal which incloses the spinal column, presents anteriorly no cranial expansion, but the spinal chord extends from one extremity to the other. This fact, in connection with others of a similar character in the invertebrate kingdom, demonstrates that the brain is but a developed portion of the spinal column. The liver is reduced to its rudimentary condition, a greenish glandular layer, lining a portion of the intestines. The imperfect development of the fluids and solids of this animal would lead us to place it below the Cephalopods.

It is remarkable that the spleen is also absent in this animal. The appearance of the spleen in vertebrate animals is accompanied by an improvement of all their organs, apparatuses, and nutritive fluids. This little organ is the herald, rather than the cause of these great changes. Its presence indicates a higher development of organization.

Traces of an arrangement of the circulatory apparatus similar to that of the Amphioxus, are found in some other fishes, especially in the cartilaginous group. It is remarkable that in some of these cartilaginous fishes, as the Stingray (*Trygon Sabina*), the pancreas, kidneys, and generative apparatus, are more highly developed than in the osseous fishes, having more perfect nervous and osseous systems. The young of the Stingray is developed in a uterus. The appearance of this organ, and the attachment of the fœtus resembles closely the arrangement of these parts in the highest mammalia.

These facts confirm what has been before asserted, that each higher animal does not pass through successively all the stages in the development of those placed below. Whilst the general plan of the development of the solids and fluids is similar in all animals, still each species, genera, and class has its own peculiar laws of development, which are immutable. The principal, or only heart, in many Fishes, has but one auricle and one ventricle. It is traversed by venous blood alone and corresponds with the right heart of the higher vertebrata. The heart is lodged within a pericardium, to the inner surface of which it is frequently attached, as in many Amphibia. In the lowest orders of Fishes, as the Plagiostomi, the pericardium communicates by openings with the peritoneum, and is bathed by the water introduced through the apertures in the peritoneum, situated near the anus. In most Fishes, especially those belonging to the osseous division, the cavity in which the heart is lodged, is separated from the peritoneum by a kind of tendinous diaphragm, and also by a capacious sinus which collects the venous blood from all parts of the body preparatory to its admission into the auricle of the heart. The auricle is more capacious and has much thinner walls than the ventricle. Between the two cavities we find generally two, and rarely three muscular valves. From the anterior part of the ventricle arises the contractile trunk of the branchial arteries, which consist of very powerful annular muscular fibres, and is situated within the pericardium. This strongly developed portion of bloodvessel is called the bulbus arteriosus, and by its contractions aids materially in the circulation of the blood. It is separated from the ventricle by strong valves, and is so muscular and capacious, that it should be considered as forming a second ventricular chamber. The venous blood from all parts of the body is collected in the auricle, and by its contractions is transmitted to the ventricle. The contraction of the ventricle forces the blood through the bulbus arteriosus into the branchial arteries, generally four in number, which pass in a groove in the convex side of each branchial arch, and ramify upon the branchial leaflets. The capillary network thus formed, terminates at its other extremity in the branchial veins, which run along in the same groove in the branchial arches behind the arteries in an opposite direction. The branchial veins run up to the base of the skull and commencement of the vertebral column, and there form an extensive circle of arterial vessels, from which arises posteriorly the aorta, the contractions of which performs the office of the left ventricle in higher animals, and propels the slow moving blood in its course through the arterial system. This great systemic artery divides and subdivides and distributes the arterial blood to all the organs and tissues of the body. The arterial blood, after having traversed the capillaries, becomes venous, and after being elaborated and purified by the action of the liver and kidney is returned by the systemic veins, into a large dilatation (*sinus venosus*), which enters the posterior part of the auricle of the heart by a large orifice, guarded by two membranous valves. In Fishes, as in many Amphibia, we find a double portal system, one for the liver, and the other for the kidneys. The venous blood from the stomach, intestinal canal, spleen, pancreas, and sometimes the generative organs, enter the liver in different parts by several branches, and rarely unite into a common portal vein. The kidneys receive blood from the tail, and partly also from the sexual organs and swimming bladder. The arrangement of the portal systems varies in different species and genera. The venous blood, after it has been elaborated by the liver and purified from certain effete compounds, empties into the great venous sinus, and from thence is conveyed to the heart. Several peculiarities of the circulatory apparatus which connect the Fishes with Reptiles and the fœtus of higher vertebrata deserve an especial notice.

The heart of the Chick, about the 65th hour of incubation, and that of the fœtus of the dog, about the 21st day of its development, resembles, in many respects, that of Fishes and the larvæ of the Batrachians. It then consists of two cavities and a bulbus arteriosus. In warm-blooded animals, this bulbus arteriosus, between the third and fifth days in the chick, and longer in the Mammalia, gives off a succession of arches which encompass the pharynx, and are true analogues of the branchial arches of Fishes. These are successively obliterated, and the bulbus arteriosus finally subdivides into two branches, one communicating with the left, and the other with the right ventricle. The former subsequently becomes the aorta, and the latter the pulmonary artery. In some Fishes, which present distinct reptilian characteristics, there is a slight indication of this division of the bulbus arteriosus. Another peculiarity exists in the circulation of Fishes which distinguishes it from that of the invertebrata, and foreshadows more important modifications in the higher classes. Two or more small arteries pass off from the branchial arches, and convey pure aerated blood to the head and brain. A similar arrangement exists in the Alligator and the embryo of higher vertebrata. In the Alligator and other reptiles, only a moiety of the blood passes through the respiratory organs, the arterial and venous blood being mixed directly in the heart, or by communications between the two systems. The partially vitiated blood of the heart would be unfit for the supply of so important an organ as the brain, and consequently special arteries supply it with purified blood, directly from the lungs. As the organism is developed, the nervous system is correspondingly developed, and greater provisions made for its maintenance and preservation. The importance of the preservation of the nervous system is farther seen in the development of the bony case in which it is contained, which is ossified just in proportion to the perfection of the organs and apparatuses. In all the invertebrate animals except the highest Cephalopods, we find no special internal framework. In the lowest Fishes it is cartilaginous. In the fœtus of mammalia it is in the earlier stages entirely cartilaginous.

In the Garfish (*Lepisósteus ósseus*), we find a still higher development of the circulatory and respiratory systems. In this remarkable fish, the only representative of the great Sauroid family of the earlier periods of the earth's history, we find a capacious lung resembling, in all respects, the structure of the respiratory organs in the Amphiúma Méans, and other reptiles. The blood is *sent to the lungs by prolongations of the branchial arteries.* The capillary network formed by the ramification of these vessels carrying arterial blood, terminates in vessels which transmit the aerated blood directly into the aorta. This singular fish has both a branchial and pulmonary respiration. I have often watched them, when lying near the surface of the water, expel the vitiated air in a rapid succession of small bubbles through the nostrils, and then quickly with a splash of the tail and flirt of the body, thrust their long bill into the air, and draw in a fresh supply.

Having rapidly traced the development of the circulatory apparatus from the Amphioxus or Branchiostoma to the most highly organized Fishes, we pass next to the class of Reptiles.

The circulatory apparatus of Reptiles presents many varieties dependent upon the peculiar organization and metamorphoses of the different orders. We can only notice those peculiarities of structure and development which have an important bearing upon our investigations.

The family Phanerobranchoidea, the members of which have permanent gills, ranks next to the class of Fishes in their modes of life, and the general development of the respiratory and circulatory systems and organs.

In the Lepidosiren, a creature so exactly intermediate between Fishes and Reptiles, that it is difficult to determine to which class it belongs, the heart consists of a single auricle, a ventricle, and a bulbus arteriosus; the venous blood from all parts of the body is conveyed by the vena cava directly into the auricle; the pulmonary vein bringing the aerated blood from the lung, enters the ventricle by a distinct orifice, guarded by a cartilaginous valvular tubercle. The continuation of the pulmonary vein prevents the admixture of the venous and arterial blood until they have reached the cavity of the ventricle. The bulbus arteriosus connected with the ventricle gives off on each side six vessels corresponding to the number of the branchial arches. Four of these arches on each side support gills, and are supplied by a corresponding number of arteries. The two remaining arteries on each side are continued around to the dorsal region, and give off the pulmonary arteries, and then unite to form the aorta. Each contraction of the ventricle of the heart, assisted by that of the bulbus arteriosus, drives the mixed blood, derived from the venæ cavæ and pulmonary veins, first to the gills, secondly to the aorta, and thirdly to the lungs. By this arrangement, whether the animal be placed in water or in air, respiration is carried on vicariously, either by the branchial or pulmonary apparatus. The only difference between the circulation of the Lepidosiren and the Garfish (*Lepisósteus ósseus*) is, that in the former, the pulmonary vein empties into the ventricle of the heart, whilst in the latter it empties into the aorta.

In the Siren and Menobranchus we have a still higher development of the circulatory apparatus by the dilatation of the pulmonary vein into a left auricle. The heart in these animals consists of two auricles, separated by a thin septum, a ventricle, and a bulbus arteriosus. Within the ventricle of the Siren there is even found a rudimentary septum. The vessels carrying venous blood, unite and form the large superior and inferior venæ cavæ, which dilate, as in Fishes, into a contractile venous reservoir (*sinus venosus*). The venous blood from all parts of the body collected into this sinus venosus is driven into the right auricle of the heart. The pulmonary veins, bringing aerated blood from the lungs, empty into the left auricle. The contraction of the two auricles sends the blood into the common ventricle, in which we have a mixture of the venous blood from all parts of the body and the aerated blood from the lungs. The contraction of the ventricle forces the blood through the bulbus arteriosus into the branchial arteries, which terminate in a capillary network upon the branchial arches. This capillary network of the gills ends in three branchial veins, which unite in a common trunk, and anastomosing with that of the branchial veins of the opposite side, form the descending aorta, which distributes the oxygenated blood throughout the system. By comparing the circulation of these animals with that of Fishes, we see at once that the only difference is the existence of a lung and a left auricle devoted to the reception of the aerated blood. Remove the lung and left auricle, and you have remaining the simple heart of fishes with its bulbus arteriosus, circulating only arterial blood.

In the Menopoma and Amphiúma, which have branchial arches without any capillary network forming gills, a farther advance is made towards that form of the circulatory apparatus which exists in the Chelonia and Sauria. The bulbus arteriosus divides into branchial arteries; but as in the adult animals there are no branchiæ, these vessels wind around the side of the neck, and again unite into a trunk on each side. The union of these two trunks forms the aorta. From the lowest branchial arch a pulmonary artery is given off, which ramifies over the surface of the lung. In the earlier conditions of the development of the Salamanders and Batrachians, the circulatory system presents successively those arrangements which we have described as permanent in the Phanerobranchoidea.

In the larvæ of the Batrachia, the heart consists of a single auricle and ventricle, a bulbus arteriosus, and a sinus venosus, and the circulatory apparatus resembles in all respects that of Fishes. The left auricle is formed as the lungs develop. In the earlier period of the development of the Tadpole, the pulmonary artery is a minute branch, derived from the aortic system, and corresponds with the rudimentary condition of the lungs. The greater portion of the blood goes to the branchiæ, whilst only a very small part passes through the lungs. Minute vessels at this period unite the branchial arteries with the branchial veins, which increase in importance during the subsequent stages of the metamorphosis. As the branchiæ with their arteries and veins diminish with the progressive development of the lungs and pulmonary arteries, the anastomosing vessels are correspondingly enlarged. When the lungs are fully developed, and the Batrachian prepared for the habitation of the land, the branchiæ entirely disappear, and the circulation is carried on as in the Amphiúma and Menopoma, through the anastomosing branches. These branchial arches exist permanently in all Reptiles, and are also found as a transitory condition in the development of the circulatory apparatus of warm-blooded animals.

In the higher orders of cold-blooded animals, the Ophidia, Sauria, and Chelonia, the circulatory apparatus is more perfectly developed, but still a mixture of venous and arterial blood always takes place in the ventricle. The heart consists of three cavities, two capacious auricles and a strong muscular ventricle. The auricular cavities are separated from the ventricle by valves. The general shape of the heart varies with the different orders. Thus, it is elongated in the Ophidia and Sauria, and short and broad in the Chelonia. The ventricle in these higher orders is generally divided by an imperfect septum, which in the heart of the Alligator is very strong and almost complete. Just at the outlet of the ventricles, however, we find a communication established between the two, and thus the vitiated and purified blood is mixed together, and the similarity with the heart of the rest of the Reptiles and the fœtus of birds and mammalia is preserved. The venous blood from all parts of the body is returned to the right auricle of the heart through the venæ cavæ, the terminations of which are guarded by strong valves. The left auricle is appropriated exclusively to the lungs, from which it receives the aerated blood through the pulmonary veins. From the single ventricle two sets of vessels are sent off, the pulmonary and the aortic. The pulmonary artery divides into two branches, one for each lung. The aorta, immediately after its origin, divides into two trunks, which, winding backwards, join and form a large vessel, the branches of which distribute the blood to all parts of the system. The contraction of the right auricle forces the venous blood into the ventricle, whilst the contraction of the left auricle transmits the aerated blood from the lungs into the same common cavity. The contraction of the ventricle distributes a portion of the mixed blood into the lungs through the pulmonary artery, and the remainder to all parts of the body, through the aorta and its branches. From this arrangement it is evident that not only is partially *aerated* venous blood diffused throughout the system, but also only a moiety of the whole amount of blood is sent to the lungs and exposed to the action of the atmosphere at each contraction of the ventricle of the heart.

These peculiarities in the structure of the circulatory apparatus in Reptiles should be attentively studied; for they will aid us materially in the interpretation of some of the most complex phenomena of life. *As the circulatory apparatus is developed, the influence and importance of the nervous system is increased, and corresponding arrangements established for its perfect preservation.* The brain of many reptiles, especially that of the most highly organized, as the Sauria, is supplied by small arteries given off from the left arch of the aorta, which is connected with the left ventricular cavity, and contains pure blood. The same condition exists up to the termination of the embryo state of the higher vertebrata, including the human species. The portal system of Reptiles corresponds with that of Fishes, in the circumstance that both the kidneys and liver are supplied with venous blood. The minute and extended description of the hepatic, portal, and renal circulations will be postponed until the anatomical and physiological description of these organs.

From the consideration of the heart of the Alligator we pass very naturally to that of warm-blooded animals. The circulatory apparatus differs in no essential respect in the two great classes of warm-blooded animals—Birds and Mammalia. In these higher animals we have a double heart, and two distinct and complete circulations of the blood. Each portion of blood which has passed through the capillaries of the system, and become vitiated, is aerated in the lungs before its distribution over the body. This is one of the most important of all distinctions between warm and cold blooded animals. The right heart is devoted to the circulation of venous blood, and the left heart to the circulation of oxygenated or arterial blood. The auricle and ventricle of one heart has no communication with the auricle and ventricle of the other, except through the bloodvessels and capillaries. The vessels of each heart are distinct, and perform distinct offices. It is unnecessary to enter into a minute description of all the anatomical details, as these are familiar to every one, or may be readily reviewed in all the works on human anatomy. The right auricle receives the venous blood from all parts of the system, and transmits it to the right ventricle. The contraction of the right ventricle distributes the venous blood to the lungs. The aerated blood is conveyed from the lungs to the left auricle, and from thence to the left ventricle, and the contractions of this distributes it throughout all parts of the system. In Birds, the portal circulation resembles to a certain extent that of reptiles. The portal trunk receives its blood, not only from the veins of the digestive apparatus, but also by branches from those of the pelvis and posterior extremities, and still communicates with the renal circulation. The portal circulation in Mammalia is limited to the liver, the kidneys being supplied with arterial blood alone.

The circulatory apparatus of warm-blooded vertebrata, during its development, passes through very nearly all the stages, which exist as permanent conditions in the lower animals. Thus the bloodvessel system is formed and a motion of the blood commenced, before the formation of a heart. The heart, in its earlier conditions, is a simple tube. At a later stage of its development, like that of Fishes, it consists of only two cavities and a bulbus arteriosus. Branchial arches in the earlier periods are given off, analogous in all respects to those of the Menopoma and Amphiúma, and Reptiles generally. Finally, the heart assumes the form of that of the most highly organized reptiles, as the Alligator, and this condition continues up to within a short period of the completion of the embryo.

We will next consider the relative size of the heart, and the rapidity of its action in different animals. I obtained the following results by carefully weighing the entire body of an animal, and then carefully ascertaining the weight of its heart upon a delicate balance capable of turning to the $\frac{1}{1000}$th part of a grain. By dividing the former by the latter, the weight of the heart in comparison to that of the body is ascertained, and may be compared with others.

Comparative Weights of the Hearts of Fishes.

		Number of times heavier than its heart.
Weight of	female Stingray (*Trygon Sabina*)	1012
"	fœtus of Stingray (*Trygon Sabina*)	1070
"	Hammerhead Shark (*Zygæna málleus*)	1156
"	Hammerhead Shark (*Zygæna málleus*)	899
"	female Garfish (*Lepisósteus ósseus*)	965

Comparative Weights of the Hearts of Reptiles.

Weight of	Bullfrog (*Rána pipiens*)	576
"	female Black Viper (*Héterodon niger*)	496
"	male Black-snake (*Cóluber constrictor*)	425
"	Coachwhip-snake (*Psámmophis flagellifórmis*)	354
"	male Corn-snake (*Cóluber guttátus*)	400
"	male Rattlesnake (*Crótalus durissus*)	441
"	Alligator Cooter (*Chelonúra serpentina*)	405
"	Loggerhead Turtle (*Chelónia carétta*)	480
"	Chicken Terrapin (*Emys reticuláta*)	420
"	Yellow-belly Terrapin (*Emys serráta*)	592
"	Yellow-belly Terrapin (*Emys serráta*)	577
"	Yellow-belly Terrapin (*Emys serráta*)	543
"	male Gopher (*Testúdo polyphēmus*)	455
"	male Gopher (*Testúdo polyphémus*)	470
"	female Alligator (*Alligátor Mississippiénsis*)	398

Comparative Weights of the Hearts of Birds.

Weight of	Wild Turkey (*Meleágris gallopavo*)	279
"	Wild Turkey (*Meleágris gallopavo*)	275
"	Hooting Owl (*Syrnium nebulósum*)	220
"	Turkey-Buzzard (*Cathártes atrátus*)	113
"	Wood Ibis (*Tantalus loculator*)	108
"	Wood Ibis (*Tantalus loculator*)	100

Comparative Weights of the Hearts of Mammalia.

Weight of	common Sheep	256
"	Gray Squirrel (*Sciúrus Carolinénsis*)	261
"	Opossum (*Didélphis Virginiánus*)	280
"	Raccoon (*Prócyon lótor*)	164
"	Raccoon (*Prócyon lótor*)	140
"	young Raccoon (*Prócyon lótor*)	142
"	common Cat	275
"	Pointer Dog	128

By comparing these tables, we see that the heart is smallest in Fishes, and largest in Birds. As the organs and apparatuses of the animal economy are developed and perfected, the necessity for a vigorous circulation of the nutritive materials becomes more urgent. As the temperature, intelligence, and activity of animals, with their corresponding physical and chemical metamorphoses of the elements of organic structure, increase, there is a corresponding necessity for a rapid supply of those materials by which the wastes may be repaired, and from which the various secretions may be elaborated and separated. The importance of the facts demonstrated by these tables will be evident when we come to treat of animal temperature, and compare the phenomena of cold-blooded animals with those of the warm-blooded.

We will next consider the rapidity of the circulation in different animals. The action of the heart may be taken as a general index of this. We are not aware that any special researches have as yet been made upon the rapidity of the heart's action in the different classes of the invertebrate animals. All comparative anatomists, however, concur in the statement that it is generally much slower than that of the vertebrata. The circulation of the blood in the tubular axis of colonial polyps is completed in about two or three minutes. The motion of the blood in all the invertebrata which are without a central organ of circulation is correspondingly sluggish.

In the Amphioxus, whose circulatory apparatus has been previously described, the contractions of the several distinct hearts succeed each other at regular intervals, in such a manner that each in turn becomes filled whilst the others contract. Each heart contracts with such violence that it empties itself entirely, and remains for some little time undistinguishable. By this arrangement each portion of blood passes the entire round of the circulation in the time which elapses between the consecutive contractions of the separate hearts. The space of time occupied in the complete circulation of a given portion of the blood of the Amphioxus is stated to be about one minute.

As the fluids and solids of Fishes become more highly elaborated and developed, the action of the heart and circulation of the blood becomes more rapid and vigorous. The same remark applies generally to the remaining vertebrate animals. These principles are illustrated by the following table, which has been drawn up from the researches of Dumas, Prévost, Müller, and Simon:—

	Number of beats in a minute.
Amphioxus	1
Carp	20
Fishes generally	20 to 24
Green toad	77
Frogs generally	about 60
Pigeon	136
Common hen	140
Duck	110
Raven	110

	Number of beats in a minute.
Heron	200
Birds generally	100 to 200
Ox	38
Horse	56
Sheep	75
Goat	84
Hare	120
Guinea-pig	140
Dog	90 to 95
Cat	100 to 110
Ape (*Simia Calitriche*)	90
Human embryo	150
" " just after birth	130 to 140
Human being during the first year	115 to 130
" " during the second year	100 to 115
" " during the third year	90 to 100
" " about the seventh year	85 to 90
" " about the fourteenth year	80 to 85
" " in the middle period of life	70 to 75
" " in old age	50 to 65
Mammalia generally	38 to 140

This table shows us that the rapidity of the circulation depends upon the structure, habits, age, and development of animals. If the vital forces are of a low grade, either from original conformation or the depressing influences of old age, the circulation is correspondingly sluggish and feeble.

We will next briefly consider the development and structure of the respiratory system in the different orders of animals. One of the essential conditions of the life of all organized beings, whether vegetable or animal, is a supply of oxygen. The modes in which oxygen is brought in contact with the fluids and solids of organized structures vary with the development and peculiar modes of life of the different classes of animals. In the lowest classes of the invertebrata, in which the digestive matters pass directly from the stomach into the different structures of the body, and become integral parts of the animal, we find no special circulatory system, and respiration is carried on by the whole surface of the body which is bathed by the water. In animals still more highly developed we find canals, carrying water into all parts of the system. In many individuals bloodvessels accompany these canals, and ramify around their walls. An incessant motion of the water through this aquiferous respiratory system is maintained by ciliæ lining their interior. These canals open upon the exterior of the body, and into the visceral cavity. In many animals of this class the digestive cavity, which is bathed continually by fresh portions of water, performs the function of respiration. The "water vascular" system of the lower articulata finds its homologue in the tracheal system of air-breathing Myriapods and Insects. In the higher orders of the invertebrata, the respiratory system is confined to a definite portion of the exterior or internal membrane, which is developed within a small space into a great extent of surface, so as to render the contact with the air or water as extensive as possible, without any loss of room or power. *According as the fluids are elaborated, and the solids correspondingly developed, the respiratory system becomes more condensed and perfected.* The branchial apparatus of the cephalopoda is similar in structure and function to that of fishes.

Our time will not permit us to enter upon the minute details of the respiratory apparatus of the different classes of the invertebrata, and we pass immediately to the consideration of the respiratory system of Fishes and the higher vertebrata. In the Amphioxus, the pulmonary apparatus corresponds with the degraded type of the cerebro-spinal system and all the organs, and, like that of many invertebrate animals, is lodged in the same cavity with the liver, generative apparatus, kidneys, and the greater portion of the alimentary canal.

In the Cyclostome Fishes the branchial apparatus presents a remarkable variation, being composed of six or seven pairs of gills on each side, not attached to the cartilaginous arches, but developed as folds from the lining membrane of as many distinct sacculi. In the invertebrate animals, and the Amphioxus amongst the vertebrata, the circulation of the water through the branchiæ is maintained principally by ciliary action.

In Fishes, however, of higher organization, whose blood is more highly elaborated, and circulates with greater rapidity, mere filamentous tufts hanging to the side of the neck will not suffice for the aeration of the blood. It is necessary that large streams of water should be constantly and forcibly propelled through the branchial apparatus, in order that the blood should be exposed as much as possible to the action of the air scantily contained in the water. This is accomplished by the connection of the gills with the cavity of the mouth, the muscles of which send rapid currents of water through the branchial passages. The structure and position of the heart also are such that it propels all the venous blood through the branchiæ before its distribution to the body generally.

At first sight, the circulation and respiration of Fishes appear to be more perfect than that of Reptiles; this, however, is not the case. By a reference to the table of the comparative weights of the heart in different animals, it will be seen that the heart of Fishes is about $\frac{1}{1000}$th, whilst that of Reptiles is about $\frac{1}{504}$th of the weight of the entire body. The heart of reptiles is relatively more than twice as large as that of fishes. The table of the comparative rapidity of the heart's action in different animals shows that the circulation of Fishes is much slower than that of reptiles. The aeration of the blood also is much slower and less perfect in Fishes, from the fact that the amount of air contained in the water is infinitely less than that of the atmosphere. The respiratory apparatus in Fishes consists of cartilaginous or bony arches suspended from the hyoidean arch. To the convex margin of each of these branchial arches is attached a double row of pointed, lanceolate, vascular lamellæ or leaflets, which project from the sides of the arch like the teeth of a comb. Each leaflet is provided with a thin fibro-cartilaginous plate, which keeps it stiff and straight. The extent of the surface is increased by numerous transverse ridges.

The branchial artery runs in a groove situated upon the convexity of the branchial arch, and sends off branches to every one of the lamellæ or leaflets, which divide into a minute capillary network, covering both surfaces of the branchial fringe. This capillary network terminates in veins which empty into a venous canal, running along the internal margin of each lamella, and these last unite to form the branchial vein situated in the same groove, but running in an opposite direction with that of the branchial artery. By these arrangements, the extent of surface covered by minute capillaries, exposed to the action of the oxygen of the air contained in the water is very great. In descriptions of this character, we should bear in mind the fact that, when the terms veins and arteries are applied to the bloodvessels of the respiratory organs of animals, the character of the blood does not correspond with the name and office of the vessel. The branchial arteries convey venous blood to be exposed to the action of the air in the water, and the branchial veins carry aerated, or arterial blood from the respiratory organs.

The objection may be urged against the assertion that the blood of Fishes receives its oxygen from the air of the water, that they die in a short time when placed in the atmosphere which contains a far more abundant supply of oxygen. This, however, is readily explained when we consider the mechanism of their respiration and the necessity for the moisture and division of their branchial fringes. The mouth is first filled with water, its muscles contracting expel the fluid through the apertures on either side of the pharynx into the gill-cavity, and, at the same time, the branchial arches are lifted and separated from each other so that the gill-fringes hang freely. After the oxygen of the air has been exhausted from this portion of water, it is expelled by muscular pressure through the external openings, its return into the pharynx being prevented by valves. When a fish is exposed to the atmosphere, the filaments of the gills being no longer moistened, separated, and, supported by the water, become glued together, and expose but a comparatively small surface to the action of the atmosphere. Their surfaces also become dry, and the circulation of the blood in the minute capillaries is diminished if not completely arrested, and as a necessary consequence, the exosmose of the carbonic acid and the endosmose of the oxygen is retarded. Those fishes which have the external opening very small, so that the gill-cavity may be kept distended with fluid, are capable of living for a much greater length of time out of the water.

In the Labyrinthibranchii, the anterior branchial arches give origin to a curious lamellated apparatus similar to that of the Land-Crab, which retains water for a considerable length of time. The gills by this arrangement being kept moist, they can exist for a length of time in the atmosphere, and are said to perform long migrations over the land in search of food.

In several remarkable fish having strongly marked reptilian characters, as the Garfish (*Lepisósteus ósseus*) and the common Mudfish (*Amia cálva*) of our southern swamps and rice fields, we find both gills and a pulmonary organ. The lung of these fishes has been considered by many physiologists and anatomists as analogous to the swimming bladder of other fishes. This organ is absent in some individuals, and its presence or absence in those which possess it, appears to make no material difference; in others it communicates externally, whilst in others again it is completely closed, and in all its offices are wholly unknown. It is, therefore, impossible with our present knowledge to decide whether or not the air-bladder of fishes should be considered as a rudimentary lung.

The lung of the Garfish (*Lepisósteus ósseus*) is a capacious fibrous sac, which opens by a short trachea high up in the throat and, extending nearly the whole length of the abdominal cavity, terminates within a short distance of the anus. It lies between the posterior surface of the liver and the anterior surface of the kidneys. When removed from the abdominal cavity and fully inflated, its diameter is nearly equal to two-thirds of that of the fish. Its structure resembles that of the *Amphiúma Méans* and other doubtful reptiles. The lungs of Serpents and Terrapins are also formed upon the same general plan, only more highly developed. The bloodvessels ramify over the walls of this sac, the internal surface of which is increased by the development of numerous sacculi. *This increased development of the respiratory system is attended by corresponding improvements in the structure and functions of the solids.* The gar is a destructive and active pirate, and consequently needs great muscular power to outstrip and capture the swift inhabitants of the watery element. It is a very difficult matter to hold a recently captured gar, two or three feet in length, even with both hands. The contortions and contractions and flirts of its body are so great and sudden, that it will often extricate itself from a powerful grasp. When removed from the water, like the mudfish (*Amia cálva*), it will live for a much greater length of time than fishes which have no pulmonary organ.

The manner in which the lung of the *Lepisósteus ósseus* is supplied with blood has been already described. Not only in this respect, but also in the general form and appearance of the viscera, this fish bears a strong resemblance to reptiles.

The Menobranchus Maculatus of our northern lakes, and the Phanerobranchoidea generally have both gills and pulmonary organs. *The relative action of these two systems varies with the comparative development of the organs.* The branchial apparatus of these animals resembles that of young Fishes during their development, and is not so perfect as that of the higher orders of fish. *As the fluids and solids of the body are elaborated and perfected, the pulmonary apparatus is correspondingly developed, and the branchial apparatus becomes more and more imperfect, until it disappears.*

These progressive changes may be studied either in the permanent states of the respiratory system of the Doubtful Reptiles, or in the transitory conditions in the development of the larvæ of the Batrachia.

In the Congo snake of our southern swamps and rice fields, and the Hellbender (*Menopoma Alleghaniensis*), we find branchial arches without any development of the gills. The lungs of the Congo snake (*Amphiúma méans*), communicate with the exterior through a short trachea, which opens by a slit in the pharynx just opposite to the base of the cranium. The trachea passes down between the divisions of the bulbus arteriosus, and a short distance below the position of the heart divides into two short branches which open into the lungs. The lungs are long slender sacs, having the general structure of these organs in the Batrachia, Reptilia, and Chelonia. Their internal surface is increased by sacculi developed in their walls, upon which ramify numerous bloodvessels. The diameter of the lungs, even in their inflated condition, is very small, being about one-half of an inch, whilst their length is very great, in full-grown individuals being about eighteen inches. Notwithstanding the absence of gills, the lungs are far smaller than the pulmonary organ of the garfish (*Lepisósteus ósseus*), which has also a large and well developed branchial apparatus. This may be due in part to the fact that its naked skin, as in frogs and naked animals generally, whether vertebrate or invertebrate, performs the office of a lung. The chief cause, however, of these discrepancies in the development of the respiratory organs of these two animals is found in their habits and vital endowments. The Gar is active and powerful, whilst the Amphiúma is sluggish and degraded in habits and appearance. *This is one of numerous instances which might be adduced to show that the consumption of oxygen and the corresponding wastes of the tissues correspond exactly with the development, habits, and temperature of animals.*

The lungs of the several orders of Reptiles are formed upon one type, being capacious sacs, whose walls are divided into sacculi and supplied with bloodvessels, according to the perfection of the organ and apparatuses, and the habits of the animal. From the internal surface membranous septa project inwards, partially dividing the interior of the organ into numerous polygonal cells, which are themselves subdivided into smaller compartments. The bloodvessels are distributed over the internal walls of the lungs and over the sides of the pulmonary cells. In Serpents, only one lung is developed, and the pulmonary cells are most numerous in the superior portion, whilst the inferior part of the long cylindrical lung is a mere membranous sac with few or no bloodvessels ramifying upon its walls. We find the greatest number of the polygonal cells, and the greatest distribution of the bloodvessels in the pulmonary organs of the higher Chelonia and Sauria, thus foreshadowing the condition of the lungs in Birds and Mammalia. In these orders, the lungs are filled more or less by a coarse and fine network, or areolar tissue, forming angular or rounded meshes which rest partly upon the walls of the lungs, and inclose lesser meshes, or air-cells. The bloodvessels ramify over the meshes, as well as over the walls of the lungs. The sacculi thus formed communicate with each other, and can all be inflated from any one point. In Amphibia and Batrachia the lungs are filled by an action that resembles swallowing.

In some Chelonia we have observed a muscle which is attached to the back and passes over the surface of the lungs. This fan-like muscle is especially developed in the Emys serrata. The expansion and contraction of this muscle aids materially in the introduction and expulsion of the air. In Serpents and Sauria respiration is assisted by the ribs and abdominal muscles.

The size of the lungs differs in the different orders, according to their structure and habits. Amongst the Chelonia we find the most capacious lungs in the Gopher (*Testudo polyphemus*). These animals burrow deeply in the ground, and need large lungs to keep a supply of air. In aquatic serpents which remain under the water for a great length of time, the lungs are capable of holding a greater quantity than those of land serpents.

We will next briefly consider the structure of the lungs in the warm-blooded animals.

In Mammalia and Birds the blood is abundant, and the circulation rapid, and the wastes and metamorphoses of the tissues correspondingly great, and hence the lungs are composed of an infinitude of minute cells, containing air, and surrounded by a capillary network. The respiratory system of Birds is more highly developed than that of Reptiles, but not so concentrated as that of the Mammalia. In this class the lungs are no longer closed bags, like those of Reptiles, but are spongy masses of great vascularity, communicating with numerous air-sacs, and the cavities of the bones. The main trunks of the bronchial tubes pass through the lungs, and open into the cavity of the thorax. The whole thoracico-abdominal cavity is divided by bands of serous membrane into numerous cells, communicating with each other, and the cavities of the hollow and spongy bones. Such is the freedom of communication between the air-cells, cavities of the bones, and the lungs, that if the trachea be tied, the animal will continue to respire, and support life, by an opening in the humerus or femur. In many birds, especially those of powerful flight, the air is admitted into the interspaces between the muscles, and between the skin and muscular system. By this arrangement, which reminds us of the tracheal system of insects, the air penetrates almost every part of their bodies, bathes all their viscera, and fills the cavities of the hollow and spongy bones. It follows as a necessary consequence, that the actions between the oxygen of the atmosphere and the organic elements of their bodies, are rapid and incessant, and the temperature correspondingly high.

The minute structure of the lungs of Birds resembles, in many respects, that of Reptiles; the cells, however, are infinitely more numerous and minute, and the surface exposed to the action of the atmosphere correspondingly more extensive. The entire mass of each lung is divided into innumerable lobules or lunglets, the walls of which are formed by a cartilaginous network derived from the bronchial tubes, and by the ramifications of the capillary vessels.

From this arrangement it is evident that the bloodvessels are suspended in the air, and exposed to its influence on every side. These cells, or sacculi, are never terminal cells as in the Mammalia, but open parietal cells, communicating freely with each other through the meshes of the capillary and cartilaginous network. The mechanism of respiration is more complete in this class than in Reptiles, but not so perfect as that of the Mammalia. From the elastic character of the cartilaginous and bony framework surrounding the thoracico-abdominal cavity, the natural condition of the lungs is that of inflation. The air is expelled by the action of those muscles which bring the sternum nearer to the vertebral column. When these muscles cease to act, the extended sternum attached to the elastic thorax, springs outward, and the air rushes into the lungs to fill the vacuum thus formed.

In the Mammalia, the abdominal cavity is completely separated from the thoracic cavity by the diaphragm, the great muscle of respiration. The lungs are closed bags, situated in the cavity of the thorax, and are surrounded by a serous membrane, which, after lining the ribs and intercostal muscles, and thoracic surface of the diaphragm, is reflected on the lungs from the point occupied by the pulmonic vessels. They are composed of innumerable cells communicating with the terminal branches of the bronchial tubes, around which ramify a delicate and closely woven network of bloodvessels. Collectively, these cells present an immense surface over which the blood circulates, and is exposed to the action of the atmosphere. It has been calculated that the number of these air-cells grouped round the termination of each bronchial tube, is about 18,000; and that the total number in the human lungs is not less than 600,000,000.

Not only are the lungs more highly developed, but the mechanism of respiration is more perfect in the Mammalia than in all other animals.

The inspiration and expiration of the atmospheric air are effected by the alternate movements of the diaphragm and the walls of the thoracic cavity.

A close relation exists between the number of the respirations and the rapidity of the circulation of the blood. This will be seen in the following table, drawn up from the researches of Dumas, Prevost, and Simon:—

Animals.	Number of beats of the heart in a minute.	Number of respirations in a minute.
Horse	56	16
Hare	120	36
Goat	84	24
Cat	100	24
Dog	90	28
Guinea-pig	140	36
Ape (*Simia callitriche*)	90	30
Man	72	18
Heron	200	22
Raven	110	21
Ducks	110	21
Common hen	140	30
Pigeon	136	34

This table shows that, as a general rule, the activity of the respiratory function corresponds with the rapidity of the circulation. Having studied the respiratory and circulatory systems, it would at first sight appear proper to consider the physiology of respiration. This function, however, being modified by the habits, food, vital, chemical, and physical constitution of animals, and the peculiar operations of their organs and apparatuses, its consideration will be delayed until we have studied the chemical and physical properties of the blood and all the organs in a normal state, and under the influence of starvation and thirst, and a change of diet.

The following important facts and principles have been derived from this review of the invertebrate and vertebrate kingdoms:—

1. *The development of the circulatory system, and elaboration of the blood, is always accompanied by corresponding improvements in the organs and apparatuses.* In those invertebrata which have no circulatory system (the nutritive fluids from the digestive cavity simply permeating the structure of the body), special organs and apparatuses are absent. In the invertebrate animals in which the circulatory system communicates directly with the digestive cavity, and contains a fluid differing in no essential respect from the digested matters of the stomach, the glandular and nervous systems do not exist, or are imperfectly developed. The closure of the circulatory system from the gastric cavity is attended by an improvement of the chemical and physical properties of the blood, and a corresponding improvement of the organs and apparatuses. *In those animals having the most perfect circulatory system, and the most highly elaborated blood, do we find the greatest perfection of the nervous, muscular, and organic systems.*

2. *As the organs and apparatuses of the animal economy are developed and perfected, the necessity for a vigorous circulation of the nutritive materials becomes more urgent. As the temperature, intelligence, and activity of animals, with their corresponding physical and chemical metamorphoses of the elements of organic structure, increase, there is a corresponding necessity for a rapid supply of those materials by which the wastes may be repaired, and from which the various secretions and excretions may be elaborated and separated.* The investigations upon the size of the heart and rapidity of the circulation, the perfection of the respiratory system, and the rapidity of its action, demonstrated conclusively that as the fluids and solids became more highly elaborated and developed, the action of the circulatory and respiratory systems became correspondingly rapid and vigorous.

3. *The bloodvessel system makes its appearance before the formation of a heart.* The same fact may be noticed in the development of the fœtus in warm-blooded animals. The motion of the fluid in this system, in some individuals of the invertebrate animals, is effected by the contraction of the walls of its vessels; in others, by the motion of ciliæ lining the walls of the vessels; in others, by the irregular contractions of the body; and in others, again, by an unknown force. The circulation of the blood in the stem of

colonial polyps cannot be explained by a contraction of the walls of the vessels, or by the motions of the animal.

These facts show that the existence of the heart is not essential to the motion of the blood. This remark applies, also, to the motion of the blood in the capillaries of higher animals. When the capillaries of a living animal are placed under the microscope, the blood corpuscles do not always move in the same direction. It is stated by physiologists, that if the blood of a warm-blooded animal be abstracted, and deprived of its fibrin, and then injected into the circulatory system, it will not circulate in the capillary system. The animal will die, and if examined after death, the capillaries will be found congested with blood. This fact demonstrates conclusively, that the circulation of the blood in the capillaries is dependent, in a great measure, on the heart's action, and a mutual reaction takes place between the blood and capillaries, and unless the circulatory fluid possess certain definite physical and chemical properties, the capillaries will not perform their office.

4. The blood, with its corpuscles, exists in many invertebrata which are without any special organs. The same fact has been noticed in the development of the fœtus of warm-blooded animals. A vascular system, circulating blood-corpuscles, exists before the formation of any special organs. *These facts show that the primary origin of the blood-corpuscles, in both invertebrate and vertebrate animals, is independent of any special organs.*

5. *A progressive development of the different constituents of the blood may be traced in the animal kingdom.* In the blood of the lowest invertebrate animals, we find simple granules, analogous to those which are found in the blood and organs of all animals, when nutrition and growth are active. In the more highly organized, granular cells, analogous to the colourless corpuscles of the vertebrata. In the most highly organized invertebrata, colourless nucleated cells, analogous to the coloured corpuscles of Fishes, Reptiles, and Birds. In the three lowest classes of vertebrate animals, the coloured corpuscles are nucleated. This form also exists in the fœtus of the mammalia; it is, however, a transient condition, and the coloured corpuscles of the adult mammalia are without nuclei. The proportion of the albumen, and the perfection of the fibrin, varies with the development of an animal.

6. The office of the blood-corpuscle in the invertebrata, appears to be rather the elaboration of the nutritive elements than the conveyance of oxygen. Mr. Newport observed, that in the insects, the blood-corpuscles are most numerous in the larva at the period immediately preceding each change of the skin. The blood, also, is more coagulable, and possesses a greater formative power. The blood, examined after the formation of the skin, contains corpuscles in much fewer numbers, and is far less rich in nutritive matters. The same increase in numbers, and rapid consumption of the blood-corpuscles, is observed in the pupa state during the active development of the new parts which constitute the perfect insect. After the completion

of the perfect insect, only a few corpuscles remain, and most of the plastic elements of the blood have been withdrawn during the formative process.

7. *The spleen is absent from all invertebrate animals, without exception. It is also absent from the Amphioxus, the connecting link between the Fishes and the higher forms of Mollusca. In the Amphioxus and invertebrate animals, the blood-corpuscles are always colourless. The appearance of the spleen is accompanied by a change in the colour of the blood.* Has the spleen anything to do with the production of the red colour of the corpuscles of vertebrate animals? The appearance of the spleen in vertebrate animals is accompanied by an improvement of all their organs, apparatuses, and nutritive fluids. This little organ is the herald, rather than the cause of these great changes. Its presence indicates a higher development of organization.

8. *The improvement in the solids and fluids of organized beings occurring simultaneously, it is impossible to determine which system was the cause of the development of the other.* In every individual of the animal kingdom, the component parts are mutually dependent upon each other. It would be impossible for a highly developed nervous system to exist without a correspondingly developed circulatory apparatus to supply it with blood, and organs to elaborate that blood, and remove from it all noxious compounds. *These facts show clearly the necessity for the existence of a force distinct from nervous, chemical, and physical forces, which presides over the molecules of matter, controlling and directing their chemical and physical laws and affinities, thus moulding shapeless masses into definite forms. The development and perfection of each organ and apparatus and individual being depends upon the peculiar endowments of this vital or organizing force.* The creation of a force, by whose modifications the physical, chemical, and vital constitution of every living being on earth, in air or water, is precisely adapted to fulfil certain definite ends, necessarily presupposes a Creator, who constructed, comprehended, and controlled all the physical, chemical, and vital laws which regulate the universe.

9. *The operations of nature are carried on upon the same great plan, no matter how simple or complex be the animal.* Cold-blooded animals are such, not from any peculiar chemical or physical endowments of the organic and inorganic molecules of their bodies, but from the peculiarity of the structure of their circulatory and respiratory systems. The perfection of these two systems may be taken as the index of the rapidity of the physical and chemical changes of the molecules of their fluids and solids; and the intelligence and activity of the life actions are exactly proportional to the rapidity and amount of the physical and chemical changes of the organic and inorganic molecules. *Modifications in the vital phenomena are accomplished by peculiar modifications of the structure and arrangements of the various organs and apparatuses, and by peculiar applications of the forces, and not by a suspension or alteration of the physical and chemical laws which govern all matter.*

III. *Blood of Vertebrate Animals in its Normal Condition.*[1]—The blood is a highly complex fluid; this will be readily seen by an inspection of this table, drawn up by Simon:

	Water.
Protein compounds	Fibrin. Albumen. Globulin.
Colouring matters	Hæmatin. Hæmaphæin.
Extractive matters	Alcohol-extract. Spirit-extract. Water-extract.
Fats	Cholesterin. Serolin. Red and white solid fats, containing phosphorus. Margaric acid. Oleic acid.
	Iron (peroxide).
Salts	Albuminate of soda. Phosphates of lime, magnesia, and soda. Sulphate of potash. Carbonates of lime, magnesia, and soda. Chlorides of sodium and potassium. Lactate of soda. Oleate and margarate of soda.
Gases	Oxygen. Nitrogen. Carbonic acid.
	Sulphur.
	Phosphorus.

Traces of the following substances have also been detected in the blood in certain pathological states of the system:—

Sugar,	Urate of soda,
Urea,	Urate of potassa,
Bilin, and its acids (?)	Uric acid,
Biliphæin,	Benzoate of soda,
Glutin (?)	Margarin,
Hæmacyanin,	Olein,
Erythrogen,	Copper,
Hydrochlorate of ammonia,	Manganese,
Acetate of soda,	Silica.

[1] Our limits will not permit an extended discussion of the various methods employed by different authors. Those who wish to investigate this subject for themselves, will find much useful information in *Simon's Chemistry of Man*, p. 142, Philad., 1846; *Lehmann's Physiological Chemistry*, translated by G. E. Day, and edited by Prof. Rogers, vol. i., pp. 541–648, Philad., 1855; *Bowman's Medical Chemistry*, pp. 145–194, Philad., 1850.

In investigations upon cold-blooded animals, it will be utterly impossible to determine all, or even a majority of these constituents, owing to the small amount of blood (often not more than 100 grains) which can, with the greatest care, be obtained from each individual.

As little or nothing has been done in the study of the fluids of these animals, it was necessary first to determine the most important constituents. The following is a brief statement of the method which I employed to determine the—

Water,
Solid matters of blood,
" " serum,
Moist blood-corpuscles,
Water of moist blood-corpuscles,
Solid matters of moist blood-corpuscles,
Liquor sanguinis,
Water of liquor sanguinis,
Solid matters of liquor sanguinis,
Albumen and extractive matters,
Fibrin,
Fixed saline constituents.

a. Receive into a porcelain capsule, capable of containing about f ℥ss, the weight of which had been previously carefully ascertained and noted, from 25 to 50 grains of blood.

b. Fill a 100 gr. specific gravity bottle carefully with blood.

c. Receive the remainder of the blood into a porcelain capsule (weight previously ascertained and noted) capable of containing about 500 grains of blood. In the majority of reptiles, and small birds and mammals, the blood will have been exhausted after the filling of the last vessel. Ascertain the weight of the capsule (*a*), with its blood, carefully, upon a delicate balance, and subtracting from this the weight of the capsule, we have remaining the weight of the blood. Place it upon a chloride of calcium bath, and subject it to a temperature of from 220° to 230° F. until it ceases to lose weight on being weighed at intervals of half an hour or an hour, the outside being carefully wiped clean and dry each time. Subtracting the weight of the porcelain capsule from the last weight, we obtain the amount of solid matters in the portion of blood evaporated; and subtracting the solid matters from the amount of blood used, we ascertain the amount of water. To ascertain the amount of water and solid matters in 1000 parts of blood, we use the following proportion:—

$$\left\{\begin{matrix}\text{Weight of}\\ \text{blood}\\ \text{evaporated}\end{matrix}\right\} : \left\{\begin{matrix}\text{Weight of}\\ \text{dry}\\ \text{residue}\end{matrix}\right\} :: 1000 : \left\{\begin{matrix}\text{Proportion of solid matter}\\ \text{in 1000 parts of the}\\ \text{blood.}\end{matrix}\right\}$$

Having obtained the amount of solid matters in 1000 parts of blood, the amount of water may be determined by simply subtracting the solid matters from 1000. Next incinerate carefully the solid residue in a porcelain or platinum crucible until all the carbonaceous matters are destroyed, and a light red or yellow ash remains behind. A high heat, and much care is needed in this tedious process. Another method recommended by Prof. Rogers, of the University, is to treat the dried residue with nitric acid, and gradually boiling down, incinerate. The organic matters pass of readily in the form of gases. A crucible of porcelain is to be preferred to one of platinum. The proportion of fixed saline matters in 1000 parts of blood may be calculated in the following manner:—

{Weight of blood evaporated} : {Weight of ash after incineration} : : 1000 : {Proportion of fixed saline matter in 1000 parts of blood.}

From this first portion of blood we have now obtained—

Water of 1000 parts of blood.
Solid matters of 1000 parts of blood.
Fixed saline matter of 1000 parts of blood.

b. Determine accurately upon the balance, the specific gravity of the blood. This should be done immediately after the porcelain capsule containing the blood was placed upon the chloride of calcium bath.

c. Ascertain the weight of the porcelain capsule and the last portions of blood, and, subtracting the weight of the porcelain capsule, we have remaining that of the blood. Set it aside until the blood is completely coagulated, and the serum separated from the clot; the length of time required for this varies with the animal. Ascertain the specific gravity of the serum in the 100 gr. sp. gr. bottle. Pour into a porcelain capsule (weight previously noted) from 20 to 50 grains of serum, and evaporate upon the chloride of calcium bath until it ceases to lose weight. The water, solid matters, and fixed saline constituents in 1000 parts of serum, may be ascertained in a manner exactly similar to that by which these ingredients were determined in 1000 parts of blood. It is also necessary to ascertain the amount of solid matters in the serum of 1000 parts of blood. Knowing the quantity of water in 1000 parts of blood, and assuming that the water of the blood exists wholly in the form of serum—knowing, also, the amount of water and solid matters contained in a given portion of serum, we may, from the quantity of water in the blood, estimate the quantity of solids held in solution in the serum, thus—

{Weight of water in the quantity of serum employed} : {Weight of solid matter in the quantity of serum employed} :: {Water in 1000 parts of the blood} : {Solids of serum in 1000 parts of the blood.}

This is not absolutely correct, and all physiological chemists have failed to ascertain with absolute accuracy the amount of solid matters in the serum of 1000 parts of blood. The error, however, is very small, and cannot be avoided.

The clot which remained after the removal of the serum, is next cut into thin slices, and inclosed in a muslin bag, and carefully washed under a stream of water until the fibrin remains in the bag, free from serum and blood-corpuscles, and almost colourless. Another method of obtaining the fibrin, is to receive into a small glass bottle (capable of containing from f℥ij to f℥iv) a portion of blood, and then dropping in some dozen small strips of lead, and closing with the stopper, agitate and shake until the fibrin coagulates around the lead-strips.

Two strong objections lie against the employment of this method in investigations upon cold-blooded animals: 1. Their blood, in most cases, cannot be obtained in sufficient quantities; and 2, the fibrin is so soft that it will not coagulate around the lead-strips. The clean fibrin is then placed in a small evaporating dish, and dried upon the chloride of calcium bath, at a temperature of 220° to 230° F., until it ceases to lose weight. If we wish still greater accuracy, it may be treated with dilute hydrochloric acid, absolute alcohol, and ether, to dissolve out the saline and fatty and extractive matters before evaporation upon the chloride of calcium bath.

After having obtained the weight of dried fibrin in the quantity of blood used in the experiment, the proportion in 1000 parts of blood may be determined by the following calculation:—

$$\left\{\begin{array}{c}\text{Weight of}\\ \text{blood}\\ \text{employed}\end{array}\right\} : \left\{\begin{array}{c}\text{Weight of}\\ \text{fibrin}\\ \text{obtained}\end{array}\right\} :: 1000 : \left\{\begin{array}{c}\text{Quantity of fibrin}\\ \text{in 1000 parts of}\\ \text{blood.}\end{array}\right\}$$

From the third portion of blood (c) we have thus obtained the following constituents:—[1]

Water in 1000 parts of serum.
Solid matter in 1000 parts of serum.
Solid matters in serum of 1000 parts of blood.
Albumen and extractive matter.
Fixed saline constituents in 1000 parts of serum.
Fibrin in 1000 parts of blood.

We have now sufficient data from which to calculate the dried blood-corpuscles, moist blood-corpuscles, and liquor sanguinis. To ascertain the weight of the dried blood-corpuscles, add together the weights of the fibrin and the solids of the serum contained in 1000 parts of blood, and deducting the sum of them from the weight of the entire solid matter, which consists of fibrin, solids of the serum, and corpuscles, the difference therefore will represent the proportion of the latter in 1000 parts of the blood. Another method is founded upon the fact that a solution of Glauber's salts possesses the property of rendering the blood-corpuscles capable of being retained upon a filter. This method has been applied by Figuier, Dumas, and Höfle.

Defibrinated blood is treated with eight times its volume of a concentrated

[1] If the fixed saline constituents of serum of 1000 parts of blood be subtracted from the solid matters of the serum of 1000 parts of blood, we have remaining the albumen and extractive matters.

solution of Glauber's salts, and filtered; the residue on the filter is rinsed with the same solution; a stream of oxygen is passed through the mass lying on the filter at the same time; and finally, the mass of blood-cells is either coagulated with hot water upon the filter, or washed off into tepid water, and coagulated by boiling. This method, although apparently practicable and accurate in theory, is not to be depended upon in practice, because some of the blood-corpuscles always pass through the filter, and it is impossible to determine whether all the serum is actually separated in this manner; and also the solution of the Glauber's salts passes into the corpuscles by endosmosis, whilst the organic constituents of the corpuscles must pass out.

Simon's method of finding the quantity of the blood-corpuscles directly, is also altogether wanting in accuracy. C. Schmidt, to whose intelligence and indefatigable researches physiological chemistry is indebted for many brilliant discoveries, first attempted to determine the relation of the moist blood-cells to the intercellular fluid, or liquor sanguinis. He found by laborious researches, that the constant factor, by which we may calculate the moist blood-cells from the dry blood-corpuscles, was 4. If we multiply the number of dry blood-corpuscles by 4, we obtain the quantity of fresh blood-cells; subtracting these from 1000, we have remaining the amount of liquor sanguinis in 1000 parts of blood.

We will now proceed to consider the results of our investigations without stopping to consider those innumerable little steps of caution and accuracy which would naturally suggest themselves to every intelligent and careful observer during an organic analysis. I have arranged the results in as condensed a form as possible, so that the facts and principles developed may be evident at a glance.

Amounts of blood in different animals.—Great discrepancies have prevailed amongst physiologists with regard to the amount of blood contained in the bodies of animals. Blumenbach estimated the quantity in an adult man at 8.5 to 11 pounds, and Reil at 44 pounds. M. Valentin, by his method of injecting water into the bloodvessels during life, arrived at the following results. The numbers represent the relations existing between the quantity of blood and the weights of the body.

Large dogs, as . .	1 : 4.5	(the mean of four experiments.)
A lean, debilitated sheep	1 : 5.02	
Cats (female) . .	1 : 5.78	(the mean of two experiments.)
Large female rabbit .	1 : 6.20	

From these data he estimated the amount of human blood to be—

Male sex	1 : 4.36
Female sex	1 : 4.93

At the present day, the blood is generally estimated at 22 pounds, which is equal to about the eighth part of the weight of the entire human body.

Lehmann determined the amount of blood in the bodies of two criminals who were decapitated, to be nearly one-eighth of that of the whole body.

By numerous careful examinations of cold-blooded animals, I have arrived at the following results, which must be considered only as an approximation to the truth:—

Amount of blood in		Ophidians	$\frac{1}{10}$ to $\frac{1}{13}$	of the weight of the whole body.		
"	"	Emys terrapin	$\frac{1}{11}$ to $\frac{1}{14}$	"	"	"
"	"	Emys serrata	$\frac{1}{13}$ to $\frac{1}{16}$	"	"	"
"	"	Testudo polyphemus	$\frac{1}{14}$ to $\frac{1}{17}$	"	"	"

These results show that the blood is far less abundant in cold than in warm-blooded animals. This fact is important, as it will aid us in the explanation of the differences which distinguish the two great classes of animals.

In all the cold-blooded animals which I have thus far examined, the portions of blood first drawn coagulate more slowly than those drawn last.

Owing to the admixture of venous and arterial blood in the common ventricle of the heart of these animals, their arterial blood is never of that bright red colour of the arterial blood of warm-blooded animals, but is of a dark red colour, intermediate between that of arterial and venous blood.

The colour of the serum in most Reptiles, as Ophidians, Batrachians, Fishes, and some Chelonians—as the Gopher—is of a light yellow colour. In the Yellow-belly Terrapin (*Emys serrata*), Chicken Terrapin (*Emys reticulata*), and Salt-water Terrapin (*Emys terrapin*), the serum is of a golden colour.

The strong smell of both cold and warm-blooded animals appears to reside especially in the serum, and may be developed by treating the serum with a little sulphuric acid, and a gentle heat. I have demonstrated this fact in numerous instances, and often in the serum of disagreeable animals, with disgusting power.

The following table represents the specific gravities of the blood of different animals, which were accurately determined upon a delicate balance; and we would here state, that the balance which was used in all my analyses was capable of turning to $\frac{1}{1000}$ of a grain.

			Specific gravity.
Blood of	Coach-whip Snake (*Psámmophis flagellifórmis*)		1036.
"	female Alligator (*Alligátor Mississippiénsis*)		1046.
"	Loggerhead Turtle (*Chelónia carétta*)		1032.5
"	Alligator Cooter (*Chelonúra serpentina*)		1025.5
"	female Salt-water Terrapin (*Emys térrapin*)		1035.3
"	Chicken Terrapin (*Emys reticuláta*)		1034.
"	female Yellow-belly Terrapin (*Emys serráta*)		1026.5
"	male Gopher (*Testúdo polyphémus*)		1030.
"	female Night Heron (*Ardea nycticorax*)		1028.
"	common Cur Dog		1043.6
"	common Cur Dog		1045.5
		mean	1051.5
"	pregnant women, by Becquerel and Rodier	max.	1055.1
		min.	1046.2

		Specific gravity.
Blood of 20 persons, by Becquerel and Rodier,	mean . .	1055.
" 10 " " "	mean . .	1056.0
" 11 men " "	mean . .	1060.2
" 8 females " "	mean . .	1057.5

Table of the Specific Gravities of the Serum of different Animals.

Serum of Loggerhead Turtle (*Chelónia carétta*)	. . . .	1014.8
" Alligator Cooter (*Chelonúra serpentina*)	. . . .	1013.6
" Salt-water Terrapin (*Emys térrapin*)	. . . .	1012.7
" Yellow-belly Terrapin (*Emys serráta*)	. . . .	1013.7
" Yellow-belly Terrapin (*Emys serráta*)	. . . .	1014.
" male Gopher (*Testúdo polyphémus*)	. . . .	1018.
" male Gopher (*Testúdo polyphémus*)	. . . .	1017.
" common Cur Dog	. . . .	1030.5
" 11 men, by Becquerel and Rodier	mean . .	1028.0
	maximum . .	1030.0
	minimum . .	1027.0
" 8 females " "	mean . .	1027.4
	maximum . .	1030.0
	minimum . .	1026.0
" 8 human (Lehmann)	. . . .	1028.

From these tables we learn that, as the organs and apparatuses, and intelligence of animals are developed, the blood becomes more concentrated.

Table showing the Amount of Water in 1000 *parts of the Blood of different Animals.*

COLD-BLOODED ANIMALS.

Blood of Invertebrate Animals.

Name of observer.	Name of animal.	Water in 1000 parts of blood.
C. Schmidt.	Pond Mussel (*Anodonta cygnea*)	999.146
Harless and Bibra.	Shell Snail (*Helix pomatia*)	985.482
" "	Cephalopods (*Loligo* and *Eledone*)	992.67

Blood of Vertebrate Animals.

FISHES.

Jos Jones.	Stingray (*Trygon sabina*)	884.20
"	Hammerhead Shark (*Zygæna málleus*) . .	861.14
"	Garfish (*Lepisosteus osseus*)	886.70
J. F. Simon.	Carp	872.00
"	Tench	900.00
Dumas and Prevost.	Trout	863.70
" "	Eelpout	886.20
" "	Eel	846.00

Name of observer.	Name of animal.	Water in 1000 parts of blood.
	AQUATIC REPTILES.	
Jos. Jones.	Bullfrog (*Rána pipiens*)	832.51
Dumas and Prevost.	Frog	884.60
Jos. Jones.	Loggerhead Turtle (*Chelónia carétta*)	879.19
"	Alligator Cooter (*Chelonúra serpentina*)	895.00
"	Salt-water Terrapin (*Emys térrapin*)	845.28
"	Chicken Terrapin (*Emys reticuláta*)	846.98
"	Yellow-belly Terrapin (*Emys serráta*)	875.41
"	Alligator (*Alligátor Mississippiénsis*)	823.86
	LAND REPTILES.	
J. F. Simon.	Bufo variabilis	848.20
Jos. Jones.	Hognose Viper (*Hetérodon platyrhinos*)	833.24
"	Black Viper (*Hetérodon niger*)	860.57
"	Coach-whip Snake (*Psámmophis flagellifórmis*)	818.30
"	Black-Snake (*Cóluber constrictor*)	788.63
"	Gopher (*Testúdo polyphémus*)	843.38
	WARM-BLOODED ANIMALS.	
	Blood of Birds.	
Nasse.	Goose	814.88
"	Hen	793.24
Dumas and Prevost.	Hen	779.90
" "	Pigeon	797.40
" "	Duck	765.20
" "	Raven	797.00
" "	Heron	808.20
Jos. Jones.	Heron (*Ardea nycticorax*)	872.89
"	Hooting Owl (*Syrnium nebulósum*)	839.66
"	Black Turkey-buzzard (*Cathártes atrátus*)	799.17
	Blood of Mammalia.	
Andral, Gavarret, and Delafond.	17 Horses { mean	810.50
	maximum	833.30
	minimum	795.70
Nasse.	Horse	804.75
Dumas and Prevost.	Horse	818.30
Andral, Gavarret, and Delafond.	14 Cattle { mean	810.30
	maximum	824.90
	minimum	799.00
Nasse.	Ox	799.59
Dumas and Prevost.	Calf	826.00
And., Gav., and Dela.	30 Sheep (mean)	818.50
Nasse.	Swine	768.94
"	Rabbit	817.30
Dumas and Prevost.	Rabbit	837.90
" "	Goat	814.60
Nasse.	Goat	839.44
And., Gav., and Dela.	16 Dogs (mean)	774.10

Name of observer.	Name of animal.	Water in 1000 parts of blood.
Nasse.	Dog	790.50
Dumas and Prevost.	Dog	810.70
Jos. Jones.	Common Cur-Dog	811.87
"	Common Cur-Dog	806.52
Dumas and Prevost.	Cat	795.30
Nasse.	Cat	810.02
	Man { maximum	853.135
M. Leeanu.	Man { minimum	778.625
	Man { mean	815.880

Table of the Solid Matters in 1000 parts of the Blood of different Animals.

COLD-BLOODED ANIMALS.

Blood of Invertebrate Animals.

Name of observer.	Name of animal.	Solid matters in 1000 parts of blood.
C. Schmidt.	Pond Mussel (*Anodonta cygnea*)	0.854
Harless and Bibra.	Shell Snail (*Helix pomatia*)	14.518
" "	Cephalopods (*Loligo* and *Eledone*)	7.33

Blood of Vertebrate Animals.

FISHES.

Name of observer.	Name of animal.	Solid matters in 1000 parts of blood.
Jos. Jones.	Stingray (*Trygon sabina*)	115.80
" "	Hammerhead Shark (*Zygæna málleus*)	138.86
" "	Garfish (*Lepisósteus ósseus*)	113.30
J. F. Simon.	Carp	128.00
"	Tench	100.00
Dumas and Prevost.	Trout	136.30
" "	Eelpout	113.80
" "	Eel	154.00

AQUATIC REPTILES.

Name of observer.	Name of animal.	Solid matters in 1000 parts of blood.
Jos. Jones.	Bullfrog (*Rána pipiens*)	167.49
Dumas and Prevost.	Frog	115.40
Jos. Jones.	Loggerhead Turtle (*Chelónia carétta*)	120.81
"	Alligator Cooter (*Chelonúra serpentina*)	105.00
"	Salt-water Terrapin (*Emys térrapin*)	154.72
	Chicken Terrapin (*Emys reticuláta*)	153.02
	Yellow-belly Terrapin (*Emys serráta*)	124.59
	Alligator (*Alligátor Mississippiénsis*)	176.14

LAND REPTILES.

Name of observer.	Name of animal.	Solid matters in 1000 parts of blood.
J. F. Simon.	Bufo variabilis	151.80
Jos. Jones.	Hognose Viper (*Hetérodon platyrhinos*)	166.76
"	Black Viper (*Hetérodon niger*)	139.43
"	Coach-whip Snake (*Psámmophis flagellifórmis*)	181.70
	Black-Snake (*Cóluber constrictor*)	211.37
	Gopher (*Testúdo polyphémus*)	156.62

WARM-BLOODED ANIMALS.

Blood of Birds.

Name of observer.	Name of animal.	Solid matters in 1000 parts of blood.
Nasse.	Goose	185.12
"	Hen	206.76
Dumas and Prevost.	Hen	220.10
" "	Pigeon	202.60
" "	Duck	234.80
" "	Raven	203.00
" "	Heron	191.80
Jos. Jones.	Heron (*Ardea nycticorax*)	127.11
"	Hooting Owl (*Syrnium nebulósum*)	160.34
"	Black Turkey-buzzard (*Cathártes atrátus*)	200.83

Blood of Mammalia.

Name of observer.	Name of animal.	Solid matters in 1000 parts of blood.
Andral, Gavarret, and Delafond.	17 horses { mean	189.50
	maximum	204.30
	minimum	166.70
Nasse.	Horse	195.25
Dumas and Prevost.	Horse	181.70
Andral, Gavarret, and Delafond.	14 Cattle { mean	189.70
	maximum	201.00
	minimum	175.10
Nasse.	Ox	200.41
Dumas and Prevost.	Calf	174.00
And., Gav., and Dela.	30 Sheep (mean)	186.50
Nasse.	Swine	231.06
"	Rabbit	182.70
Dumas and Prevost.	Rabbit	162.10
" "	Goat	185.40
Nasse.	Goat	160.56
And., Gav., and Dela.	16 dogs (mean)	225.90
Nasse.	Dog	209.50
Dumas and Prevost.	Dog	189.30
Jos. Jones.	Common Cur-Dog	188.13
"	Common Cur-Dog	193.48
Dumas and Prevost.	Cat	204.70
Nasse.	Cat	189.98
M. Leeanu.	Man { maximum	221.37
	minimum	146.86
	mean	184.12

A careful comparison of these results leads to the following conclusions:—

1. *The proportion of water is greatest in the invertebrata.* The blood of those animals has a specific gravity not much above that of common water. The specific gravity of the blood of *Limulus Cyclops*, according to Genth, is only 1010.317.

2. *Amongst vertebrate animals, the amount of water existing in the blood is*

greatest in Fishes and aquatic Reptiles, and least in Serpents, Birds, and Mammalia. As a necessary consequence, the solid matters of the blood are less in the invertebrata, fishes, and aquatic reptiles, and greatest in serpents, birds, and mammalia.

3. *It may be laid down as a general law, that as the organs and apparatuses of the animal economy are developed, and the temperature and intellect correspondingly increased, the blood becomes richer in organic constituents.* The blood of Serpents appears at first sight to form an exception. The large amount of solid matters, however, existing in their blood, is readily accounted for when we consider their habits. These reptiles seldom or never drink water; consequently the fluids of their bodies are derived from the animals which they consume. In all animals, the water of the blood and tissues is continually evaporating from the surface of the lungs and body. The amount of evaporation is in proportion to the structure, habits, and temperature of animals, and the temperature and moisture of the atmosphere. It is greatest in warm-blooded animals, and in hot and dry climates. Amongst cold-blooded animals it is greatest in those having naked skins, and least in those covered by scales, bone, and horn. No matter how slow and small this evaporation, if it be not counteracted by a corresponding supply of water, the blood necessarily becomes concentrated, and yields a larger proportion of solid constituents upon analysis.

4. Our knowledge is as yet too limited to develop any laws respecting the amount of water and solid constituents which characterize the blood of each species and genus. By comparing the analyses of the blood of the Mammalia, we see that the proportions of its constituents vary as much in individuals of the same species as in individuals of remotely separated genera.

We will next consider the amounts and constitutions of the moist blood-cells, and liquor sanguinis.

Table of the Moist Blood-Corpuscles, and their Constituents in 1000 *parts of Blood.*

Name of animal.	Moist blood-corpuscles in 1000 parts of blood.	Water in moist blood-corpuscles in 1000 parts of blood.	Solid matter in moist blood-corpuscles in 1000 parts of blood.
Shark (*Zygæna málleus*)	293.44	220.08	73.36
Garfish (*Lepisósteus ósseus*)	229.00	171.75	57.25
Trout	275.20	206.40	68.80
Eelpout	192.40	144.30	48.10
Eel	240.00	180.00	60.00
Bullfrog (*Rána pipiens*)	450.12	337.59	112.53
Frog	276.00	207.00	69.00
Hognose Viper (*Hetérodon plat.*)	444.84	333.63	111.21
Black Viper (*Hetérodon niger*)	270.40	202.80	67.60
Coach-whip Snake (*Psámmophis flagelliférmis*)	488.80	366.60	122.20

Name of animal.	Moist blood-corpuscles in 1000 parts of blood.	Water in moist blood-corpuscles in 1000 parts of blood.	Solid matter in moist blood-corpuscles in 1000 parts of blood.
Black-Snake (*Cóluber constrictor*)	469.20	351.90	117.30
Turtle (*Chelónia carétta*)	289.52	217.14	72.38
Alligator Cooter (*Chelonúra serpentina*)	235.40	176.55	58.85
Salt-water Terrapin (*Emys térrapin*)	447.28	335.46	111.82
Chicken Terrapin (*Emys reticuláta*)	372.00	279.00	93.00
Yellow-belly Terrapin (*Emys serráta*)	336.76	252.57	84.19
Gopher (*Testúdo polyphémus*)	393.56	302.67	90.89
Alligator (*Alligátor Mississippiénsis*)	364.08	273.06	91.02
Goose	485.80	364.35	121.45
Hen	579.00	434.25	144.75
Hen	628.40	461.30	157.10
Duck	600.40	450.30	150.10
Pigeon	622.80	467.10	155.70
Raven	586.40	339.80	146.60
Heron	530.40	367.80	132.60
Heron (*Ardea nycticorax*)	315.84	236.88	78.96
Hooting Owl (*Syrnium nebulósum*)	427.36	320.52	106.84
Black Buzzard (*Cathártes atrátus*)	626.88	470.16	156.72
17 Horses, mean	411.60	308.70	102.90
17 Horses, maximum	448.40	336.30	112.10
17 Horses, minimum	326.00	244.50	81.50
Horse	468·52	351.39	117.13
30 Sheep (mean)	404.40	303.30	101.10
Sheep	369.68	277.26	92.42
14 Cattle, mean	398.80	299.10	99.70
14 Cattle, maximum	468.40	351.30	117.10
14 Cattle, minimum	340.40	255.30	85.10
6 Swine, English breed (mean)	422.80	317.10	105.70
16 Dogs, mean	593.20	444.90	148.30
16 Dogs, maximum	706.40	529.80	176.60
16 Dogs, minimum	509.20	387.90	121.30
Common Cur-Dog	363.64	197.73	65.91
Common Cur-Dog	322.76	242.07	80.69

Table of the Liquor Sanguinis and its Constituents in 1000 *parts of Blood.*

Name of observer.	Name of animal.	Liquor sanguinis in 1000 parts of blood.	Water in liquor sanguinis in 1000 parts of blood.	Solid matter in liquor sanguinis in 1000 parts of blood.
Jos. Jones.	Shark (*Zygœna malleus*)	706.56	641.06	65.50
"	Garfish (*Lepisosteus osseus*)	771.00	714.95	56.05
"	Bullfrog (*Rána pipiens*)	549.88	494.92	54.96
"	Hognose Viper (*Heterodon platyrhinos*)	555.16	499.61	55.55
"	Black Viper (*Heterodon niger*)	729.60	657.77	71.83
"	Coach-whip Snake (*Psámmophis flagellifórmis*)	511.20	451.70	59.50

Name of observer.	Name of animal.	Liquor sanguinis in 1000 parts of blood.	Water in liquor sanguinis in 1000 parts of blood.	Solid matter in liquor sanguinis in 1000 parts of blood.
Jos. Jones.	Black-Snake (*Cóluber constrictor*)	530.80	436.73	94.07
"	Turtle (*Chelónia carétta*) . . .	710.49	662.05	48.43
"	Alligator Cooter (*Chelonúra serpent.*)	764.60	718.45	46.15
"	Salt-water Terrapin (*Emys térrapin*)	552.72	509.82	42.90
"	Chicken Terrapin (*Emys reticuláta*)	628.00	567.98	60.02
"	Yellow-belly Terrapin (*Emys serráta*)	663.24	622.84	40.40
"	Gopher (*Testúdo polyphémus*) .	606.44	540.71	65.73
"	Alligator (*Alligátor Mississippiénsis*)	635.92	550.80	85.12
"	Heron (*Ardea nycticorax*) . .	684.16	636.01	48.15
"	Hooting Owl (*Syrnium nebulósum*)	572.64	519.14	53.50
"	Black Buzzard (*Cathártes atrátus*)	373.12	329.01	44.11
"	Common Cur-Dog	736.36	613.14	125.22
"	Common Cur-Dog	677.24	564.45	112.79

The following general facts and conclusions have been derived from a careful comparison of the results of the examination of the important constituents of the blood of different animals:—

In the invertebrata, the number of blood-corpuscles is very small in comparison with the number which exists in the blood of the vertebrata. In this class, we find only colourless corpuscles. In the Branchiostoma, or Amphioxus, the connecting link between the highest orders of the invertebrata and Fishes, the blood, like that of invertebrate animals, contains only colourless corpuscles, is exceedingly rich in water, and correspondingly poor in solid constituents. *As the organs and apparatuses are developed, the blood is correspondingly improved. The increased development of the cerebro-spinal system, and the organs of vertebrate animals, is attended by a corresponding increase in the number of the solitary gland-cells of the blood.* In this class, the number of blood-corpuscles is, as a general rule, lowest in cold-blooded animals, and highest in Birds and Mammalia. There are, however, exceptions to this rule. I have found the number of blood-corpuscles in some cold-blooded animals, especially Serpents, higher than that of some Birds and Mammals. This statement, however, will be modified somewhat by the fact, that the whole amount of blood, and the absolute number of blood-corpuscles existing in the blood of cold-blooded animals, is much less than that which exists in the blood of warm-blooded animals.

The following table contains some striking facts:—

Blood-corpuscles in 1000 *parts of blood.*

Bullfrog (*Rána pipiens*)	108.68
Salt-water Terrapin (*Emys térrapin*)	103.82
Alligator (*Alligátor Mississippiénsis*)	86.39
Hognose Viper (*Hetérodon platyrhinos*) . . .	102.22
Coach-whip Snake (*Psámmophis flagellifórmis*) . .	118.34
Black-Snake (*Cóluber constrictor*)	112.22

Heron (*Ardea nycticorax*)	74.91
Owl (*Syrnium nebulósum*)	101.08
Horse	81.50
Horse	102.90
Goat	86.00
Goat	102.00
Cur-Dog	62.72
Cur-Dog	78.04
Dog	123.80
Cow	85.10

Notwithstanding the differences in the number of blood-corpuscles, the difference of temperature was preserved, not only between the warm and cold-blooded animals, but also between the individual species of each class. The thermometer indicated a temperature of over 100° F., in the Heron having 74.91 parts of blood-corpuscles, whilst in the Frog, Serpents, and Chelonians, having nearly double the number of blood-corpuscles in a given quantity of blood, the thermometer indicated a temperature several degrees below that of the surrounding medium.

Several physiologists assert, that the sole office of the blood-corpuscle is to carry oxygen in, and convey carbonic acid gas out, of the animal economy. If this be true, the temperature of an animal should be determined, in great measure, by the number of its blood-corpuscles, for the temperature of the body is proportional to the amount of oxygen which enters the animal economy, and combines with the organic elements of its nutritive fluids and tissues. Many other facts might be mentioned, in addition to those which we have just mentioned, to prove that the sole office of the blood-corpuscles is not the introduction of oxygen, and the carrying out of carbonic acid. The following considerations will show that the serum of the blood is also active in the performance of these important offices:—

In the capillaries and bloodvessels, the coloured corpuscles rush along in the centre of the streams, whilst pure serum, alone, is in contact with the walls of the vessels. In the capillaries of the lungs, the oxygen, from this arrangement, must necessarily be absorbed first by the serum. Again, in no case do we find the organic cells—the active agent in all secretion and excretion—in immediate contact with the blood-corpuscles. They are separated from them by the coats of the capillaries, and a structureless basement membrane. The same is true of the anatomical elements of the muscular tissue. From whence do they derive oxygen, a continuous supply of which is absolutely necessary for the life and activity of every living molecule of organic matter?

The same arguments will also prove that the blood-corpuscles are only secondary agents in the conveyance of carbonic acid gas out of the organs and tissues to the lungs. These conclusions can be sustained by numerous examples. Do we find blood-corpuscles in plants? Do we find blood-corpuscles in the lowest orders of invertebrate animals? Spallanzani has long since demonstrated that all organized bodies, whether living or dead, possess the property of absorbing oxygen, and giving out carbonic acid.

What, then, are the principal offices of the blood-corpuscles? and what does an increase in their number denote? These questions can only be answered by a consideration of their constitution and their relations with the liquor sanguinis by which they are surrounded.

Each corpuscle is a cell, resembling in its nutrition, growth, and general structure the active agents in the formation, elaboration, and separation of all secretions and excretions. Their cell-walls possess the power of separating from the surrounding medium certain peculiar mineral and organic compounds. If a blood-corpuscle be placed in water, it swells up, and finally bursts. If it is placed in a dense solution, its contents pass out, and the cell-wall shrivels up. The same physical laws of endosmose and exosmose are at work in the animal economy. A mutual action and reaction is incessantly carried on between the interior fluid contents of the blood-corpuscles and the exterior liquor sanguinis. Whenever water, or liquids of low specific gravity, are introduced, they dilute the serum, and immediately there is an endosmose of the exterior less dense fluid into the denser contents of the corpuscle. When water is withheld, the liquor sanguinis continually loses this element by evaporation from the surface of the lungs and skin, and by the action of the kidneys, and becomes denser than the contents of the corpuscles, and exosmose takes place into the surrounding medium. The cell-wall modifies the physical and chemical properties and constitution of every molecule of liquor sanguinis that passes through its structure. *The office, then, of the blood-corpuscles, taken collectively, is that of an immense gland, which elaborates the constituents of the blood.*

In the Mammalia we have an increase, not only by weight, but also an immense increase in numbers, of the blood-corpuscles, owing to their greatly diminished size, and the amount of secreting surface exposed to the intercellular fluid is correspondingly increased. This being the case, the blood of these animals must be more highly elaborated, and all their organs and apparatuses correspondingly developed.

The solid residue of the liquor sanguinis is very small in the invertebrata. Amongst vertebrate animals it varies without reference to the species, genus, and class, and appears not to be influenced in its amount or chemical constitution by the development of animals. It is reasonable to suppose that it is dependent more immediately upon the character of the food.

The fibrin presents a remarkable index of the vital organic and intellectual endowments of animals. In the whole of the invertebrate kingdom it is absent, except in a few of the most highly organized, in whom its appearance is accompanied by a corresponding improvement of the cerebro-spinal system, and all the organs.

In the lowest orders of the vertebrata, as Fishes and Batrachians, it is soft, unstable, and readily convertible into albumen.

In the Ophidians and Chelonians, although it is stable and does not dissolve, still its structure is soft, inconsistent, and resembles in many respects the fibrin which is formed when the vital forces of warm-blooded animals have been exhausted by copious and continued bleedings.

Here we have a beautiful demonstration of the fact that the animal kingdom is constructed upon one great plan. Pathological conditions of the most highly organized animals are found to exist as the normal and permanent conditions of those placed below in the scale of creation. If the forces of a warm-blooded animal be reduced, it presents a condition in many respects similar to that of a cold-blooded animal. We will illustrate this by one other example. Warm-blooded animals, in health, are able to maintain their temperature at a fixed standard, regardless of that of the surrounding medium. As the surrounding temperature descends, the efforts of nature to sustain a definite degree of heat, increase. If, however, the forces of the animal economy be impaired, the efforts of nature are no longer sufficient to keep the body heated to the definite normal standard, and gradually the body assumes the temperature of the surrounding medium. The intellect and all the organic forces become torpid; the chemical actions cease, or are performed in a feeble or perverted manner; and finally, the once active and warm-blooded animal is reduced to the condition of a sluggish cold-blooded animal. The following table represents the amount of fibrin in 1000 parts of the blood of different animals:—

Name of observer.	Name of animal.	Fibrin in 1000 parts of blood.
C. Schmidt.	Pond Mussel (*Anodonta cygnea*) . . .	0.033
Jos. Jones.	Stingray (*Trygon sabina*)	unstable
"	Hammerhead Shark (*Zygæna málleus*) . .	unstable
"	Garfish (*Lepisósteus ósseus*)	unstable
J. F. Simon.	Carp	unstable
"	Tench	unstable
Jos. Jones.	Bullfrog (*Rána pipiens*)	unstable
J. F. Simon.	Bufo Variabilis	unstable
Jos. Jones.	Black Viper (*Heterodon niger*) . . .	2.16
"	Coach-whip Snake (*Psámmophis flagellifórmis*)	1.88
"	Black-Snake (*Cóluber constrictor*) . . .	5.06
	Loggerhead Turtle (*Chelónia carétta*) . .	2.61
	Alligator Cooter (*Chelonúra serpentina*) . .	0.35
	Salt-water Terrapin (*Emys térrapin*) . .	4.15
	Chicken Terrapin (*Emys reticuláta*) . .	2.51
	Yellow-belly Terrapin (*Emys serráta*) . .	1.04
	Gopher (*Testúdo polyphémus*)	5.73
"	Alligator (*Alligátor Mississippiénsis*) . .	3.07
Nasse.	Goose	3.46
"	Hen	4.67
Jos. Jones.	Heron (*Ardea nycticorax*)	2.20
"	Hooting Owl (*Syrnium nebulósum*) . . .	4.69
"	Black Turkey-buzzard (*Cathártes atrátus*) .	0.41

Name of observer.	Name of animal.		Fibrin in 1000 parts of blood.
Andral, Gavarret, and Delafond.	17 Horses	mean	4.00
		maximum	5.00
		minimum	3.00
Nasse.	Horse		2.41
Andral, Gavarret, and Delafond.	14 Cattle	mean	3.70
		maximum	4.40
		minimum	3.00
Nasse.	Ox		3.62
And., Gav., and Dela.	30 Sheep (mean)		3.00
Nasse.	Swine		3.95
And., Gav., and Dela.	6 Swine (English breed), mean		4.60
Nasse.	Goat		3.90
And., Gav., and Dela.	16 Dogs (mean)		2.10
Nasse.	Dog		1.93
Jos. Jones.	Common Cur-Dog		3.04
"	Common Cur-Dog		3.15
Nasse.	Cat		2.42

In addition to the observations which we have previously made, this table also shows that the fibrin is one of the most variable of all the constituents of the blood. This arises, in great measure, from imperfections in our methods of analysis.

We will next consider the amount of fixed saline constituents existing in the blood of different animals.

Table of the Fixed Saline Matters in 1000 *parts of the Blood of different Animals.*

Name of observer.	Name of animal.	Fixed saline matter in 1000 parts of blood.	
C. Schmidt.	Pond Mussel (*Anodonta cygnea*)	0.256	Inverte-brated animals.
Harless and Bibra.	Shell Snail (*Helix pomatia*)	6.12	
Bibra.	Ascidans and Cephalopods	2.63	
Genth.	Limulus Cyclops	3.327	
Jos. Jones.	Stingray (*Trygona sabina*)	14.70	Salt-water Fishes and Reptiles.
"	Hammerhead Shark (*Zygœna málleus*)	8.36	
"	Garfish (*Lepisósteus ósseus*)	10.27	
	Salt-water Terrapin (*Emys térrapin*)	10.74	
	Alligator (*Alligátor Mississippiénsis*)	8.65	
	Loggerhead Turtle (*Chelónia carétta*)	3.58	
	Bullfrog (*Rána pipiens*)	5.78	Fresh-water Reptiles.
	Alligator Cooter (*Chelonúra serpentina*)	4.39	
	Yellow-belly Terrapin (*Emys serráta*)	5.22	
	Chicken Terrapin (*Emys reticuláta*)	7.79	
	Hog-nose Viper (*Hetérodon platyrhinos*)	13.47	Land Reptiles.
	Black Viper (*Hetérodon niger*)	7.04	
	Coach-whip Snake (*Psámmophis flagellifórmis*)	5.57	
	Black-Snake (*Cóluber constrictor*)	8.77	
"	Gopher (*Testúdo polyphémus*)	5.83	

Name of observer.	Name of animal.	Fixed saline matter in 1000 parts of blood.	
"	Black Buzzard (*Cathártes atrátus*)	8.33	Birds.
"	Heron (*Ardea nycticorax*)	6.59	
"	Owl (*Syrnium nebulósum*)	8.06	
Nasse.	Goose	7.92	
"	Hen	8.79	
"	Sheep	7.76	Mammalia.
	Horse	7.85	
	Ox	6.95	
	Calf	7.87	
	Goat	7.84	
	Rabbit	6.28	
	Cat	7.84	
"	Dog	7.33	
Jos. Jones.	Common Cur-Dog	6.04	
"	Common Cur-Dog	6.11	

From this table we learn that the proportion of fixed saline constituents in the blood, is remarkably uniform throughout the whole animal kingdom. This fact, in connection with others, which will be mentioned hereafter, demonstrates their importance.

In the invertebrata they exist in largest amount, relatively to that of the organic constituents of the blood, than in vertebrate animals. Thus, in the blood of the Shell Snail (*Helix pomatia*), there were 6.12 parts of mineral, and only 8.39 parts of organic substances. In the blood of Ascidans and Cephalopods, Bibra found 4.7 parts of organic, and 2.63 parts of mineral substances. When we consider the character of the shells of these animals, it is not wonderful that the blood should contain so large a proportion of mineral substances. Schmidt found the albumen of the blood of the Pond Mussel (*Anodonta cygnea*) combined with lime. This fact shows that these mineral bodies are chemically combined with the organic constituents of their bodies.

Amongst vertebrate animals, we find the largest amount of mineral constituents in the blood of Fishes and Reptiles inhabiting the salt-water. The only exception to this rule was found in the blood of a Loggerhead Turtle (*Chelonia caretta*), which had been kept, for forty-eight hours previous to the analysis, in a tub of fresh water. It is probable that an interchange may have taken place between the exterior water and the salts held in solution in the blood. The blood of the hog-nose viper (*Heterodon platyrhinos*), yielded a larger amount of ash than that of any other animal. This is accounted for by the fact that the reptile had been starved for a length of time, and the blood was in a concentrated condition. The Alligator is classed amongst the salt-water Reptiles, because it had resided in a small salt-water stream, in a salt marsh, for about a year. This reptile inhabits, most generally, the brackish and fresh-water rivers, lakes, swamps, and rice-fields.

A knowledge of the constitution of the ash of blood is of great interest and importance, not only in a chemical, but also in a physiological point of view.

The researches of C. Schmidt have shown that the fluid contents of the blood-corpuscles contain, in addition to peculiar organic matters, a preponderance of the phosphates and potash salts; whilst the liquor sanguinis contains the chloride of sodium in large amount, with a little chloride of potassium and phosphate of soda. In the blood-cells, the fatty acids and globulin are combined both with potash and soda; whilst in the plasma, the organic materials are combined only with soda. The researches of Liebig, confirmed by those of Schmidt, have shown that the fluid contained in the tubules of muscles, is like that of the blood-corpuscles, exceedingly rich in the phosphates and potash salts. The phosphates, also, exist in large amount in the structure of the brain. From these facts it is probable that one of the most important functions of the blood-corpuscles is the separation and elaboration from the liquor sanguinis, of those organic and inorganic compounds which constitute the most important part of the structure of the muscles and brain.

Iron is a peculiar and constant constituent of the coloured corpuscles. Its office, in the animal economy, is entirely unknown. The assertions of several chemists and physiologists, concerning its power of combining with oxygen, and thus aiding in respiration, can at present be considered nothing more than a beautiful hypothesis.

That the fixed saline matters are absolutely necessary, not only for the formation of the different structures, but also for the maintenance of life itself, was conclusively demonstrated by a series of experiments performed in France. It was found that when animals were fed upon grain, from which only one element (the phosphate of lime) had been abstracted, they rapidly lost their forces, and died in the course of a few weeks.

We hope to be able to continue this subject in a future number of this journal.

ART. II.—*On Œdema Glottidis resulting from Typhus Fever.* By THOMAS ADDIS EMMET, M. D., late Visiting Physician to the New York State Emigrant Hospital, Ward's Island.

As a secondary affection of typhus fever, œdema glottidis occurs under two distinct conditions.

The most frequent form met with, is that following laryngitis—the result of reactive ulceration of the mucous membrane of the air-passages, in consequence of typhus deposit. In this condition, general and profuse bronchitis is persistent throughout the course of the fever, and is often accompanied by pneumonia. The infiltration takes place gradually, before convalescence has been established—usually between the second and third week, and does not reach its height for several days.

The other variety, is a consequent alone of the debilitated condition in which the patient is left, after the primary disease has subsided. Convalescence has been slowly taking place, when coincident with some exertion, or on suddenly assuming the upright position, asphyxia occurs, and death results in a few moments.

The areolar or cellular tissue is very abundant throughout the glottis, and terminates almost abruptly along the under border of the larynx; at this point, when resulting from a debilitated condition (the cellular tissue being pervious), the œdema gravitates, and is usually found most extensive. The effusion gradually accumulates to a certain point, without producing much or any irritation, until, by muscular action, the quantity is suddenly increased, and spasmodic closure results. Occasionally, at the upper border of the glottis, or on the epiglottis (when depending upon a slight local inflammation), the serum accumulates under the mucous membrane in a vesicular or cellular form, the vesicle not seeming to communicate freely, the one with another. Several of these closing together by accident or gravitation, will form a valve-like arrangement, becoming the more perfect with each effort of inspiration.

When infiltration is the result of the reactive inflammatory action of laryngo-typhus, the surface of the mucous membrane is more generally elevated, smooth, and unyielding—thus equally closing the course of the passage throughout.

Before entering into a consideration of the cases presented, the only point of diagnosis which will engage our attention at present, will be that in reference to a modified condition of the act of respiration. To a certain extent, this can be relied upon as indicative of the locality involved. Bayle and many others have stated that, in œdema of the larynx the respiration is alone difficult and sonorous in character, while the expiration, on the contrary, is free and easy. This statement is partially true, and in such cases only, where the œdema exists principally about the epiglottis and superior portion of the larynx, resulting from an extension of inflammation from the fauces, or in consequence of the inhalation of steam, irritating substances &c. Thus, as a result of situation, and the prominent or vesicular form of the œdema, with each act of inspiration (as we have already seen), a valve is formed, closing from above downwards. When the infiltration is more general, and caused by acute laryngitis, syphilitic ulcerations, tubercular or typhus deposit, it may extend or not to the epiglottis and neighbourhood, while a more equable diminution in caliber is produced. Thus both the inspiration and expiration will be very nearly equally affected. In the asthenic form, the accumulation having gravitated (which it will always do when existing independently of an inflammatory obstruction), it hangs free, as a sac into the trachea. While this condition also materially lessens the area, it offers comparatively but little obstruction to inspiration; the expiration, on the contrary, is, I believe, in every case unnaturally prolonged, and difficult in proportion to the extent of the accumulation. This seems to be in consequence of the upward pressure from behind, in the outward passage of the air—as closure of a semilunar valve is produced by regurgitation. In Case V., cited, the sac in its free diameter was quite sufficient to have produced complete closure in this manner. As the difficulty increases, it is easy to conceive that, beyond a certain point, the sac would cease to be movable as a valve, and both acts of respiration (if complete asphyxia has not already supervened) would be equally affected, while the application of the stethoscope, in a case of doubt, would determine with much certainty the exact point involved.

Case I. A male, aged 18, a native of Ireland, and ten days from shipboard, was admitted to the fever ward of the hospital, under my charge, Nov. 20, from the city. His general appearance was phthisical, with light hair, blue eyes, and of a spare habit. The previous health had been good; he never had contracted syphilis, and his parents were healthy. After a loss of appetite, and general lassitude for several days, he was seized on the 17th inst. with a chill, followed by headache and fever, and on the second day with cough and pain in the chest. He was admitted, on the third day of his indisposition, with the typhus eruption out, and the fever well marked in every respect. A profuse double bronchitis, with pneumonia, existed—more extensive on the left side. Nothing of note occurred during the actual course of the disease, which was rather of a more severe type than usual. The pneumonia did not advance beyond the first stage, and disappeared in a few days; while the bronchitis was never entirely absent, often rapidly increased in severity, and would sometimes as suddenly subside in intensity on the same day. During the night of the fifteenth day of the disease, and on the 2d inst., a marked remission took place. In the morning, the pulse had lowered in frequency, and the fever lessened, while the tongue became moist at the edges. The expression of the face, as well as the general appearance, was indicative of convalescence about being established. The quantity of brandy (of which he had been taking some ten ounces a day) was now decreased. During twenty-four hours the condition remained nearly stationary. About bedtime of the evening of the 3d, he complained of a sore throat, followed by some difficulty in swallowing. During the night, the inspiration was first impeded, afterwards the expiration became principally so, while dyspnœa, with slight hoarseness came on, accompanied by tenderness of the larynx on pressure. The fauces were found injected, and the epiglottis felt distinctly tumid, elevated and smooth, while the voice sank to a whisper, as the parts lost their elasticity. He assumed the upright position from choice, and became restless. The lower extremities were being constantly flexed, and extended in turn; the hands were often applied to the region of the pomum Adami, and apparently without any definite object for doing so. On being questioned, he seemed too much occupied with his condition to give a satisfactory answer. The skin was hot and dry, becoming afterwards cold and clammy; the neck and face suffused and puffy in appearance. The eyes became prominent and injected, and the nostrils tremulous. The pulse at first increased rapidly in frequency, but afterwards became weak, small, compressible and irregular, until it intermitted and ceased. The epiglottis was freely scarified; a blister applied to the upper part of the sternum, with dry cups to the nape of the neck, and along the root of the lungs, on each side of the vertebral column. Calomel, quinia, and Dover's powder, in combination, were taken, and repeated every two hours. On the morning following, his condition was worse in every respect, with the expiration much prolonged, and with a croupy sound. A solution of argent. nitras (ʒss–f℥j) was applied freely to the fauces and epiglottis, which was followed by some temporary relief. During the day, the calomel was stopped, but I continued the use of the quinia and Dover's powder, and ordered wine whey. The operation of tracheotomy was proposed, which he refused—wishing (in his own words) to die in preference to having his throat cut. Through the night he sank rapidly. Suffocation was inevitable on the morning of the 5th inst.; the lungs were being blocked up from venous accumulation; the brain was already suffering in consequence, and the patient sinking into an insensible condition. The trachea was opened about 11 o'clock A. M., with the full conviction that a different issue might have resulted, could the operation have been performed earlier. Before its completion, life apparently had ceased. The lungs were inflated, and the ribs depressed in turn; soon the heart's action was again perceptible, and was followed by reaction in the course of fifteen or twenty minutes. With the return of consciousness, he seemed much relieved, and in half an hour afterwards sank into a sound slumber, for the first time during thirty-six hours. He took a moderate quantity of stimulants and beef-tea during the day, with large doses of the muriated tinct. of iron. The pulse sank to 90 per minute, after having been, previous to the operation, too rapid to count. He breathed regularly through the tube, yet but little change took place in the dulness, which was extensive at the posterior and inferior portion of the lungs, with quite an accumulation of mucus in the bronchial tubes. He suddenly awoke about 7 o'clock P. M., with a return in the difficulty of breathing; no obstruction existed in the tube; the lungs were found to be becoming engorged; the bronchi filled; while the dulness on percussion had sensibly increased over nearly the whole chest, from below upwards. The temperature of the trunk augmented, that of the extremities diminished, while the features became pinched in appearance. The pulse was soon countless from its frequency, wanting in volume, and afterwards irregular and intermitting. Stimulants, frictions, counter irritation, and a stimulating enema, together with dry cups, were resorted to without relief. He sank slowly into a profound coma, and died eighteen hours after the operation, on the fourth day of the attack, and the nineteenth of the fever.

Post-mortem examination seven hours after death.—General œdema, and thickening of the submucous structure of the glottis, was found terminating along the under border of the lower vocal ligament. Some infiltration of the epiglottis existed, but its surface was corrugated. A large, deep ulcer, with blackened edges, existed in the posterior part of the ventricle on each side, together with a few superficial ones scattered here and there in the neighbourhood. The lining membrane of the trachea above the bifurcation was partially injected, below this point it was very much so; several small and empty ulcers were found, and the bronchi filled with a thin, frothy mucus. Both lungs were engorged with venous blood, which flowed freely with each incision made. Not a trace of tubercle existed. The heart was softened, and of a dark colour, from venous congestion of its capillaries; the right side with its vessels was greatly distended, while the left was nearly empty. The spleen was enlarged and friable, the liver congested, and all the veins of the portal system were distended, in consequence of the retarded circulation. The larger vessels on the surface of the brain were in the same condition, while quite an extensive effusion of serum had taken place under the investing membranes. Some opacity and thickening of the dura mater was found principally along the course of the longitudinal sinus on both sides, with a few points of effused fibrin scattered over the surface. A cross section into its substance showed the congestion to be general; on extending it into the lateral ventricles, they were found filled with serum. The substance of the brain was in consistence somewhat softer than natural, although not sufficiently so to be regarded as a pathological condition. About two ounces of fluid were contained in the spinal canal. The blood of the general system was in a fluid state, and presented the "claret sediment" appearance, often found in typhus fever. Nothing further of interest was noticed, and especially no ulcerations of the glands of Peyer existed.

Case II. James Hogan, 30 years of age, was admitted on the 2d of January. The case was early marked by great deafness and stupor, from which condition he could at all times be partially roused; no eruption appeared. Bronchitis came on after the first week, and was persistent; it was accompanied by the crepitant rhonchus of pneumonia, which disappeared entirely in a few days. On the 18th day of the disease, symptoms of laryngitis were noticed; the fever remitted somewhat on the 21st day, but the local difficulty increased. About 9 o'clock A. M. of the 23d day it was evident (after the occurrence of the symptoms detailed in the preceding case) that the general system was rapidly failing from an inadequate supply of oxygen, and the consequent accumulation of carbonic acid. As a last resort, the trachea was opened, which was followed by general prostration. By means of artificial respiration, partial reaction was established, with much relief. During eighteen hours the patient's condition was comfortable, but he became conscious that only temporary relief had been obtained. The circulation was very incomplete, as a large portion of the lungs remained clogged up. In twenty-four hours the bronchitis became general, the lungs slowly congested, and the bronchi filled. He sank from a gradual stupor into a comatose condition, and died forty-eight hours after the operation, on the twenty-sixth day of the fever, and on the eighth day of the laryngitis.

The *post-mortem* appearances were characteristic. A deep empty ulcer, with dark edges, was found occupying a similar position in the ventricle of the larynx, but somewhat smaller than that of the preceding case. The œdema and thickening of the submucous structure was general throughout the glottis. The mucous membrane of the trachea and bronchi was much congested, while the superficial ulcerations in the latter were more numerous. The condition of the brain, heart, lungs, and intestines, was in every respect similar. It is worthy of remark, that of two or three other cases occurring in the service of the gentlemen connected with the institution, the same unhappy result followed the operation.

It is a fortunate circumstance, that, in comparison, the occurrence of laryngitis in this form is a rare complication in typhus fever, and still more so that it does not invariably produce, in consequence, a sufficient œdema of the glottis to require the trachea to be opened for its relief. When laryngotyphus is so severe in its effects as to endanger life, the operation of either tracheotomy or laryngotomy is of doubtful efficacy, while we have no better means of relief to offer. The only hope for success in this disease, as in all others where the operation is resorted to, lies in acting without delay, as soon as the first indication of a stasis in the circulation through the lungs is detected. The following condition results: the *vis à tergo* continues, while the venous blood thus sent to the lungs, will not pass readily on to the left side of the heart, until the proper functional changes have been fully effected. Stagnation gradually takes place in the minute radicles of the pulmonary veins (which probably require to be stimulated to action by the presence of oxygen), until a large portion of the lungs becomes completely destroyed in function. The result is, that nothing is gained by an operation at so late a period, from the fact that the obstruction will remain, and too small a portion is left in its integrity for the purposes of maintaining life. Even on the other hand, if the condition has not advanced so far, it is greatly to be feared that the irritation consequent upon the operation will be sufficient (if it has ceased), to re-establish the bronchitis, which has already subsided but a short time previously. The reactive inflammatory action of the larynx rapidly descends, the bronchitis becomes profuse, and results invariably in an intense congestion of the lungs; general infiltration takes place; the bronchi soon become filled with a fluid accumulation, which the patient is now unable to remove, and death results from suffocation. The cause, then, of œdema glottidis in laryngo-typhus, is to be regarded as resulting from a local inflammatory obstruction, and is more pathognomonic of typhus fever than that of the other variety, which is considered (as we have seen) an effect alone of a diminution of the vital forces, and independent directly of the original disease. We now pass to a consideration of this condition.

Case III. William Daly, aged 20; eleven days from ship; was admitted from the city on the 12th of March, with the eruption just fading. The fever was of a grave type, but ran its course uncomplicated. The case slowly convalesced for several days, when, on the nineteenth of the disease, between 5 and 6 o'clock P. M., suffocation came on in consequence of suddenly sitting up in bed, for the purpose of receiving his food. I obtained the assistance of my colleague, Prof. Carnochan, and the trachea was opened some five minutes after the occurrence of the accident. But, before the operation was completed, the patient was pulseless and insensible; all attempts at respiration had ceased, while the heart's action was no longer perceptible. In a few minutes after artificial respiration had been commenced, the livid appearance about the neck and face began to disappear, and soon a feeble action of the heart was again detected. At the end of some ten minutes, complete consciousness and gradual reaction were established. From this time, the necessity for inflating the lungs artificially ceased; but, for a period of five hours and several minutes after the operation, coincident with each expiration, I depressed the ribs. The muscular or contractile power of the respiratory apparatus appeared completely paralyzed. After depressing the ribs, the air, of course, readily passed in to fill the partial vacuum thus produced; but, when I ceased doing so (as I did several times from fatigue), suffocation was almost immediately produced, the face and neck became livid, and the patient soon insensible. So dependent did he feel on me for this assistance, and so fearful was he I might leave him, that my wrists were severely bruised in consequence of his grasp during nearly the whole time. At midnight, all danger was removed; and ten grains of Dover's powder, with two of quinia, being administered, he slept well during the night, and no further difficulty arose. The tube was removed on the eighth day, and the wound soon healed, but it was not until the one hundred and third day after admission that he had recovered his strength sufficiently to be discharged.

Case IV. Thomas Goffrey, aged 40, was admitted on the 4th of February. The course of the fever differed but little from that of the preceding case, with the exception that no eruption appeared. The convalescence was slow, with some œdema of the feet, while he was up and about the ward for several days. On the 26th inst. he called my attention to his throat, which was sore, and at the same time I noticed some hoarseness in the tone of voice. As he arose from the bed for the purpose of examination, he became suffocated, and in a short time insensible. Dr. George Ford, my senior, being present, opened the trachea; this was followed, after depressing the ribs several times, by almost immediate relief. The tube was removed on the ninth day, and the case discharged on the fifteenth after the operation, and on the thirty-fifth day after admission.

Case V. Shortly after the discharge of the above case, a man under my charge, as house physician in the service of Dr. Henry G. Cox, became similarly affected on the twenty-eighth day after admission. He was 31 years of age, and had almost entirely recovered his strength, after a serious attack. As in the other cases, without any premonitory difficulty in breathing, the accident was preceded by a sudden change in position. I was absent from the ward at the time; thus an unfortunate delay occurred before the trachea could be opened, and although life was not quite extinct, no reaction followed the attempt at resuscitation. I was informed afterwards by the nurse, that he had mentioned, the day previous, having a tickling or disagreeable sensation in the throat, which had been attributed to taking cold. At the *post-mortem* examination, some slight œdema of the superior portion of the glottis existed. On the left side, along the under border of the lower vocal cord, the œdema had accumulated in a pendulous sac, nearly closing the opening below. The mucous membrane of the respiratory organs was not injected, and no evidence of inflammatory action existed anywhere. The lungs were perfectly sound, and only presented the usual appearance resulting from asphyxia. The other organs were also in a healthy condition, while the venous congestion was not so extensive, and principally confined to the lungs and larger vessels of the brain. The left side of the heart was nearly empty; the right side, with its cavities, distended; and, in fact, the organ presented the general condition already described. It is not unreasonable to suppose a happy result would have followed an immediate operation, could it have been possible.

Case VI. came under my charge while a house physician in the service of my late friend and colleague Dr. Macneven. A female, aged twenty, was admitted with fever on the 14th of April; on the 10th of May following, after convalescence had been established some eight days, suffocation suddenly occurred. Tracheotomy was promptly performed, and followed by a complete recovery. The tube was removed on the sixth day, and the case discharged on the eleventh after the operation, having been thirty-seven days under treatment.

Case VII. occurred also in a female, aged 23, who was admitted on the 10th of December. The fever was uncomplicated, and abated on the twelfth day. The convalescence (with œdema of the feet), was tedious up to the 5th of January, when symptoms of œdema glottidis were manifested. Complete asphyxia did not at any time take place, but a certain amount of difficulty in expiration existed during some eight days; it was sudden, spasmodic, and increased by muscular exertion—sometimes even while speaking. The application of the stethoscope in the neighbourhood of the thyro-cricoid space, indicated beyond doubt the existence of a constriction at this point, which gradually disappeared, and at the time of discharge, the sounds were of a normal character. With the exception of an occasional occurrence of dyspnœa and hoarseness, all the other symptoms were negative in character. On examination, neither the fauces nor epiglottis presented any change from a healthy condition. There was no interruption to the circulation, and consequently no change was produced in the lungs. The pulse increased in frequency as the dyspnœa was augmented, but otherwise, was alone indicative of a debilitated system. Preparations for operating were early made, but happily the exigencies of the case did not require it. The treatment consisted in maintaining perfect rest in the horizontal position so long as danger existed, extra diet, and a moderate quantity of stimulants. Quinia and iron in combination, were freely administered, with Dover's powder at night when required. A number of dry cups were repeatedly applied on each side of the vertebral column, along the root of the lungs; while an application of the tinct. of iodine was made externally over the region of the larynx, and the temperature of the extremities regulated by artificial means. The discharge took place on the 20th of January, the case having been forty-one days under treatment.

CASE VIII. A male, aged 47, was admitted in March, having been five days indisposed. The typhus eruption appeared the day after admission, and was present until about the twelfth day. Slight bronchitis came on during the first week and soon subsided. The case was of a very low type, so much so that a large bed-sore formed on the right buttock between the second and third week, and the cornea sloughed on the nineteenth day. Between the third and fourth week the fever abated, leaving the case perfectly prostrated; from this condition, together with the irritation of the bed-sore, no reaction followed, and death occurred forty-three days after admission. Post-mortem examination: emaciation was extreme; nothing worthy of note was detected, with the exception of some infiltration of serum in the inferior portion of the larynx, while there was no appearance of inflammation whatever. I regarded the quantity at the time, as being too small to have materially influenced the termination; since then, with more experience, I have satisfied myself that a very slight obstruction at this point is sufficient to influence and gradually lower the tone of the general system, without giving any evidence of its existence during life. I was somewhat surprised to find that no tuberculous infiltration had taken place in the lungs, as his general appearance, some days previous to death, had led me to suspect such would be the case.

CASE IX. Also a male, aged 29, was admitted in January, on the second day of the attack, with the eruption just out. It was a malignant case, but uncomplicated; for several days (between the second and third week) sixteen ounces of brandy were administered during the twenty-four hours. On the twentieth day an abscess was opened, which had formed under the scapula, and from which some five ounces of pus were evacuated. At what time the typhous influence subsided, it was impossible to note, as it ran into a low irritative fever in consequence of the great discharge from the abscess; this condition lasted until death, which occurred on the 39th day after admission. The œdema was similarly situated in the larynx, but more extensive than that in the preceding case, yet gave no indication of its existence during life.

I am convinced, when reaction does not readily take place, that œdema of the glottis exists after many diseases, as a consequence of the extremely debilitated condition resulting, and may be the immediate cause of death oftener than is suspected. Since my attention has been directed to this subject I have met with this condition in two other cases; the one after death from chronic diarrhœa, and the other after a long protracted case of Chagres fever, both being without tubercular deposit. As there is so little indicated which cannot, in these cases, be accounted for, as a result of the disorder of the general system, the condition may be easily overlooked even after death. We must suppose, in consequence of its gradual accumulation, the system becomes to a certain extent accustomed, and adapts the want to the supply, until, eventually, the vitality of each organ becomes so much lowered that death gradually takes place. This explanation is identical with that which occurs in many cases of phthisis, where, after death, so small a portion of the lungs is found unaffected by disease, that it is a matter of surprise how life, often, under such circumstances, could possibly have been maintained so long. It will be a matter of interest for future observation, to examine the condition of the larynx in those cases of sudden death after typhus, which sometimes occur on placing a patient in the upright position; under such circumstances it is the custom to attribute the cause of death to anæmia, or some disturbance of the circulation in the brain; an explanation which is convenient only as a cover to our ignorance on this point.

After a review of the cases presented, it is evident that a more favourable issue is likely to follow the operation of tracheotomy, or laryngotomy, when employed for the relief of the asphyxia following simple œdema, than that resulting from the local cause. In the table exhibited, it will be observed, that, in every fatal case of laryngo-typhus, bronchitis existed; and, furthermore, that it invariably recurred after operating, as soon as reaction was established. The result was different where convalescence had already taken place, as the reactive inflammatory tendency had subsided, while there seems but little likelihood of its being again established from this cause, even if bronchitis had previously existed.

In reference to a choice of locality for operating (in the latter condition especially, where the least delay is of such vital importance), the opening should be made through the thyro-cricoid space. From experience, I am satisfied nothing is to be gained by tracheotomy; the other operation is more simple and as effective, while, at the same time, being also below the terminating point of the œdema, the risk of establishing an inflammatory action is not thus materially increased. But in either variety, if tracheotomy is decided upon, after the first incision made through the integument (as the veins are always enormously distended), the instrument should be laid aside. The subjacent structure can be rapidly separated by means of the thumb-nail or handle of the scalpel; if this is not done, even with the greatest care, the hemorrhage will often be fearful, and so far delay the opening that death will result. After a removal of a portion of the trachea has been effected, it is advisable at first not to introduce the tube, as the mucous membrane is in an exceedingly irritable condition; unfortunately this exists principally in the posterior portion of the trachea, and where the muscular structure is most abundant. At this point, with the least displacement of the instrument, and with each act of swallowing the saliva, a spasmodic condition is being constantly excited, which is doubtless transmitted to the minutest subdivision of the bronchial tubes, thus diminishing the extent of surface available for respiration. This irritability usually passes off after reaction has been fully established, provided bronchitis has not occurred; the tube may be then used or not, as may be deemed advisable. It is decidedly safer to rely upon some mechanical contrivance to keep the lips of the wound apart, because the largest tube which can be introduced cannot equal the natural capacity of the trachea; the mucus, which appears in large quantities at the opening, can be more easily removed, while a larger quantity of air seems able to pass in a given time through a simple incision, with the lips well separated, than through a tube which the cut will receive; this is naturally inferred as the number of inspirations decrease within a short time after the removal of the tube.

After the operation, artificial respiration, a stimulating enema, frictions, with the application of artificial heat to the extremities and other means, must be persevered in, until no possible hope remains of resuscitation. The patient must not be left until the circulation has been completely re-established, and the extremities become of a comfortable temperature. This is obviously necessary, as we have seen already, the respiratory power does not completely recover its tone, sometimes for many hours after the operation. Occasionally, within the first twelve hours, this difficulty will occur again, even after the function has been carried on for some time unaided; if, under such circumstances, assistance be not at hand immediately, to depress the ribs for the moment until the danger is again removed, the result will be fatal. As the air passes directly into the lungs almost entirely unchanged, the temperature of the room, must be regulated with care and kept as nearly as possible of an equable degree, as either bronchitis or congestion of the lungs will be likely to result in consequence of any sudden change. Perfect rest must be maintained in the horizontal position, until all irritability of the system has ceased. The circumstances of the case can alone indicate when the tube, if used, can be removed and the wound closed with safety. In the mean time it is obvious, that every means must be employed for the purpose of building up and improving the general system, as rapidly as possible.

During a service of five years in the institution, one thousand nine hundred and thirty-one cases of typhus fever came under my charge. Of so large a number, only twenty-three were of the laryngo-typhus form, and seven were.

cases of simple œdema glottidis, from debility without inflammation, and with the following result:—

Typhus fever and œdema glottidis, with the complications in order as they occurred.	TOTAL NUMBER.			NUMBER AND RESULT OF OPERATION.		AVERAGE NUMBER OF DAYS UNDER TREATMENT.	
	Cured.	Died.	Treated.	Cured.	Died.	Cured.	Died.
Feb. typhus, broncho-pneumonia, laryngitis, et œdema glottidis .	7	6	13	...	2	57	$21\frac{1}{6}$
Feb. typhus, broncho-pneumonia, laryngitis, glosso-pharyngitis, et œdema glottidis	...	1	1	...	...	...	43
Feb. typhus, broncho-laryngitis, et œdema glottidis	4	1	5	...	...	$35\frac{1}{2}$	19
Feb. typhus, diarrhœa, laryngitis, pharyngitis, et œdema glottidis .	1	...	1	...	...	95	...
Feb. typhus, laryngo-pharyngitis, parotitis, et œdema glottidis .	2	...	2	...	...	28	...
Feb. typhus, laryngo-tonsillitis, parotitis, et œdema glottidis . .	1	...	1	...	...	122	...
Total result from the local cause .	15	8	23	...	2	54	24
Total result from the general condition	4	1	5	2	1	$53\frac{1}{2}$	28
Total result from the general condition (discovered after death) .	...	2	2	...	...	...	41
Total	19	11	30	2	3	54	$25\frac{4}{11}$

The average age of the whole number (30) was 24 years—the ages ranging from 12 to 47 years; of 20 cases, the average duration of disease previous to admission, was exactly five days and twelve hours—the time ranging from 2 to 10 days. The complications occurred in different months as follows:—

	Jan.	Feb.	March.	April.	Nov.	Dec.	Total.
Cases	7	4	8	4	1	6	30

The word angina, or quinsy, was used by the early writers to express any obstruction occurring in respiration or deglutition, seated above the lungs or stomach. Hippocrates, Celsus, and Aretæus treat of two forms of obstruction—the one situated within the larynx or upper portion of the trachea, and only recognized by producing sudden suffocation; the other in the fauces, or about the epiglottis, and visible. Aretæus regarded the former variety as being so suddenly fatal in character, that he compared its effects to that produced by carbonic acid; or, in other words, to "vapours inhaled from pits or caverns," and that death resulted before any means could be employed for its relief.

Boerhaave, in *Aphorism* 784, states: "Of this disease there are observed two kinds. The first appears without any manifest sign of tumour or swelling, either external or internal; but the other kind is constantly found with some tumour in one part or other," &c. Again, in the next aphorism: "The former of these happens mostly in the end of lingering diseases, especially after profuse and often repeated evacuations. It is attended with a paleness, dryness, and shrinking of the fauces at the same time, and therefore the nerves and muscles are commonly paralytic in this case; it is almost constantly a sign of death approaching, being very seldom curable, and then only by such remedies as fill the empty vessels with good juices, and which warm and corroborate at the same time." *Aphorism* 786: "This first kind of the disorder sometimes arises suddenly without manifest signs of any disease preceding; it hardly admits of a cure; and it almost constantly, after death, demonstrates a suppuration in the lungs." Van Swieten, in his commentaries on this aphorism, also states: "But observations teach us that, sometimes, even in healthy people without any signs of diseases preceding, the deglutition or respiration, or both, are suddenly impeded, and death follows soon after, though there is no tumour in the fauces or external parts." Again: "But, in the mean time, it is certain that this very rarely happens, since we do not here treat of an inflammation suddenly arising about the upper parts of the larynx, which, indeed, very speedily kills by suffocating the patient, but may be known and distinguished by the acute pain and other signs preceding or attending the disease." According to the same author, Schenckins relates a case of "suffocating catarrh," which occurred in a man who had no disease except a "weariness or lassitude," was seized suddenly and suffocated before any assistance could be rendered. He also states such cases are rare, and that the lungs after death are found "suppurated." The word catarrh does not imply that an inflammatory action existed; we have just seen that Van Swieten states distinctly in this form—"we do not here treat of an inflammation," &c., while in this connection we find the following: "Many authors have called the like disorder a suffocating catarrh, because they constantly believe it to arise from a sudden distillation of dissolved humours upon the lungs and fauces. For when they saw in the disorder called a coryza, that there often happens such a sudden and copious flux of a sharp serum through the nose; and that the Schneiderian membrane suddenly swelled so as to impede all the passage of the air through the nostrils, which are naturally so large, they with good reason believed that something of the like nature might happen in the membranes investing the larynx or windpipe, from whence must follow the most sudden suffocation and death." Sydenham also relates a case which suddenly occurred after "a continued intermittent fever;" he regards the disease as being rare and very fatal, while the lungs are found "engorged after death." Boerhaave treats particularly of "the watery œdematous or thin catarrhous quinsy," and non inflammatory (in *Aphorism* 791), which is caused, as he states, by "a too weak circulation of humours." Van Swieten describes the watery quinsy as being found "in the larynx or windpipe, by which free respiration is disturbed, and that it occurs in weak, pale, and leucophlegmatic patients, who have almost their whole body swelled with a cold sluggish tumour." He recommends, as a treatment to strengthen their solid parts, by the salutary use of chalybeates, more especially dissolved in vegetable acids, to increase the languid motion of the humours.

We now pass to a consideration of the condition of the larynx where, from inflammation, the diameter is more nearly equally diminished throughout, and extending from the body towards either extremity of the organ, or to both. (Boerhaave, *Aphorism* 801): "If the windpipe only is inflamed in the muscular membrane which lines it internally without injuring other parts, then there follows a tumour or swelling therein, with heat, pain, and an acute, ardent fever, but without any signs externally; the voice becomes shrill, squeaking, and wheezing or whispering; inspiration is attended with an acute pain; the respiration is small, frequent, performed with great labour and with an erect or raised posture of body; hence the circulation of the blood becomes difficult through the lungs, the pulse waves or trembles very swiftly, and in a surprising manner; great anguish and oppression attend, and death soon follows;" "the nearer the disorder is seated to the glottis and epiglottis, so much the more fatal is it." Van Swieten, in describing the same condition, remarks: "Thence this inflamed membrane is stretched, and thus an acute pain is produced in the act of inspiration. But expiration is likewise impeded, as the air cannot pass from the lungs but in a less quantity through the windpipe, now straitened by an inflammatory tumour, whence it is obliged to pass with a greater celerity;" and again, "the air cannot conveniently pass into, nor out from the lungs, as it used to do in health." Hippocrates observed this form of the disease, and states that death from suffocation takes place on the same day, or on the second or third, or fourth.

Of the third variety, Hippocrates, Aretæus and others, observed that when the inflammation is situated about the epiglottis and fauces, the difficulty is in the inspiration. Thus, Arctæus states: "But they draw their breath very short, until they are suffocated, the passage into the lungs being intercepted." Death, according to Hippocrates, occurred in these cases on the fifth, seventh, or ninth day.

Morgagni, at a modern date, was the first to enter into detail in describing this disease. Bichat followed, locating the affection in the superior portion of the larynx, and described it as a peculiar species of serous engorgement found in no other portion of the body, producing death by suffocation; but, in many respects he was vague and indefinite. Bayle, early in the present century, with more accuracy detailed the disease and circumstances under which it was found. He distinguished two forms in which the œdema occurred—one idiopathic, and arising spontaneously; the other secondary, or subordinate to some local laryngeal affection. He noted also its occurrence in the non-inflammatory form during convalescence from typhoid fever, and that its existence, up to the moment of suffocation, was unsuspected. M. Thuilier, a few years afterwards, advocated Bayle's views, and regarded the non-inflammatory form as a distinct condition. Bouillaud, in 1825, denied the occurrence of œdema glottidis from any other cause than that resulting from local inflammation. Cruveilhier's views agree with those of Bouillaud, while he describes the disease as a submucous laryngitis. Legroux, Trousseau and Belloc, Bricheteau, Vidal (de Cassis), and in fact nearly every writer on the subject, seems only to have met with the inflammatory form. Ryland defines œdema glottidis as a variety of laryngitis, in which the submucous tissue of the superior part of the larynx becomes œdematous by the inflammatory process, whilst the external surface of the mucous membrane is found free from any signs indicative of the existence of inflammation. Two cases are given as types of this condition—in one an ulcer existed, with vascular edges; in the other the mucous membrane was congested, with an infiltration of pus in the sub-cellular tissue. In both œdema existed at the superior portion of the larynx, resulting from the inflammatory obstruction below; indeed, they may well have been classed under the head of laryngitis, from which cases they differed but in a degree. M. De Lesiauve, in a memoir on œdema glottidis (reviewed in *Ranking's Abstract*, 1845, art. 4), subscribes to the opinion advanced by Bayle, and regards one form of the disease as idiopathic and independent of inflammatory action. Dr. Thomas Watson (*Lectures on the Principles and Practice of Physic*), states: "A distinction has been made between laryngitis and œdema of the glottis, and it is a just and real distinction. Œdema of the loose areolar tissue subjoined to the mucous membrane of the glottis, is indeed one common consequence of inflammation of that membrane, but it may occur independent of inflammation."

Dr. Horace Greene, of New York (*Polypi of the Larynx and Œdema Glottidis*), remarks, in treating of this affection: "When the disease occurs independent of any other local affection, it is termed idiopathic; and secondary, when it follows diseased action of the larynx, or of any of its neighbouring tissues. Not unfrequently the affection arises during convalescence from typhus and other forms of fever. It originates, also, from inflammation and from ulcerations of the lining membrane of the larynx." M. Valleix (*Guide du Médecin Praticien*) enumerates, as a cause of œdema glottidis, typhoid fever, and admits that it occurs in persons debilitated by acute or chronic diseases; while he regards this circumstance as being "the only one that observation has placed completely beyond doubt." Again, we find in contradiction, "a last question which regards the nature of this disease, is to know if œdema of the glottis can develop itself without previous inflammation; in other words, if there is an essential œdema of the glottis." And: "It is at least doubtful whether there exists an œdema glottidis purely passive, for the facts cited to prove this occurrence are very few and incomplete." M. Valleix, in explanation as to the cause which misleads, maintains "that traces of slight inflammation in the laryngeal mucous membrane, sufficient under certain circumstances to produce œdema, may disappear after death." What these circumstances may be, by which traces of inflammation, with the consequent œdema are removed, it is not easy to conceive. A moment's reflection on the mode of death and over-distended state of the venous system, would be conclusive that this is impossible. It is theoretical, for the arterial capillaries are never found empty, although the character of the blood may have been changed, the difficulty occurs at this point early, and is accumulative; we would, therefore, find, if arterial congestion had existed previous to the first difficulty in respiration, the condition would be actually increased. The same reasoning applies to the examples given by MM. Trousseau and Belloc, in the disappearance, after death, of redness in parts previously affected by erysipelas, the exanthematous eruptions, &c. These gentlemen also cite cases in which the white colour from infiltration of pus, with œdema at the superior portion of the larynx, may deceive. There can be no differing in opinion with them, as to this circumstance being proof positive of the previous existence of inflammation somewhere, even in the absence of all congestion of the parts.

Such cases are not in question, as there is no interruption of the general circulation previous to death—while the locality of the œdema is demonstrative of the cause. If it takes place in consequence of debility, it will gravitate to the most dependent part; on the contrary, when inflammation has existed by adhesion, the permeability of the areolar tissue is destroyed, and the infiltration, which is uniform, cannot be removed by puncture at any one point. As MM. Trousseau and Belloc have truly stated, after inflammation the infiltration below the œdema is found to be pus or sero-purulent in character; such is not the case in simple œdema. In the cases of œdema which have come under my observation, the areolar tissue became soon greatly emptied and corrugated in consequence of the incision made through the organ, for the purpose of examination; and while the œdema remained, it could be without difficulty displaced by pressure. On the contrary, several specimens in my possession of infiltration from inflammation, in consequence of typhous ulcerations, have but little changed (after being in alcohol several years), except in the superior portion of the larynx, where simple œdema existed. Whenever it is thus situated, or on the epiglottis, it is invariably the result of inflammation at some point below, with infiltration of pus throughout the areolar tissue involved. The only exception to this rule which can be conceived, might exist in some case where, at an anterior date, inflammation had existed and permanently destroyed the character of the tissue involved. Except under such circumstances, it would be impossible for œdema to accumulate sufficiently, from below upwards, to extend to the epiglottis without producing suffocation, from complete closure of the glottis below. Of forty cases of sudden death, given in the Guy's Hospital Reports for April, 1855 (*London Lancet*, N. Y. edit.), one occurred from simple œdema glottidis, which terminated fatally within five minutes after the first difficulty arose; no mention is made of any inflammatory appearances having been detected. Several cases are on record of non-inflammatory œdema of the glottis occurring after scarlet fever; one has been given by Bayle, which MM. Trousseau and Belloc regard as the only case (previous to their day), in which the œdema could be regarded as resulting from a non-inflammatory cause. M. De Lesiauve has given two, which occurred towards the close of cardiac disease, and of thirty-four other cases which had the affection developed during convalescence from different diseases, seven had suffered from a continued fever. Sestier collected one hundred and ninety cases, of which number eighteen had had typhoid fever; it would be interesting to know what proportion of these resulted from ulceration of the larynx in consequence of typhus deposit. Those given by M. De Lesiauve seem to have occurred after the primary disease had subsided; this is not the case, as we have seen in laryngo-typhus, although occasionally asphyxia takes place as suddenly as in the other form. M. Valleix remarks: "Furthermore, œdema of the larynx is most frequently only the termination of ulceration of the larynx, the process of the one necessarily occasioning the other." There are some writers who have expressed a doubt as to the occurrence of ulceration in the larynx from any other cause than those produced by syphilitic and tuberculous deposit. Copland, in his *Dictionary*, under the head of Laryngitis and œdema glottidis, states: "There are five cases, however, quoted by MM. Trousseau and Belloc, in which it is supposed to have arisen from an affection of the larynx, attended with ulcerations of its investing mucous membrane, while the lungs were free from tubercles. M. Valleix and Louis question the authenticity of these cases. It is, moreover, worthy of remark that Trousseau and Belloc do not appear to have themselves observed a single case of laryngeal ulceration without pulmonary tubercles." In *Rokitansky's Pathological Anatomy* we find: "Laryngo-typhus is with us an unusually common and extremely unfavourable symptom in many epidemics of typhus." In an article on laryngitis of typhus fever (*Ranking's Abstract*, 1847, art. 4), by Dr. Frey, mention is made of the very frequent occurrence of lesions of the larynx, threatening fatal obstruction to the glottis from mucous inflammation, fibrinous exudation, deposit of typhus matter, &c. The editor writes: "We do not call in question the accuracy of the above remarks, suggestive of the frequent occurrence of laryngeal complications in fever in Edinburgh, but they are certainly (such at least as would require laryngotomy) far from common elsewhere."

The earliest description of œdema glottidis I have been able to meet with, in any of the journals to which I have had access, is a case in a boy, which came under the care of Dr. Farre, in 1806, and was reported by him (with several others) in the 3d vol. of the *Medical and Chirurgical Transactions* of London.

In describing the case of "cynanche laryngea," he states: "A noise attended every respiration, which she (the mother) expressed by the monosyllable—flip-flap. It seemed to her that something was *lifted up every time he breathed*, and in striving to breathe, his head, body, and limbs worked," &c. "At the *post-mortem examination*, the œdema was general. The sacculi-laryngei were completely concealed, the greatest deposition of lymph having taken place at this part of the windpipe, by which it was so much narrowed that there was scarcely room for the point of a crow-quill to enter," &c. This case is interesting in connection with the explanation I have given in reference to the difficulty in expiration, when the œdema existed below the ventricles of the larynx. No mention is made as to the time at which the noise ceased, but as the boy became gradually insensible several hours before death, it is likely, as the effusion continued to increase, it did so as the parts became immovable from distension. No traces of inflammation seemed to have been noticed in the case.

Among the Guy's Hospital Reports, published in the *London Lancet* (June 1, 1850, p. 670), is found the following, the only one on record, to my knowledge, presenting that curious and interesting condition after the operation of tracheotomy that existed in Case III, where artificial respiration was steadily maintained during five hours, before the function of respiration could be carried on unassisted. Although the primary exciting cause was different, the case is no less instructive, while it illustrates, by a second attack, the existence of difficulty in expiration, with œdema, resulting most likely from a debilitated condition. A boy, aged 4 years, swallowed some boiling water on the 5th of March. A few hours afterwards, he was admitted to the hospital, under the care of Mr. Alfred Poland, with symptoms of œdema glottidis. The difficulty increased to such an extent, that tracheotomy was performed before morning. "No benefit followed the operation; indeed, it appeared to have extinguished the little flickering of life left in the child. No natural effort at respiration ensued; no air rushed in when the trocar was withdrawn from the canula; the pulse had already ceased to beat for some time; the surface of the body was perfectly cold, the face of a deadly hue, and the child lay a motionless and apparently lifeless body." Artificial respiration was performed at the rate of twenty-five inspirations per minute. In four or five minutes the pulse began to beat, and the surface of the body became warm, but still no other signs of life manifested themselves, and no effort was made at natural respiration. As soon as the artificial means were suspended, to ascertain if any inherent vital power was rekindled, the pulse ceased, and the child became cold. At the end of five hours and a half: "At last the child gave one natural gasp, drew in a long unaided respiration, and slowly expired the air. Then succeeded a short interval of repose, and a similar movement was repeated; when again came a very long pause, when the child was assisted by a puff down the canula. This happily succeeded; respiration became slowly established; the little patient began to rally, open his eyes, and become conscious." After forty-eight hours the tube was removed, but the opening was not closed until some twenty days or more after the operation. Soon after recovering, the child "took cold"—"great difficulty of breathing ensued, requiring efforts *in expiration*, which were chiefly made by the abdominal muscles. *A peculiar crowing noise attended each expiration, and it seemed as if there was some obstruction in the larynx about the vocal cords,*" &c. In consequence of the dyspnœa becoming so urgent, at one time the question was raised in reference to operating again; the patient, however, improved, and finally recovered, having been forty days under treatment. In the first attack, the inflammation was very violent, with œdema in the superior portion of the larynx most likely—where it is usually found under such circumstances. At this time, if any difference existed between the inspiration and expiration, it was doubtless in the former act, although in the history of the case no mention is made in reference to this point. The exigencies of the case, it was thought, required an active treatment. Seven leeches were applied to the throat soon after admission, and calomel and antimony freely administered during the course of the disease. With the prostration consequent upon the operation, and remaining probably at least thirty days in the hospital before the second attack occurred, it is not unreasonable to attribute it to the same condition as existed in the cases after typhus—in fact, simple œdema about the inferior portion of the larynx, from general debility, independent of any inflammatory condition. This is most likely true, as the case is reported with such precision in every respect that, had any other condition existed apart from the intermitting dyspnœa (probably increased by muscular action), it would have been mentioned. The existence of difficulty in expiration, with the seat of affection, must not be overlooked as a coincidence, if not a diagnostic mark of this condition.

In the *London Lancet* (for July 17, 1830, p. 619) mention is made of a case which has also a bearing on the preceding one. M. Roux, in his practice at the *Hôpital de la Charité* in Paris, operated for a case of œdema glottidis, the particulars of which are not given, further than the fact, that artificial respiration was maintained for several hours after the operation, before reaction was established. The necessity for this course was attributed to the circumstance of some blood passing into the trachea and bronchi during the operation. This is evidently a case in point, for had the quantity been sufficient to have endangered life so long from this cause, artificial respiration could neither have maintained it nor removed the difficulty.

Œdema glottidis in connection with typhus fever, except as a result of inflammation, seems to have been entirely overlooked by all writers on this subject. The literature therefore on this point could have been dismissed in a few words, but it would have been incomplete, without considering in connection the occurrence of the affection under similar circumstances in other diseases. We have seen how large a proportion of the writers on this subject have maintained its existence as resulting alone from an inflammatory cause. Œdema glottidis, by comparison, is indeed a disease of rare occurrence under any circumstance, and in a large majority of the cases which have been recorded, it resulted doubtless from this cause. But that the other form, proportionately scarce, has never been met with by those who deny its occurrence, cannot, on this ground alone, be received as evidence that it never exists, while the testimony of the more fortunate minority, certainly is entitled to the greater weight. It is remarkable, under the circumstances, that so much labour should have been expended in endeavouring to prove that simple œdema cannot occur in the larynx, as it does undoubtedly from debility in other portions of the body, while the arguments advanced in proof, without exception, are either wanting in force, contradictory, or unsustained on true physiological grounds.

113 Fourth Avenue, New York.

Art. III.—*Cases of Rupture of the Womb, with remarks: being a Sequel to a Monograph upon this subject, in this Journal for January and April,* 1848. By James D. Trask, A. M., M. D., of White Plains, New York.

In a paper published in the Nos. of this Journal for January and April, 1848, we presented an analysis of three hundred and three cases of rupture of the womb. Since its publication, we have obtained access to some authorities which were not then within reach, especially the essay of Duparque; and we have gathered, from this and other sources, over a hundred cases additional to those embraced in our previous communication. We have thought that a brief analysis of such of these cases as have been already published, and a somewhat more extended history of several cases which have been communicated to us, might prove useful as an addition to what has already been presented. We propose to give a summary of the results of these and of the cases in the former paper, taken as a whole. It is possible that, in some instances, the same case may be reported more than once, in consequence of the occasional imperfections of the references, though great care has been taken to avoid this source of error.

Rupture during Pregnancy. Recoveries.

Case CCCIV. A woman had the abdomen and womb torn open, transversely, by the horns of a bull. The child escaped from the aperture, with a large quantity of blood. It was not until an hour afterwards that the funis was cut. It lived eight hours, and the mother recovered perfectly in six weeks. (*Lechaptois,* par M. Deneux, *Essai sur les ruptures de la Matrice,* p. 35. See *Duparque,* p. 20.)

Case CCCV. In a case similar to the above, it was necessary to increase the size of the opening, in order to extract the contents of the uterus. Recovered completely in less than forty days. (Schmucker, *Melang. de Chirurg. Ancien. Journal de Méd.,* t. lxvi. p. 354. See *Duparque,* p. 21.)

Case CCCVI. At seven months she fell from a tree; motions of child ceased, and she suffered for a month. Four months afterward, felt a movable body in the abdomen; soon had bloody discharges, with some portions of hair; health good. Thirteen months from the fall, she was confined. Following the accouchement, an abcess formed, from which the remains of the first child escaped. Recovered perfectly. (M. Bochard, in *L'Ancien. Journ. de Méd.,* t. v. p. 42. See *Duparque,* p. 72.)

CASE CCCVII. Æt. 27. Fifth month; second pregnancy; fell from a tree, and felt a tearing pain in the lower part of the abdomen; was confined to her bed for two months, and for five years had great irritation of the bladder. When fifty years old, she expelled a calculus from the bladder, formed around a bone; and soon after, twelve similar ones were withdrawn from an abscess below the neck of the bladder. She recovered. (M. Lessieux, *Extr. des Bull. de la Soc. Méd. d'Emulation*, 1822. See *Duparque*, p. 92.)

CASE CCCVIII. Æt. 24 years. Had undergone Cæsarean section about three years previously. Was found with symptoms of bilious colic; five hours afterward, complained that she was "tearing in two," and said something had torn inside of her; the os was slightly patulous, and there was some hemorrhage from it. Upwards of forty-eight hours afterward, the fœtal heart was distinctly heard. In three weeks was about the house; vaginal discharges came on, with great constitutional irritation, and the fœtus was removed, by gastrotomy, three months and six days from the rupture. There was an opening through the uterine walls. Recovered. (H. A. Bizzell, *Amer. Journ. Med. Sci.*, Jan. 1856, p. 79.)

Rupture during Pregnancy. Deaths.

CASE CCCIX was hurled into the air by the horns of a bull, her abdomen and uterus having been torn open. The child, escaping from the womb, fell upon the ground at the same instant with the mother; the child lived a month, the mother died in thirty-six hours. (Sue, *Essai Historique sur l'Art des Accouchement*, t. i. p. 209, from *Duparque*, p. 19.)

CASE CCCX. Æt. 26 years. For three hours had had violent colic pains, with great restlessness; the face pale; skin covered with cold sweat; the pulse small and intermittent; belly not hard or tender. Her husband reported that she had missed her catamenia for three months, and had lately been indisposed; in the evening she ate cauliflowers, and at night was taken with colic, vomiting, &c. During this conversation she turned upon her side and died.

Post mortem.—Great effusion of blood; a fœtus of about *two* months had escaped from a rent in the left cornu of the uterus—edges of the rent thin and brittle—walls were four or five lines thick, excepting at the rupture, where, for the space of an inch, they were very thin. (M. Collineau, *Journ. Gen. de Méd.* See *Duparque*, p. 49.)

CASE CCCXI. Æt. 30 years; mother of five children and had several miscarriages. When three months pregnant, made a misstep, and, in the effort to recover, felt violent pains in the womb and sinking; great prostration. After five days' repose, she got up, and was about the house for a month, when similar depressions returned, and she died in three days.

Post mortem.—A rent of one inch at the fundus, near the insertion of the right tube, corresponding with the situation of the placenta; womb contained a fœtus of three to four months. (J. B. Puzin, *Thèse*, 1809. See *Duparque*, p. 51.)

CASE CCCXII. Æt. 30 years; three months pregnant; always had good health. While at her needle-work, she became faint and sick with sudden, intense pains in the stomach. When called, at 9 P. M., she was in extreme pains; nauseated; pulse small and feeble; had eaten heartily of tripe, a few hours before. Gave a full dose of opium. 11 P. M. Excessive depression; almost pulseless; dying evidently from internal hemorrhage; *now*, had occasional pains in back, but chiefly in stomach; no vaginal discharge. Died six hours from the attack.

Post mortem Immense coagula; a *perfect ovum* protruding through a rent in the uterus, which was firmly contracted; was about four months gone; uterus "excessively pale and soft, indeed, I could easily tear it asunder; rent antero-posterior, as regards the fundus; no cause could be ascertained." (F. H. Warren, *Lond. Med. Gaz.*, 1851, vol. ii. p. 1103.)

Case CCCXIII. Æt. 28 years; a single woman; slightly indisposed for some days; for last few hours had complained of pain in abdomen, and sickness, which became suddenly aggravated, when the physician was sent for, who found her in *articulo mortis*.

Post mortem.—About seven months pregnant; much blood in the cavity of the peritoneum; rent in fundus of womb four inches long, and gaping—the placenta prevented escape of the fœtus; womb "no thicker than a sheet of writing-paper for at least a distance of two inches around the rent; liquor amuii had not escaped. (J. Watson, *L. Lancet*, 1853, vol. i. p. 267.)

Case CCCXIV. Æt. 28. Admitted at full term; second pregnancy; good health. At seventh month she fell and shook herself violently, but no disturbance followed. Two weeks after admission, got vomiting, with restlessness; pretty strong pains followed, during one of which she felt a severe "crack in the back," as if something had given way inside; os nearly closed; pains ceased; died next day; no expulsive pains.

Post mortem.—In abdomen, blood; and a full-grown fœtus, dead several days. Rent from centre of fundus, posteriorly along whole length to the os; uterus seemed to be perfectly healthy; no softening; no appearance of previous inflammation; surrounding parts healthy; usual predisposing and exciting causes absent. (T. F. Brownbill, *Lond. Lancet*, 1848, vol. ii.)

Case CCCXV. Æt. 25. Eighth month; fell on a step, and struck the abdomen; she felt as if something had burst. Now the movements of the child could be felt on the right side, very close to the skin. Died on fourteenth day.

Post mortem. Rent at the fundus, on anterior surface, one inch below the summit, extending transversely from side, and from four to five inches in length, and great loss of blood; uterus and peritoneum of a dark green colour. (*Ingleby's Obstet. Med.*, p. 217.)

We have *eleven* additional cases of rupture during pregnancy, which, added to the *thirty-eight* previously reported, make *forty-nine* cases. Of these, Cases CCCIV, CCCV, CCCVI, CCCVII, CCCIX, and CCCXI, were of traumatic origin; in the remaining four, the accident was spontaneous. These, added to *six* among the above, make thirteen of traumatic origin.[1]

In Case CCCVIII, the remarkable fact is stated, that two days after the apparent occurrence of the rupture, the pulsations of the fœtus ceased to be heard.

Recoveries at full term of Pregnancy.

Case CCCXVI. Sixth labour; contracted pelvis. Seven hours and a half after escape of waters, the uterus was fully dilated; pains very powerful; and she complained of pains at right sacro-iliac junction. In a half hour, pains ceased entirely. Four hours after this, some hemorrhage; perforation attempted; delivery completed at end of four hours. Rent oblique, in direc-

[1] In Case XXVI, as we are informed by Dr. Bond, in a private communication, the patient's foot slipped, while she was leaning against a barrel, and that she came with a good deal of force against the barrel.

tion of right sacro-iliac junction; but little collapse. Recovered after many weeks. (*Dr. Ingleby's Obstet. Med.*, p. 212.)

CASE CCCXVII. Was first seen after being in strong labour thirty-six hours; pains had suddenly ceased; os dilated; the fœtus partly in the peritoneal cavity, and high up. Delivered at once by turning. Rent on right side, from the cervix nearly to the fundus; placenta and coagulà removed; very considerable depression; menstruation returned at the end of five months. (*Ibid.*, p. 214.)

CASE CCCXVIII. Æt. 35. Primipara; extreme rigidity of os; pains strong for thirty-six hours, when the os being dilated to half a crown, and "hard as marble," with excessive violence of pains, the cervix was felt suddenly to give way to the touch, and to split asunder; delivery took place in a few minutes. (*Perfect's Cases*, vol. ii., CXLII.)

CASE CCCXIX. After delivery in the usual way, the intestines could be very distinctly touched, having descended through a rent in the fundus. The surgeon replaced them, and held the hand in the womb until it was sufficiently contracted to prevent any further hernia of the bowels, and she recovered perfectly. (Rungius, *Instit. Chirurg.*, pars sec., p. 728. See *Duparque*, p. 167.)

CASE CCCXX. Æt. 16½ years. Primipara. After three days of severe labour, the os partially dilated. Forceps were applied. After forcible traction, the head was suddenly forced into the pelvis. The cervix was torn from the vagina upwards. Recovered. (*Duparque*, p. 187.)

CASE CCCXXI. The entire ovum passed into the peritoneal cavity. After many months, portions began to escape by the anus. After her death the remainder was found in contact with an ulceration into the colon. The rupture of the womb was nearly cicatrized. (M. Fleury, *Rec. pér de la Soc. de Méd. de Paris*, t. iv. p. 268. See *Duparque*, p. 235.

CASE CCCXXII. Æt. 32 years; delicate; third pregnancy. Somewhere about twenty-four hours from beginning of labour, three accoucheurs separately attempted the application of forceps and version, occupying several hours. Eight hours after this, delivered by perforation, occupying three-fourths of an hour, with but slight fatigue. A rent detected to the right, and behind, at the junction of the vagina; recovered in a month. (*M. Lachapelle*, t. 111, p. 179. See *Duparque*, p. 288.)

CASE CCCXXIII. Æt. 28 years; strong, well formed, primipara; had been in labour five days; waters escaped four days; many attempts at delivery by forceps and version; extreme prostration; perforation, with much difficulty in extraction; vagina separated from uterus in the whole of its posterior half. Recovered. (*Ibid.*)

CASE CCCXXIV. In April, 1847, I was summoned in great haste to meet Dr. M. The patient was very fat, about 30 years old, and in labour with her seventh child. The pains had been severe, and then ceased, with a cry from the patient that something was the matter. The head receded; the pulse was 124, and she became restless. I passed my hand to the head; attempted to bring it down with forceps, and failed. I then passed in my left hand, and discovered a rent in the uterus opposite the *linea ileo pectinea*, of about four and a half inches, and the nates and feet had passed through it and among the abdominal viscera. I reached the feet, and delivered her. The placenta came away with the child. She recovered, and continued well for years, and died a year since in consequence of erysipelas. (*Communicated by Prof. Willard Parker.*)

CASE CCCXXV. Æt. 42 years; large and corpulent; mother of nine;

unusual pain in uterus from one to two months; labour slow; pains strong, at long intervals. When os fully dilated, and head almost in perineum, she suddenly exclaimed, "What a cramp I have in my belly!" Expulsive pains ceased; an opiate given; great prostration; the head receded, and the child could be felt in the abdomen; was delivered with considerable difficulty. Rent oblique, from near the fundus toward the left; inflammation; recovery. (James Church, *L. Lancet*, vol. i., 1849.)

Case CCCXXVI. Æt. 37 years; muscular. When in labour six or eight hours, on getting into bed had a tremendous pain, and a loud-cracking sound heard; pains ceased, and she was believed to be dying, but as she was living six hours afterwards, Dr. P. was sent for. Extreme prostration, and child felt through the abdomen; delivered her easily by forceps. There was *hernia* of the intestines; intense inflammation followed, and she recovered with apparently but little care. (Dr. Prassart, from *Caspar's Wochenschrift*, 1847. See *Brit. and For. Med.-Chir. Rev.*, 1848, p. 279.)

Case CCCXXVII. Æt. 30 to 35 years; strong, primipara. The edges of the os thin, hard, and very rigid posteriorly; anteriorly congested, and an inch thick. After *thirty-five* hours of energetic labour, the neck was torn almost entirely off, and the head descended. A year afterward she had a second child, after a labour of ten minutes. (Dr. W. P. Johnston, *Amer. Journ. Med. Sci.*, April, 1851, p. 342.)

Case CCCXXVIII. Æt. 30; apparently very feeble; for two months had extreme anasarca; sixth child; os well dilated at the end of six hours; the back presenting, the breech was brought down, and after two hours of "very hard labour," the feet could be brought down; every prudent effort to deliver by the feet; attempts to perforate failed. The fœtus was dissected to the axillæ, occupying two hours, severe labour continuing Rupture was suspected; as she was rapidly sinking, *gastrotomy* was performed. The head and placenta were in the peritoneal cavity; inflammation treated by cal. and op. By the eighteenth day the wound was healed, and by the twenty-ninth day could attend to domestic duties. (Dr. H. M. Jeber, from *South. Med. and Surg. Journ.* in *Am. Journ. Med. Sci.*, April, 1851, p. 538.)

Case CCCXXIX. Primipara; æt. 30 years; bilious temperament; good health; eight months and one week gone. After twenty-eight hours of labour, head pressed on perineum; one hour after this she was restless, and got up; on returning to bed, she fell back into the chair, screaming "O, nurse!" Put her hand to the pit of the stomach, and gasped for breath; could not bear a recumbent posture; uterine tumour ill defined, and a swelling above it; the head impacted; delivery completed in forty minutes, the child living. The placenta was removed, "tremendous hemorrhage" followed, and the hand, when introduced, detected a *rent* at the upper right side of the fundus, antero-posteriorly admitting three fingers; no hernia; after thirty-five days, well. (Mr. Thomas, *Prov. Med. Journ.*, 1846, p. 613.)

Case CCCXXX. Æt. 38 years; fifth child; all previously born dead, and "cross-births." Called in consultation at 10½ A. M.; labour began at 4 A. M. She was seen immediately; the os was fully dilated; the pains regular, without any excessive strength. The breech presented to the left. About 8 A. M. the female genitals of the child were visible, and delivery was expected after a few pains. Suddenly he noticed the entire disappearance of the presenting part; the head had escaped into the peritoneal cavity. Dr. Gardner turned, the head was detained at the brim, the child was dead, and he perforated and delivered. The patient, by the great care of the attending physician, recovered. The laceration extended through the neck of the uterus upward, and the *bladder* downward, and she will be shortly treated by Dr. Sims. Dr. G. attributed the recovery to the application of ol. terebinth. to the abdomen, which seemed to exert a magical effect. (*Communicated by Dr. A. K. Gardner, New York.*)

CASE CCCXXXI. Æt. 30 years; delicate; third labour; previous labours severe and protracted. After something over twelve hours of moderately severe labour, the os was found rigid, and equalling a quarter of a dollar; head at superior strait. Two hours after this, after a pain of great severity, she complained suddenly of great abdominal distress, and the pains ceased. She was left from midnight till morning, when she was somewhat exhausted, and the head could not be felt. Ergot and stimulants given. Dr. G. was called in late in the afternoon; and found a rent upward and backward, the womb contracted, and no part of the child to be felt. He performed *gastrotomy*, the child having escaped twenty-one hours previously. Was about the house in seven weeks. (Dr. John T. Gilman, *Amer. Journ. Med. Sci.*, April, 1854, p. 401.)

CASE CCCXXXII. Excellent constitution; sixth labour; pains came on about 8 P. M.; had been in labour about two hours and a half, with pains of increasing severity; the os fully open, and but slight advance of the head, when she went to stool, and there had two pains, the second causing intense agony and a burning sensation in the right side. She was certain that something had given way within her; head receded; rupture diagonal; all but the placenta was in the peritoneal cavity. Turning declined. Next morning, *gastrotomy*. Child hydrocephalic; rent enormous, and womb uncontracted. She was convinced that she should recover, and at the end of just a month she was at the wash-tub. (Dr. Mason, *Am. Journ. Med. Sci.*, Jan. 1855, p. 281.)

CASE CCCXXXIII. Reached her after she had been in labour three days. She was pale and exhausted; had suffered no pain for more than twelve hours. The shoulder presented; there was a laceration of the neck of the womb, through which the head only had passed. Delivered her immediately, with little difficulty; expected she would die soon; she recovered, and in eighteen months afterwards was delivered of a living child without assistance. See Case CCCXCVI. (Dr. H. A. Hartt, *New York Journ. Med.*, Nov. 1850, p. 330.)

CASE CCCXXXIV. Æt. 29 years; medium stature, strumous habit, good health, third child. Labour set in at 1 A. M.; it went on favourably; between 6 and 7 P. M. head began to press on perineum. On the passing of a pain not unusually severe, she exclaimed she had a "queer cramp" in the belly, different from anything before, and that she must rise up. She walked across the room three or four times, scarcely lamenting. On touching her pulse, found it 120. She lay down, but was restless; the head had receded; was surprised at the few symptoms of rupture. She said, that as the last pain passed off, the child gave three kicks, followed by the cramp; there was no hemorrhage, anxiety, or prostration. She remained sitting in a rocking-chair for twelve hours, without any marked decline. At 9 A. M. next day the child was turned, and delivered with ease to the head; this could not be delivered even by forceps. Child was then detruncated, and a hook passed into the foramen magnum without success; eventually delivered after perforation and removal of bones of the head. The omentum and intestines were distinctly felt, but there was *no hemorrhage* or *clots;* has been much prostrated, and not expected to live an hour. On eighth day put upon calomel and Dover's powder, blisters and tonics. The rent was at the juncture of the neck and body. In four weeks from the accident she was in the street, and in nine weeks menstruated. (Dr. W. H. Maxwell, *N. Y. Journ. Med.*, May, 1851, p. 328.)

Dr. Maxwell has kindly favoured us with the subsequent history of this patient, which will be found in Case CCCXCVI.

Case CCCXXXV. Æt. 32; robust; third labour. Labour began December 30, at 3 P. M.; foot presentation; pains slow at first, became strong and frequent toward 9 P. M. About 11 P. M. a pain of great violence came on; a free flow of blood; labour ceased immediately, and foot no longer to be felt. She remained that night, and the following day and night, with acute pain in the abdomen. "Late in the evening of January 1 (about forty-eight hours from rupture), *gastrotomy* was performed. The child could be felt high in abdomen; a rent could be felt on a level with the brim of the pelvis, remaining open for a quarter of its length in the left side, and elsewhere obstructed by clots, &c." Child dead; but little fever followed; nothing remarkable occurred; she resumed her work in forty days. (M. Mazier, *Journ. de Méd. et Chirurg. Pratique*, quoted in *Edin. Month. Journ. Med. Sci.*, Feb. 1854.)

Case CCCXXXVI. An oblique, contracted pelvis; had borne two dead children; head became impacted at the brim. The pains, which were very strong, suddenly ceased; pulse sunk very low; a rupture felt at posterior part of the uterus; *gastrotomy;* child dead, with a greatly enlarged head. Recovered completely in five weeks. (J. F. Halder, *Nederland Weekbl.*, Aug. 1853, in *Edin. Month. Med. Journ.*, Feb. 1854.)

Case CCCXXXVII. Sixth labour; learned she had been in labour twenty-four hours; pains had been regular, but not severe; the membranes had ruptured a few hours before his arrival; head had pressed on perineum, and just on eve of expected delivery she felt something give way; the child's head had receded beyond reach, and pains had ceased. He found her with intense suffering; pulse rapid and feeble; respiration difficult; no pains; a large rent in front of uterus; the *head* remaining in the uterus; passed in his hand, and turned without difficulty; child dead; a large dose of laudanum. (Dr. Thos. Christie, in *Canada Med. Journ.*, 1853; in *Assoc. Med. Journ.*, Nov. 1853, p. 969.)

Case CCCXXXVIII. July 6, 1851, was sent for by midwife about 5 P. M., who had been with the patient since 11 o'clock A. M. The pains were then strong; os uteri quite dilated; the head did not descend, but rested on the brim of the pelvis. Saw her again at 8½ o'clock; found the head in the same position, the expulsive pains having ceased completely, although she complained of great cramps in the abdomen. I prescribed tinct. opii gtt. l. and left her for an hour and a half. On my return was informed that the laudanum had been rejected; she complained of excessive pain in the abdomen. On examining, the head of the child had disappeared, and could not be reached by the fingers. On examining the abdomen externally, the child appeared high up, close to the diaphragm. From these facts I inferred, that when the expulsive pains suddenly ceased, a rupture of the uterus had taken place. I therefore introduced the hand, and having secured the feet, extracted the child. It gave no signs of life; the placenta was extracted without difficulty. She was extremely ill for several days; pulse small and rapid; constant vomiting; abdomen distended, and very painful; a very fetid discharge from the uterus, and considerable irritation of the bowels. I gave up all hope of saving her, but she finally was restored to health. (Dr. F. Chatard, Baltimore; *communicated through Prof R. H. Thomas.*)

CASE CCCXXXIX. The wife of W. C., a milkman, 4th mo. 27th, 1852, with her second child. She had been delivered by forceps several years before, and had suffered severely from vaginal inflammation. Dr. W. had been in attendance two days. The labour had been regular and natural until the os uteri was dilated, and the head descended into the pelvis. It was then discovered that the further advance was prevented by two firm bands, almost semi-cartilaginous, nearly closing the outlet of the pelvis. The pains being strong and forcing, the doctor hoped the bands, thick as they were, would gradually soften and yield. In the course of the night the pains left her; he could not learn whether very suddenly or not. At 6 o'clock this morning, Dr. K. being called, they agreed to send for me. I found her at 7 A. M. with feeble pulse, little or no labour pains, tender abdomen; head down against the two thick semi-membranous bands. As agreed upon, I passed a sharp-pointed bistoury through the bands on each side of the vagina, dividing them freely from without inward. There was not much blood lost. Without delay I put on the forceps, and delivered her easily of a dead child. The placenta came down in a few minutes, and being withdrawn, rather more hemorrhage followed than was thought compatible with her safety. I passed my hand into the vagina, and at once encountered a knuckle of intestine, the descent of which was being promoted by a sense of bearing down. Taking the bowel between my fingers and thumb, I carried it through a rent which was found readily between the vagina and uterus. Upon attempting to withdraw the support of my fingers, the bowel again came through; I therefore prevented it by the fore and middle fingers within, while by gentle friction without I induced the uterus to contract so much as to close the rent. I withdrew first one finger and then the other, and the bowel did not follow. A large opiate, with calomel, was given. She said she was much relieved, and though we thought it right to tell her husband how desperate was her condition, and he did not conceal it from her, she boldly said, "I shall certainly recover." For two days, no very serious symptoms occurred; on the third day, a chill, followed by high fever, tumid and tense abdomen, tenderness and pain, obstinate constipation—in a word, severe peritonitis. Without detailing the treatment, which was much as usual in such cases, it will be sufficient to say that she quite recovered in a few weeks, and has continued well. (*Communicated by Dr. Richard H. Thomas, Professor of Obstetrics, University of Maryland.*)

CASE CCCXL. Fourth child; had been in labour twelve hours, but for four hours pains had ceased; shoulder presented; turning effected with slight difficulty and delay; child dead. On introducing the hand on account of hemorrhage, "a transverse rent in the walls of the uterus, about three inches above the cervix anteriorly," was discovered, through which three fingers could be passed. Sero-sanguineous and purulent discharges continued for several weeks, with irritative fever and diarrhœa. Recovered, and has good health. (W. W. Duvall, M. D., *Amer. Journ. Med. Sci.*, Oct. 1855, p. 542.)

Deaths from Rupture at full term.

CASE CCCXLI. Æt. 35; seventh child; had been in hard labour ten hours; os equalled a half-crown piece; hydrocephalic fœtus diagnosed; pains violent; was about to perforate, when, on being allowed to stand up, she had a singular sensation, with pain below the heart, with fainting and vomiting, and pains ceased; head receded; great prostration; child found among the intestines; feet brought down. She died before delivery of the head, twenty minutes after getting out of bed. Rent from side to side of womb. (W. H. Borham, *Lond. Lancet*, 1848, vol. ii. p. 551.)

CASE CCCXLII. Æt. 32; stout, sixth labour; had pain in right side since last confinement, and not generally so well as before; drinks hard; had acute pain in right side and back four days before labour came on. Pains began at 3 A. M.; at 6½ A. M. os larger than a shilling; soon membranes ruptured, but in half an hour the head had receded beyond reach; she had felt a sudden cramp, or something snap, with a tearing, and distinctly heard it; had frequent returns of the cramp, with an effort to strain; pains subsided *gradually*, and ceased at 8½ A. M. Slept quietly; got up through the day two or three times. At 5 P. M. severe pains after oil; no complaint of debility; voice firm; slight sanguineous discharge; venesection, &c.; turning, apparently at night; delivery difficult; head partly through the rent. Death in thirty-six hours from rupture. (Dr. Reid, *Lond. Med. Gaz.*, 1845, Part I., p. 685.)

CASE CCCXLIII. Æt. 28; fourth child; narrow pelvis; had been in labour twenty-four hours, and turning unsuccessfully attempted; found in a state of collapse, without pain. The breech could be felt in the peritoneal cavity; the head presented *per vaginam;* head opened. The rent had been felt in passing in the hand. Died on fourth day. (Dr. Smallwood, St. Martin, Canada, in *Brit. Amer. Journ.*, 1848, quoted in *Prov. Med. Journ.*, 1848, p. 138.)

CASE CCCXLIV. Sixth child, all preternatural; distorted pelvis; shoulder presentation; arm had been amputated after ineffectual attempts to turn; womb ruptured; I brought down the feet. Rent in back part of body of the womb, obliquely up toward right broad ligament. Died on fourth day. (F. Ramsbotham's Reports, *Lond. Med. Gaz.*, 1843, iv. p. 463.)

CASE CCCXLV. Twelfth child; foot presentation; uterus did not act violently, and no force used in extraction. Child dead; lived three hours after delivery. (*Ibid.*, p. 486.)

CASE CCCXLVI. Had a family; head; died some time before help arrived; child and placenta in peritoneal cavity. (*Ibid.*, p. 519.)

CASE CCCXLVII. In expulsion of a blighted ovum suffered transverse rupture at the cervix, above the os. Believed herself near full time, and had hemorrhage for two weeks previous. A surgeon removed the ovum from the vagina, and detected the rent. The uterus had not exerted itself greatly. The rent almost across the womb, and did not involve the peritoneum. (*Ibid.*)

CASE CCCXLVIII. Contracted pelvis; fourth child; membranes had been broken forty hours, but no strong pains. Symptoms of exhaustion occurred rather suddenly, and found her cold, with extreme depression. Laceration felt in anterior part of cervix; feet presented, and child was extracted after perforating the head; placenta and body among the intestines. Head had originally presented. Dr. Ramsbotham has known this evolution in another instance; time of rupture unknown.

Post mortem.—Rent transverse; six inches in length; walls of uterus around it easily tore, and the whole organ much softened; evidence of inflammation in abdomen of some standing. (*Ibid.*, p. 330.)

CASE CCCXLIX. Tenth child; labours always lingering; pelvis distorted at the brim; head presented; rupture eight hours after membranes broke; pains not strong; no tearing sensation at the rent; child and placenta in the abdominal cavity; delivered by the feet; rent horizontal in anterior part of cervix; child dead; she died in twenty-four hours. (*Ibid.*, p. 369.)

Case CCCL. Eighth child; head presentation; died in forty minutes after delivery. (*Ibid.*)

Case CCCLI. Pendulous abdomen; head rested on pubis out of midwife's reach; was delivered after use of ergot; at the end of forty-eight hours, feverish, with vomiting, swelling, &c.; "the black vomiting, soft but tumefied abdomen, the absence of pulse, and the coldness of the body, led me instantly to hazard the opinion, that the symptoms were the result of laceration." She died almost immediately. An opening in the vagina behind, communicating with one in the uterus, probably made by a finger. (Dr. Ingleby, *Obstetric Medicine*, p. 206.)

Case CCCLII. Had several very difficult labours. Before twelve hours the os was fully dilated, and a consultation held previous to perforation; the head receded, laceration having taken place. Turned. Died.

Post mortem.—Cervix and vagina lacerated extensively just opposite the promontory of the sacrum. Brim measured three inches. (*Ibid.*, p. 207.)

Case CCCLIII. Third labour; strong pains; soon after rupture of membranes, they grew weaker. Arm presentation; turning under very feeble pains. A laceration detected in a few hours. Died about twelve hours after rupture.

Post mortem.—Rent from cervix upward, for five inches; uterus thin and weak at rupture, but thick and strong elsewhere. (*Ibid.*, p. 208.)

Case CCCLIV. Third child. Turning, effected with much difficulty, several hours after unsuccessful attempts at delivery. Rent of cervix into the vagina detected, and the peritoneum found extensively detached. (*Ibid.*, p. 209.)

Case CCCLV. Eighth child. Labour began at 1 A. M.; 10 A. M. of next day, very much exhausted with vomiting, &c. Head had been impacted the day before; now free; perforated, but could not be extracted. Died in a few minutes.

Post mortem.—Rent anteriorly, for two-thirds the length of the womb. The edges were not thinner than the surrounding parts; the contents of the womb in the abdomen; contracted pelvis. (*Ibid.*, p. 215.)

Case CCCLVI. Fifth child. Six weeks before labour, she fell down stairs, and got a violent blow upon the left side of the belly, and she exclaimed that *something had given way and broke within her.* From that time, had acute pains in hypogastrium. On the eighth day of labour, the os was somewhat dilated, the membrana broken, the pains weak and few. After being "nearly a week in labour," she was delivered by turning—fœtus long dead. Died on third day.

Post mortem.—Uterus ruptured, within an inch of its internal orifice, to extent of nearly four inches. (*Perfect's Cases*, vol. ii., Case 78.)

Case CCCLVII. Æt. 27 years; good health; second child. At the end of twenty hours, the pains having been very severe, even when under the influence of ether, there was cessation of the pains, and vomiting of greenish fluid, and a knee projecting directly under the integuments, near the fundus. Pulse small, and not to be counted. Perforation. The *head* did *not recede.* Delivery very difficult. Died on fifth day.

Post mortem.—Rent across the anterior wall of the cervix, just below the os internum. (Dr. Cabot, *Amer. Journ. Med. Sciences*, July, 1851, p. 70.)

Case CCCLVIII. Æt. 40 years. Had repeated hemorrhages of late. Premonitory symptoms of labour during the day; waiting for real labour, when she had a single, most violent pain, which felt as if something had given way within her; great prostration ensued; the os was slightly dilated;

the placenta presented. The head and arm could be distinctly felt, as if projecting through. No part of the child could be felt per vaginam. The rent was in the uterus. Died in ten hours from rupture, undelivered. (Dr. Wm. Rankin, *Amer. Journ. Med. Sciences*, Oct. 1853.)

CASE CCCLIX. Sixth child. Suddenly felt a violent pain, and immediately the waters escaped with a great quantity of blood, from a rent in the inferior and right side of the womb, by which the body escaped into the peritoneal cavity while the head descended into the pelvis. The edges of the rent were firmly contracted about the neck. She died undelivered, in twenty-four hours. (Leclerc, *Ancien. Journ. de Méd.*, t. xxv. p. 522, from *Duparque*, p. 125.)

CASE CCCLX. Æt. 40. Sixth pregnancy; all her previous labours severe. Died after three days of suffering; the fundus was rent; the fœtus, which was very large, had passed into the abdomen, with prodigious hemorrhage. (*Obs. Var. de Méd.*, ii., *Obs.* xxx, from *Duparque*, p. 128.)

CASE CCCLXI. Æt. 27 years; third labour; died after a severe labour of forty-eight hours, having presentation of the placenta; rent of uterus and vagina; child entirely in abdomen; womb at the rupture very thin, and torn into strips, much distended; the rest of the womb contracted and entire. (Nauche, *Des Malad. de l'Uterus*, p. 216, from *Duparque*, p. 129.)

CASE CCCLXII. Arm in the vagina. On introducing the hand for turning, a rent was felt, two inches in length; but, as no part of the fœtus was engaged in it, turning was completed. Died on the fiftieth day, when an opening, at the left cornu, communicating with an abscess. (B. M. Planchon. See *Duparque*, p. 132.)

CASE CCCLXIII. A tearing felt during labour, and the pains instantly ceased. A living child was delivered by the "usual means." A large rent in the side of the womb, which was apparently in a scirrhous state. Died in a few hours. (Mad. Lachapelle. See *Duparque*, p. 137.)

CASE CCCLXIV. Contracted brim; pains severe; *head* advanced. There was excessive sensibility of the abdomen. In about twelve hours there was suspension of pains, and while she was carried on a bed, she complained of a tearing and extreme oppression; the head could not be felt; the placenta was expelled, and the *feet* felt in the womb, by which it was extracted. Hernia of omentum. Died in six hours.

Post mortem.—Oblique rent; downward and forward; the edges of the rent in a scirrhous state. (Mad. Boivin, *Obs. No.* 111. See *Duparque*, p. 137.)

CASE CCCLXV. Dr. Just. Frid. Ling, cited by Sue, speaks of a womb of which the fundus was extremely thick, while the right side was very thin and pierced by the feet. (*Duparque*, p. 143.)

CASE CCCLXVI. A case by Camper, in which the womb was so thin as to be pierced by the feet of the child. (*Duparque*, p. 143.)

CASE CCCLXVII. Æt. 40 years; ninth labour; at full term, fell from a ladder; felt no more motion; labour-pains eight days after. Os dilated, fœtus unfavourably placed. Next day, immediately after a very strong pain, seconded by violent efforts, an arm came down, and, at the same time, a noise as of a body bursting, was heard. On the third day of labour, the child could not be felt. She died next day. A very long rent was found in the right side, from which the head and one arm had escaped." The uterus could not have been healthy. (*Duparque*, p. 153.)

CASE CCCLXVIII. A rupture at the fundus was recognized; the child born; no bad symptoms followed, and she nursed the child. Enlargement of the abdomen ensued, and in a few weeks she died. A rent was found in the fundus. (Chambon. See *Duparque*, p. 163.)

Case CCCLXIX. In carrying the hand into the womb, to detach the placenta, a rent was felt, and a large hernia through it. The intestines were returned, womb contracted, and she lived a month. (From *Duparque*, p. 168.)

Case CCCLXX. Æt. 28 years; strong; had natural delivery two years ago. After three days' labour, repeated attempts with forceps. Turning attempted, causing frightful suffering; and, after two and a half hours' trial, she was abandoned, and sent to the hospital. Pains had ceased; uterus could be felt in front of the fœtus; head at the superior strait; the cervix contracted around the child's neck. On attempting to seize the feet, the entire child passed into the abdomen. She was abandoned. She retained her consciousness, and awaited the fatal moment.

Post mortem. A longitudinal rent, starting at the vagina, inclining to the right side. Its edges were thick, and deeply ecchymosed. (Mad. Lachapelle, t. iii. p. 159. See *Duparque*, p. 180.)

Case CCCLXXI. Had rupture of the membranes at 5 A. M.; at noon she ceased to feel the child move. For five hours repeated fruitless attempts were made, by three practitioners, to apply the forceps, and to turn, and she was sent to the hospital. Delivered by perforation, after failure to apply forceps. Died twenty-four hours after delivery.

Post mortem.—A longitudinal rent, from cervix upward; the edges ecchymosed. (*Ditto.*)

Case CCCLXXII. Mad. Lachapelle relates a case of a woman who died, undelivered, from hemorrhage. It proceeded from a vein beneath the peritoneum which had been only slightly broken. The region of the rupture was remarkably thin, the rest of the womb thick. (*Duparque*, p. 185.)

Case CCCLXXIII. Æt. 25 years. Lost blood, with the premonitions of labour. At the end of three days, was confined, in great pain, and died that day; uterus torn in its left side, with laceration of uterine arteries and veins, from which there had been great hemorrhage. (*Mém. de l'Acad. de Chir. Rech. sur l' Oper. César.*, P. M. Simon. See *Duparque*, p. 185.)

Case CCCLXXIV. Good constitution; third pregnancy; head; after two days' labour, version, with much difficulty. In the neck, to the left and behind, was a deep fissure, *which did not involve the peritoneum.* Died, after a few weeks, having phthisis. (Mad. Lachapelle. See *Duparque*, p. 185.)

Case CCCLXXV. Obliquity of the os; pains directed against the pubes. Death at the end of twenty-four hours.

Post mortem.—The placenta and almost the whole fœtus in the abdomen, with only part of the head in the uterus. The body of the womb was very thick, but around the rent it was scarce two lines in thickness. (Muller, in *Collect. des Thèses de Haller*, from *Duparque*, p. 202.

Case CCCLXXVI. Breech presentation. When in labour twelve hours, the os not being completely dilated, the anterior part of the neck separated from one side to the other, and the child passed immediately into the abdomen. It was withdrawn with much difficulty, in less than two hours. She died five hours after delivery.

Post mortem.—The pelvis was a little narrow; the point of the os sacrum passed through the posterior part of the womb. The inner and prominent edge of the pubis and ilia resembled an ivory paper-knife. (See *Duparque*, p. 206.)

Case CCCLXXVII. Æt. 26; delicate; third pregnancy; hydrocephalic fœtus; rupture within twenty-four hours after commencement of labour. Hernia through the rent. Rent transverse, near the union of the vagina and uterus. Delivered by forceps; died almost immediately. (*Duparque*, p. 219.)

Case CCCLXXVIII. Death after five hours of labour, with oppression, nausea, &c. The body of the child and the placenta were in the abdomen, while the head was still in the pelvis. Rent in posterior part, at junction with vagina. (Thibaut, *de l'Acad. de Rouen*, from *Duparque*, p. 222.)

Case CCCLXXIX. Æt. 28 years; third pregnancy; labour had not made sensible progress for twenty-four hours, when bloody mucous discharges took place; inexpressible uneasiness, and coldness of limbs. Twelve hours after this, she had a violent pain, followed, at once, by general sinking and cessation of pains. Rupture detected twelve hours after, but she was left undelivered for more than twelve hours, and died before it could be accomplished by forceps.

Post mortem.—Rent in inferior, posterior, and lateral parts of the womb, involving the vagina to a great extent; child hydrocephalic. (M. Haime, *Journ. Gén. de Méd.* See *Duparque*, p. 227.)

Case CCCLXXX. Delicate; had three severe labours. After several hours of moderate labour, the os not being fully dilated, suddenly, without having had any severe pain, was seized with vomiting, &c. The presenting parts (the foot and head) had disappeared, and the uterus was empty. M.M. Devreux, Gardien, and Roux being called in, found rupture of cervix at its union with the vagina. Turning was agreed upon in preference to gastrotomy, and done with little effort. Child dead. She died two days after. (*Duparque*, p. 265.)

Dr. Brainard, of Chicago, writes: "I have met with two cases of ruptured uterus. In one of these,[1] Case CCCLXXXI, there was a firm cicatrix across the vagina. The womb was torn transversely in front above the attachment of the vagina. After three days' labour the woman died, and being then called in to examine the body, I found the child in the abdomen. I have also ascertained, pretty certainly, that the cicatrix was produced by attempts to procure abortion.

"The other case, Case CCCLXXXII, occurred in a young woman, with, I think, her third child. She had very tedious and severe labours, and after several hours' pains, the head was well down in the pelvis. * * I found all the fœtus, but one foot, escaped from the uterus; by that I delivered. She lived four days, when she died, apparently from strangulation of the intestines."

Case CCCLXXXIII. Æt. 28 to 30 years. In the first labours the woman was delivered by taking the child from her by craniotomy. In the second labour, I was called in consultation on the third day of labour, and delivered the child, dead, of medium size, from above the superior strait, with the long forceps. I advised, in case of a third pregnancy, premature delivery. My advice was not adopted by her; and the two physicians who attended her in the third labour permitted the natural violent throes to continue three days without assistance, or even attempting to deliver her. The womb ruptured; the child passed into the cavity of the abdomon; mother and child were both lost.

The *post mortem*, which I witnessed, demonstrated what I had rendered evident with the long forceps in her previous labours, that there was capacity enough in the pelvis, but in consequence of excessive curvature of the lower

[1] See this Journal for 1848, vol. ii. p. 113, Case LXIV.

part of the spine, prominence of the sacro-lumbar junction, and non-conformity of the axis of the pelvis with the axis of the womb, the child's head could not be directed in and forced through the pelvis by the natural efforts. The expulsive action being directed toward and upon the pubis, ruptured the womb at that point. (*Communicated by Dr. Lewis Shanks, Memphis, Tenn.*)

CASE CCCLXXXIV. Æt. 38 years; fourth labour. When called at 5 P. M. all pains had ceased an hour and a half before. Up to that time, pains regular and vigorous from the commencement of labour on the preceding night; abdomen a little tender; pulse 85, warm; os very high, dilatable; felt what was thought to be the head; suspected rupture; there was *no tendency* to collapse, or any marked symptom of so formidable an injury; child could not be felt under the integuments. By consent was left till 8 P. M.; head no longer felt; condition the same; pulse 92; had not had a single pain since 2 P. M. She refused to be delivered; some slight pains in about an hour. At 10 A. M. next day, she was dead. The abdomen at once opened; child and placenta among intestines; extensive rent of cervix. (Dex. Bean, Esq., Halifax, in *Lond. Loncet*, 1853, vol. i. p. 30)

CASE CCCLXXXV. Fifth pregnancy; delivered after about five hours' labour; no hemorrhage; child long dead; was left well and cheerful. Two hours after this he found her *in articulo mortis*. She had, in the meantime, been very angry, and just after this excitement, collapse ensued.

Post mortem.—She had had uterine disease for years; uterus uncontracted; dark, extravasated appearance on the right side, at the right lateral ligament. Two pounds of blood had escaped; nothing unusual on the inner surface; cervix rugged and ulcerated. (J. Berncastle, M. D., *Lond. Lancet*, vol. ii., 1851.)

CASE CCCLXXXVI. Wretchedly destitute; had a stillborn child after a most protracted and severe labour; considerable hemorrhage, but no alarming symptoms followed till the tenth day, when profuse bleeding came on and recurred, and she sank in five days.

Post mortem.—Rupture in anterior and superior portions of uterus near the cervix; also an abscess at upper part of vagina. (G. J. Squibb, "*The Institute*," Lond., Dec. 1850.)

CASE CCCLXXXVII. Was seen by a student at 3 P. M. In the evening, the right foot and hand brought down by a physician. Efforts at delivery ceased at about 11 P. M.; after this she had no pains, but began to vomit, and sank rapidly. At 11 A. M. Dr. C. was called in, and finding the leg protruding through the vulva, discovered a laceration of the womb. We "proceeded to turn," and delivered her of a dead child in half an hour, without much inconvenience to the patient, who felt relieved. Died in twenty-four hours, or thirty-six hours after the rupture. Hernia followed; placenta had passed into the abdomen.

Post mortem.—Rent three inches up the cervix, and the same distance down into the vagina. (*Reported by Dr. Conant to N. Y. Patholog. Soc.* See *N. Jersey Med. Rep.*, May, 1855.)

CASE CCCLXXXVIII. Delivered previously by craniotomy; narrow pelvis. Was called in consultation at 11 A. M. on the 4th. She was taken in labour on the 1st; pains slight till evening of the 3d, when Dr. G. was sent for. Pains had been strong all night, but suddenly almost entirely ceased about 6 A. M.; abdomen tender, not tumefied; constant grumous discharge; head felt presenting very high up. Brought down a foot, and delivered her in a few minutes of a semi-putrid child. Shoulders and head delivered with some difficulty; the flattened head indicated great pressure; placenta came, and womb contracted well; prostration followed; soon fell asleep; bid fair to convalesce till she expired suddenly at 6 A. M. next day.

Post mortem.—Slight peritonitis; a rent in anterior surface, almost severing the cervix from the body. Diameters of superior strait 2¾ in. and 4⅛ in. (Dr. A. K. Gardner, in *Amer. Med. Monthly*, 1854, vol. ii.)

CASE CCCLXXXIX. Robust; ninth labour. Found child delivered, and mother prostrated from profuse hemorrhage. Labour had been rapid, but, as the head passed the vulva, there was a copious dash of blood, which still flowed; placenta not yet come away. In search of this the hand suddenly slipped through a jagged strictured orifice, and touched the intestines. She soon expired. For two or three months, though in apparently good health, she believed she would not survive this labour. "Could there have existed a softened or diseased spot—say of ulcerative inflammation in the fundus—which, during gestation, without giving rise to much general disturbance, could yet, through nervous depression, account for the woman's prescience, and which caused so weakened a state of the parietes as to cause them to give way during labour?" (Dr. H. R. Worthington, in *Amer. Journ. Med. Sci.*, Oct. 1854.)

CASE CCCXC. Æt. 40 years. Called at 10 P. M. She had for two or three months been subject to uterine hemorrhage, and for two weeks almost constantly. Had premonitory symptoms in the morning, and during the day, but no real labour until a short time before the visit, when she had a single most violent pain, and felt something give way. Great prostration, followed with tendency to vomit; great tenderness of abdomen, and coldness of whole body; pulse was imperceptible; constant sighing and restlessness; os was slightly dilated; presentation could not be felt. The head and arm could be distinctly felt through the parietes of the abdomen, as if projecting through a rent in the uterus. Fearing to deliver in her depressed condition, she was left to her fate, and died at 8 A. M. (Dr. Rankin, *Amer. Journ. Med. Sci.*, Oct. 1853, p. 393.)

CASE CCCXCI. Healthy; æt. 40; second gestation; labour pains came on in afternoon of 9th inst., when they became quite strong, and continued so till midnight, when she had one unusually severe, followed by a chill, and then ceased; 3 A. M. physician sent for, who found her cold and nearly pulseless; at 9. A. M. she was moribund; the child's head had remained down nearly to the external organ, but was not immovable.

Post mortem.—Breech protruded four inches from the rupture; uterus contracted; placenta loose in abdomen; rent extended from the os laterally to within an inch of the fundus. Thickness of walls at the rent was half an inch; at the opposite side one inch and a quarter. (Dr. Putnam; see *Amer. Journ. Med. Sci.*, July, 1855, p. 50.)

CASE CCCXCII. Multipara; after a labour of twelve hours, had sudden excruciating pain, followed by distress at scrobiculus cordis, with vomiting, and rapid, feeble pulse. Delivered by forceps; placenta easily removed. Died in forty hours from rupture. There was in this no retrocession of head, nor external hemorrhage. (*Ibid.*)

CASE CCCXCIII. Fourth child; afternoon, found os pretty well dilated; head could be reached only by an effort, by which membranes were ruptured; pains regular, and tolerably vigorous till midnight, when, as head was little inclined to descend, gave from half a drachm to a drachm of ergot in three doses. The pains became powerful, then less severe, then ceased; head receded, and body passed out of the uterus, and could be felt there. The delivery of the head required the crotchet, as the head was large and firm.

Died on third day. (*Transact. New Jersey Med. Soc.;* see *Dr. Storer's Rep. to Amer. Med. Assoc.*)

Case CCCXCIV. After labour had lasted several hours, pains almost entirely ceased; forceps failed; pains subsided; patient died in twelve to thirteen hours after first seen.

Post mortem.—A rent four inches long in anterior part of fundus; the most of the child had escaped; the head unusually large. (Dr. J. M. Pugh, in *Philad. Lancet*, vol. i. See *Dr. Storer's Report to Amer. Med. Assoc.*)

Case CCCXCV. Under care of midwife. Twenty-six hours after labour began she suddenly exclaimed that something *had given way internally*. Pains at once subsided; soon after a physician sent for, who remained all night, and *bled* her for *rigidity of the os uteri*. Dr. H. was called in the morning. The head had receded from the perineum beyond reach, and the child had escaped from the womb. She was sinking rapidly, and was left undelivered.

Post mortem.—A rent several inches in length through the cervix. (*Reported by Dr. H. A. Hartt, N. Y. Journ. Med.*, Nov. 1850, p. 330.)

Case CCCXCVI. The same patient as in Case CCCXXXIV of recoveries. About three and a half years after first rupture Dr. H. was sent for, and reached her in the fourth day of her labour; was very weak; pulse 118, and feeble; respiration hurried. The hand had presented with severe pains, and twenty-four hours after they began, a snap was distinctly heard by her friends around her, the hand receded, and from that moment labour had been suspended. Found a large opening in the seat of the former rupture, and felt the child in the peritoneal cavity. Dr. H. turned and delivered, with great gentleness. She gradually sunk, and died thirty-six hours after delivery. (*Ibid.*)

Case CCCXCVII. Æt. 35 years, seventh child. Labour progressed favourably for four or five hours, when the pains suddenly ceased. She complained of chilliness and of great pain in the left iliac region; great prostration ensued. Death twenty-four hours after labour pains ceased. The head was low down, and an attempt to apply forceps was made just before her death; the head did not recede after the rupture.

Post mortem.—Fœtus in peritoneal cavity; head firmly impacted in the inferior strait, and "it required no small amount of force to dislodge it;" placenta also had escaped. The rent was through the left portion of the neck, near its union with the vagina; edges irregular, and softened "from inflammation following the accident;" extensive marks of peritonitis. (Dr. S. S. Purple, *N. Y. Journ. Med.*, Nov. 1852, p. 338.)

Case CCCXCVIII. Fifth child; called in consultation at 3 A. M.; taken in labour near 6 P. M. the preceding evening; labour went on well till one hour ago; membranes ruptured at midnight; head advanced steadily till 2 A. M., when she got a sudden cramp, and said something had given way within her. Expulsive pains ceased; cramps continued; pulse feeble, irregular; respiration hurried; sense of suffocation; jactitation; green vomiting came on, and collapse, followed by death, a few moments before he reached her. The head was low down the vagina, and had not receded.

Post mortem.—Fœtus in peritoneal cavity with placenta, &c.; body of womb contracted; on right side, near union with the vagina, was a large ragged rupture. "The parietes were softened, and required no great force to produce separation." (*Ibid.*)

Case CCCXCIX. Same patient as Case CCCXXXIV. "Eighteen or twenty months after previous rupture, I attended her in labour of about eight hours. The labour progressing, and the head descending, I was at the bedside with the finger in the vagina, when suddenly there was a complete cessation of the labour; the head of the child receded. Up to this time there were no symptoms to indicate any but a favourable termination of the labour. I was watchful for the opportunity to aid my patient in her delivery by the use of the forceps. Before, however, the child, which was dead, could be removed from the mother, the latter expired. No post mortem could be obtained." (*Communicated by Dr. W. H. Maxwell, New York.*)

CASE CCCC. Æt. 32 years; well made, pelvis well formed, and no obstruction in passage; presentation natural; head of average size; seventh labour. Labour began at 4 P. M.; until 5½ P. M. only ordinary pains, when the membranes broke after a violent pain, and about a gallon of water escaped. After this, there was no pain till 8 P. M., when she had two peculiar pains, and the head descended somewhat, according to the midwife; no pains afterward; low and anxious, with great tenderness. At 10 P. M. she gave ergot, but with little or no effect; 4 A. M. first seen by a surgeon. She was restless, exhausted, weak; rapid pulse; great pain and tenderness; forceps cautiously tried at 6 A. M., but failed to apply them; ergot given without effect. 9½ A. M. I was sent for; great and immediate danger; perforated with considerable difficulty, from its mobility. Removed the placenta, and found extensive rupture of posterior part of womb; the hemorrhage slight. Died at 10 P. M., about eleven hours from removal of child. (W. Sedgwick, *Lond. Lancet*, 1853, vol. i. p. 54.)

CASE CCCCI. After long-continued pains, the os very slowly dilating, she had a peculiarly acute pain, followed by collapse; os not found more dilated than before, and a fissure extended from it; a dead child was extracted by forceps, and the mother did not survive the operation.

Post mortem.—A rent on left side, four inches in length; a *cyst* in *left ovary* of the size of a child's head, had prevented the descent of the head. There was no rupture of the peritoneum. (Dr. Ogier Ward, *Lond. Lancet*, 1853, vol. ii. p. 487.)

CASE CCCCII. Æt. 38 years; twelfth labour. Visit at 4 A. M.; os equalled a crown piece; head presented; membranes ruptured; roomy pelvis; pains slack, but much complained of, and occasional vomiting. Up to 7 A. M. labour progressed very slowly; the first stage completed, and as pains did not improve, gave ergot, repeated in a half hour; as little effect was produced, gave no more. The pains were not like labour pains, but much harder to bear, and confined to lower part of abdomen. About 8½ A. M. found head well down toward the perineum; pains moderate; but she now became violently excited; cried out that the "pain was dreadful, of an intense burning character, which never left her, and which she could not live under." She persisted in getting out of bed, when she became suddenly pale and quite calm. Instantly suspected rupture; placed her on the bed; the head had receded; was almost pulseless; gave stimulants, and sent for forceps. It was now 10 A. M.; fell asleep, awaking occasionally. All pain had left her. About 12 she asked, "What was that crack?" Immediately applied forceps; she complained again of the burning pain, and became very violent. In about half an hour, after much labour, just as I delivered the head, she expired. The shoulders defied all efforts to extricate them.

Post mortem. Breech and legs of child, with placenta, in peritoneal cavity; contracted womb low down in left iliac region, hid from sight; the rent extensive in the anterior wall; child occupied entire pelvis, and could not be moved; probably a quart of coagula. As far as I could ascertain, there was no thinning of the uterus, or disease of the walls. (James Barron, *Lond. Lancet*, 1853, vol. ii. p. 587.)

CASE CCCCIII. Æt. 32 years; always healthy; ninth child; all had presented unnaturally; pelvis roomy. Called at noon; had been in labour twenty-seven hours, and waters escaped for twenty-five hours; her whole appearance choleraic; pulse small and quick; great thirst; vomited coffee-ground coloured matter; had pains about once in fifteen minutes, crying out loudly at the accession of each; os equalled a crown piece; presentation of something soft, could not be made out; excessive tenderness of bowels; uterus felt contracted to size at three months. The collapse was constantly increasing, and she was not delivered. She died at 6 P. M.

Post mortem.—Child weighed twelve to thirteen pounds; in the peritoneal cavity; placenta in the vagina; coagula in abdomen; the rent obliquely forward from near the broad ligament down to the os; the vagina not torn; at the upper part the walls were two inches thick, at the mouth six-eighths of an inch.

She had been seen by a quack seven hours after labour began, who introduced his hand, and during his manipulations she felt a sudden great pain, exclaiming something had burst, and that she was killed. Soon after this, vomiting commenced, and she continued to grow worse. (Chas. Vaudin, *Lond. Lancet*, 1854, vol. ii. p. 273.)

CASE CCCCIV. Thirty five years, strong and healthy, tenth pregnancy; had been in labour twenty-four hours, and the waters had escaped twelve hours; the os equalled a crown piece; vertex presentation; pains frequent, trifling, and ineffectual. She remained thus "without further evidence of completion of labour" for twelve hours. Turning was then performed, but, owing to some unknown difficulty, delivery could not be effected; collapse ensued; she died in twelve hours from his first visit.

Post mortem.—Child a female, weighing eleven pounds, which had been extruded from the uterus, excepting the feet and legs; rent in right side, close up to the os, and almost half through its circumference, the edges jagged and shreddy, the whole organ very dark, very flabby, and much softened; pelvis rather small, with a prominence of sacrum, which diminished the sacro-pubic diameter. (*Ibid.*)

CASES CCCCV, CCCCVI, CCCCVII. "I have seen three other cases of rupture of the uterus, which all terminated fatally. One under the care of Dr. R., the rupture having taken place while the patient was attended by a midwife; she lived for several days. The second occurred to the late Dr. M.; the case terminated fatally in an hour after the accident. The third I saw with the late Dr. B.; she lived two or three days." (Dr. F. Chatard, Baltimore. *Communicated.*)

CASE CCCCVIII. Æt. 19 years, with her first child. She had a severe labour, and was constantly making immense efforts when her pains were present—greater than I ever knew to be made—so violent, that I repeatedly told her she would rupture her womb if she persisted. In the midst of a violent pain she shrieked out vehemently, and the pains became almost instantly less severe. She soon gave birth to a *living child*, but gradually collapsed, and in three or four hours died. The neck of the womb presented a rupture through its *muscular coat* an inch and a half to two inches in extent; the peritoneal coat was safe. (*Communicated by Prof. D. H. Storer, Boston.*)

CASE CCCCIX. Æt. 40 years; had eight or ten children. Dr. T. had visited her repeatedly the day before in a slowly progressing labour; vertex presenting at the upper strait. The doctor left her at 10 P. M., directing the friends to send for him if the pains increased in strength and frequency. At 4 A. M. he was sent for. While leaning with her pendulous abdomen upon a wooden stool, she had a violent pain, and cried out something had given way; some blood was lost from the vagina, and the pains did not return. The head of the child, which was very evidently at the upper strait at 10 P. M., had now disappeared, and the pulse very feeble. I was sent for, and found the patient, between 5 and 6 A. M., almost pulseless, countenance sunken, skin bathed in sweat, steady pain in the abdomen, and almost moribund. Child's limbs could be felt through the abdominal walls. Having prepared myself for turning, and directed the frequent administration of brandy—the woman being quite sensible and able to swallow—I introduced my left hand into the vagina, and discovering a large rent on the left and upper part of its connection with the uterus, passed my hand into the peritoneal cavity, found the feet, and brought them without difficulty into the vagina and pelvis. Some bearing-down pains (abdominal muscles) now came to my assistance, and a large dead child was without any improper delay delivered. The placenta, and perhaps a pound or two of coagula and fluid blood, followed. The uterus was found to be contracted, and the hemorrhage ceased. The pulse rallied; she expressed great relief; pain ceased; she took some laudanum, brandy, &c. In about eight hours she sank and died.

Autopsy.—Flaccid, pendulous abdomen; cellular tissue loaded with fat; leucophlegmatic appearance of skin; uterine walls unusually thick—softened and diseased in the right side, where a laceration, even in the semi-contracted state of the organ, measuring two and a half inches, had occurred; the vagina also forming a large part of the aperture. (*Communicated by Dr. Richard H. Thomas, Prof. of Obstetrics, University of Maryland.*)

Case CCCCX. Called to Johns, a coloured woman, 11th mo. 30, 1849, by Dr. K. She had been several days in labour, under the care of a midwife, who had repeatedly given her medicine. When Dr. K. saw her last evening, the pains had ceased suddenly, after having been very strong. She appeared much fatigued, but nothing very unusual attracted the Dr.'s notice. He directed refreshments and rest. He left her in charge of a midwife. About 4 A. M., Dr. K. was summoned. She had rested none; constant pain in the uterine region. She had been growing weaker, almost fainting; sick stomach and vomiting; if not relieved must die. Stimulants were given, and I saw her at 8 A. M. Pulse very feeble; countenance depressed and sunken; skin cool, and bathed in sweat; abdomen and uterine globe tender and painful; mind clear, anxious for relief. Shoulder presented above the superior strait, and entirely in utero; os very dilatable; diagnosed rupture of uterus, without escape of child. The midwife prevaricated, and did not acknowledge what we afterwards ascertained to be the fact, that she had given ergot freely, before the pains ceased so suddenly. While we endeavoured to sustain, by brandy and water, Dr. R. proceeded to turn; the feet were easily found, and the pelvis readily came down; but the shoulders and head were large, and much delay and difficulty took place in their disengagement. She was very much exhausted. The placenta soon followed, with little hemorrhage. She continued to sink, and died in two hours.

Autopsy.—Uterus contracted to nearly the usual size, twenty-four hours after delivery. A large rupture extended from the vagina, nearly half its length; part of the vagina also lacerated. (*Ditto.*)

Case CCCCXI. Æt. 32 years; had five premature confinements. Fourth mo., 1853, Dr. K. was called, at 7 P. M., on 26th. Vertex presenting, membranes gave way at 11½ P. M. Copious discharge of waters; head slightly advanced, "pains severe and expulsive;" great restlessness. About 1 o'clock A. M., while on close-stool, patient suddenly cried out with excruciating pain in epigastrium; faintness; vomiting; total cessation of all labour pains; and frightful prostration ensued. Dr. K. at once concluded a rupture of the uterus had taken place; had her properly placed, and sent for a medical man, who, with him, wishing my assistance, I saw her at 4 A. M. She was greatly depressed; almost pulseless; extremities cold; brandy was being administered freely; the head of the child being still within reach, I was able to use the perforator, and, after evacuating the contents of the cranium, to deliver the child with the crotchet, about 5 A. M. Hemorrhage, to a considerable extent, took place during the delivery, but ceased very much upon the delivery of the placenta. A rupture, large enough to admit the hand, was detected on posterior wall of the vagina and neck of the uterus. The patient continued very prostrate until 8 o'clock A. M., when reaction came on, and the pulse returned at the wrist, and warmth to the extremities; strict quiet; anodynes. 28th. Rested well; no febrile excitement; a dose of oil. 29th. Rested well; pulse frequent; tongue brown; abdomen greatly distended; uterine region tender; was bled and leeched with relief. 30th. Better. From this time she improved until 5th mo. 9th, when she was declared to be convalescent, and the Dr. took his leave. On the 12th, Dr. K. found her suffering with throbbing pain in the right iliac region; tympanitic abdomen; small, thready pulse. May 13. Pain was relieved yesterday; followed by four or five dejections, containing blood and pus. She is now sinking. She died at 8 A. M., about twenty-four hours from the first complaint of pain in the iliac region, and eleven days after the occurrence of the rupture. "The patient clearly recovered," remarks Dr. K., "from the ruptured uterus, as she had been for some days without fever, had good appetite, &c. She succumbed at last to the pelvic abscess, which discharged into the rectum." (*Ditto.*)

Case CCCCXII. Æt. 28; admitted into Emigrant Hospital, June 22, 1853; second child; labour commenced some hours prior to admission; the head presenting in the first position; pelvis of normal size, and the os uteri well dilated. The pains were extremely severe, until the head had passed through inferior strait, when they suddenly ceased; the countenance became anxious, the lips livid, the patient complaining of dizziness only; pains soon recurred slightly, with very moderate expulsive force, and her strength began to fail; the pulse to increase in frequency; and, as the axilla could be reached with the finger, it was introduced, and delivery completed by very slight traction. Child stillborn; head large and tumefied; liquor amnii greenish; placenta in vagina; the uterus was contracted sufficiently for the bandage. The lividity of countenance remained, without any complaint of pain. Soon she became restless, with increased anxiety, and great exhaustion; there was no hemorrhage; ice and brandy were given freely, but she died without reaction in an hour after delivery.

Autopsy, twenty-four hours after death.—Body well nourished; muscles pale and flabby.

Abdomen.—Uterus firmly contracted. In the centre of the posterior portion of the neck of the uterus there was a rupture, from the os, an inch and a half in length on the internal surface, and an inch externally. The walls were flabby, of normal thickness. About two ounces of blood were found in the peritoneal cavity. The liver was large, and had a fatty appearance, as in cases of pulmonary phthisis, and quite friable; kidneys exsanguined and soft.

The lungs were healthy; the heart was flabby, with some fatty deposits on the exterior surface. There had been nothing peculiar in her condition, until the moment after her pains had ceased.

The small extent of rupture, and the fatty appearance of the liver and heart, are worthy of regard, in connection with the occurrence of death so soon after so slight a lesion. (*Communicated by Henry G. Cox, M. D., Prof Theory and Practice Med. N. Y. Med. Coll.*, and formerly *Clin. Lecturer on Dis. of Women and Children in State Emigrant Hospital.*)

Case CCCCXIII. Was seen after about two days' labour. For thirty-six hours after the rupture of the membranes, there was little or no pain; pains then came on, and early delivery expected; but the pains ceased, vomiting came on, skin cold and clammy, pulse feeble, but the head did not recede, nor had any sharp, sudden pain been noticed. Was seen by Dr. C. seven hours afterward. A soft, fluctuating tumour, not the bladder, could be felt over the hypogastrium. The forehead was felt per vaginam; forceps slipped off the head; head perforated; found hydrocephalic. She lived four hours after delivery, and eleven after rupture.

Post mortem.—A half pint of blood in abdomen; the peritoneal coat supposed to be torn in removal; for, in the vicinity of the rent, the uterus was softened; some lymph upon the uterus, and some pus between bladder and pubes. On opening the uterus, which was large, dark, and somewhat softened, a rent was discovered on the right side, anteriorly and near the neck; vagina intact. (Dr. Thos. F. Cock, *N. Y. Journ. Med.*, 1855.)

Case CCCCXIV. Æt. 20 years; third pregnancy; one stillborn after severe labour; labour favourable until head had descended into the pelvis, when, about forty-one hours from the beginning of labour, the contraction ceased, but abdominal pains and vomiting were present. Forceps were applied, but head receded. When seen by Dr. C., seven hours after supposed rupture, she was livid, distressed, restless, vomiting; pulse 150; fœtus felt through the parietes, abnormally distinct. There was a perforation in the perineum, and a band in the vagina, from a former labour. The finger could reach the head above the pubes; forceps and perforation inadmissible; gastrotomy mooted; died undelivered, three hours afterward, or about ten hours after rupture.

Post mortem.—Fœtus entirely escaped from the uterus; a knuckle of intestine and a part of peritoneum showed marks of inflammation. A large transverse rent anteriorly, one inch above the os. The anterior vaginal wall extensively lacerated. *Pelvis.* Antero-posterior diameter at brim, four inches; transverse, four and a half inches. Inferior strait, transverse, three and a quarter inches; antero-posterior, four and a half inches. The pubic arch resembled that of the male; the *linea ileo pectinea* "quite sharp." (*Ditto.*)

Case CCCCXV. Multipara; æt. 35; sixth child; previous labour easy. Labour progressed slowly, with inefficient pains for thirteen hours; pains then ceased. There was *no outcry*, or *sensation of tearing*, and the head did not recede. In about seven hours after this, she was found with a sunken, haggard, and pale countenance; jactitation; with pain over whole abdomen; pulse feeble, and 160; the head had not receded; portions of fœtus distinctly felt on left side, but not on right; forceps tried, but bent, and head opened. She lived one and a half hours, or about eight and a half after rupture. (*Ditto.*)

Case CCCCXVI. Æt. 37; seventh labour; good health. Labour began at noon; doctor called at 7 P. M.; pains expulsive, regular, and everything favourable. At 1½ A. M., during a strong contraction, she complained of acute pain in the back and abdomen to the umbilicus. Contractions ceased suddenly; she felt, during the pain, as if she should burst; she got upon her feet and fainted; countenance pale and sharp; surface cold and clammy; pulse rapid, wiry, and fluttering; head had not receded; vomiting of dark red fluid soon occurred; forceps applied, and child delivered stillborn, followed by two or three quarts of blood. Child weighed 12 to 13 pounds. Previous to delivery, the uterus had broken away, and occupied the right upper abdomen, and the fœtus the lower and left—the head not having receded. Death in less than two hours after rupture.

Post mortem.—Uterus excessively large and firm; rent of two and a half inches of cervix and vagina, posteriorly; uterine walls more than double usual thickness. Hence it is inferred the rupture occurred from immense muscular power, the fœtus being large. (*Ditto, communicated by Dr. E. W. Owen.*)

CASE CCCCXVII. Æt. about 30 years; had had an instrumental labour, the second natural, the third fatal. Labour pains began in the morning. In the afternoon labour seemed near its close, but suddenly the contractions ceased, and had pain in epigastric region, with dyspnœa; forceps used with great difficulty; head drawn down with difficulty by perforator. By successive efforts of three operators, fœtus drawn down by a handkerchief around the neck. She died in an hour.

Post mortem.—Large clots, and some blood in abdomen; transverse rent anteriorly, at junction of uterus and vagina, three inches long, with ragged edges, and greatly ecchymosed; antero-posterior diameter of brim of pelvis $3\frac{1}{4}$ inches; transverse, $5\frac{1}{2}$ inches; promontory very prominent. (*Ditto; seen only after death.*)

Causes of Rupture.—The cases now presented afford still further confirmation of the views urged more especially by Dr. Murphy, and supported by our previous statistics, that a diseased condition of the womb is frequently met with in cases of this accident. Thus the uterus was thin and brittle in Case CCCX. It was thin in *seven*, viz: in CCCXIII, CCCLXI, CCCXV, CCCLXVI, CCCLXXII, CCCLXXV, CCCXCI. It was softened in *seven*, CCCXII, CCCXLVIII, CCCXCVII, CCCXCVIII, CCCCIV, CCCCIX, CCCCXIII. In Case CCCLIV the peritoneum was extensively detached. In Cases CCCLXIII, CCCLXIV, it was in a scirrhous condition. In Case CCCLXXXV the womb had been long diseased. In Cases CCCLXX, CCCLXXI, it was deeply ecchymosed. In Case CCCCXII the walls were flabby, and of natural thickness. In Case CCCCXVI there was great development of muscle. In Cases CCCLV, CCCCII, there was no disease. Of *twenty-two* of these in which the point is distinctly stated, in *nineteen* there was positive disease, and in *three* there was no appreciable disease. These *twenty-two*, added to the *forty-five* previously reported, we have *sixty-seven* in which the condition of the womb happens to be reported. In *thirteen* only is it reported as healthy; in *twenty* softened; in *twenty-one* thinned; in *one* both thinned and softened; in *three* both thinned and thickened; in *eight* "diseased;" in *one* thin and brittle. The larger proportion of instances in which the condition of the womb is stated, among the cases now presented, is probably due to the fact that attention has been only quite recently turned to this point. Observations in this particular are of the highest importance in enabling us to determine the causes of this accident, and it is very desirable that attention should be especially directed to it in future examinations when the result proves fatal.

The above are, we believe without exception, cases of *spontaneous* rupture of the womb. Lacerations of the cervix and vagina may, of course, take place in consequence of rude violence in attempts at delivery, as our cases abundantly show. When there is no such morbid condition, if it can be shown, as would seem from our statistics to be very probable, that spontaneous rupture is generally associated with, and we may therefore say due to an appreciable morbid condition of the womb, the practitioner is relieved of a degree of the responsibility which is attached to him.

In a few cases, not included among those enumerated, the parts around the rupture are described as "deeply ecchymosed;" others as "flabby;" these conditions are most probably due to some decided alteration of structure, though there was no appreciable softening or loss of substance. In Case CCCCXII, Dr. Cox suggests that the "small extent of the rupture, and the fatty appearance of the liver and heart, are worthy of regard, in connection with the occurrence of death so soon after so slight a lesion;" we would still further suggest that the condition of the uterus, predisposing to rupture, might possibly be due in such a case to a fatty degeneration of the muscular fibre similar to that found in the heart. This point may be worthy of notice in future examinations of those dying from a ruptured womb. Whatever the cause may be of the softening and thinning which is found in so large a proportion of the cases of this accident in which the condition of the womb has been hitherto noted, we certainly, as yet, know little of it. Do these lesions take place during the last few months of pregnancy, or do they take place during parturition? Some light may yet be thrown upon this point by examining the uterus of puerperal females dying from other causes than this accident, to ascertain if these lesions ever exist in such. That thinning of the inferior segment of the womb may occur from long-continued pressure of the gravid uterus, we may conceive possible; but if this be a cause of rupture, it is remarkable that the accident is of such rare occurrence, since in every pregnant woman the pressure exists. Moreover, we have instances in which the thinning was of the body of the womb, and others in which it was confined to a limited portion which had become dilated before rupture. Thus, in Case CCCLXI, the right side was entire and contracted; the left side "much distended, very thin, and torn into strips." In Case CCCXIII, at the seventh month, the rent was in the fundus, and the surrounding parts were of the thickness of writing paper. Of the cases of softening, in CCCXLVIII there was evidence of inflammation of some standing. In CCCXCVIII, "the parietes were softened, and required no great force to produce separation." Rupture occurred after eight hours' labour, and death apparently within one hour after the accident. The changes in the uterine structure, it would seem, must have been antecedent to labour, as they could scarcely have come on during labour, and certainly not after the accident occurred. On the other hand, in Case CCCCIV, in which the pains had been feeble, and she died thirty-six hours from the beginning of labour, the organ was "very dark, very flabby, and much softened," and yet she is reported as strong and healthy, and in her tenth pregnancy.

These alterations of structure doubtless take place in some instances, antecedent to labour, from causes not well understood; and in others during labour, from long continued muscular exertion

Contractions of the pelvis have always been prominent among the causes enumerated by authors. We have already quoted the remark of Ramsbotham, that he had never known a case in which there was not some contraction. The most obvious modes by which a contracted pelvis may lead to this accident, are the thinning of the lower segment of the womb from pressure, and the resistance presented to the progress of the child under the impelling power of the uterus. Disproportion between the head and the pelvis, from whatever cause arising, would seem to produce similar results. That there is an intimate relation between such disproportions and the occurrence of the accident, will appear from what follows.

In Cases CCCXLIII, CCCXLIV, CCCXLVIII, CCCXLIX, CCCLII, CCCLV, CCCLXXVI, CCCLXXXVIII, CCCCIV, CCCCXIV, CCCCXVII, total *eleven*, the pelvis was more or less contracted. These, added to *sixty-three*, make *seventy-four* as the total of contracted pelves in about four hundred cases of rupture. But, as the histories of many of our cases are brief and imperfect, the existence of contraction may have been omitted in some, so that it is proper to state it thus—that there were *at least* seventy-four in *four hundred and seventeen;* or 18 per hundred.

The head was impacted from disproportion in Cases CCCLVII, CCCCII; and in CCCXIV the head was unusually large. There was obliquity of the os, the pains being directed against the pubis, in Cases CCCLXXV and CCCLXXXIII. In Case CCCCI, the descent was prevented by an enlarged ovary.

In Cases CCCXXXII, CCCXLI, CCCLXXVII, CCCLXXIX, CCCCXIII, the fœtus was *hydrocephalic.* These *five*, added to *seven* previously reported, make *twelve*, so that there were *at least* that number of instances of this complication in about four hundred cases, or *three* per hundred.

Rigidity of the os.—In cases CCCXVIII, CCCXXVII, CCCXXXI only, did the obstinate rigidity of the os appear to be the *cause* of rupture; adding *three* previously reported, gives *six.*

Obstructing bands in the vagina.—In Cases CCCXXXIX, CCCLXXXI, CCCLXXXII, CCCCXIV, the resistance of these apparently caused the rupture; adding *two* previously reported, gives *six.*

We have, then, as *conditions obstructing the progress of the child*, and therefore leading to rupture:—

In 417 cases of this accident, *at least*	74	cases of	contracted pelvis.
" " " "	12	"	hydrocephalic fœtus.
" " " "	6	"	rigidity of the os.
"	6	"	bands in the vagina.
	1	case of	enlarged ovary.
Total,	99		

The proportion of each of these complications, compared with the whole number of cases, must be regarded as relatively very large, especially in the instance of contracted pelvis. We see that in at least one-fourth of the whole number of cases there is a disproportion between the head and the pelvis, or an obstruction from organized adhesions of the vagina. This estimate is exclusive of cases in which the head is noted as large and firmly ossified. We cannot, therefore, err in regarding this relation as one of cause and effect. That such obstructions existed in many cases in which it is not alluded to in the histories given, is rendered probable by considering the duration of labour previous to rupture.

Time from beginning of labour to rupture.—Taking the whole of our cases in which this is specified, we find that rupture occurred in—

6 hours and less	from the beginning of labour in	38	cases.
12 " and over six	" " "	36	"
18 " and over twelve	" " "	10	"
24 " and over eighteen	" " "	20	"
36 " and less	" " "	16	"
48 " and less	" " "	14	"
Three days and less	" " "	11	"
Four days and less	" " "	2	"

Comparing these with the *duration* of labour in the 15,850 cases reported by Dr. Collins, we find that 13,412, or eighty per cent., terminated within six hours; 1,672, or sixteen per cent., in from six to twelve hours; and that in corresponding periods of six hours beyond this, they were but from one to two per cent.

The table above embraces 34 cases of contracted pelvis, but, after deducting these, the relative periods remain but little changed. It will be seen that the duration of labour previous to rupture is very much greater on the average than the entire duration of ordinary labours, according to Dr. Collins. The obstacle to delivery presented by the disproportion between the head and the pelvis, &c., explains this fact; and the probability that such hindrances to the progress of the child existed in many of our imperfectly reported cases, in which it is not noted, is strengthened by a consideration of the protracted character of the labours as a whole. But while the protracted character of the labour, under a continued succession of unavailing efforts to drive the head of the child through the pelvis, explains the frequent coexistence of such disproportion and rupture, there are not a few instances in which the duration of the labour was so short, or the character of the labour so little severe, that we cannot so readily trace any necessary connection between these and the relative size of the head and pelvis. In not a few instances, the first labour-pain was that causing the rupture. Thus, among contracted pelves, in Case XLII the head had passed the superior strait at which contraction existed, before rupture took place. In Case XCI, pains were feeble. In CCXVIII pains were feeble, and of but six hours' duration. In CLXIX pains feeble, and four hours. In CCCXLVIII they were not strong; in CCCXLIX, no strong pains; in CLXVI, moderate pains; in CXCVII, common labour.

Inordinate voluntary exertion deserves to be enumerated among the causes of rupture. It is prudent to persuade the patient to abstain from voluntary efforts, provided there be resistance to the progress of the child from any cause. We believe that no case of rupture has yet been published in which chloroform[1] was used, which may be due to the fact, that voluntary effort is for the most part suspended under its influence. In Case CCCCVIII, Dr. Storer warned his patient of her danger, but the accident occurred.

Dr. Tyler Smith, in his work on Parturition, p. 225, Amer. edit., remarks, "in ordinary labour, some amount of voluntary or instinctive action of the muscular system, and particularly of the expiratory muscles, is quite natural during the stages of propulsion and expulsion. In acute or severe labour, these voluntary exertions are productive of great mischief," as lacerations of the uterus and perineum, and exhaustion.

Then we have another class in which rupture was induced by violence, or from artificial stimulus of the womb. In Cases LXIII, CXLI, CCXCIV, CCCXCIII, CCCCX, ergot[2] was given; and in Case CCLXIII, alcoholic stimulants.

Among the cases of hydrocephalus, we have Case CCCXXXII, a labour of but two and a half hours; and Case XLVII, which lasted five hours. The remainder of these, with those in which there was rigidity of the os and bands in the vagina, were in labour, with scarce an exception, over thirty-six hours.

Situation of the Rupture.—During pregnancy four involved the fundus; these, added to thirteen in the fundus and body, before reported, make *seventeen* of the fundus and body, and *eight* involving, more or less, the cervix.

During labour: Of the entire number of cases, *one hundred and ten* are distinctly spoken of as involving the cervix; seventeen the fundus; and *seventy-one* the body of the womb. Of these seventy-one, by far the larger part are reported as ruptures of the anterior or posterior part, or of the right or left side; and in some of these, it is highly probable that the rupture involved the cervix also.

[1] This consideration, which is certainly an inducement to the use of chloroform in severe labours, is suggested by our respected friend, Dr. J. P. Batchelder, of New York.

[2] Dr. James Fountain, of Peekskill, writes, "I have seen one case only of rupture of the womb. It was the effect of a dose of *ergot.*"

In Cases CCCXLVI, CCCLXXIV, CCCCI, CCCCVIII, the peritoneum was not involved.

It appears to be a fair inference, from the above, that labours in which rupture occurs are, as a class, protracted; that the lesions of softening and thinning generally precede the rupture, and are, for the most part, a consequence of the delay; but that, in a certain proportion of cases, as in those occurring during pregnancy and early in labour, these lesions must have existed before the expulsive action of the womb was set up; while in certain other cases, rupture appears to occur in the womb unaltered by morbid changes.

We copy the *table* of *ages*, with the additions, from the new cases:—

16 years,	2 patients.	26 years,	9 patients.	37 years,	8 patients.
17 "	1 patient.	27 "	5 "	38 "	8 "
18 "	1 "	28 "	20 "	39 "	1 patient.
19 "	1 "	29 "	3 "	40 "	12 patients.
20 "	5 patients.	30 "	24 "	42 "	2 "
21 "	3 "	32 "	15 "	43 "	2 "
22 "	1 patient.	33 "	6 "	44 "	4 "
23 "	1 "	34 "	4 "	47 "	1 patient.
24 "	5 patients.	35 "	13 "	40–45 "	1 "
25 "	11 "	36 "	17 "		

The largest number were at the age of 30 years.

The largest number of cases delivered under Dr. Collins' Supervision, was also at the age of 30 years; viz: 2,346 in a total of 16,414 cases.

The table showing the number of the pregnancy in which the rupture occurred:—

No. of pregnancy	1st	2d	3d	4th	5th	6th	7th	8th	9th	10th	11th	12th	13th	Multiparæ.
No. of patients	31	25	30	27	21	25	14	7	7	12	8	5	2	25

Symptoms of Rupture.—The total, in which the character of the previous labour is stated, is 156. Of these

In 46, or 29.5 per cent., it was very severe.
" 39, or 25 " " strong.
" 46, or 29.5 " " moderate.
" 11, or 7 " " feeble.
" 14, or 9 " " "tedious."

In *fifty-five* the pains ceased suddenly; in *seventeen* they ceased gradually.

From this, it appears that liability to rupture is not confined to cases in which the labour is of great severity, and that it may sometimes happen when the pains from the outset are feeble. Its occurrence in the course of a labour of moderate severity, appears to be quite as common as when the pains are very severe. We have also the contrast of extensive rupture and escape of the child with few and feeble pains, and a simple laceration of the muscular coat after labour of great severity, as in Case CCCCVIII.

The sudden cessation of the pains is one of the most characteristic symptoms of the accident; but we learn that this is not of invariable occurrence, but that, in a small proportion of cases, the cessation of pains is gradual.

Again, the *recession of the presenting part* of the child takes place, as a general rule, upon the occurrence of the accident; but the exceptions are of sufficiently frequent occurrence to deserve especial notice. Among the cases now presented, in CCCXXXIX, CCCLVII, CCCLIX, CCCXCI, CCCXCVII, CCCCX, CCCCXIII, CCCCXV, CCCCXVI it is stated that the head did not recede; and among those previously reported, there are several of which the same is affirmed. In a few, not included among these, the head remained within reach, permitting delivery by the forceps or perforation; and, in a few instances, the head did not recede until the application of the forceps was attempted.

In addition to the instances quoted before, in which the rupture was accompanied by a peculiar *sensation* experienced by the patient, the same is noted in Cases CCCXXIV, CCCXXV, CCCXXXI, CCCXXXII, CCCXXXIV, CCCXXXIX, CCCXLI, CCCXLII, CCCLVI, CCCLVIII, CCCLXIII, CCCLXIV, CCCLXVII, CCCLXXXIX, CCCXC, CCCXCV, CCCXCVIII, CCCCI, CCCCII, CCCCIX, CCCCXI, CCCCXVI.

In CCCXXVI a loud cracking noise was heard, and in Cases CCCXLII, CCCLXVII, CCCXCVI the rupture was heard by the patient or bystanders.

In CCCCXIII, CCCCXV there was no sudden acute pain, or tearing sensation. In CCCCIII, pains continued once in fifteen minutes, the patient crying out at the accession of each, but the womb empty and contracted.

Exceptions also occur to the early appearance of extreme depression after rupture, as is seen, in a remarkable degree, in Cases CCCXXXI, CCCXXXIV, CCCLXXXIV, &c.

While the cessation of the pains, the sudden outcry of the patient, and the recession of the child, followed by symptoms of great prostration, in general render the diagnosis of the accident easy, the absence of any one of these is, as we have seen, not incompatible with the existence of rupture, and the knowledge that such exceptions occasionally exist, may, in some cases, aid in the diagnosis.

Influence of Delivery on Mortality.—Total of all cases delivered, 207. Of these, 77 recovered, or 37 per cent.

Total of all cases undelivered, 115. Of these, 27 recovered, or 23.5 per cent.

But among the cases previously reported, were many in which the foetus having escaped into the abdomen, was subsequently discharged after decomposition, and were reported as remarkable cases of recovery. Among the cases now related, of 26 undelivered, only three recovered, or about 11 per cent.

We repeat what was distinctly stated in our first paper, that these results are to be regarded only as approximating the relative proportion of cases saved and lost in actual practice; since we would naturally expect to find the larger proportion of cases published to have been cases of recovery.

But, if our statistics did not clearly exhibit a diminished mortality among those delivered, they show that life is prolonged by this measure, even in cases that do not recover.

We formerly showed that the average duration of life, after rupture, with those *delivered*, was *twenty-two* hours; and that of the *undelivered*, but *nine* hours. By adding to those the new cases, we find that, of those *delivered*, *fifty-four* per cent. survived beyond *twenty-four hours;* while of those dying *undelivered*, *twenty-seven* per cent. survived beyond the same period.

Relative success of different modes of Treatment when the Head and the whole or part of the Body has escaped into the Peritoneal Cavity.

SUMMARY OF ALL THE CASES.

Gastrotomy saved	16,	lost 4,	or 20	per cent. lost.
Turning, &c. "	23,	" 50,	or 68.5	" "
Abandoned "	15,	" 44,	or 75	" "

Relative success of different modes of Treatment when the Pelvis is Contracted.

SUMMARY OF ALL THE CASES.

Gastrotomy saved	6,	lost 3,	or 33	per cent. lost.
Perforation, &c. saved	15,	" 30,	or 65	" "
Abandoned "	0,	" 11,	or 100	" "

Adding together these two classes, we get, as the comparative results of the different modes of treatment—

Gastrotomy saved	22,	lost 7,	or 24	per cent. lost.
Turning, perforation, &c. saved	38,	" 80,	or 68	" "
Abandoned "	15,	" 55,	or 78	" "

Result as effected by facility or difficulty in Delivery.—Taking all the cases together in which this circumstance is alluded to, in *seventy* cases of *recovery*, *forty-eight* were delivered with ease, or 68.5 per cent. In *ninety-one* cases resulting in *death*, delivery was accomplished with ease in but *thirty-eight*, or 41.7 per cent.

We have included under *easy* deliveries those in which gastrotomy was performed; the term *easy* having reference to time occupied, as well as facility of execution. In all the cases of gastrotomy in which allusion is made to the point, delivery was accomplished very rapidly, and with comparatively little suffering.

If we deduct from each class just enumerated the cases of gastrotomy, we still find a preponderance of easy deliveries among recoveries, and of difficult deliveries among those who were lost. Thus, among *recoveries*, we get *twenty-six easy*, and *twenty-two difficult*, or 54 per cent. delivered with ease; and, among the deaths, *thirty-one easy*, and *fifty-three difficult;* or 37 per cent. delivered with ease.

Case CCCVIII has not been included in the enumeration of cases of gastrotomy, as the operation was peformed several weeks after the accident.

We have already discussed at some extent, in the former part of this paper, pp. 411, 412 (April 1848), the conditions under which gastrotomy commends itself as the proper resource. It is evident, we think, that this operation is now regarded with more favour by the profession than formerly; at least five cases having met our eyo as reported within the last five or six years. These additional cases, in connection with those delivered by other methods, confirm in every respect the conclusions to which we arrived, after a study of the cases embodied in our first paper. Those conclusions were briefly as follows:—

1. When rupture occurs, where there is no disproportion between the pelvis and the head of the child, and the head remains in the cavity of the pelvis, the child being ascertained to be living, the careful employment of the forceps should be attempted; if the head retreat, perforation will probably be required; if the child is dead, perforation is to be preferred. An impaction of the head in the hollow of the pelvis would of course require the use of the perforator.

2. Should the fœtus have escaped into the peritoneal cavity, the feet may be sought, and the child delivered by turning, *provided there be a pelvis beyond doubt ample, a head of moderate dimensions, and the edges of the uterus uncontracted, or the rent confined chiefly to the vagina.*

3. But as contraction of the uterus almost uniformly takes place upon the escape of the child, it will prove an obstacle to delivery in almost every case of escape of the child, in which the vagina is not also involved to a very considerable degree. The performance of gastrotomy will then offer the best chance of success.

We believe that a neglect of this mode of delivery has contributed much to the exaggerated estimates of the mortality of the accident, which are so generally entertained. It is an operation requiring no little resolution and true courage under the trying circumstances in which the physician is placed, and consequently arises the need of settled principles of practice to guide one in this extremity.

Although, as we have distinctly repeated, we do not believe that our cases give the actual proportions of recoveries and deaths under any one course of management, yet we maintain that the principal circumstance which vitiates one class is the same that renders the remainder imperfect, viz: an undue proportion of recoveries; and inasmuch as we have shown that, in some respects, our statistics conform with the experience of standard authorities, and that in others they conform with acknowledged principles of general practice, we have confidence that they are worthy of a degree of reliance in elucidating points upon which we have no other standard wherewith to compare them. The relative success of gastrotomy is, as we have seen, greater than that of any other mode of delivery, and we believe that a more frequent resort to it would result in a diminished mortality to the accident. In short, *as a gene-*

ral rule, from whatever cause we might be led to anticipate a protracted and difficult delivery by the natural passages, gastrotomy will afford the best chance of recovery. The only exception we would make is, when there is impaction of the head in the pelvic cavity or in the inferior strait.

There is a total of twenty-four cases of *hernia of the intestine* through the rent in the womb. In Case CCCLXIV, it was of the epiploon. In Case CCCLXXXII, death was attributed to the strangulation of the bowel.

In one instance, the placenta only disappeared through the rent.

In Cases CCCXLVI, CCCLXXIV, CCCCI, CCCCVIII, the peritoneum was not involved.

Case CCCLXI was complicated by presentation of the placenta.

In Cases CCCXCVI, CCCXCIX, rupture occurred in wombs previously ruptured.

Several instances of injudicious interference, or unjustifiable violence in delivery, will be observed on a careful perusal of the cases.

Case CCCXLVII is an instance of spontaneous evolution; the head which had presented, retreating, and the feet descending within reach. Dr. Ramsbotham has observed this evolution.

In Cases CCCLXV, CCCLXVI, the womb was pierced by the foot of the child. In Case CCCLI it was pierced by the fingers of the midwife. In Case CCCLVI, rupture occurred from a fall weeks before labour came on.

ART. IV. *Description of a Valve at the Termination of the Right Spermatic Vein in the Vena Cava, with Remarks on its Relations to Varicocele.* By JOHN H. BRINTON, M. D. (With a plate.)

THE pathology of the venous system has of late years been carefully investigated by numerous and accurate observers; and although by their efforts much light has been shed upon subjects hitherto imperfectly comprehended, there still remains much to be explained in this important class of affections.

Of all the lesions to which the veins are subject, none perhaps has attracted more attention than phlebectasis or varix. In this condition the vein is said to be varicose, its walls become unnaturally dilated, and its calibre consequently increased. The veins most frequently affected are those of the rectum, the spermatic cord, and the inferior extremity, although doubtless every portion of the venous system is liable, under certain circumstances, to become the seat of varicose dilatation.

The causes of the varicose condition of the veins are various, and are as yet not fully elucidated. The older surgeons were in the habit of invoking, as the sole cause, the existence of simple mechanical impediment to the return of the venous blood; but more recent observation has shown that explanations other than of a purely mechanical nature must be sought for.

That pressure upon a vein—the existence of tumours—the weight of a gravid uterus—the presence of a ligature—or a position of the body, by which the current of venous blood is directed contrary to gravitation—may all act in producing varix, is incontestable. Cases, however, constantly occur in which it is evident that none of these predisposing circumstances exist; and on these grounds, therefore, the explanation is impossible.

Hasse, in his treatise on general pathology,[1] advocates the doctrine that the varicosities of the veins are due to "a peculiar habit of the body, a morbid predominance of the venous system, which manifests itself through the intervention of influences at once mechanical and dynamical"

Rokitansky[2] also seems disposed to teach that the doctrines which ascribe the origin of phlebectasis to mechanical obstruction alone are untenable; for, he states, that "we have, therefore, after much experience, adduced other causes in explanation of the dilatation of the veins. There are, however, always cases occurring in which these cannot be detected; and as varicose veins present many symptoms which are hitherto perfectly unexplained, the theory of phlebectasis is still deficient in an important part."

It has been affirmed, and is generally supposed, that the superficial veins alone are subject to a varicose enlargement. Sir Benjamin Brodie,[3] in his Clinical Lecture on Varicose Veins of the Leg, explains the fact by stating that the deep-seated veins are exposed to uniform pressure on every side by the surrounding muscles, which is sufficient to prevent their dilatation. Recently, however, M. Verneuil read before the Academy of Medicine at Paris a paper, in which he contends that whenever varicose veins occur spontaneously on the lower limbs, the deep-seated veins are also affected; and also, that the deep muscular veins may be dilated without the superficial veins being in any way involved. These results, should they be verified by future observations, would doubtless go to weaken the explanation of the occurrence of the affection, as the result of purely local accidental causes.

The views already expressed with regard to the general causes of varix, apply with especial force to the dilatation of the veins of the spermatic cord, constituting varicocele or circocele.

This affection is generally met with, according to the statistics of Landouzy and Curling, about the period of puberty, and is of far more common occurrence than is generally supposed.

An interesting point with regard to the etiology of varicocele is this: Has the affection any direct relation to the varices of the veins; and does it occur synchronously with them in the same patient? Mr. Curling states that in patients suffering under varicocele, he has often found weakness in other

[1] Sydenham edition, p. 37.
[2] Rokitansky's Pathological Anatomy (Sydenham), p. 366.
[3] Brodie's Clinical Lectures on Surgery, Amer. ed., p. 113.

portions of the venous system, especially of the inferior extremity. Hasse, on the contrary, is inclined to consider that whenever one form of varix occurs, it is to the exclusion of all others.

The occurrence of varicocele is insidious and gradual, and is productive at first of little or no inconvenience. In fact, the patient is unaware of the existence of the disease until some time subsequent to its development. When discovered, the swelling in the scrotum resembles, as has been well said, a bundle of earthworms, of greater or less size; but it must be observed that the size of the mass is by no means an indication of the inconvenience sustained by the patient. A large varicocele will often give rise to but little pain; whilst one of small size may sometimes be attended with very great suffering.

The disease once developed, the changes which take place both within and without the walls of the vein, are exactly similar to those observed in every instance of phlebectasis. The vein, besides being increased in calibre, becomes tortuous, and increases in length; its walls at first somewhat thinned, become eventually thickened and hypertrophied, and insufficiency of the existing valves follows.

A most striking peculiarity with regard to this disease is the frequency of its occurrence upon the left side of the body, and its very great rarity upon the right. This circumstance, although it has attracted the attention of every observer, has never as yet been satisfactorily accounted for. The fact, however, is incontestable, and in explanation the following reasons have been adduced.

1. The difference in the direction of the venous current through the spermatic veins upon the two sides of the body. It is asserted that, as the spermatic vein of the right side empties into the vena cava, in a direction nearly parallel with the course of the blood in this latter vein, no impediment is offered to the discharge of its contents. Upon the left side, however, the anatomical relations of the veins vary. Here the spermatic vein throws its blood into the emulgent vein in, as we are told, a nearly perpendicular direction; and the renal vein then empties itself into the vena cava in a similar manner. Hence it is supposed that the course of the blood through this double rectangular channel is sufficiently impeded to give rise to the disease in question.

2. The pressure of the viscera upon the left renal vein as it passes across and rests upon the aorta.

3. The position of the testis, which hangs lower upon the left than upon the right side.

4. The pressure of the sigmoid flexure of the colon, especially when charged with accumulated feces, upon the spermatic veins.

A careful study of the anatomy of the veins in question will, however, I think, clearly show that the frequent occurrence of varicocele upon the left side, and its non-occurrence upon the right, is not in reality due to the causes ordinarily assigned; indeed, the reasons before alluded to have already been discarded by a most accurate observer, Nélaton.[1] Sir Astley Cooper, in his remarks on this disease, also conveys an idea of the insufficiency of the previously quoted causes of varicocele.[2]

Desirous of investigating this subject more fully, I have, during the past year, made a series of examinations upon the dead body, and with the following deductions:—

1. That the causes hitherto assigned are insufficient to account for the rare occurrence of varicocele upon the right side.

2. That the cause of the non-occurrence of varicocele upon the right side is referable to the existence of *a very perfect valve hitherto unnoticed, at the termination of the right spermatic vein in the vena cava.*

3. That *no* such valve exists upon the *left* side at the termination of the spermatic in the emulgent vein.

4. That a similar valve exists in the *analogous vein* of the female, the *right ovarian vein,* but none upon the left side.

The examination of this valve may be best conducted in the following manner: Remove the vena cava, emulgent, and spermatic veins from the body; pin them upon a board, in position, and then lay open the vena cava anteriorly by a longitudinal incision. Pass a probe gently up the right spermatic vein, and it will then be found to emerge into the vena cava through a slit-like aperture, not corresponding in size or direction with the apparent opening of the spermatic vein, as viewed from the interior of the vena cava. This apparent orifice is in reality a large, deep, and very perfect sinus, across which the delicate transparent valve floats. This sinus serves to receive regurgitating blood, and thus effectually to close the valve. The presence of this valve may be also demonstrated by an injection thrown up the vena cava; the injected matter will pass freely into the left spermatic vein, but not into the right; unless an undue amount of force be exerted, and the valve thus forced. The length of the valve, measured upon its free border, is about the one-fifth of an inch. Microscopically examined, it proves to be formed by a prolongation forwards of the internal and middle tunics of the spermatic veins, and

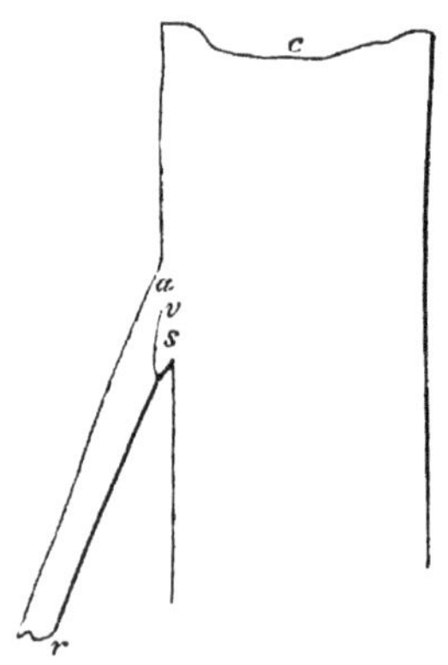

c. Vena cava.
r. Right spermatic vein
a. Aperture between right spermatic vein and vena cava.
v. Right spermatic valve.
s. Sinus.

[1] Nélaton's Clinical Lectures on Surgery. Atlee, p. 644.

[2] Testis, p. 231, Amer. edit.

is composed chiefly of elastic and connective tissues. The former is arranged in thick, wavy, longitudinal bands, crossed here and there by transverse striæ of the same structure. These transverse bands are more developed towards the free margin of the valve. The connective tissue is also arranged so as to form thick fibrous bands. The surface of the valve is lined by the ordinary epithelium found in the interior of the veins. Examination of the left spermatic vein has not revealed, as far as my experience goes, the existence of a similar valve.

I am not aware that the attention of anatomists or of pathologists has ever been called to the existence of the valve. Valves have, it is true, been said to exist in the spermatic veins, but they have always been described as occurring below the abdominal rings. In most works on anatomy no allusion is made to them whatever.

In the anatomical plates of Fabricius, published at Leipsic, in 1687, no spermatic valves are described, although the plates of the venous system are full and for the most part accurate. Cheselden also fails to notice them.

Morgagni, in his description of varicocele, merely observes that the disease is more frequent upon the left than upon the right side. This he attributes to the angle formed by the left spermatic vein. (*De Sedibus et Caus. Morb.*, Epist. 43, Art. 34.) The Elder Monroe, in his remarks upon the anatomy of the spermatic vessels and cord, and in his article "Varicocele," denies the existence of valves in the spermatic veins.[1]

In the posthumous works of Petit, vol. ii. p. 498, varicocele is described at length, and the following passage as to the causes occurs: "Ex vitiis hepatis . . . . . frequentiores esse in latere sinistro, quod fæces in colo sinistro morentur." Jourdan[2] denies the existence of valves, but mentions that Monroe *pretends* to have found them.

In *Fyfe's Anatomy*, Edin., 1810, the spermatic vein is described as furnished with valves, but more particularly *without* the abdomen.

Sir Astley Cooper[3] states that the veins of the cord *below* the external ring have valves, but that owing to their anastomoses they may be injected contrary to the course of the blood.

In Quain's plates, vol. ii., the same remark is made concerning the existence of the valves below the abdominal ring.

Mr. Curling[4] describes the spermatic veins thus: "Many anatomists speak of the spermatic veins as being destitute of valves, which they assign as one of the reasons for the occurrence of varicocele. I have several times injected these veins with alcohol, and, on laying them open, have observed valves in

[1] The works of Alex. Monroe, M. D., published by his son, Alex. Monroe, M. D., Ed. 1781, pp. 542 and 582.

[2] Encyclopædie Anatomique, tome iii. p. 646.

[3] Testis, Amer. edit., p. 38.

[4] Diseases of Testis, London, 1843, p. 28.

the large vessels, and I have also found injections thrown into the veins arrested by the valves. They are seldom, however, seen very near the testis, or in the smaller veins, forming the plexus; *nor* have I observed them *within* the abdomen."

Jamain,[1] in his anatomy, describes the veins, and assigns as the cause of varicocele on the left side, the angular direction of the current of blood.

Sappey[2] speaks thus minutely of the course of the spermatic veins: "En penétrant daus l'abdomen les veines du testicule sont le plus souvent réduites a deux troncs, qui cheminent entre le peritoine et le fascia iliaca; celles du côté gauche passent sous l'Siliaque du colon, dont le poids les comprime, et explique au moins en partie le siege presque constant du varicocele à gauche."

Professor Hyrtl, of Vienna,[3] describes the spermatic veins as "valveless" (*klappenlosen*), and attributes the development of circocele to the length and great calibre of the veins, and to the fact of their being destitute of valves. In the several treatises on anatomy by Wistar, Wilson, Knox, and Sharpey and Quain, I find no mention of the valve I have described at length; nor is the existence of any such arrangement alluded to in the recent treatises on surgery by Chelius, Fergusson, Pirrie, or Erichsen.

Hasse[4] ascribes varicocele of the left side to the causes previously stated, and also "to the general practice of carrying the scrotum upon the left side, whereby the left testicle and spermatic cord are obviously more compressed than the right, and at the same time exposed to a degree of warmth favourable to the production of the evil."..

In the pathological anatomy of Drs. Jones and Sieveking, the usual circumstances are assigned as the causes of varicocele upon the left side in preference to the right. In an article on the diseases of the veins,[5] Mr. S. J. A. Salter is even more specific in the description of the anatomy of the spermatic veins; for after the usual enumeration of the proximate and dynamical causes of varicocele, he adds: "It cannot be said that there is any difference in structure or constitution between the two veins in the same individual."

From the careful examination of works of the above mentioned authors, and of others, I feel convinced that the presence of the spermatic valve of the right side has hitherto escaped the attention of observers; a circumstance somewhat singular when we consider the peculiar pathological fact presented in the varicose condition of the left side. I am also inclined to believe that a careful consideration of the import of the right spermatic valve may tend to place the pathology of varicocele before us in a new point of view. Hitherto writers upon the subject have been in the habit of considering varicocele as an affection of the left side of the body, produced by local causes peculiar to that

[1] Paris, 1853, p. 442.

[2] Traité d'Anatomie Descriptive, tome 1er, p. 566.

[3] Handbuch der Topographischen Anatomie, Wien, 1847, Bd. 2, p. 42.

[4] Hasse, *loc. cit.*, p. 45.

[5] Todd's Cyclopædia of Anatomy and Physiology, vol. iv. p. 1397.

region alone, and not existing upon the other side. That such, however, is not the case will be evident if each of the hitherto received causes of varicocele be examined in detail.

In the first place, does the perpendicular direction of the venous current upon the left side, in reality, act in producing the disease? In regard to this M. Nélaton states, that he has made many dissections for the purpose of examining the direction of the spermatic veins, and that rarely did he find "the vein emptying perpendicularly; that the spermatic veins curved, so that the blood in both veins, the spermatic and renal, had nearly a parallel direction before joining." This observation I have had frequent opportunities of verifying by dissection; and the fact is, moreover, in analogy with the termination of the other veins of the body.

2d. Are the spermatic veins liable to compression by the sigmoid flexure of the colon? Such a view is at least rendered improbable when we examine the exact position of the spermatic vessels in the abdomen. We here find them placed behind the peritoneum, and securely invested by a fibrous sheath. This involucrum has been described at length by the elder Monroe, who even assigns to it the office of protecting the subjacent vessels from the pressure of the viscera. The high authority of Nélaton can also be adduced upon this point. This latter observer denies the influence of such pressure in producing varicocele; and he states, moreover, that the dilatation of the vein continues high up the abdomen. A specimen of a dilated ovarian vein of the left side, now in my possession, substantiates the truth of this assertion; the varicosity extending up to the emulgent vein. In this preparation, the valve which I have described exists upon the right side, which is unaffected.

That the accumulation of feces in the colon does not act as a predisposing cause to varicocele, will be rendered evident when we reflect for a moment upon the epochs of life in which these different states exist. Varicocele is a disease almost peculiar to puberty, whilst constipation occurs as a rule at a later period of life. In all instances I have failed, upon inquiry, to trace any clinical connection between the affection under consideration and the accumulation of feces which has been assigned as its cause.

3d. The position of the testis—lower upon the left than upon the right side—certainly cannot play a very prominent part in the production of the disease. The greatest difference in the length is not more than half an inch. In this connection it may be observed, that whilst the ovarian veins are of precisely the same length, the left one is always the seat of the varicose dilatation.

From the consideration of the foregoing facts it seems probable that the causes of varicocele hitherto adduced are insufficient to account for the presence of the disease. May we not, with at least equal justice, believe, that the causes of the affection are more general than is commonly imagined; and that in reality the dilatation of the spermatic veins is simply a symptom of engorgement of the great internal venous trunks? It will then be easily understood what influence may be exerted by the right spermatic valve in preventing the development of the disease upon that side; and may not the same law obtain, in the explanation of varix of the left ovarian vein, since we have in the female an analogous locality to the valve?

EXPLANATION OF PLATE.

Dissection of the vena cava, emulgent, and spermatic veins, showing the right spermatic valve, and its accompanying sinus.

c. Vena cava.
e. Emulgent vein.
r. Right spermatic vein.
l. Left spermatic vein.
a. Aperture by which the right spermatic vein empties into the vena cava.
v. Right spermatic valve.
s. Sinus, across which the valve is stretched.
f. Termination of the left spermatic vein, in the emulgent vein.

ART. V.—*Case of Spinal Apoplexy.* By ISAAC G. PORTER, M. D., of New London, Conn.

So rarely do we meet with cases of this nature, or even of spinal congestion terminating fatally, that the following example, though deficient in some of its details, may be interesting.

"Spontaneous effusion of blood into the cervical, dorsal, or lumbar portions of the cord, is an occurrence of extreme rarity, and its history is, consequently, very defective. The cases recorded by Abercrombie, Chevalier, Stroud, Cruveilhier, and others, show that the attack is always characterized by acute and sudden pain in the back, corresponding with the seat of the effusion. Sometimes there are precursory symptoms of shivering, and in others there is sudden paralysis of one or more of the lower extremities, below the seat of pain. The other symptoms that have been observed are similar to those we have noticed while treating of myelitis, affecting the cervical, dorsal, or lumbar portion of the cord."—*Tweedie's Lib. of Med.*, vol. ii. p. 324.

In 386 recorded cases of apoplexy, Andral notices the effusion as occurring eight times within the spinal canal.

A talented and opulent merchant, largely engaged in commerce, was busily engaged from early dawn until afternoon of an intensely hot day in September last, in getting to sea one of his ships. He was forty years of age, and his general health good, although there is in the family a proclivity to plethoric, congestive, and paralytic diseases. He had drank freely, though prudently, of cold liquids, and, after the ship had sailed, went into a barber's

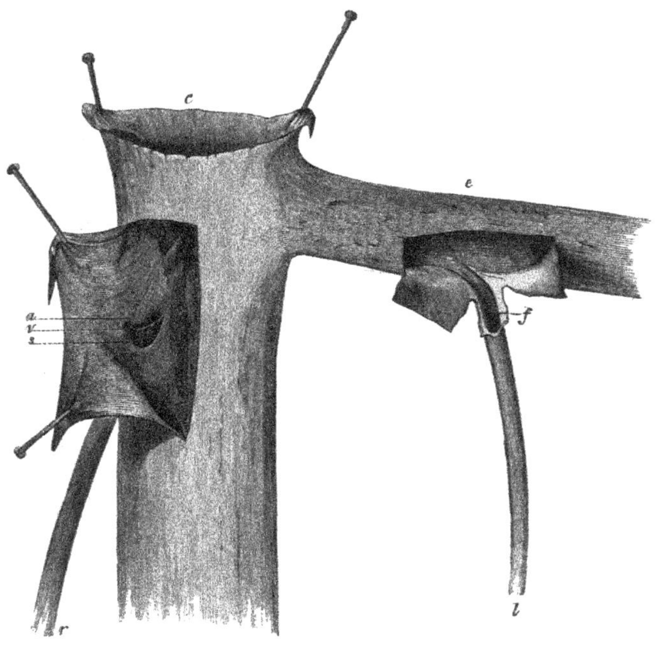

Dissection of the vena cava, emulgent and spermatic veins,

showing the right spermatic valve.

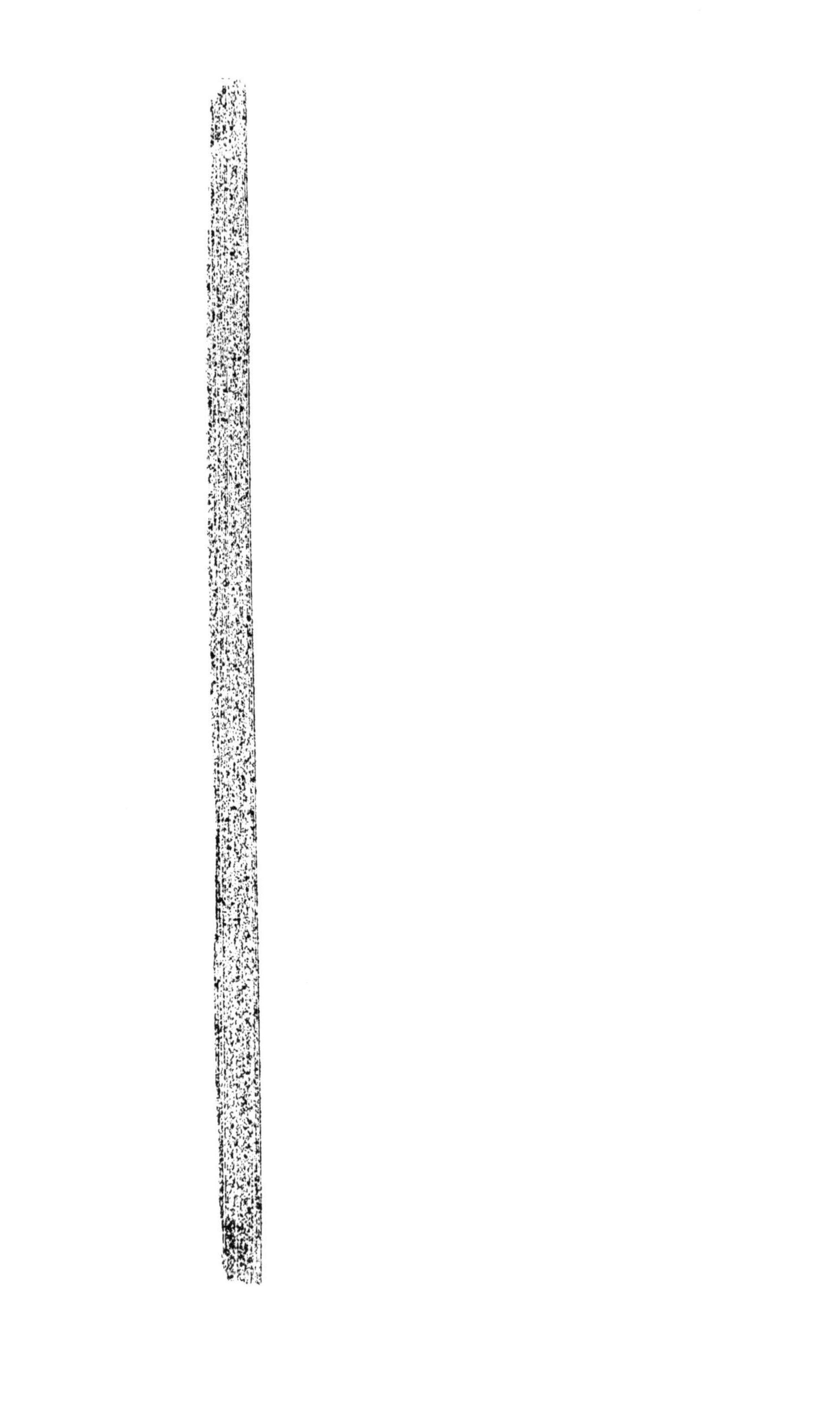

shop about 5 o'clock P. M., and had his head "shampooed," as he had occasionally done before. Heated and exhausted as he was, the irrigation of the water, as it flowed over the back of his head and neck, was, for a time, very grateful, though it had been standing, as was said, the most of the day in the room. He soon, however, became chilly, and was seized with a violent pain in the lower part of his back, and, on attempting to leave the shop, became partially paralyzed; and he was obliged, soon after, to stand motionless in the street for some minutes. The powerlessness then seemed gradually to leave him, and he was able to walk, though with difficulty, his gait being noticeably changed, as observed by his friends. About half an hour after, he was again seized with pain in the back and numbness, and loss of power in the lower limbs, attended with a very severe chill; yet the palsy was not severe enough to prevent his walking home at 6 P. M., when he went immediately to bed. By advice of friends, he took hot stimulant drinks and teas, hot pediluvia, and had bottles of hot water placed around him. He soon emerged from the chill, and moderate reaction came on, but complained greatly of pain in the back, and numbness of his extremities. A little before 10 o'clock P. M. I saw him—intellect perfect; countenance anxious, though disposed to think lightly of his disease, saying he should be at his store in the morning; shaking with the cold at the slightest motion of the bedclothes; gentle perspiration, but the hands cold and clammy when exposed to the air. The pain in the back, and numbness, still continued, and new distress, like colic, had lately manifested itself in the abdomen, with a most urgent desire for a passage from the bowels. A free motion had occurred just before the attack, and, previous to my arrival, he had endeavoured to use the close-stool, but immediately on rising, with help, into the upright position, he had fainted. Insisting on making a second attempt, he arose with help, but rather *fell* than *sat* in the chair. Immediately his head dropped on his chest, his breathing became stertorous, and the muscles began to show convulsive action. Contrary to my express command, he afterwards made another attempt, with the same result, and on coming to himself he said: "I am truly in a critical situation, and will make no further effort." There was desire to pass water, but it was by no means so urgent, and none passed him during life. From 11 o'clock P. M. of Tuesday night until 4 P. M. of the following day, when he expired, he maintained the horizontal position, except as he vomited twice in the night, and slightly turned from side to side, with restlessness and jactitation from pain in the bowels and back. His pulse, as I entered the room, was a mere thread, contrasting strongly with his flushed and congested countenance. The slightest pressure annihilated it, and after effort on his part it was entirely gone.

The aspect of the case, at the outset, was almost hopeless, and the symptoms progressed with rapid strides towards a fatal termination. About 4 o'clock in the morning his acute distress left him; the pulse slightly rose in volume and power under the use of stimulants and nourishment, and by crowding them it was for a short time maintained, but soon either the stomach rejected them, or they ceased to have anything more than a momentary influence. He soon after became somnolent, though he was aroused without difficulty until within an hour or two of his death, and always showed a good share of intelligence, and answered questions promptly and properly. While apparently asleep, he occasionally uttered incoherent expressions, but on being aroused, was perfectly conscious. Showing how naturally and spontaneously our thoughts flow in their accustomed channels, shortly before he expired he said in a firm voice, "I believe that everything is aboard," which were his last words. "Even in our ashes, live their wonted fires."

Soon after dissolution, remarkable evidence of venous engorgement presented itself. The entire surface of the body appeared as if deeply cechymosed or cyanosed. The colour was uniform and permanent.

There were unusual reasons for preserving the body as long as possible, and the weather was very hot and oppressive. Much as a *post-mortem* examination was desired, yet these reasons, and the mechanical difficulties to be overcome being so great in exposing the vertebral canal, and the want of suitable instruments, all conspired to render it impracticable.

The treatment in this case was directed, at the outset, to obviating the alarming prostration. Ignorant, at that time, of the cold douche, the chills in the barber's shop, and the subsequent loss of muscular power, the debility was referred to some unknown *functional* derangement, and alcoholic drinks, sulph. ether, and aromat. spts. ammo. were freely used with animal broths; and externally, fomentations were applied to the abdomen, and Granville's lotion, sinapisms, and a blister to the back. Leeches were proposed to the medical gentlemen in consultation, but declined on account of the adynamia. The influence of medication was momentary and trifling.

This case, so rapid in its progress towards dissolution, possesses some peculiarities which may repay examination. Deprived, as we are, of the positive testimony of a *post-mortem* examination, we are compelled to examine it *per vias exclusionis,* and much in the same way as if the patient, after having been exceedingly ill, had finally recovered. Was it, then, a case of cerebral congestion, or apoplexy? This latter supposition must be excluded by the existence and continuance of consciousness and intellect until just before death. Was it a case of acute myelitis? The symptoms, in some respect, pointed to that affection, but the attack was much more sudden and violent than is usual in that disease, and the termination more speedy—myelitis proving fatal, usually, from the fifth to the tenth day; and, at no time, were symptoms of active inflammation present. Spinal meningitis is also excluded by the absence of tonic rigidity and increased sensibility, which characterize that affection.

Was it a case of simple venous engorgement of the medulla spinalis? or was this state accompanied or succeeded by serous or sanguineous effusion within the canal? The leading symptoms, at the outset, were pain in the back, and paralysis of the lower extremities. These conditions, however, disappeared after a few minutes, so that the patient was able to walk home. Had effusion occurred at the first appearance of these symptoms, it is not possible that the pressure on the medulla spinalis could have been so speedily removed as to have allowed the use of his limbs. But the symptoms returned with renewed violence, and proceeded uninterruptedly to a fatal termination by an apparent extension of an effusion (which then first occurred) upward toward the brain. The severe colic pains in the abdomen will be remembered. These are very common in myelitis of the lumbar portions of the cord, and according to Tweedie, also occur in spinal apoplexy. In the upward progress of the paralysis, the cardiac and pulmonary nerves were finally involved. The powers of the circulation, however, were easily affected, doubtless through sympathy, and the violence of the nervous shock. It is, therefore, my opinion, that so intense became the congestion in the last attack, that it resulted in a gradual effusion into the spinal canal.[1] "When the symptoms come on slowly, and in an imperfect degree, without anything like a sudden shock, or fit, the effusion is generally of serum." (*Cyc. Med.*, art. Cerebral Apoplexy.) It may have been serous, but from the intense engorgement of the surface of the body immediately after death, and which was doubtless to be attributed, in part, to rupture of the capillaries, we have reason to believe from the condition of the bloodvessels, as thus evinced, that it was sanguineous.

It is a question of some interest, how far the cold douche, on the base of the brain, exerted a noxious influence. The power over the circulation of the blood, by the application of heat and cold, is shown by the influence of sinapised foot-bath, and the cold douche, or the ice-cap to the head in congestive headache, threatening apoplexy, or in convulsions, with strong determination of blood to the head. The objection may be offered, that granting a remedial influence in this case, it does not prove the converse, viz: that the same agent may operate at one time as a *cure*, and at another as a *cause*, of a similar affection. Another instance, then, more in point, may be adduced. The very injurious effects on the organism of currents of cold air operating on *limited* portions of the surface, will not be denied—nor the pernicious influence of wet feet on an individual not inured to it by habit, more especially if he be fatigued at the time, and constitutionally infirm. This is probably owing, primarily, to a depressing influence thus exerted on the "automatic nerve force," which, succeeded by irregular circulation in the capillaries, finally results in internal congestions.

Todd, however, in his late valuable work on diseases of the nervous system, has the following words: "It is unsatisfactory in a scientific, and dangerous in a practical point of view, to refer paralysis to local congestion. The vessels of a part, all important as they are to its nutritive and other vital actions, are nevertheless only secondary elements in the condition of the organ, and unless in themselves *diseases*, they can play only a secondary part in the production of organic or functional derangement. Congestion of bloodvessels, or hyperæmia of a part, must be an *effect* either of some disordered state of the intrinsic elements of the tissue or of the blood, or of the forces by which the blood circulates." These are doubtless correct pathological principles, and two of the conditions specified I think we have in the foregoing case—"the disordered condition of the bloodvessels, and of the forces by which the blood circulates." In ordinary health, the cold douche, even when operating on the base of the brain, may have been harmless, but not so when the vital energies were at a low ebb, through a long and exhausting day's exertion in a hot sun. It is under similar circumstances that a draught of cold water

[1] See a case recorded by Walsh, *Lancet*, July, 1849, p. 7.

sometimes proves fatal. The same thing is shown by a fact familiar to "gentlemen of the turf." A horse, although quite warm from exercise in the early part of the day, may drink cold water with comparative impunity, while one-half the amount, if drank at the close of a summer day's travel, would cause his death.

Having thus shown that the forces by which the blood circulates were disordered and enfeebled, as a part of a general affection, a few words only remain in relation to the condition of the bloodvessels. That they were in a morbid state appears from the aspect of the surface of the body immediately after death. Should this be referred to incipient decomposition, the question arises; why does not the same appearance always occur in early decomposition? The innervation and nutrition of the capillaries were doubtless affected at the same time that the congestion occurred in the medulla spinalis, of which softening of these vessels, and ultimate effusion, were the consequence.

ART. VI.—*Obstetrical Memoranda.* By RICHARD MCSHERRY, M.D., of Baltimore.

Labours Complicated by Accidental Shortening of the Cord.—Death of the Child from an unusual cause.—During the past year I attended several cases of labour, protracted for hours after the child's head had reached the perineum, when there was no manifest cause of delay either in the size of the head, or in the condition of the mother. In every case the delay was owing to accidental shortening of the cord. In two cases the children died before delivery, of strangulation, from double folds of the cord closely investing the neck. In another case the cause of death was different, and very uncommon.

On the 18th of Sept. I was called to Mrs. H., rather a delicate young woman in labour with her first child. I found her suffering pretty severely, and vomiting freely of mucus and greenish bile; she told me she had been long very costive, troubled with headache and general *malaise.* In a reasonable time the head began to distend the perineum, the soft parts were relaxed, and the pains were sufficiently active. I promised her a speedy termination of her sufferings, but finding pain after pain fruitless, little gained by each pain and that little lost directly after, I determined to use the forceps. At the expiration of two hours, however, from the time when I first expected each pain to bring the head, it came into the world unassisted, with a single turn of the cord around the shoulders. No effort was required to disengage it; the body followed immediately. Upon looking at the child I observed a large bluish mass overlying the abdomen, which upon examination proved to be the intestines deeply congested. By careful tracing I found they had escaped by a rent at the side of the umbilical cord. They were much distended with meconium, but after some patient manipulation I succeeded in restoring them within the abdominal cavity. Compresses and bands were applied immediately to the tumid abdomen; the child lived feebly for half an hour, when it expired. The contents of the stomach issued from the mouth in a thick stream.

In the other two fatal cases the expulsion of the shoulders was retarded by the turns of the cord; I found it impracticable to disengage them without violence, and resorted to the scissors, by which the labour was expedited though the children were lost.

The instructions of authors are uncertain and contradictory in such cases; the use of the forceps is commonly advised, but if I had resorted to the instrument in the case of the rupture at the umbilicus, the friends would have thought the operation the cause of death, and indeed, the same suspicion may have fixed itself upon my own mind.

Other cases terminated favourably.

Considering the difficulties of treatment, it appears to me that the practitioner does best who confines his active assistance before the birth of the head to keeping the fundus of the womb depressed, and to supporting the perineum. Caseaux says, "If the head be at the inferior strait, at the time when the alternate movements of elevation and descent begin to manifest themselves during and after the contraction, the forceps should be applied." (See his treatment of *Dystocia*, from shortness of the cord.) Bonnet says, in his *Cours d'Accouchement*, *"Il est difficile de suivie un traitement qui met fin à un tel etat."* So I have found it. He continues, "cependant, si on parvient à le reconnaître, et si l'accouchement en est empêché, il faut couper le cordon, et le lier, sil est accessible aux doigts, on tout au moins, aussitôt que l'enfant sera sorti des organes maternels." A single turn of the cord may be relaxed by the application of the accoucheur's fingers drawing upon the placental extremity, when sufficiently in reach, but a double turn is unmanageable, and slipping it over the head is often quite impracticable. The scissors then must be our principal assistance.

And what of the forceps? Bonnet says, "On devrait appliquer le forceps sil survenait quelque accident pressant." Possibly such occasion may arise, but Cascaux makes use of the following remarkable language, under another head (General considerations on employment of forceps): "Lastly, it has been shown how a brevity of the cord may become a cause of dystocia. When this happens the forceps is a hazardous resource, that ought to be avoided; but the real source of the delay is generally unknown, and even if it were not I know of nothing better to be done."

Such conflicting statements certainly justify the expectant practice, and reduce our agency to depressing the fundus of the womb when circumstances require it, and of using the scissors when the natural efforts bring the coils of the cord in reach, provided we cannot slip them over the head or shoulders without violence.

Subsidence of the Womb eight weeks before labour.—On the 7th of May I was called to Mrs. ——, who complained of severe pains in the loins after some unusually active exercise the day before. During the night the womb had subsided, as it usually does shortly before labour. She had previously engaged my services for the early part of the month of June. I advised rest, and mild counter-irritation, telling her the labour was nearer than she anticipated. Her husband, a very active man of business, was about going to the West for two or three weeks, but as he did not wish to be absent during her confinement, I counselled him to remain at home. The lady soon became tired of restraint, finding herself generally comfortable, and she was not confined until the 5th of July, when her second child was born. There was some tendency to uterine hemorrhage in excess, which was soon brought under control—otherwise things were as usual. I do not know if this early subsidence is often observed by gentlemen in large obstetrical practice, but authorities generally assign it to the last two weeks, if not to the last few days of utero-gestation. Duges, indeed, says that "the subsiding is generally observed only in the last months of pregnancy;" other authors pretty uniformly allow weeks or days only.

Hydrocephalus protracting Labour.—Mrs. M., æt. about 40, was confined with her first child on the 12th of May, 1855. The waters broke during the first hour of labour pains, after which the pains kept up well for twenty-three hours more before the child was born. I attributed the delay to the age and *embonpoint* of the mother. The child's head was not excessively large, though I observed a peculiar sponginess or elasticity of the cranial bones, before the birth. This was the only indication of a then existing disease, which some six or seven weeks subsequently displayed itself very manifestly—the head had become enormously large, with distinct sense of fluctuation under the anterior fontanelle, &c. The general health did not seem impaired. I commenced a course of treatment which did not arrest the continued progress of the disease, whereupon the parents consulted, in turn, several other physicians with no better results, for it still lives in the same condition.

Leather Pessaries.—In January, 1855, I was consulted by a poor woman, a widow, the mother of several children, for a complete prolapsus of the womb. That organ was enlarged to the dimensions of a good sized orange, and protruded considerably from the vulva. There happened to be in my office at the time some leather rings or disks, intended for a very different purpose (washers), but it occured to me they would give temporary support until some more permanent instrument should be applied. I accordingly restored the womb, and introduced one of the rings after oiling it, but as it appeared too flexible, I introduced a second. Both together made a very firm support. The woman, who earned her daily bread by hard labour, had been long suffering, but had not sought relief until that time, when she had become quite disabled. I directed her to report progress to me from time to time, and found her soon again at the wash-tub, suffering little or no inconvenience from her disease. There was no reason to change an instrument which answered so well, so she wears it still, and gets on very comfortably.

The entire diameter of the ring is two inches eight lines; of the circular space within, one inch eight lines.

The above cases, perhaps, present nothing new to many of your readers, but they appear to be sufficiently different from the routine of every-day practice to be worthy of being recorded.

BALTIMORE, *March* 15, 1856.

ART. VII.—*On Wire Splints.* By J. C. NOTT, M. D., of Mobile, Ala.

I HAVE recently been using in fractures of the extremities *wire splints,* which I do not recollect to have seen recommended elsewhere, and which possess manifest advantages over those of any other material heretofore used.

The objections to wood, pasteboard, gutta percha, and other solid materials, are that they keep the inflamed parts too warm, and *do not admit the application of cold water.*

The "*wove wire*" is the lightest material out of which a firm splint can be made, and being malleable, may be moulded with the fingers to the shape of the limb.

Being porous, no obstruction is offered to the entrance of cold lotions, and the parts may be subjected, if necessary, to a stream of water.

The material out of which these splints are made is easily procured and easily cut into proper shapes. The hardware stores all keep what is called "*wove wire*" of various qualities, coarse and fine, and with a pair of strong shears it is readily cut into any form we may desire. The edges should be turned over to prevent the wires from sticking into the flesh, and to give more strength to the splint. It is well also to give them a coat of asphaltum or other varnish, to keep them from rusting. The material does not cost more than from fifty cents to one dollar a yard.

Figures 1 and 2 will give an idea of these splints.

Fig. 1.

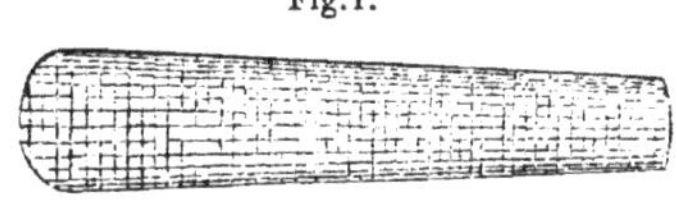

Fig. 2.

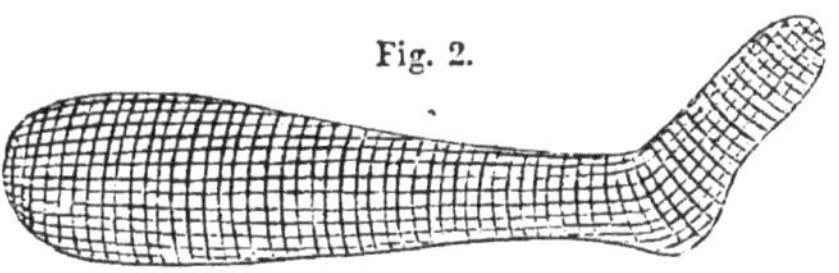

Suppose, for example, we have a common fracture of the bones of the leg. Two splints of the shape of Fig. 2 are selected, and being well padded with lint or old soft rags, they are applied on each side of the leg, and nicely moulded to its shape. A bandage is then rolled from the toes up to the knee over it, or what is more simple, pieces of bandage are tied around at short spaces from toes to knee. We at once have a solid fixture, having all the advantages and none of the inconveniences of the starch bandage, and the patient may move the limb about as he pleases, or get up on crutches.

ART. VIII.—*On Liquidambar Styraciflua.* By CHARLES W. WRIGHT, M. D., Professor of Chemistry in the Kentucky School of Medicine.

LIQUIDAMBAR Styraciflua, commonly called *sweet-gum*, is indigenous to nearly every part of the United States, and constitutes one of our largest forest trees. When an incision is made through the bark of this tree, a resinous juice exudes, which possesses an agreeable balsamic odour. When this substance first exudes, it is of the consistence of turpentine, and possesses a stronger smell in that condition than it does after it has become resinified. Contrary to the statements made by Wood and Bache, in their *Dispensatory*, this tree furnishes a considerable quantity of resin in the Middle States, particularly in the States of Ohio, Indiana, and Kentucky, bordering on the Ohio River. It is annually collected in those States, and sold under the name of *gum-wax*. It is a much more agreeable masticatory than the spruce-gum, and is chewed in the West by nearly all classes. By proper incisions, one tree will yield annually about three pounds of the resin.

The chemical composition of the specimens collected in this latitude correspond with that given by M. Bonastre, of specimens gathered elsewhere, viz: benzoic acid, a volatile oil, a semiconcrete substance separated by distillation and ether, an oleo-resin, a principle insoluble in water and cold alcohol, termed *styracine*. The bark of the tree contains tannic and gallie acids, to which its astringency is due.

What I wish more particularly to call attention to is the employment of a syrup of the bark of this tree, in diarrhœa and dysentery, and more especially the diarrhœa which is so prevalent among children during the summer months in the Middle States, and which frequently terminate in cholera infantum.

The best formula for the preparation of this syrup is that given in the *United States Pharmacopœia*, for the preparation of the syrup of wild-cherry bark, of which the following is a copy, the sweet-gum bark being substituted for the wild-cherry bark.

"Take of sweet-gum bark, in coarse powder, *five ounces;* sugar (refined) *two pounds;* water *a sufficient quantity*. Moisten the bark thoroughly with water, let it stand for twenty-four hours in a close vessel, then transfer it to a percolator, and pour water upon it gradually until a pint of filtered liquor is obtained. To this add the sugar in a bottle, and agitate occasionally until it is dissolved."

The dose of this syrup for an adult is about one fluidounce, to be given at every operation, as long as the operations continue to recur too frequently.

One advantage which this medicine possesses over most astringent preparations is that of having an exceedingly pleasant taste, and of being retained by an irritable stomach when almost every other substance is rejected. Children never object to it on the score of bad taste. The resinous and volatile bodies which it contains, no doubt enhances its value. My brother, Dr. J. F. Wright, of Columbus, Indiana, has employed this preparation for the past three years in a great number of cases, with the most satisfactory results. He prefers it to any other article where there is an indication for astringent medication in the class of diseases before referred to. In the bowel complaints of children it has a decided advantage over all preparations containing opium, and I am always pleased with the happy results which follow its employment in that class of patients.

ART. IX.—*Inversion of the Uterus, replaced on the Third Day.* By ISAAC G. PORTER, M. D., of New London, Conn.

CASES of this accident are, it is well known, extremely rare in hospital practice; less so, doubtless, for obvious reasons, than in the experience of practitioners at large; a late article in this journal showing, from the statistics of certain English lying-in establishments, that they occur scarcely less frequently than once in 85,000 labours. Always alarming, and frequently fatal, a certain amount of interest always attaches to them, but the point especially inviting attention in the following case, is the length of time that elapsed after the inversion before its replacement. It would not be difficult to surpass it, in this respect, by a reference to recorded experience of remarkable cases; but if this notice shall encourage perseverance in similar instances, its object will be attained.

A lady, thirty years of age, of delicate organization, though of uniformly good health, was confined in the country, at 4 o'clock A. M., Tuesday, March 18th, under the care of a neighbouring practitioner. The labour was not severe, lasting but little over four hours, but the delivery of the placenta was delayed one or two hours, doubtless owing to atony of the uterus. It came away somewhat disrupted, although the physician disclaimed having used any undue interference. Previous, and subsequent to its delivery, there was much flooding, attended with great faintness, prostration, nausea, &c. Some hours after, she partly arose in bed, to urinate, when the uterus made a complete descent, through the external parts, forming a tumour the size of "two fists." Increased prostration, and much alarm and distress followed the shock which the system sustained from the abnormal displacement and the downward pressure of the contents of the abdomen, as well as from an entire inability to pass water. This function was not performed, after the accident, until the re-inversion of the uterus, except as the mass was crowded upwards by manual assistance, thus relieving the pressure on the urethra; and on my arrival, I found the protruded body partially returned, within the vagina, where it was supported by a pessary, or tampon, resting externally on the bed. The physician and patient both informed me, that great relief followed this partial reposition, she being enabled thereby to pass water, yet with difficulty, while, by the same means, the traction of the uterus, on its ligaments, was considerably lessened.

The patient resided about twenty miles distant, and I did not see her until Thursday eve, at 8 o'clock, almost three days after the accident. The foregoing account I received from the physician in attendance. At this time, moderate reaction had come on—countenance anxious and deadly pale, pulse 120 and irritable. There was much distress and tenderness in the abdomen, flooding not severe, since the complete inversion, and immediate danger to life did not appear imminent. An examination confirmed the suspicion of inversion. The vagina was filled with a firm, yet compressible, globular, and sensitive mass, answering the usual description of books—no os tineæ was discovered, but there was a marked fold of the vagina encircling the tumour, which is mentioned in this place as being confirmatory of the opinion that this constitutes a valuable diagnostic between inversion of the uterus and polypus. Gentle, but gradually increasing force with the back of the flexed fingers caused the mass to diminish in size, and slowly to ascend in the direction of the superior strait. As it grew less in dimensions it was more easily grasped, and ultimately, the uterus, with the hand encircling and compressing it, was used as a *stem*, with which upward pressure was exerted. Under this compound action of compression and elevation, the restoration became much more rapid. Owing to extensibility of the soft parts, considerable counter-pressure on the abdomen became necessary. The sensation communicated to the hand was very different, when the parts were returned as far as the os tincæ and the uterus, in which latter, the regular process of involution had evidently commenced. There was less resiliency in the uterus at the last stage of the operation than is common, immediately after delivery—but rather a spontaneous yielding to slight force, with one or two fingers; these were retained in the cavity for some minutes after the completion of the operation, which occupied about twenty-five minutes. Immediate relief followed, the uterus resumed its place in the hypogastrium, and the abdomen became much less tender on pressure. Under the influence of a stimulant, and an opiate, the patient enjoyed her first sleep since her confinement. The horizontal position for a week was strictly observed, and there being incontinence of urine for a few days, the catheter was uncalled for. Some febrile excitement existed in the form of thirst, frequent pulse, and much pain in the back. The lochia were sparing, and the secretion of milk never occurred. The countenance was blanched and leucophlegmatic, and there was anæmic headache.

On the 13th day, while attempting to sit in a chair for the first time, a severe pain in her right hip and leg seized her, which was the commencement of a mild attack of phlegmasia dolens. For two days the pain was extreme, as was the tenderness in the tract of the femoral vessels. The case, however, speedily yielded, verifying the principle, that the later the attack after parturition, the more amenable to remedies. Laxatives, alternated with opium, and fomentation, repeated every four hours, and followed with gentle friction, with warm tinct. of aconite, and tinct. of opium, āā 1 part, and ol. oliv. 2 parts, were speedily successful in relieving the pain. Contrary to my expectation, a flannel bandage, reaching from the toes to the hips, was, even at an early stage, conducive to comfort, and she continued to wear it, for support, until she passed from my observation.

REVIEWS.

ART. X.—*Physical Exploration and Diagnosis of Diseases affecting the Respiratory Organs.* By AUSTIN FLINT, M. D., Professor of the Theory and Practice of Medicine in the University of Louisville, &c.

THE time was when a medical man could, within the covers of a single volume, find almost all that was to be found of medical science; and he was, indeed, a happy man and a painstaking student who was able and willing to consult more than the one author, whose theories he had learned and whose disciple he had become. Within the memory, indeed, of not a few of our profession, a single treatise upon the theory and practice of physic was all that most practitioners ever cared to read. Experience was the one dependence of our profession, and years were supposed to bring wisdom. The man of largest experience was he who had seen the most cases, and he oftentimes resigned practice, only confirmed in the notions which he had erroneously acquired while *riding* with his instructor.

To-day we have the profession cut up into specialties. For every region we have treatises, and for every disease a monograph. There are many who doubt the expediency of so dividing our labours and our studies; who think a man a better physician for being a good surgeon, and a far better surgeon for being a good physician. This is, to a very great extent, true. But the truth does not so appear from anything inherent in the practice of physic or surgery, but because men who practice one branch are so apt to consider every other as secondary to their own. To act promptly and efficiently, a physician should neglect the reading of no part of medical science. He is not fit for a physician unless he understands physiology, nor for a surgeon unless he has a practical acquaintance with mechanical laws.

The same train of thought is applicable to the diagnosis of diseases of the chest. Men are still in successful practice who ridicule the idea of physical exploration; and it is to be feared, that many of our younger brethren pay such perfect deference to physical signs, that they allow rational signs of the utmost importance to escape them entirely.

Such men are not followers of the school to which the author of the treatise on Physical exploration and diagnosis of diseases affecting the respiratory organs, belongs. He has given us over six hundred pages upon this single subject. And they are six hundred pages of very readable and most instructive matter, in a clear and comprehensive style. We wished, on seeing the book, that it had been more condensed; but, after reading it through, we are unable to point out anything which should have been omitted. The book is founded upon facts, which have come under the author's own patient observation, and which have been judged by careful comparison with each other, and with the experience of other labourers in the same field with himself.

But, it may be asked, why write this book at all? Is not the literature of the chest already ample? Is not the field already crowded? The answer is very easily given; not so long as any careful and intelligent observer has any observations and opinions to communicate. And no one, in our opinion, can read Dr. Flint's treatise, without feeling satisfied that he has contributed to our medical literature a work of original observation of the highest merit.

We always read a preface, because we can learn from it whether a book is worth our study. We do not think it any vanity in a writer who finds that he disagrees with others, and tells us that he does not hesitate to follow a rule "which, in matters purely of observation, should not lead to the imputation either of egotism or presumption, viz., not to be more ready to distrust one's own accuracy than that of others." Dr. Flint tells us, in his preface, that "questions have so frequently arisen which are to be settled only by an appeal to the results of observation, that I have sometimes been tempted to lay aside the pen, and have resumed it only under the conviction that such questions must for a long period continue to arise; and that to wait for the means of meeting promptly every inquiry, is equivalent to an indefinite postponement."

The writer of this review is thankful that the author continued his work. With all the merit which belongs to the treatise of Professor Walshe, that book is very hard reading. The work of Skoda, which has come to us at a later day, we read without carrying off anything which gave us pleasure. The latter reminded us too forcibly of the painful studies of our collegiate course, which we were too glad to finish.

The work of Dr. Flint is eminently a readable one.

The introduction is devoted to the consideration of preliminary points pertaining to the anatomy and physiology of the respiratory apparatus. The modifications caused by sex and age, the differences of motion and of sound in different portions of the same side, and the *comparatively* similar, but not like parts of the two sides are fully examined. To the neglect of precaution in testing these differences, the examiner of moderate practice has occasionally condemned a patient to a fatal disease, whose recovery in other hands has caused him to lose confidence in the usefulness of physical exploration; or, more happily, has taught him to review his studies and correct his errors. To the one, experience is of no value; to the other, its value is inestimable. Some such experience probably induced Dr. Flint occasionally to amplify, "somewhat after the usual mode of oral teaching," and occasionally to repeat where otherwise he would have consulted brevity.

The words *bronchi*, *bronchia*, *bronchiæ*, are frequently used throughout the book. It seems to us that physicians are not sufficiently careful to adhere to the true words. The Latin *bronchus* and Greek *βρογχος* have neither neuter nor feminine plurals. To be sure, gentlemen make the distinction of *bronchus* and *bronchia* between the primary and secondary divisions of the trachea, and we believe some medical dictionaries have done the same, but the distinction is arbitrary. If it were the universal custom to make such distinction, it might perhaps be allowable, but the same writer will frequently use the different words to express the same idea, and thus cause confusion. Primary, secondary, ultimate bronchi, would be a better and more accurate nomenclature. We may be accused of being hypercritical in relation to this matter, and certainly if we can find no greater fault with the book than this, it can hardly be deemed a very venal one.

Except in the original paper of Dr. Dalton, we have not before seen any notice of the experiments upon the respiratory movements of the glottis. These experiments, showing that "during normal respiration there is a constant and regular movement of the vocal chords, by which the size of the glottis is alternately enlarged and diminished, synchronous with the inspiratory and expiratory movements of the chest," will be of much service to us in the treatment of those spasmodic symptoms which we see so frequently in true and false croup. We may learn the propriety of putting young patients under the influence of narcotics or anæsthetics, sufficiently to enable us to destroy the irregular innervation by local or constitutional remedies.

The first part of Dr. Flint's book, to the three hundred and forty-sixth page, is taken up with the Physical Exploration of the Chest. This is the scientific part. It teaches how to examine the causes of the sounds we hear, the reasons why they differ, the methods of comparing them with each other, and indirectly the dangers of trusting too confidently to what has been written, without careful comparison of the examinations of others with our own observations.

Percussion and auscultation are the means mostly made use of, to discover what are called the physical signs. There are other means of less value in most cases of respiratory disease, but occasionally the practice of inspection, palpation, mensuration, and even succussion, will give us aid in the greatest degree. It is not necessary that we should all understand the science of acoustics; and should we at the outset consider such knowledge essential, we should find but few of our profession capable of conducting the simplest examination. There are certain principles of acoustics, however, which every man of moderate abilities may learn, which no physician of our day should be ignorant of, though he may not even know the meaning of the word. To the same extent a mechanic may be able to build his wall, who knows nothing of the gravity which keeps his plumb-line perpendicular.

"It is a common impression with those ignorant of the subject, that the signs generally represent uniform and definite morbid conditions; in other words, that each sign possesses its own special significance; and therefore, for the practice of physical exploration, that it is simply necessary to be able to recognize and appreciate certain abnormal sounds. According to this view, physical exploration is merely a mechanical art. This is implied when *symptoms*, as distinguished from *signs*, are called *rational*. The inference is, that to determine the value of signs, processes of reasoning are not required: that they express in themselves their full import, and that the ability to discriminate different diseases thereby depends mainly on manual tact and the cultivation of the senses. The student should, as soon as possible, dispossess the mind of this error. Few signs, individually, are pathognomonic. Their diagnostic signification depends on their combination with other signs, and on their connection with symptoms. Hence, something more than delicacy of hearing and skilful manipulation is requisite. Thought and the exercise of judgment are needed, not less than in determining the nature and seat of diseases by their *vital* phenomena. In short, physical exploration develops a series of facts which are to be made the subjects of ratiocination in their applications to diagnosis, as much as facts obtained by other methods.

"To be convinced of the great benefit which practical medicine has derived from the introduction of physical methods of exploration, it is only necessary to contrast the facility of discriminating the most common pulmonary affections at the present time, with the difficulty which confessedly existed prior to the employment of these methods. If the reader will turn to the works of Cullen, or the more recent writings of Good, he will find that these authors acknowledge the inability of the practitioner often to distinguish, by means of symptoms, pneumonitis, pleuritis, and bronchitis from each other, so that for practical purposes it was deemed sufficient to consider these three affections as one disease. At the present time, with the aid of signs, it is very rarely the case that the discrimination cannot be made easily. And that this improvement is mainly due to physical exploration, is shown by the fact, that to distinguish these affections by means of symptoms alone, is still nearly as difficult as heretofore. But to realize the importance of the subject it is not necessary to institute a comparison of the present with the past. It is sufficient to refer to the mistakes in diagnosis daily made by practitioners who rely exclusively on symptoms, which might be easily avoided by resorting to physical signs. It may not be amiss to cite some illustrations from instances that have fallen under my own observation. Examples of confounding the three affections just named are sufficiently common. Of these affections, pneumonitis and pleuritis are not unfrequently latent, so far as distinctive vital phenomena are concerned, and consequently are overlooked. Chronic pleurisy is habitually mistaken for other affections by those who do not employ physical exploration. Of a considerable number of cases, the histories of which I have collected, in a large proportion the nature and seat of the disease had not been ascertained.[1] Yet nothing is more simple than to determine the existence of this affection by an exploration of the chest. Acute pleuritis and pneumonitis are sometimes completely masked by the symptoms of other associated affections, and thus escape detection. This is observed in fevers, and when head symptoms become developed, especially in children. Under these circumstances, the practitioner who avails himself of physical signs is alone able to arrive at a positive conclusion as to their existence. Emphysema is an affection which cannot be recognized by symptoms alone, and hence, they who neglect signs have no practical knowledge of it. Acute tuberculosis I have known repeatedly to be called typhoid fever; on the other hand, I could adduce numerous examples of different affections erroneously considered to be phthisis, and a still greater number of instances in which patients with this affection were incorrectly supposed to be affected with some other disease than tuberculosis. Were we to dwell upon these, and other mistakes which might be added, it would be easy to show that they are unfortunate, not merely in a scientific point of view, but with reference to practical consequences involving the welfare, and it may be the lives of patients." Pp. 66–68.

Physical signs and symptoms have each their value. Taken together, they tell us all that can be of avail in treatment. Separate them, and we are in constant danger of making mistakes. Who does not recall cases of hæmoptysis, which would once have divided a man from his family, perplexed him in his business, condemned him to expensive travel, and a regimen which, if it did not kill him, would have rendered his very existence a burthen? The use of physical signs enables us to tell him that he has no disease incompatible with a long and useful life, and teaches us to look elsewhere for a cause that may be removed. But these signs alone are of little value. They must be detected repeatedly in the same case, but they must be compared with the rational.

"By thus directing attention," says Dr. Flint, "to some of the points of contrast between symptoms and signs, it is not to be concluded that these two classes of phenomena hold conflicting relations in the practice of medicine. Neither is to be employed in diagnosis to the exclusion of the other. They are not to be disconnected save for abstract consideration. They are always to be brought to bear conjointly in clinical investigations; combined, they lead to conclusions which neither may be competent to establish alone. They mutually serve to correct or confirm deductions drawn from either separately. It is never to be lost sight of in the study or practice of physical exploration, that to devote too exclusive attention to signs, is as much a fault as to ignore their value, and rely entirely on symptoms." P. 69.

We have often wondered that so little attention has been paid to this comparison even by physicians in city practice. It is their fault, not their misfortune, which prevents their acquiring a reasonable knowledge of physical exploration. Some men learn very easily to detect differences in sounds, and some require untiring labour; but with a single patient a practitioner can learn, if he is willing to use the means nature has given him. One of the

[1] Vide Clinical Report on Chronic Pleurisy, by the author.

greatest merits of Dr. Flint's treatise is, that it teaches us as much about healthy as diseased signs. Writers have generally been satisfied to say, that in one part of the chest we shall find vesicular respiration and resonance, in another blowing respiration and resonance; again dulness, and here tympany. But a large part of this book tells us, what students do not always know how to find and where to find certain sounds in health as well as in disease. One who never examines a chest, unless he suspects disease there, throws away the most essential means of discovering disease. In the hospital, almost every student listens for bronchial respiration and friction sound in pneumonic and pleuritic patients; but a few take every opportunity to listen at those chests, where they know that there is no other sound than that of healthy respiration. It is needless to say which become the most correct auscultators. He who studiously reads Dr. Flint's book, and examines the healthy chest will, at all events, learn that most important part of our professional knowledge, when *not* to treat a patient.

Before entering upon the study of abnormal sounds, it is desirable that one should be familiar with percussion in health. After guarding against the effect of irregular posture, and making allowance for the sounds produced by bodies against which the subject leans or reclines, the examiner is to bear in mind the fact, that the sounds elicited in the particular case are to be compared immediately with each other, secondarily with the sounds obtained in other cases. His own position must be such that, in passing from one point to another, upon the two sides, his relative position to the patient should be the same. This is of more importance than we are at first inclined to think. But no one can fail to be convinced of this who will invite a friend to percuss for him, while he is content to be an auditor only. Indeed, we are a little surprised that this course is not more frequently pursued; and we should have considered it another excellence in Dr. Flint had he laid stress upon it. We never should have been able, in any great degree, to appreciate Skoda's remarks upon the tympanitic sound of dull chests, if we had not listened to the exercise of a friend upon one of our own patients.

There were twenty subjects selected, apparently free from disease, whose chests were symmetrical in conformation. In only eight was the percussion sound, over the infra-clavicular regions, equal on the two sides in all respects. In ten there was greater resonance on one side. In all these the resonance was greatest on the left. In one of these it was greatest over a certain portion of the right side. In eleven, the pitch of resonance was higher on the right side. In four instances, the vesicular quality of the resonance was greater on the left side; never on the right. After showing other disparities in these apparently healthy cases, Dr. Flint says :—

"Theoretically, in view of the greater capacity of the right chest, it would seem perhaps more reasonable that the difference between the two sides should be the reverse of that which is found to exist. The larger development of the right pectoral muscle, in consequence of the greater use of the right upper extremity, may account for the fact in some instances, but the disparity exists in cases in which there is no apparent difference in the muscular covering, in this situation. Possibly the different physical conditions at the base of the thorax may afford an explanation. On the right side the lungs repose, with the diaphragm intervening, on the liver, which occupies the whole of the base on that side. The presence of this solid viscus may slightly deaden the sound. On the left side below the lung is situated the stomach, frequently more or less distended with gas, and the effects of this, it may be supposed, is to increase the sonorousness on that side, even at the summit, independent of the transmission of the tympanitic gastric sound which is sometimes observed." P. 82.

The explanations are deserving of consideration. The author might have asserted his supposition without much danger of its being controverted.

Over the scapular regions, in the same twenty patients, there was less disparity. In thirteen no difference was detected. In the remaining seven there was difference in pitch, intensity, &c. The scapular regions are less attractive to percussors, on account of the difficulty which many have of producing sounds, where the muscles are so thick. The ground has been taken that this region is of little value in physical exploration by percussion; but Dr. Flint truly says that, "like the infra-clavicular, it is an important region with reference to the physical signs of phthisis." With an assistant to percuss, it is remarkable how much light may be obtained even over this region of bone and flesh. Late in disease, there may be no necessity for noticing the sounds here; but it may be that the first confirmatory sign of chronic disease will be found here. The same remarks will apply to the mammary region in the female.

When the student has gained expertness in the study of healthy chests, he is fitted for the study of percussion in disease; and by this time he has acquired so large a part of the desired knowledge, that percussion in disease will have but few difficulties to contend with.

Percussion in disease gives us not merely a new set of sounds, but we recognize those previously heard, but often in new situations. The abnormal sounds are divided into I. *Exaggerated vesicular resonance;* II. *Diminished vesicular resonance;* III. *Absence of Resonance;* IV. *Tympanitic resonance.* Under these four heads, with as much clearness as can be expected, are included all the sounds we have been accustomed to call by the terms clear, dull, flat, amphoric, tubular, &c.

The importance of understanding the indications of percussion sounds, is illustrated, on page 105, by the supposed instances of pneumonitis and tubercle.

Tympanitic resonance under peculiar circumstances is the percussion sound, to which our attention has been more than usually attracted of late. It must be remembered that there is a tympanitic dulness as well as a tympanitic clearness; just as there is a tympanitic sound from tapping on a tenor drum, or by pounding on an eighteen inch wall. The examination of a pleuritic or pneumonitic patient often ends with detecting a level for the fluid, or the limit of probable hepatization. Many are still not aware, that the master's hand can bring sounds from many a dull spot, and these will find in Dr. Flint's book a description of tympanitic dulness.

Tympanitic resonance may mislead the careless. Without particular attention to the facts, it is said that mistakes may be and have been made; that the diseased side has been taken for the healthy one and *vice versâ,* because a morbid resonance was used as a standard of health.

"The rationale of the foregoing interesting and important facts is a matter at present *sub judice,* and inasmuch as I have no fruits of personal experiments or researches to offer, I shall not engage in a lengthened discussion of the subject. To account for an exaggerated tympanitic resonance under circumstances in which it is clinically exceptional, and apparently opposed to the laws of physics, viz., when the lung is compressed by the presence of liquid, or rendered more dense than natural by solidification, the doctrine has been advanced by Skoda that "if the lung contains less than its normal quantity of air, it yields a sound which approaches to the tympanitic, or is distinctly tympanitic."[1] He bases this doctrine on experiments made upon the pulmonary

[1] Markham's translation, Am. edition, page 47.

organs in the dead subject, and also removed from the body, taken in connection with the facts pertaining to disease which have been presented. Clinically this doctrine cannot be considered to hold good in the light of a general law, for abnormal sonorousness in cases in which the lungs are to a greater or less extent deprived of their normal quantity of air, in other words rendered more dense by disease, is by no means an invariable sign, but, on the contrary, occurs only as an exception to the general rule. The sign, therefore, cannot be due simply to the mere deprivation of air, or any constant condition, but to some contingent circumstances. The question, then, is, what are these contingent circumstances? In cases of effusion within the pleura, the natural effect is to condense the lung by compression of the liquid; but it is not certain that in all instances the proportion of air to the solid tissues above the level of the fluid is diminished. By the force of the inspiratory movements causing greater dilatation of the cells, the ratio of air may perhaps even exceed the limits of health. It is not improbable that the origin of the emphysema and dilatation of the bronchiæ which sometimes succeed pleurisy may have a date anterior to the absorption of the effused liquid. These are points which claim investigation." P. 117.

We believe it to be much more easy to acquire facility in reading auscultatory than percussion sounds. The one requires a correct ear only; the other, to be of value in doubtful cases, requires a musical ear and a nicety of touch which a large number of our profession never obtain. This seems to be the opinion of Dr. Flint. The several methods of auscultating respiratory sounds are fully described by him. Like the generality of examiners he concludes, that neither mediate nor immediate auscultation should be cultivated or practised to the exclusion of the other. Our own opinion is, that the immediate application of the ear to the chest is to be preferred by practitioners generally. Those who make the treatment of respiratory diseases a specialty, acquire by practice an ability to vary their course, and their instruments, which others never can. The ability to hold a stethoscope, so as not to make a noise with one or the other end of it, is an elegant accomplishment. Cammann's flexible stethoscope with double tubes, is recommended by Dr. Flint, in cases where a delicate examination is necessary. But we are inclined to the opinion, that, unless constantly used, it will fail to be of any service except to specialists, and to those whose sense of hearing is impaired. The author states, that in using the instrument "it is to be borne in mind, that it conducts sounds produced exterior to the chest, in no less a degree than those emanating from within." It is by no means certain, that even muscular sounds, within the body of the examiner or of the patient, might be metamorphosed into respiratory sounds.

The rules for auscultating are well laid down, and it is advised to accustom one's self to the use of either ear, if the hearing be equally acute in both, that change of position on the part of the explorer may not be necessary.

As percussion sounds in health are described at length, so are the auscultatory sounds. The sections devoted to auscultation in health, we consider the most valuable portion of the book. So important is this part of our study, that we should take frequent occasions for examining those whom we believe to be in normal condition. "Incongruous as it may at first appear, it will be found to be true, that certain of the most valuable of the physical signs involved in diagnosis, may be studied in persons entirely free from disease."

The examinations of forty-four healthy persons furnished the material for analysis. Like percussion sounds, auscultatory sounds are only valuable when properly compared. Any one by itself means nothing, or it may mean anything. Subjects must be compared with each other, and the two sides in each subject. Due allowance must be made for the size, age, sex, fulness of flesh, temperament, &c., and in disease, even the time of day must be noted; else we may find dulness and absence of respiration or coarse rales, where, at another hour, another physician would positively and truly assert, that there was abnormally increased resonance and tubular respiration.

The two sides are different in formation. One lung has three lobes, the other two. One has the liver below it, the other the stomach. The heart occupies more of the left chest than of the right. These differences were not in the course of our early studies so forcibly placed before us as of late, and still less were the variations in sounds. We have not space enough to review, even slightly, all that is said of the different sounds heard in the healthy chest. The following extracts from the sections upon VESICULAR RESPIRATION, will sufficiently illustrate Dr. Flint's method of making his analysis, as well as the style of the book.

"1. *Inspiratory Sound.*—In sixteen of twenty-four cases, more or less difference as respects *intensity* between the two sides was appreciable. In all but one of these sixteen instances the inspiratory sound was more intense on the left side. This result is in direct opposition to the statements of some authors;[1] but the matter is purely one of observation, and as the comparisons were made with care, and with no expectation of arriving at such a result, I am bound to assume its correctness. I can only account for the opinion of observers that the inspiratory sound on the right side is frequently more intense than that of the left, by supposing that elevation of pitch has been mistaken for increased intensity. The disparity in intensity was in some instances very marked. An inspiratory murmur was occasionally tolerably developed on the left side, and scarcely audible on the right. A striking difference was also in some cases observed in the effect of forced respiration on the intensity of the inspiratory sound, the intensity on the left side being proportionately increased, without any augmentation on the right side.

"In the relative amount of vesicular quality a difference was appreciable in a large proportion of the cases. And in all the instances in which a disparity in this particular existed, the greater amount of vesicular quality was on the left side. This was true in fourteen of twenty-four examinations of different individuals. The disparity in some instances was slight, but in several strongly marked; in not one instance was the vesicular quality greater on the right side.

"Compared as respects the pitch of the inspiratory sounds, a difference was apparent in a large majority of the observations. Excluding a few cases in which attention was not directed to this point, of nineteen examinations, the pitch was higher on the right side in twelve, and no disparity was appreciable in seven; in not a single instance was the pitch higher on the left side. The difference here as with respect to the preceding characters, was in some instances striking, and in other instances slight. This numerical result does not vary much from that obtained by an analysis of the series of previous examinations. The latter numbered fifteen, and of these fifteen examinations the inspiratory murmur was higher in pitch on the right side in eleven, and no disparity was observed in the remaining four.

"So far as the data just presented, then, furnish ground for deductions, a disparity between the inspiratory sounds at the summit of the chest in front, exists in a large proportion of individuals free from all symptoms of thoracic disease, this disparity pertaining to the intensity, vesicular quality, and pitch. Variations in these three characters obey certain rules, viz., the greater relative intensity is almost uniformly on the left side. The same rule holds good with respect to a greater relative amount of the vesicular quality. On the other hand the greater elevation of pitch is always on the right side.[2]

[1] Gerhard, Barth, and Roger.

[2] The relative duration of the inspiratory sound on the two sides is another point of comparison, to which attention was not directed in making the examinations.

"2. *Expiratory Sound.*—Facts relative to the *intensity* of the expiratory sound on the two sides are contained in the notes of nine examinations. Of these nine comparisons, in three instances an expiratory sound was appreciable on the right side, and none on the left side; in two the development on the right side was greater than on the left, and in three the intensity seemed equal on the two sides.

"In several instances the expiratory sound on the right side was prolonged, sometimes being nearly or even quite as long as the inspiratory; on the contrary, the expiratory sound, when present on the left side, was always short, never exceeding one-third of the duration of the inspiratory. It is noted in several instances that the expiratory sounds on the right side seemed distant from the ear.

"In several instances, on the right side, a brief interval separated the sounds of inspiration and expiration. In every instance, on the other hand, on the left side, the two sounds were continuous.

"The pitch of the expiratory sound was higher than that of the inspiratory on the right side in eleven instances, and on the left side in a single instance. It was lower on the left side in six, and on both sides in four instances.

"According to the foregoing results, an expiratory sound exists on the right side in a certain proportion of cases in which none is appreciable on the left side. It is frequently prolonged on the right side, appears distant, and is separated from the inspiratory sound by an interval, and is higher in pitch.

"The facts presented in the foregoing comparative account of the summit of the chest in front, may be seen at a glance by reference to the subjoined table.

"*Comparison of Right and Left Infra-clavicular Regions. Whole number of examinations twenty-four.*

INSPIRATORY SOUND.

Right.	*Left.*
Greater intensity in 1 case.	Greater intensity in 15 cases.
Vesicular quality more marked in no case.	Vesicular quality more marked in 14 cases.
Higher pitch of sound in 12 of 19 examinations.	Higher pitch of sound in no case.

EXPIRATORY SOUND.

Right.	*Left.*
Present on this side, and not on left side, in 3 cases.	Present on this side, and not on right side, in no case.
More intense on this side in 2 cases.	More intense on this side in no case.
Prolonged in several cases.	Prolonged in none.
An interval between the sounds of inspiration and expiration in several cases.	The two sounds continuous.
Pitch higher than that of the inspiratory sound in 11 instances.	Pitch higher in 1 instance.
Pitch lower than that of inspiration in 4 instances.	Pitch lower in 10 instances.

"Reviewing the facts pertaining to both the inspiratory and the expiratory sound, it is perceived that the several elements which have been seen to compose the bronchial respiration are manifested at the summit of the chest, in front, on the right side. This is a practical conclusion arrived at by means of the foregoing analysis. Assuming this conclusion to be correct, its importance will be apparent hereafter, in connection with the diagnosis of tuberculosis of the lungs in the early stage. In that connection, without knowledge of the facts which have been presented, it can hardly be otherwise than that error of diagnosis will be committed, by mistaking for the physical signs of disease, the several characters of the bronchial respiration which may exist at the summit of the right chest, not proceeding from a morbid condition. I am free to state that my own experience would supply illustrations of error from this source." Pp. 153–155.

In like manner are the sounds of the healthy chest followed through the different regions.

Auscultation in disease is for the purpose of determining morbid sounds and their differences from healthy sounds; to ascertain the connection between these and their causes, and to explain the morbid physical conditions. Explanation of the mechanism of these sounds is not necessary. However much we may differ as to the manner of production of a particular morbid sound; in our treatment of the case, as based upon its particular cause, we should not differ. The explanation Dr. Flint has, therefore, wisely omitted from his book, as tending only to provoke useless discussion, which would lead to differing conclusions.

Auscultation in disease furnishes modified and adventitious respiratory sounds; exaggerated, diminished, and suppressed vocal resonance; modified cough; abnormal transmission of the heart sounds. When we say that one hundred and twenty pages are usefully occupied with these subjects, every one will understand, that the limits of this paper will not permit even a brief recapitulation which would do justice to the author.

We shall, therefore, give a sketch of Dr. Flint's remarks upon a few of the more common and best known of the diseases of the respiratory organs. From these the readers of the Journal will be enabled at once to decide whether the work of the author has been properly done.

As far as the three hundred and fiftieth page there is very little mention of, no dissertation upon, any distinct affection of the chest. Thus far, it is a work complete in itself. If the latter part of the book had not been published, the profession would still have a work of great value, and one which must hereafter be looked upon as a standard in auscultation. Had the first part been published a year in advance of the second, we think it would have met with a ready sale, would have found more readers, and created a demand for the second.

This is aside from our work, however. We are informed, in the preliminary remarks, that we are not to make our diagnosis at the bedside by signs alone. There are physiological laws and symptoms which must guide us in our studies. Symptoms and signs must be balanced and compared. In pointing out the diagnosis of particular diseases, Dr. Flint bears this rule constantly in mind.

No disease comes under our observation in which an early diagnosis is more necessary than pulmonary tuberculosis. From a careful examination of one hundred cases of this disease, Dr. Flint has drawn his conclusions. The examinations of healthy chests are carefully considered in this connection. It is to be remembered, that there is a difference in the percussion and auscultatory sounds in the two sides of healthy well-formed chests. Distinct dulness in the left infra-clavicular region is of great significance; on the right side, that same dulness is to be considered, but, as a morbid sign, taken with great reserve. There is a difficulty in percussing the post-clavicular regions, which most auscultators never entirely overcome. A disparity in this region is, therefore, to be distrusted when it is slight. Dr. Flint has noticed it, however, when it was not appreciable in the clavicular and infra-clavicular regions. Percussion over the scapula has been considered of secondary importance. He attributes great value to it, because, from percussion in health, it is found that a natural disparity in the two sides behind is much less frequent than in front. It is necessary to percuss at different hours in the day; because, when a cavity has formed, percussion early in the day will detect dulness, where, after an abundant expectoration, there will be a change to clearness of resonance. The auscultator is warned against deep percussion in cases of hæmoptysis, because profuse hemorrhage has followed it so closely as plainly to show that accident to be a direct consequence of the violence used.

There is no auscultatory sound which we may not find in phthisis. An attention to auscultation in health is, therefore, demanded. The presence or absence of prolonged expiration, we know, is often considered a sufficient evidence of the presence or absence of tubercle. We are taught that either inspiration or expiration may be absent to the ear. Occasionally, except with Cammann's stethoscope, the inspiration is inaudible; sometimes that alone is to be heard. There are other abnormal modifications which must then enter into the calculation. As the expiratory sound is *sometimes* wanting, so in others it is the only sound to be heard. Considering the signs discovered in health, it must be borne in mind that the character of the broncho-vesicular sound should be strongly marked at the summit of the right side, for it to be considered, in itself, an evidence of disease. On the other hand, if situated at the summit of the left side, it is much more significant of disease.

"Moist crackling or mucous rales may, however, be produced by the escape of softened tuberculous matter into the tubes without necessarily involving the coexistence of circumscribed bronchitis. The development of moist or bubbling sounds is generally regarded as a circumstance distinctive of the fact that softening has taken place. Undue significance, as it seems to me, has been attached to this circumstance. It is impossible to determine from the characters of the sounds whether they proceed from the presence of softened tuberculous matter, or from mucous secretions, or (as must be the case frequently) from both combined. And inasmuch as circumscribed bronchitis may undoubtedly exist before softening of the tuberculous matter ensues, mucous rales are heard before the disease has advanced to this stage. Not indicating necessarily softening, moist rales limited to the summit of the chest are highly diagnostic of tuberculosis, and in cases of doubt it is useful to auscultate repeatedly, and especially in the morning before expectoration has taken place, in order to discover them, if they exist." P. 474.

The diagnosis must, to a considerable extent, be made out from the previous history. It is based on positive evidence. But its differential diagnosis requires more than we are enabled to discover by auscultation alone.

"A cough, not originating from a distinct attack of acute bronchitis, and not preceded by coryza, but frequently commencing so impereeptibly that the date of its first appearance cannot be definitely ascertained; in degree slight, moderate, or violent, but persisting for some time with little or no expectoration. Dryness of the cough, continuing for a greater or less period, according to my experience, obtains in a larger ratio of cases than is estimated by Walshe, viz., one-tenth. I should say that careful inquiry of patients will show it to be the rule. An expectoration at first small, transparent, and frothy; becoming gradually more abundant, solid, opaque, yellow, and non-aerated, subsequently consisting of sputa streaked with yellow lines, particoloured, and frequently presenting irregular ragged edges; occasionally including small particles resembling boiled rice, and a grumous-looking substance contained in a thinner fluid, like the deposit in barley water. According to Walshe, from whom is borrowed the description of the appearance last named, such a deposit occurs only in cases of phthisis. At a more advanced period purulent matter, in greater or less abundance, running together and forming an ash-coloured mass, with a nauseous and occasionally fetid odor. Small fibres, supposed to be exfoliated elastic tissue, discovered by microscopical examination: also detached fragments of other of the anatomical elements of the pulmonary structure, and possibly, in some instances, the tubercular corpuscle. Acute stitch-pains at the summit of the chest, sometimes in front, oftener beneath the scapula; recurring from time to time; at times severe, and lasting for several days; in other instances slight and of brief duration; experienced more frequently on one side than on the other, but often occurring successively, or in alternation, on both sides. These pains generally denote repeated attacks of circumscribed pleuritis. Chills, or shiverings, sometimes observing an approach to periodicity, and liable to be attributed to an irregular or imperfectly developed intermittent. Hæmoptysis,[1] frequently the first symptom to create alarm in the mind of the patient; sometimes preceding other symptoms, and all appreciable physical signs."[2] P. 489.

We are told, with much truth, we believe, that dyspepsia is not a frequent cause of phthisis, and the same is said to be true of chronic pleurisy and pneumonitis.

Acute phthisis is treated of in a few pages. More might have been said upon this subject with benefit, for we have reason to think that physicians have been, sometimes, unjustly blamed for not diagnosticating this affection in some short cases, where it was easily detected by other physicians a very few weeks or days subsequently.

The diagnosis of pneumonitis and pleurisy are sufficiently easy to be made. Yet how frequently do we have cases come under our care where the previous diagnoses have been inaccurate. How frequently is it the case, that we are doubtful whether the young patient has a pneumonitis or an encephalitis? How frequently do we say that this patient has lung fever, while we cannot help a feeling of mixed doubt and certainty, whether it may not turn out to be a functional derangement after all. When fresh from the school, we feel vastly more competent to diagnosticate disease than we are found to be ten years later. This is in part owing to the fact, that each new class of graduates has a partially new and more perfect system of diagnosis. It is in part due, also, to our having been oftentimes deceived and having learned caution. In the work before us, we believe that the signs of these two diseases are well laid down.

"If a person be seized with a chill, which is followed by high febrile movement, and lancinating pain in the chest, referred to the neighbourhood of the nipple; accompanied by cough, with an adhesive, rusty expectoration, and a well-marked crepitant rale is found on auscultating the posterior surface of the chest on one side, it is at once evident that he is attacked with pneumonitis seated in an inferior lobe." P. 421.

No one can doubt the truth of this description, particularly when it is added that "a viscid expectoration, containing a variable quantity of blood in intimate combination, is a symptom belonging exclusively to inflammation of the pulmonary parenchyma."

But we are told that the crepitant rale may be obscure; "the characteristic expectoration is by no means uniformly present in cases of pneumonitis, and, if not altogether absent, it is not always among the earlier symptoms of the disease;" there may not be an excess of pain which can be fixed in any one part of the chest. These cases are not common, but they do sometimes occur; and it so happens that the writer of this article, by that strange coincidence which every practitioner will notice as having happened with some particular diseases, has seen this want of *signs* in a large number of his cases of pneu-

[1] The subject of hæmoptysis in its relation to tuberculosis, has been elaborately investigated by Dr. Walshe; *vide* British and Foreign Medico-Chir. Review, January, 1849.

[2] In 91 of the 100 cases which I have analyzed, as respects physical signs, the histories contain information concerning hæmoptysis. It had occurred in 53 cases prior to the time of my examinations. Of 22 cases of small tubercular deposits, it had occurred in 13. Of 11 cases in which the existence of cavities was ascertained, it had occurred in 6. Of 58 cases of abundant deposit, it had occurred in 34.

monitis within the few years past. It is almost unnecessary to say, that there is something peculiar which prevents a practitioner from diagnosticating anything but pneumonitis in such cases. He of course gives a guarded diagnosis to the family. At length perfect dulness, unchanged by change of position, and bronchial respiration and voice, mixed with crepitus in some near spot, enables him to say that his mind is fully made up.

We wish that more had been said concerning these latent cases of pneumonitis.

The *crepitant rale* is the earliest and most characteristic of the positive signs, and Dr. Flint correctly differs from Skoda, we think, in saying, that it is present in a very large majority of the cases of pneumonitis.

"It is probable that examinations repeated, and made at an earlier period, would not have been negative as regards this sign in the greater proportion of the few instances in which it was not discovered. Of 149 examinations, in forty-five cases, made at different periods in the progress of the disease, the presence of the rale is noticed in eighty-five, and its absence in sixty-four. The collection of cases analyzed did not embrace cases of lobar pneumonitis occurring in infancy. My observations led me to concur with others in the opinion that the crepitant rale is much less constantly present in children than in adults. It is perhaps oftener absent than present in infant life. The constancy of the rale in acute primitive pneumonia, affecting the adult, is shown by the much more extensive researches of Grisolle." P. 409.

We should be glad to extend our notice of this book, for we have not alluded to a large part of it. The chapters on bronchitis and pleuritis will bear much study, and from them the physician in large practice will find much that is valuable, much that he will recognize as true, but which he has not read. To do the book justice, to point out what is new, or stated in a new form, would require us to quote the whole book.

In closing, we recommend the treatise to every one who wishes to become a correct auscultator. Based to a very large extent upon eases numerically examined, it carries the evidences of careful study and discrimination upon every page. It does credit to the author, and, through him, to the profession in this country. It is, what we cannot call every book upon auscultation, a readable book. C. E. B.

ART. XI.—*Statistics and Treatment of Typhus and Typhoid Fever, from Twelve Years' Experience gained at the Seraphim Hospital, in Stockholm* (1840—1852). By MAGNUS HUSS, M. D., Professor in the Medical Clinic at the Caroline Institute; Member of the Royal Academy of Science at Stockholm; Laureate of the Institute of France, etc., etc. Translated from the Swedish original by ERNST ABERG, M. D. London: Longman, Brown, Green and Longmans. 1855. 8vo., pp. 200.

THE publication of the great work of Louis on the "Typoid Affection," aside from its influence on clinical investigations in general, and the intrinsic value of its facts and results, was an important event as a point of departure for entering anew on the study of continued fever in different countries. Analyzing the phenomena faithfully recorded at the bedside, together with the morbid appearances noted in the dead-room, Louis established the individuality of a disease which previously had not only been designated by different names, but which embraces affections that had been considered as quite different from each other. The form of the febrile disease so admirably elucidated, as regards its natural history, by the researches of Louis, has since been generally known by the title of *typhoid* fever. The publication of these researches at once gave rise to the inquiry whether continued fever in other countries presents the same pathological laws and lesions which had been found to belong to the disease in France? It was soon ascertained by Dr. Lombard, of Switzerland, and our countryman, Dr. Shattuck, who, after verifying the descriptions of Louis in the Parisian hospitals, prosecuted their investigations in the capitals of Great Britain, that the peculiar intestinal lesions constantly found in Paris were frequently wanting in London, Edinburgh, and Dublin. In the mean time, the observations of Drs. Gerhard and Pennock, of Philadelphia, during the prevalence of an epidemic fever among the Irish immigrants arriving in that city, established not only the absence in this epidemic of the lesions just referred to, but the existence of striking points of dissimilarity in symptomatic phenomena from those belonging to the typhoid affection as described by Louis. Regarding these variations as a sufficient basis for a nosological division, it has been customary by those who take this view of the matter to employ the term *typhus*, to designate a form of fever presenting certain distinctive characters first clearly pointed out by Gerhard, and since more fully studied and compared with those belonging to typhoid fever, by other observers. Since the publication of the papers by Dr. Gerhard, in 1837,[1] it has been a mooted point whether a form of fever, to which has been restricted the name *typhus*, being the predominant fever in Ireland, but frequently observed in other parts of Great Britain, and met with in this country chiefly among Irish immigrants, should be regarded as a disease essentially distinct from the *typhoid* fever which prevails in France, and which has been shown to be an indigenous fever in certain portions of the United States; or whether the latter form of fever is in essence identical with the former, but presenting modifications due to extrinsic circumstances, or to individual peculiarities of constitution. The non-identity of typhus and typhoid fever has been maintained by distinguished clinical observers and medical teachers in this country, from the time that the point just mentioned first began to be mooted. This doctrine has been steadily gaining ground, and probably we are correct in asserting that at the present moment it is accredited by the majority of the well-informed members of the American Medical Profession. It has also been adopted for the most part by French writers. The German pathologists appear to hold to the identity of typhus and typhoid fever, regarding the latter as a variety of the former, and distinguished by them by the title *abdominal typhus*. In Great Britain, of late years, the unity of continued fever has been the commonly received doctrine. It is only since the recent publication of the very valuable researches of Dr. Jenner that the non-identity of typhus and typhoid fever has found much advocacy with the British medical press.

The foregoing brief sketch of opinions relating to a question recently said by an English reviewer to be "emphatically the question of the day," is given by way of introduction to a critical notice of a work, the title-page of which is prefixed to this article. The object of the work, as stated in the preface, is to present the results of the scientific experience acquired from the

[1] American Journal of the Medical Sciences, vol. xix., p. 289. It is due to the memory of the late Dr. Hale, of Boston, to state that in an account of the fever of Massachusetts, published in 1839, he foreshadowed, as it were, the distinctions between typhus and typhoid fever.

author's connection for a period of twelve years, with a hospital which received during that time more than 3000 cases of continued fever. These cases, it may be here remarked, were not all under the observation of Prof. Huss, a proportion of about one-fourth coming under the charge of his colleague, Prof. Malmsten. A small proportion only were recorded and subjected to analysis, viz: 250 cases which occurred during the last months of 1843 and the beginning of 1844. The histories of these cases were obtained with the aid of several medical attendants at the clinic, who at that time were students of medicine, but in whose accuracy and fidelity the author had full confidence. It is proper to cite these statements as tending to show the nature and extent of the author's experience, the more so because it will be seen that the conclusions purporting to be derived from it do not in all respcots accord with those based on observations made in other parts of Europe and in America.

The name of Prof. Huss will to many of our readers not be new. He is known by his previous publications on the diseases of Sweden, and especially by his description of certain effects of the abuse of alcohol, under the title of *acoholismus chronicus.* In a late publication[1] he is referred to as "a most philosophical, practical-minded physician, standing deservedly at the head of the profession in Northern Europe."

The work preper is devoted to the statistics and treatment of typhus and typhoid fever. In the introduction to the work, however, Prof. Huss declares his belief in the identity of typhus and typhoid fever, and states the grounds on which this opinion is founded. Now, the importance of the statistics which occupy a considerable portion of the volume, in a great measure depends on the correctness of this doctrine of the identity of these two forms of fever. The cases received at the Seraphim Hospital in Stockholm in all probability embraced cases of typhus and typhoid fever, as these terms are now generally applied. Prof. Huss regards these two forms of fever as essentially one disease, and accordingly his statistical researches and therapeutical conclusions for the most part have reference indiscriminately to both forms. Let it be admitted that typhus and typhoid fever are distinct affections, and the deductions from his experience it is clear cannot be applied to either affection to the exclusion of the other, more than the results of an investigation collectively, of a series of cases of rubeola and scarlatina could be made available either for extending or giving greater precision to our knowledge respectively of these different eruptive fevers. The value of Prof. Huss' work as contributing facts pertaining to the natural history of typhus and typhoid fever, thus hinges on the mooted point stated in our introductory remarks. We propose, therefore, to notice at some length the grounds adduced by Prof. Huss for his belief in the identity of typhus and typhoid fever. We prepose to do this, not because the arguments are new, ncr because they have not been already satisfactorily refuted; but the author claims that his opinion is founded on a long and extensive clinical experience, and it is due to him as well as to the importance of the subject, to institute a critical examination of the evidence which he offers in support of this opinion, while others, in different countries, who have carefully studied continued fever at the bedside, have arrived at a different conclusion.

Before entering on the discussion of the question of the identity or non-identity of typhus and typhoid fever, let us clearly understand the point concerning which opinions are divided. By those who take the ground of

[1] Transactions of American Medical Association, vol. viii. p. 583.

identity, it is not denied that certain cases of continued fever are characterized by the symptoms and lesions belonging to typhoid as distinguished from typhus. The question relates not so much to facts as to the inferences from facts. We shall presently see that Prof. Huss bears testimony to many of the facts upon which rests the doctrine of non-identity. But it is contended that the characteristics of typhoid fever, as contrasted with those of typhus, instead of denoting an intrinsic difference in the disease, proceed from extrinsic circumstances pertaining to season, place, individual peculiarities, and variations in epidemic influences. On the other hand, the advocates of non-identity contend that the points of dissimilarity in the natural history of the two forms of fever are of a nature not to be thus disposed of; that the distinctive features of either form show an essential difference inherent in the disease; and, hence, that the two forms are different diseases. Now on what conditions does the individuality of a disease depend? With our present knowledge of pathology and etiology, it is rarely the case that we are able to discriminate different affections after what we positively know of their essential nature or their special causes. We should be able to do this were medical science perfect. As it is, our nosological divisions are of necessity based on logical inference, not on demonstration. Many diseases which are justly regarded as essentially distinct, have not a few phenomena in common. This is true of all the essential fevers. Take rubeola and scarlatina for example; they often bear to each other a close resemblance, and, in fact, it is only in modern times that they have been nosologically separated. Why do we now regard them as different diseases? Clinical observation has shown that they are respectively characterized by certain peculiarities which each preserves with such constancy that the existence of distinct pathological laws may be thereon predicated. An eruption belongs to each. This eruption, although in both an efflorescence, is found to present certain features as respects sensible characters, the time of its appearance, its diffusion over the body, and its immediate effects, which are as uniformly in contrast in the two diseases as they are in accordance in successive cases of the same disease; hence they denote the existence of different laws in the two affections. In scarlatina, the pharynx is the seat of an inflammatory process; a catarrhal affection of the mucous membrane lining the air-passages, enters into the natural history of rubeola. The laws determining the anatomical characters of the two diseases are thus different. Both affections are contagious; but the miasm emanating from the body of a patient affected with scarlatina never gives rise to the phenomena which characterize rubeola, but invariably to those which belong to scarlatina, and *vice versa*. Hence it is certain that the special cause which produces each affection is peculiar to it. Moreover, when a patient has experienced either affection he is rendered thereafter, as a rule, exempt from its recurrence; but having passed through one furnishes no exemption for the future against the other. These facts, established by clinical observation, are sufficient to show that whatever may be the phenomena which are common to scarlatina and rubeola, the two affections are not merely varieties of the same species of disease, but are intrinsically and essentially distinct from each other, albeit the precise nature and extent of the difference, owing to the imperfection of medical science, cannot be defined. If in the several points of view in which scarlatina and rubeola have just been contrasted, clinical facts lead to a contrast not less striking between typhus and typhoid fever, can there be any reasonable ground for denying that, in the same sense, they are distinct diseases; in other words that they are non-identical?

Proceeding to review the grounds on which Prof. Huss founds the conclusion that typhus and typhoid fever are identical, or, as he expresses it, "different varieties of one and the same pathological process," the first point referred to is the concurrence of cases of both forms during the same epidemic. We quote his remarks under this head.

"I have endeavoured to follow with attention two rather considerable epidemies of typhus, one of which commenced in September, 1841, and continued until July, 1842, the other in December, 1845, to July, 1846. 503 typhus patients were received in the wards of the Seraphim Hospital during the course of the former, 414 during the latter epidemic. In neither instance were the cases exclusively typhus or typhoid fever, on the contrary there were some of both; so that in the beginning and to the height of the epidemic the cases were for the most part typhus, and at the end the typhoid fever almost entirely prevailed. This statement is founded not merely on the symptoms each individual case presented, but also on the results of the post-mortem examinations. With the exception of four, all who died were examined; there were 55 fatal cases in the former epidemic, 33 in the latter; of the former 55, 36 presented those alterations of the intestinal tube and mesenteric glands, which are peculiar to typhoid fever, and 19 no such alterations; of the latter 33, only 29 were examined; of these, in 19 the glands were changed in different degrees, the remaining 10 showed no change." Page 7.

The author adds in a note that another epidemic, in 1852, had every character of the exclusively abdominal form (typhoid), all the post-mortem examinations, with the exception of one only, exhibiting the usual changes in the intestinal glands.

The simultaneous prevalence of typhus and typhoid is a matter of frequent observation: on this point Dr. Jenner remarks, "a fact which has greatly contributed to typhus and typhoid fever being confounded is that often both prevail at the same time, similar circumstances favouring their propagation, the miasm of both appearing to be subject to the same laws of evolution, so that whenever one prevails the other will be likely also to prevail. This will serve to explain the contradictions which apparently exist in the descriptions of camp and jail fever, to be found in the works of old authors as well as in those of our own day."[1] In certain situations, for example in Paris, and in certain portions of our own country, typhoid fever is the species which exclusively prevails, and cases of typhus are not expected, of course, to occur; but wherever typhus prevails, cases of typhoid fever are frequently, if not generally intermingled in greater or less proportion. This is verified by observations at London, Dublin, and Edinburgh. In our own experience during several years that we were engaged in studying clinically the two fevers, cases of each were at the same time under observation, sometimes those of typhoid fever, and at other times those of typhus predominating, the cases of both occurring for the most part among foreign immigrants from Ireland and Germany.

It is simply a matter of fact that both typhus and typhoid fever may prevail at the same time and place. Certainly, in itself, the fact proves nothing with respect to the identity of the two affections. The author himself does not attach much importance to the fact, candidly saying, "experience tells us that two epidemic diseases may appear simultaneously at the same place; for instance, scarlet fever and the measles; nay, it has been said that the two diseases may occur at the same time in the same person."

[1] It is proper to state that in making quotations from the writings of Dr. Jenner, a French translation is resorted to, copies of his publications in English not being accessible to the reviewer during the preparation of this article.

A vastly stronger point would be to show community as respects the special causes of the two affections. Will the same miasm produce indifferently typhus and typhoid fever? When propagated by contagion, is typhus found to follow exposure to the miasm emanating from the bodies of typhoid patients, and *vice versa?* If the affirmative to these questions were to be proved, assuredly it would go far to establish the identity of the two forms of disease; and, on the other hand, proof of the negative is not less direct and cogent in behalf of their non-identity. The author cites two instances in which both forms of fever were supposed to spring from the same source. We quote the account of each instance in full.

"A man had died, *it was stated*, of typhus. The brother and his wife went to live in the house of the deceased, and used his clothes without previous airing and cleaning; they were soon taken ill and brought to the hospital, where they both died. The husband had violent delirium and a profuse petechial eruption, the post-mortem examination showing no change of the intestinal glands; the wife had milder cerebral symptoms and a very scarce crop of eruption; but on examination swollen mesenteric glands and swollen and ulcerated Peyer plagues were found in abundance."

We have italicised the evidence which this account affords that the primary case was typhus, although perhaps this is not of much moment so far as concerns the argument. The account is defective in other important details. How long after taking possession of the house and wearing the clothes of their deceased kinsman, were the husband and wife attacked? Were they attacked simultaneously or successively, and, if the latter, after what interval of time? Did typhus or typhoid fever, or both, prevail at that period? These inquiries have obvious bearings on the inference to be drawn from the facts stated. The husband, it appears, had typhus fever, and it is presumable that the infected clothes were worn by him alone, inasmuch as the deceased kinsman whom it was said had died of typhus, was of the male sex. So far the facts favour the doctrine of the non-identity rather than that of the identity of the two forms. The development of typhoid fever in the person of the wife may have had no connection with the occurrence of the cases of typhus. So far as details are given, it is fair to suspect, to say the least, that the concurrence or succession of the two cases of the different forms of fever in this instance was due to coincidence, in other words accidental. This suspicion is, of course, the more allowable if (what is undoubtedly true) the facts given in the foregoing account are exceptions to a general rule.

The other instance was communicated by a medical practitioner in the country, and is as follows:—

"A traveller came to a small island situated on the western coast of Sweden. He was sick when he arrived, and was the same day laid up with a fever. The disease showed all the marks peculiar to typhus petechialis, viz: clearly marked alteration of the blood, and a very copious typhus eruption (cechymotie petechiæ), and ended on the ninth day fatally. Seven persons were successively taken ill on the island; only one of these presented the marks characterizing typhus; the remaining six cases, of which one was fatal, were all clearly distinct typhoid. The course of this limited epidemic made it evident that it was produced by infection from the first diseased person who came ill, before whose arrival no case of typhus or typhoid had been seen for several years, either on the island or in the neighbourhood, and that the same contagion produced both typhus and typhoid fever."

We have the same objection to bring against this as against the preceding account, viz: it is deficient in important details. The imported case was held to be a case of typhus in consequence of *an alteration of the blood, and an eruption of ecchymotic petechiæ.* What the evidence was of an alteration of the blood peculiar to typhus we are left to conjecture. From the terms used to indicate the character of the eruption, there is room for a strong suspicion that it consisted of true petechiæ, *i. e.* minute extravasations, which are widely different from the characteristic maculæ of typhus, and by no means peculiar to the latter fever. Of the subsequent cases all but one were regarded as typhoid. The excepted case did not prove fatal, so that the evidence of its being a case of typhus rests solely on the phenomena during life. No description of these phenomena is given. The reader must rely exclusively on the judgment of the observer, and inasmuch as not a single case of either species had been known to occur on the island for several years before, it is not unfair to entertain some distrust of the ability of the practitioners residing there to discriminate practically between the two fevers. At all events, the evidence of the statements made in the report of the country practitioner is inadequate to secure for them any weight in opposition to well ascertained facts from which other conclusions are deducible; especially when it is considered that, in all probability, the observations were made under the bias of belief in the identity of typhus and typhoid fever.

With the researches of Dr. Jenner on the non-identity of the special causes of the different forms of continued fever, we presume many of our readers are familiar. Professor Huss could not have been acquainted with them, else he would hardly have attached much importance to the unsatisfactory, and, we may add, unscientific reports which have just been quoted. Dr. Jenner took pains to trace to their respective localities all the cases of continued fever received into the London Fever Hospital during the years 1847, 1848, and 1849. In 1848, one quarter of all the fever patients received into the hospital were affected with typhoid fever; and out of forty-four localities which furnished one hundred and one typhus cases, there was but a single instance in which one patient affected with typhus, and another affected with typhoid fever, came from the same house. Of five localities, which during the same year furnished nine cases of typhoid fever, the same statement holds good. In 1849, fifty-one typhus patients came from eighteen localities, and ten typhoid patients from four localities. During this period in no instance did the same house furnish a case of each fever. This rule was found to exist without an exception in 1847; but the number of cases traced in this way to their source was less during this year than the two following years.

We look upon these results of the researches of Dr. Jenner as very valuable, showing the nature of the special causes producing typhus and typhoid fever to be not identical, and, inferentially, the non-identity of the diseases themselves.

In a single instance among the large number collected by Dr. Jenner, in which two or more patients were traced to the same habitation, it was found that one house had furnished a case of typhus and a case of typhoid fever. This shows that the rule is not without exceptions. Prof. Huss, as we have seen, adduces an exceptional instance. He cites it in proof that the special cause is the same in both fevers—overlooking, however, the importance of either establishing or disproving the rule of which the instance cited was an exception.

The most rational explanation of these exceptions is to attribute them to mere coincidence. With reference to scarlatina and measles, we can cite a curious occurrence, which no one will doubt was purely accidental, but which, taken alone, would go to show identity of the contagious miasm producing these two diseases. In a family embracing two children (girls), one aged seven, and the other four years, the latter was attacked with rubeola March 28. Measles were prevalent at the time, but it was not known that the child had been exposed to the contagious miasm of this disease. On the 5th of April medical attendance was discontinued. On the 28th of April the sister was attacked with scarlatina, and was convalescent on the 9th of May. The histories of both cases were recorded. There had been no known exposure to the contagion of scarlet fever, and the child had never had measles. The exposure to the contagion of the latter disease, during the illness of her sister, was as complete as possible. We give this simply as an illustration of the risk of drawing inferences from isolated instances. As regards the point under consideration, the argument for or against the identity of typhus and typhoid fever is to be based on the law which regulates the causation in the vast majority of cases. If we may logically conclude that the special cause, whatever it may be, or whence derived, of typhus, is peculiar to it—*i. e.*, that it never gives rise to typhoid fever—and conversely with respect to the special cause of the latter, it must be admitted to constitute a very cogent argument in favour of the non-identity of these affections. The facts developed by the researches of Jenner appear to warrant such a conclusion, but it is undoubtedly desirable that the same method of examination should be still further prosecuted.

Prof. Huss states as a ground for his belief in the identity of typhus and typhoid fever that they are often with difficulty discriminated from each other; and, indeed, he asserts this to be in many instances utterly impossible. He also declares that intermediate forms are of frequent occurrence; in other words, the features said to characterize each form may be variously intermingled. The latter point he considers with reference to some details to which we shall presently advert.

These statements are opposed to the results obtained by a careful study of the two fevers in other countries. Their characteristic phenomena are found to be singularly constant, bearing numerically about the same ratio in the relative frequency of their occurrence in widely separated situations. The results of the analyses of recorded histories of typhoid fever in Paris, London, and in America, present few discrepancies. The same is true as respects England and America of typhus fever. For proof of the correctness of this position we refer the reader to the statistical researches of Louis in France, Jenner in London, Jackson and Flint in different parts of this country. Evidence is afforded in the publications just referred to of the fact that, in the same situation, in successive years, these diseases maintain a remarkable uniformity in their phenomena and laws. We have shown this to be the case by bringing into comparison the results of three distinct analyses, made in three successive years, of separate collections of histories gathered during these years.[1] So far from the statement of the author respecting the difficulty of discriminating clinically the two diseases from each other being in accordance with our experience and that of others, we should say that the

[1] *Vide* Clinical Reports on Continued Fever, etc. Dr. Jenner's testimony on this point is explicit. He says: "During the three years that nearly all the patients admitted into the London Fever Hospital were the subjects of careful observation, I did not discover any variation in the symptoms, general or local, either in the cases of typhus or in those of typhoid fever; notwithstanding that there prevailed during this period epidemics of relapsing fever, of typhus and cholera, denoting different modifications of the epidemic constitution."—*On the Non-identity of Typhus and Typhoid Fever*, Bruges, 1853, p. 164.

cases are rare in which a physician, accustomed to observe both, need hesitate in arriving at a diagnosis. Dr. Jenner remarks, that even the hospital nurses at the London fever hospital are seldom at fault in distinguishing between the two fevers; and on being asked by the attending physician whether any new cases have been admitted since the last visit, they say without hesitation, "Yes, a case of typhus," or typhoid, as the case may be. We can make the same remark. The intelligent sister of charity who had charge of the fever ward at the hospital in which our histories were mostly collected, was accustomed to designate cases as typhus or typhoid with almost uniform correctness.

In view of the learning and experience of Prof. Huss—according to him, as we are bound to do, sincerity in his statements—how are the latter to be reconciled with the opposite conclusions at which other clinical observers have arrived? We may suppose that the *signa diagnostica* of typhus and typhoid fever are uncertain in Sweden, although sufficiently reliable elsewhere. This is not probable, inasmuch as these affections are found to retain their distinctive traits, as has been seen, in different and widely separated countries. Moreover, we confess that we are skeptical as regards extensive modifications of disease by climatic influences. We do not by any means deny that modifications may proceed from this source, but there is reason to believe that diseases vary much less than it has been customary to imagine. We look upon the notions commonly held on this subject in somewhat the same light as we do the opinion so often uttered, that certain affections will not of late years bear the same measures of treatment which were formerly demanded. The true explanation of this opinion we believe is, that it is so difficult to determine with precision the success of therapeutical measures, and accordingly it was perhaps less in past time, or at the present time, than it suits our self-complaisance to suspect. In other words, the opinion is simply founded on the fact that our present views of treatment differ from those formerly practised. So with regard to the phenomena and laws of diseases; they are thought to fluctuate much more than they do, because the natural history of but few diseases is as yet settled by means of analyses of a sufficient number of recorded cases. Judging from the extent to which those affections that have been most studied are found to preserve their individual characters unchanged in different seasons and places, it may be anticipated that a more complete knowledge of the phenomena and laws of different diseases will be likely to lessen the importance which, since the time of Sydenham, has been attached to the "constitution of the year."

Another, and we are forced to conclude a truer, mode of accounting for the views of Prof. Huss, is derived from the fact that he has not taken pains to record and analyze cases of both forms of fever separately, bringing the results into contrast with each other; nor does it appear from his work that the researches of others within late years, conducted after this plan of investigation, have fallen under his notice. His convictions are based on unrecorded experience, not on conclusions educed by analysis from facts noted at the bedside. The statistics to which a considerable portion of the volume is devoted, as already stated, relate to both fevers indiscriminately.

The characters and laws pertaining to the eruption in typhus and typhoid fever are of great importance, not only with reference to the differential diagnosis, but as affording evidence of non-identity. The lenticular rose-coloured eruption in typhoid cases, as regards its sensible characters, differs in several striking particulars from the maculated eruption, called by Jenner the mulberry rash, or, as it is frequently but with doubtful propriety designated, the petechial spots belonging to typhus. Prof. Huss does not enumerate the features regarded as distinctive of the two fevers by those who hold to the doctrine of non-identity; he assumes that they are well known to others as well as to himself, and asserts that he has frequently observed the typhus and typhoid eruptions to become developed simultaneously, and also the former, not uncommonly, to appear first and disappear, the latter taking its place. Here his experience is at variance with the results of analyses of large collections of cases in which, by different observers, the appearances have been carefully noted day after day at the bedside during the whole career of the disease. What is to be said of the above assertions of the Swedish professor? Frankly, we must avow that, without impeaching his honesty, we cannot give credence to his statements. Inasmuch as he does not profess that they are based on other data than those which the memory is capable of retaining, we must believe him to be mistaken unless we adopt the improbable hypothesis, that the phenomena and laws of these diseases are widely different in Sweden from those established by recorded observations in other countries. A fair examination of the difficulty, nay, the impossibility of recollecting the facts pertaining to a series of cases sufficiently for accurate deductions, would justify the disbelief just expressed; especially when belief involves a repudiation of results obtained by different observers, without concert, who have resorted to a method of investigation requiring much care and patience, but which has the recommendation of being in a great measure free from the liability to error incident to the weakness and imperfection of the mental faculties.

We do not wish to be understood as contending that the two eruptions never present any variations in their distinctive appearances. These appearances are more strongly marked in some cases than in others. In a few of the typhus cases which we have recorded, with the characteristic *maculæ* were intermingled others bearing more or less resemblance to the *taches rosées*, but the predominant character of the eruption was unmistakable. Dr. Jenner points out certain changes which the typhus eruption undergoes in different stages of the disease which may possibly have led, in some instances, to the error of supposing that the two kinds of eruption are frequently found in combination. He states, that at first the spots have a rose hue, are slightly elevated, and the redness disappears momentarily on pressure, but they acquire soon the dusky hue, lose their elevation, and only become paler on pressure.[1] The variations, however, in sensible characters which are observed in different cases of typhus and typhoid fever, are not greater than in all the eruptive fevers, for example, in scarlatina and rubeola. The scarlatinous eruption varies in colour, and sometimes assumes the form of minute isolated dots instead of being diffused, or presenting irregular patches of greater or less size. The appearance of the eruption in measles is not less variable. But, notwithstanding these diversities, the distinctive traits belonging to each are

[1] In nearly all of the few instances among the cases recorded by the writer, in which the eruption presented mixed characters, this peculiarity was observed during the early part of the eruptive period. Prof. Huss curiously makes a statement directly the reverse of that by Dr. Jenner referred to above. He avers that it is not uncommon for an eruption of *petechiæ* to occur during the first four or six days, which disappear after the lapse of two or three days and gives place to the lenticular spots. He says, the primary petechial eruption is "sometimes of a bright and sometimes of a more dusky red," but "very seldom ecchymotic." In another place he defines the typhus eruption to be "ecchymotic petechiæ." The language just quoted suggests a doubt whether the author has a clear idea of the distinctive characters of the two eruptions. He should have guarded against this doubt by describing the appearances of the eruption. This is an omission to which the reader has a right to take exceptions.

very rarely, if ever, so confused that it becomes difficult to distinguish the one affection from the other by the sensible characters of the eruption alone. This statement we believe to be not less applicable to the cases of typhus and typhoid fever, in which an eruption is developed. But, in these fevers as in those of the eruptive class, for example, scarlatina and rubeola, the circumstances pertaining to the eruption which furnish diagnostic criteria, by no means relate solely to the sensible characters. The eruption appears earlier in typhus than in typhoid, the former, in this respect, sustaining a relation to the latter similar to that of scarlet fever to measles. In typhoid fever spots successively appear, taking the place of others which disappear during the eruptive stadium; in typhus the spots once developed are permanent during the period of the eruption. In cases of typhoid fever which prove fatal while the eruption is present, no traces of the spots are discovered after death; while in cases of typhus the eruption is observable on the cadaver. These facts not only furnish means of discrimination, but have an important bearing on the question of identity. If observation have established that the eruption in typhus and typhoid fever differs not only in obvious sensible characters, but as respects the laws regulating the time of its appearance, the mode of its perpetuation, and its duration; does not this, in itself, constitute sufficient ground for regarding the two affections as non-identical in the same sense in which scarlatina and rubeola are considered as distinct diseases?

Next in importance to the distinctive characters pertaining to the eruption, are the intestinal lesions peculiar to typhoid fever and the abdominal symptoms therewith connected, in their bearing on the question under discussion. In fact, the latter are, perhaps, even more important than the former in this relation. Both, however, are to be taken conjointly in the endeavour to determine whether typhus and typhoid fever are identical or not. Are cases which are characterized by a well-marked typhus eruption, as well as by other traits peculiar to this fever, as a rule wanting in certain abdominal symptoms, viz: diarrhœa, meteorism, tenderness in the iliac fossæ, and gurgling, which are observed in the great majority of cases presenting the characteristic typhoïd eruption; and in fatal cases are the Peyerian patches and mesenteric glands found on dissection to be very slightly or not at all affected; if the eruption and other symptoms have denoted typhus, while notable lesions in these parts are as constantly discovered, provided the eruption and abdominal symptoms have indicated typhoid fever? If the affirmative be proved, then, in addition to the different laws governing the eruption which have been referred to, other laws determining a marked difference in anatomical characters are established; a difference certainly greater than that which exists between scarlatina and rubeola. We must presume our readers to be familiar with the typhoid intestinal lesions, which, although not unobserved prior to the researches of Louis, were by him more fully described than by any previous observer, and their significance as an anatomical characteristic of a species of fever first pointed out. The absence of these lesions was the grand negative point of distinction, so far as relates to morbid anatomy, developed by the investigations of Gerhard and Pennock, which have resulted in establishing, as we think, the individuality of typhus and its essentially distinct nature. The facts contributed during the few past years by observers in different countries, to the elucidation of the points involved in the above inquiry, the reader is also supposed to be acquainted with. If not, we must refer to publications already mentioned. We could not reproduce them here in any detail without exceeding the limits appropriate to this article. Suffice it to say, that the analysis of a host of cases collected in different quarters of the world, the recorded histories embracing the appearances found after death, and the phenomena noted during life, have shown, on the one hand, constancy of connection between the eruptive and other symptomatic characters peculiar to typhoid fever and the so-called typhoid intestinal lesions; and, on the other hand, absence of these lesions when the eruption and other symptoms were unequivocally those which belong to typhus. This can be said in behalf of the non-identity of typhus and typhoid fever. Now can the advocate of their identity assemble from any or all authentic sources a group of fatal cases in which, the data being in like manner placed on record, the eruptive and other symptomatic characters of typhus were found to be associated with the typhoid intestinal lesions, or, conversely, in which the eruption and other symptoms of typhoid fever were present, and these lesions found to be wanting? It is now twenty years since the uniformity of certain intestinal lesions in well-marked cases of typhoid fever, and their uniform absence in cases of typhus began to be mooted. During this time the amount of positive evidence in support of these positions has been constantly accumulating, while there have been ardent advocates, as there are still, of the identity of the two fevers. It would obviously go far toward establishing the correctness of the latter doctrine were these positions to be disproved. Have there been any sufficiently authenticated instances reported in which typhoid lesions have been found when the diagnostic criteria of typhus were clearly present during life? This question, in fact, covers the whole ground, for the occasional absence of these lesions in well-marked typhoid cases would not invalidate their relationship to the disease more than the absence of the eruption or the throat affection in some cases of scarlatina is sufficient to impair their significance, when present, as criteria of this fever. In an able and candid article, published in 1851, in the *British and Foreign Medico-Chirurgical Review*, the writer cites as the only instances which had been offered, up to that time, of the typhoid lesions having been found in well-marked typhus cases, those reported by M. Landouzy in the *Archives Générales de Médecine.*[1]

These cases were observed during the prevalence of an epidemic in the prison in Rheims, in 1839–40. They have been often referred to in discussions of the subject under consideration. A critical examination, however, of the facts as they are reported by M. Landouzy, divests them of any value in their bearing on the identity of typhus and typhoid fever.

It appears not only as an inference from the histories of the cases, but from the statements of Landouzy himself, that both typhus and typhoid fever prevailed at Rheims when his observations were made. Of the fatal cases, six only were examined, and the morbid appearances recorded in but two instances. In one of the latter the eruption and other symptoms were undoubtedly those which are distinctive of typhus. The evidence in this case of the existence of typhoid lesions is not only insufficient, but from the description it is almost certain that they were not present. The small intestines were pronounced healthy by three physicians who examined them; but M. Landouzy "detected what he considered evidence of an incipient change in Peyer's patches, with general slight tumefaction of the solitary glands."[2] The appearances, if morbid, were in all probability those which are frequently seen in cases of typhus, consisting merely in moderate or slight hypertrophy, with perhaps the "shaven-beard" aspect.[3] The fact that the

[1] Vol. xii. pp. 1 and 306.

[2] We are indebted for these facts to the article in the British and Foreign Medico-Chirurgical Review already referred to.

[3] Our observations lead us to concur with Dr. Jenner in regarding the appearance thus designated as not distinctive typhoid fever.

patches of Peyer are not entirely unaffected in typhus fever we have endeavoured to impress in connection with our own researches. It is a fact not to be lost sight of, but it does not diminish in the least the significance of the true typhoid lesions, which are so different from the alterations just mentioned that the contrast is scarcely less than if the patches were never in the least degree altered in typhus. The morbid deposit, softening, sloughing, and ulceration, are peculiar to typhoid fever.

In the second case, the evidence of the characteristic typhoid lesions was complete, but the ante-mortem history in this case renders it pretty certain that the disease was typhoid fever. The eruption consisted of rose spots, intermingled with others which resembled flea-bites; and whereas the latter bear little or no resemblance to the maculæ of typhus, they were probably either veritable flea-bites or an eccentric variety of the *taches rosées.*

Since the publication of these famous cases of M. Landouzy, which, if they prove anything, go rather to support than invalidate the doctrine of non-identity, the importance of discovering instances in which the typhus phenomena during life are found to be associated with the typhoid lesions has certainly not been less than previously; but if such instances have been reported they have not fallen under our notice.

In the foregoing remark, I do not refer, of course, to loose general statements made by physicians who may have seen more or less of typhus and typhoid fever, but who do not take pains to record their cases, and compare the phenomena noted during life with the post-mortem appearances. The evidence in behalf of the constancy of the relation between the typhoid lesions and the diagnostic criteria of typhoid fever is based on cases, the histories of which were noted at the bedside, and it is but fair to require the same condition in admitting opposing evidence. It is sometimes asserted by practitioners that they have found the typhoid lesions in cases presenting during life the phenomena of typhus; but in view of the mass of facts which render this assertion improbable, we have a right to call for proof that there has not been an error of diagnosis; and this proof to a non-observer of the cases can only be afforded by their fully recorded histories. Taking this ground we shall find no difficulty in disposing of the statements of Prof. Huss relative to the point under consideration. He says:—

"We find, as a rule, the changes of the intestinal and mesenteric glands wanting in the graver forms of typhus petechialis, but, as exceptions, enlargement sometimes both of the solitary and Peyerian glands. It has, however, by no means been uncommon to see as well enlarged glands as spread ulcerations in milder cases, although with a distinctly pronounced petechial eruption."

Now, in accordance with the views which we have just expressed, we feel justified in attaching little or no importance to the author's assertion respecting the occurrence of exceptions to the general rule, notwithstanding his experience. The statement is not based on a comparison of the phenomena recorded during life, and the appearances noted in the dead-room. He does not profess to have made such a comparison. No evidence appears in the portion of the volume devoted to statistics that even the 250 cases whose histories were noted, with the help of five medical students, were analyzed with reference to the relation existing between the symptoms and intestinal lesions. We therefore deem it perfectly fair to assume that in the exceptional cases of the graver forms of *typhus petechialis* in which enlargement of the Peyerian and solitary glands were discovered after death, the morbid alterations did not exceed those which undoubtedly do occur in typhus as already mentioned; and that the author is mistaken in asserting ulcerations to have been found in milder cases in which a distinctly pronounced petechial eruption existed.

As already stated, Prof. Huss does not appear to have examined those of his recorded cases which proved fatal, in order to determine whether intestinal lesions were found in typhoid cases and in these cases only. His statistics, however, embrace certain data which will enable us to form, approximatively, conclusions with respect to these points. We will avail ourselves of these data, and endeavour to ascertain whether his facts are consistent with the statements of which we have just expressed an opinion. Of the 250 cases which are analyzed, an eruption was observed in 192. In 51 of these 192 cases the eruption is stated to have been petechial, and in 141 lenticular or typhoid. The ratio of the former is, then, a fraction below 26, and of the latter a fraction over 73 per cent. Now, we will assume that the cases with the petechial eruption were cases of typhus, and those with the lenticular eruption were cases of typhoid fever. This being assumed, on the supposition that in typhus cases the intestinal lesions were wanting, while they were present in the typhoid cases, it follows that these lesions existed in 73-100, and were absent in about 27-100 of the whole number, viz. 192. How do these results compare with the relative proportion of instances among the fatal cases examined after death, in which the intestinal lesions were, on the one hand, present, and, on the other hand, absent? The number of fatal cases, all of which were examined after death, was 25. Of this number the Peyerian glands were found more or less affected in 72-100, and unaffected in 28-100. Thus it appears that the ratio of instances in which a petechial eruption was noted, compared with the ratio of instances in which the Peyerian glands were unaffected, is as 27-100 to 28-100; and the ratio of instances in which intestinal lesions existed compared with the ratio in which the typhoid eruption was noted, is as 72-100 to 73-100.[1] In these calculations, we assume the number of fatal cases of both forms of fever to be equal. To this the author cannot take exceptions, as he does the same in determining approximatively the proportion of cases of petechial and abdominal typhus in the hospital cases not noted. It is evident, however, that the mortality in the two forms of disease may not have been the same, and perhaps the disparity in this respect may account for the small variation in the numerical results in the comparisons just made.

These results, to say the least, render it highly probable that had the author taken pains to have ascertained, in the 25 fatal cases, from the recorded histories, whether those in which intestinal lesions existed were characterized by the typhoid eruption, and, *per contra*, whether those in which the lesions were absent presented the typhus eruption—an undertaking not very laborious—he would have found that his opinions were disproved by his own facts. We cannot forbear expressing astonishment that it did not occur to him to institute such an examination. In the 250 recorded cases, 25 of which proved fatal and were examined after death, he had the data for testing, on a limited scale, the correctness of the opinions to which it is sufficiently clear his mind was committed prior to collecting these histories. Instead of doing this—a work of an hour or two—he contents himself with an enunciation of his opinions purporting to be based on his unrecorded experience. From this, as well as from the general tone of the work, it would

[1] The correspondence in the amount of difference in the two comparisons is worthy of notice.

seem that the analytical method of clinical investigation is either but little known, or imperfectly appreciated in Sweden.

Assuming that the abdominal symptoms associated with the typhoid intestinal lesions, denote only a variety of one form of fever, Prof. Huss accounts for their existence from the fact that the eruption is generally much less copious than when these symptoms and lesions are wanting. To quote his words: "It is true that these ulcerations (intestinal) occur less spread and less in copiousness in the petechial than in the abdominal form, which seems to me to be occasioned *by the existing antagonism between the skin and the intestinal mucous membrane, so that the more copious the eruption is on the skin the less are the intestinal glands affected and the contrary.*"[1] The opinion expressed in this quotation is not new. It was advanced several years ago in an able article in the *British and Foreign Review* (vol. xii.), and was adopted by Prof. Watson. Its correctness is abundantly disproved by the occasional occurrence, on the one hand, of cases in which the typhoid eruption has been copious, and the intestinal lesions are found to be marked; and, on the other hand, the occurrence of cases in which the typhus eruption is not abundant, and, nevertheless, the intestines are unaffected. These facts are alike applicable to the appearances after death and the abdominal symptoms during life.

In arguing for the identity of typhus and typhoid fever, Prof. Huss lays much stress on the point, that the differences on which is based the doctrine of their non-identity are not greater than are presented in different cases of other affections which confessedly retain their individuality. He instances scarlet fever as a disease offering a wider range of variations than belongs to cases, collectively, of typhus and typhoid fever. In a certain sense this statement is true, but, as an argument, it involves a fallacy which, on a superficial examination, may not be obvious. We have already, in the course of these remarks, had occasion to inquire into the circumstances which give to any disease its individuality, and we have seen that they consist of peculiarities from which are deduced laws of the disease distinct from those belonging to other diseases, which govern its external characters, its causation, its anatomical changes, etc. These laws of the phenomena, over which they preside, compose the natural history of a disease. Now, different cases of the same disease may present very great differences without material deviation from its fixed laws. These differences may be due to the greater or less intensity of certain symptoms. Here the variation is simply one of degree, not of kind, but it may give rise to a marked contrast, especially as respects the severity or danger of the disease in individual cases. Others arise from accidental complications; for example, pneumonia developed in the course of continued fever introduces a train of superadded symptomatic phenomena, yet the laws which invest the primary affection with its individuality remains. Scarlatina affords a remarkable instance of exceedingly great diversities arising from variations in intensity and complications. Its identity is not lost, because these variations do not abrogate the laws regulating its causation, distinctive characters, etc. Typhus and typhoid fever have many features in common. They have long been confounded in consequence of these points of similarity. Yet if the facts referred to in this article are admitted, these laws must be so distinctive that the individuality of each cannot be denied. Applying the argument of Prof. Huss to prove the identity of scarlet fever and measles, it would assuredly be stronger than in its application to typhus and typhoid fever.

[1] The italics are the author's.

We have now passed in review the several grounds adduced by Prof. Huss, for his belief in the identity of typhus and typhoid fever. In so doing we have presented several of the leading points in the argument for the non-identity of these affections. We have seen that, contrary to the assertions of the author, facts, so far as they have as yet been collected, go to show the existence of distinct special causes, causes which separately will produce but one and the same disease, never giving rise to the other; that the distinctive phenomena of each are preserved with a remarkable uniformity in different cases occurring not only at the same time and place, but in successive years, and in widely separated quarters of the globe; that the characters pertaining to the eruption serve to distinguish the one from the other, not less than in the two eruptive fevers, scarlatina and rubeola; and that certain intestinal lesions, which are of a peculiar character, are found nearly, if not quite, constantly in fatal cases of typhoid fever, and are invariably wanting in typhus. Contrasted in these points of view, the natural history of the two forms of fever involves a disparity as respects important pathological laws which is inconsistent with their essential identity.

A full exposition of the argument for the doctrine of non-identity would embrace several points which are merely referred to, or overlooked entirely by Prof. Huss. Our present limits will admit of only a brief notice of the more important of these.

It is abundantly proved that an attack either of typhus or typhoid fever, as the rule secures an exemption from the disease thereafter. Is this true only of each disease separately; in other words, will an attack of typhus exempt from typhoid fever, and *vice versa?* This is an important point in its bearing on the question of identity or non-identity. It is to be settled by facts which are not easily collected, and at the present moment they have not accumulated sufficiently to authorize a positive conclusion. Researches directed to this point are desirable. We have reported a single instance in which a patient entered hospital with typhoid fever, the characteristic eruption being well marked, and was convalescent on the twenty-third day after taking to the bed. Twenty-six days after the date of convalescence he was attacked with typhus, contracted, probably, from patients in the same ward, the distinctive eruption being well marked, and convalescence occurred on the seventeenth day. He died soon afterwards with tuberculosis of the lungs, and the traces of the typhoid intestinal lesions were apparent at the autopsy.[1]

An isolated case, or a few cases only of this description, would not suffice to settle the point, for exceptions to the rule, that either form of fever is experienced but once, are occasionally met with. An instance of two attacks of typhoid fever, the second succeeding the first about a fortnight after convalescence, has fallen under our observation during the last winter. In both attacks the typhoid eruption was well marked. Dr. Jenner has reported an instance in which a similar relapse took place.

Statistics have established a difference of susceptibility to the two diseases pertaining to age. Of the persons affected with typhoid fever the vast majority are under 40, but persons above this age are not less susceptible to typhus. In nearly one-third of the cases of typhus analyzed by Dr. Jenner, the patients were 50, or upwards. Prof. Huss gives statistics, as respects age, in 3,186 cases of both fevers. He states, that of 27 among these cases in which the age exceeded 50, eight had the abdominal form, *i.e.* typhoid fever. These results, while they confirm the rule, show an unusual number of excep-

[1] Clinical Reports on Continued Fever, etc., p. 312.

tions. One cannot avoid the suspicion that, inasmuch as the two diseases were believed to be identical they were not discriminated always with accuracy. This suspicion is strengthened by recalling the author's assertion that often the discrimination is impossible. Moreover, the histories of only 250 cases were recorded, and it is not stated that these 27 cases were included among the latter.

The two diseases observe different laws as respects duration. Statistical researches show that typhus runs a more rapid career, either to convalescence or death, than typhoid fever; that the former stage, or the period from the commencement of illness to the time of taking to the bed, is shorter in the former than in the latter. Prof. Huss' statistics confirm this distinction. They show, also, that in typhus convalescence oftener commences by a crisis than in typhoid. He is peculiar in enumerating *sleep* among the critical events, the others being perspiration, epistaxis, and diarrhœa.

The two diseases prevail together, as a rule, only in certain countries. Typhus fever does not occur in France except in certain rare epidemics. It is very rarely seen in this country save among foreign immigrants, or when it has been derived by contagion from imported cases. It is an indigenous fever in Ireland. In this country it is vastly more common among Irish immigrants than those coming from Germany. The disease, however, appears to prevail to a greater or less extent in Germany. It is observed in London and Edinburgh; and from the work of Prof. Huss it appears to exist in Stockholm, but the proportion of cases to those of typhoid fever is small. By an approximative calculation, he arrives at the conclusion that out of 3,186 cases, 892 were cases of typhus, and 2,294 cases of typhoid fever.[1]

It would seem to be a rule that typhoid fever exists wherever typhus is liable to prevail, but the former may prevail in localities in which the latter is never seen.

Repeated analysis of cases collected in France, Great Britain, and America, have shown that the two diseases do not observe the same laws as respects the season of the year when they are most likely to prevail. Typhoid fever in the countries just named manifest a decided predilection for the autumnal months, while typhus prevails indifferently at any period. On this point, the statement of Prof. Huss is remarkable. He says: "The season, also, has, in this matter, shown a decided influence; sporadic typhus occurring during autumn and winter, while spring and summer have introduced the typhoid cases." If this statement be correct it shows a variation in the law of typhoid fever as respects this point in Sweden. We regret to make use of this qualification, but the author here, as in other instances relating to the phenomena and laws which distinguish the two diseases from each other, merely enunciates the statement without professing to base it on the results of analytical investigation. Even the 250 cases collected "during the last months of 1843, and the beginning of 1844," are not analyzed with reference to this more than to other matters involved in the question of identity or non-identity. In this as in other instances, prudence dictates that something more solid and reliable than general impressions purporting to be founded on recollected experience should be required to invalidate laws confirmed by statistical researches in different quarters of the world.

[1] The basis of this calculation is the proportion of instances in which the typhoid intestinal lesions were found out of twenty-five fatal cases which occurred within a few months. This basis is quite inadequate to furnish correct results, inasmuch as in places where both fevers prevail together, great variations are observed in different years as respects the predominance of the one or the other.

The subject of contagion is hardly touched upon by Prof. Huss.[1] An important point of distinction between the two diseases is involved in this subject. The contagiousness of typhus is unquestionable, and that typhoid fever may be diffused by contagion, we regard as not less conclusively proved.[2] The two diseases, therefore, do not present so striking a difference as would exist were it true that one is contagious and the other non-contagious. The difference, however, is striking in the degree of contagiousness. The communicability of typhoid fever, under ordinary circumstances, is so rarely exemplified that decisive proof of its being ever diffused in this way has, with difficulty, been collected. On the other hand, the proof that typhus is transferred from one person to another is abundant. In our hospital experience, when cases of typhus and typhoid fever were under treatment at the same time and in the same ward, we have seen every attendant who nursed these patients contract successively typhus, while in not a single instance in hospital cases has typhoid fever been communicated. The vastly greater contagiousness of typhus is then a highly distinctive feature of this fever.

Other distinctive circumstances might be cited pertaining both to the symptomatology and anatomical characters of the two diseases, but a complete discussion of the question of their identity or non-identity would lead us beyond proper limits. Our object has been to review the grounds taken by the author in support of their identity, and in connection therewith to present points sufficient, if established, to show a dissimilitude as respects the phenomena and laws peculiar to each, that the two must be deemed essentially distinct from each other, on the same principle that other diseases are regarded as non-identical; for example, rubeola and scarlatina.

One half of the work by Prof. Huss is devoted to the *treatment* of typhus and typhoid fever. The pathological views from which he deduces rational principles of management are set forth in the following:—

"The primitive cause of the typhus process, as far as it is accessible to our understanding, seems to be a peculiar change in the blood. The chemical characters of this change are: diminished proportion of fibrin and increased proportion of several inorganic salts, especially carbonate of soda. This change in the blood is carried by the introduction into the system of some foreign matter, sometimes a miasm, sometimes a contagion, sometimes a decided poison (putrid water, putrid food). It is this foreign matter introduced by means of the respiratory or digestive act, that alters the blood in its chemical composition and vital power. We apply, consequently, the term zymotic to diseases generated in the said way. * * * In one the disease assumes the form of typhus petechialis, in another of typhus abdominalis, in still other cases it takes an intermediate form between these two extremes. The fever process, with all its different phases in whatever form they occur, is a manifestation of

[1] The only reference to this subject which he makes is contained in the following quotation: "During both these epidemics a contagion, or noso-comical miasma, developed itself within the hospital, which attacked a few patients who had entered the hospital with other complaints, as well as some of the nurses and medical students. These got what is called noso-comical fever, but this fever agreed in every respect with the prevailing epidemic. Some cases exhibited the petechial form, others the abdominal." The same looseness which characterizes other statements is here apparent. Judging from the facts observed in other hospitals with reference to the difference in contagiousness between typhus and typhoid fever, it is probable that analytical examination would have shown the disease developed within the hospital to have been typhus and not typhoid.

[2] For facts coming under our own observation, on which this conclusion is based, we will take the liberty of referring the reader to appendix to "Clinical Reports on Continued Fever, etc."

the endeavour of the system to render innocuous, or to throw off the foreign and noxious matter received into the body." P. 98.

The general indications for treatment deduced from the foregoing views are embodied in several propositions, as follows:—

"*a.* Remove all causes by whose influence the typhus process is generated, and all conditions which experience teaches might promote its malignancy. Hence, all the hygienic prescriptions, change of abode, strict attention to ventilation, &c. &c., to which we shall return in another place.

"*b.* Counteract the assumed primitive cause of the disease, the altered state of the blood, so that it may be kept within the limits necessary to render the preservation of life possible.

"*c.* Act upon these symptoms from whatever organ they may proceed, which are developed with such intensity as to require special attention, and which may not be comprised under the preceding indication.

"*d.* Promote convalescence, when once commenced, to which it also belongs to treat the sequelæ, and endeavour as far as possible to prevent their development." P. 100.

The plan of management which the author adopts is thus eminently expectant. He has no confidence in abortive measures, nor in our ability by any mode of treatment as yet discovered, to shorten the career of the disease.[1] The cases which prove abortive he explains by "the supposition that the power of resistance in the system is strong enough to eliminate the noxious matter in some way or other without the aid of a complete pathological process."

In recommending particular measures or remedies, Prof. Huss does not undertake to furnish numerical results. To this, however, we are not disposed to take exceptions. The eduction of therapeutical principles from statistical researches in many diseases is attended with difficulties which render this method of investigation but little available; but its applicability to continued fever is especially limited for the following reasons. Statistics show that the mortality, both from typhus and typhoid fever, varies greatly at different times and places when patients are situated under precisely the same circumstances, so far as the latter are appreciable, and treated in precisely a similar manner. The tendency to a fatal issue is great in some seasons, or during particular epidemics, and slight in others, without our being able to account for the disparity in this respect. Hence, the rate of mortality is not reliable evidence of success or failure as regards the influence of medication on the termination of the disease. Duration does not afford a test of the superiority, or otherwise, of particular methods of treatment, for it is generally conceded that we cannot expect to abridge the career of these diseases. So far as any inferences may be drawn from mortality or duration, they are negative rather than positive. We are warranted in concluding from a small number of deaths, and a duration falling below the average, that our therapeutical measures have not exerted an unfavourable influence. There is, however, a way in which numerical investigation may lead to certain positive conclusions, viz: enumerating the instances in which the apparent *immediate* effects of remedies denote either benefit or injury. In other words it would be practicable, with due care and patience, to determine by means of the ana-

[1] It is an interesting fact that medical science has discovered means of arresting fevers which have not a limited career, viz., the periodical fevers, while we are unable to cut short or abridge those which end after a certain period from intrinsic limitations. In the latter class are the eruptive and continued fever, to which may be added yellow fever.

lysis of recorded cases the *juvantia et lædentia* with greater precision than belongs to merely the general impressions based on recollected experience. This application of statistical research has been hitherto not sufficiently appreciated.

Of the therapeutical details contained in the portion of the work under reviewal, we shall enumerate the more important, stopping to notice, briefly, certain points which, from their novelty or the emphatic testimony of the author, we may presume will be of interest to our readers.

Emetics, which were formerly much in vogue in the treatment of the early stage of continued fevers, have, we believe, in this country, nearly passed out of use. Prof. Huss regards them as injurious in most cases, being indicated only when the stomach happens to be overloaded at the time when the patient is attacked with the disease. He has found no favourable results, in general, from the purgative method of treatment. Cathartics are indicated only when there is evidence of a considerable congestion of brain, together with more or less violent delirium, and under these circumstances only during the first three days. The cathartics which he is accustomed to employ are castor oil, calomel, and the sulphate of soda.[1]

After a fair trial of general bleeding, he states that his experience entirely condemns its use. He has not found it to relieve violent delirium, nor to be useful when the disease becomes complicated with pulmonary inflammation. Topical bleeding by leeches or cupping, on the other hand, he regards as often beneficial when congestion of the brain or spinal marrow is supposed to be marked; in capillary bronchial catarrh, and when considerable tension and tenderness exist over the ileo-cæcal region. Local bleeding, however, as a rule, is not judicious after the fifth day, in consequence of the liability to produce undue prostration of strength.

In cases characterized by determination to the head, and active delirium in the early stage, he has found the ice-cap frequently highly serviceable. If the patient be conscious he is guided in its use and continuance by his sense of relief, or otherwise. When cerebral symptoms are prominent, mustard poultices to the thighs, calves, neck, or back, often afford relief. Hot embrocations of turpentine constitute an eligible means of revulsion over the abdomen when the abdominal symptoms are prominent, and over the chest when pulmonary complications occur. Blisters, as a rule, are to be condemned; they are only indicated when grave cerebral symptoms are present, applied, under these circumstances, to the back of the neck.

He attaches considerable importance to the application of compresses wetted in cold water over the abdomen in cases of typhoid fever. He says: "I do not hesitate to assert that it is one of the most important remedies in treating abdominal typhus." Following the application of mustard or hot turpentine, he thinks they counteract the tendency to meteorism, lessen the diarrhœa, and even render perforation of rarer occurrence than when they are omitted. The compresses may be covered with oiled silk to restrain evaporation, or with several thicknesses of dry linen, and are to be wetted as often as they become dry. They are applied over the chest with advantage when bronchitis or pneumonia become developed in the course of the fever.

[1] From a limited trial in cases that have, within the past eighteen months, fallen under our observation, we are disposed to think favourably of the use of saline laxatives when the abdominal symptoms, especially tympanites, are prominent. We witnessed their apparently salutary effects in several instances in Paris during the summer of 1854, and we were informed that they are generally employed, under the circumstances mentioned, in the Parisian hospitals.

The administration of the mineral acids, more especially the phosphoric, is regarded as a highly important part of the treatment. Of the phosphoric acid the author says:—

"The physicians of France and England [and America may be added] seem very seldom to make use of this acid in treating typhus. In Germany, its use is often spoken of, and in Sweden it is at present the remedy which the physicians most commonly employ. Swedish experience certainly does not weigh much in the balance of science. I think, however, that in this matter it merits being tried as well by the physicians of France in treating typhus abdominalis, as by those of England in the treatment of typhus petechialis."

Theoretically, he regards the mineral acids as indicated by alterations of the blood consisting in diminished fibrin[1] and increased carbonated salts, especially soda. The blood undergoes in these fevers changes similar to those found to take place in animals which have for a long period taken alkalies, and, under these circumstances, it is supposed that acids concur in restoring it to a natural state. As the phosphoric acid in the treatment of typhus and typhoid fever will be to many of our readers a new remedy, we subjoin the author's mode of administration. ℞. Solut. acidi phosphor. ʒii–iii; decoct. althææ, ℥iv; syrup, ℥iii. M. S. A tablespoonful to be taken every other hour.

The *solutio acidi phosphorici* of the Swedish Pharmacopœia contains 25 per cent. of the phosphoric acid. The muriatic and sulphuric acids may also be employed, but the author gives a decided preference to the phosphoric.[2]

Turpentine is extolled as a valuable remedy in cases in which bronchial catarrh is prominent, and when pneumonia becomes developed. It may be administered in emulsion or in capsules. The author remarks, "Before one has tried the turpentine under these conditions it would seem *à priori* that it ought to act as an irritant as well on the mucous membrane of the stomach and intestines as on the circulating and nervous systems. Experience shows us the reverse, or if its action be irritating, this irritation must be beneficial, as I never saw it do harm, where the contra-indications stated above" (redness of the tongue, active delirium and determination to the head) "had been observed, but in a considerable number of cases it has acted advantageously in the most marked manner." Our readers need not be reminded of the fact that in this country turpentine is by many considered as a highly useful remedy with express reference to the typhoid intestinal affection. For this object it is strongly recommended by Prof. Wood.

Active delirium, which the author attributes (but incorrectly as we suppose) to congestion of the brain, is treated by ice to the head, cupping on the neck, mustard poultices to the extremities, and the tartrate of antimony. The remedy last named, more particularly since the strong testimony by Dr. Graves, of Dublin, to its efficiency, in combination with opium, in relieving the delirium of fever, has been much employed by physicians for that end. We can testify from our own experience to its usefulness. We have found the remedy efficacious in less doses than those advised by Dr. Graves. In this respect, our practice coincides with that of the author, who gives from $\frac{1}{4}$ to $\frac{1}{2}$ grain in aqueous solution every other hour. The author cautions against its being too long continued, advising to withhold it after two or three

[1] According to Lehmann, diminution of the fibrin of the blood does not constantly obtain in essential fevers.—*Physiological Chemistry*, vol. i. p. 320, Am. edition.

[2] A medical friend of ours, a practitioner of considerable experience, relies mainly on the administration of alkalies in the treatment of typhoid fever, and claims that the excellence of this method is proved by its success.

days. Generally we have found it sufficient to administer it during the evening or night when the delirium is most apt to be manifested, or when, if constantly present, it is increased.

During the latter part of the disease, or, as the author terms it, the *stadium depressionis*, excitant remedies are often required. He attaches great importance to the sounds of the heart as furnishing an index of the state of the muscular system and vital forces. We quote his remarks on this point.

"To study the sounds of the heart, and especially the first sound, I consider to be very important and very useful in determining the use as well of camphor as of the other excitant remedies. The state of this sound is certainly closely connected with that of the pulse, but I think the ear a more accurate observer of the strength of the heart than the finger of that of the pulse. * * * The weakness of the muscular system in general being a sign of the general *depressio virum*, the weakness of the action of the heart, measured by the change of its sounds, is an accurate, nay the most accurate measure of the general depression, and indicates most exactly the use of excitantia. In cases where the sounds do not undergo any alteration, these are neither indicated nor necessary." P. 147.

The importance of auscultation of the heart, as our readers are aware, has been emphatically inculcated by Dr. Stokes, with whose writings American physicians are familiar, but we suspect that it is less resorted to in practice than its importance claims.

Among the remedies of the excitant class which may be usefully administered, when the indications are present, the author notices camphor, the carbonate of ammonia, musk, and phosphorus.

Of diffusible or alcoholic stimulants wine only is mentioned, and this is very sparingly given. He says: "I allow only so much to be mixed with the drink as to give to it a slight taste, the whole quantity allowed in a day being one or two wineglasses. Port and sherry are the kinds I have used; its effect must, however, be closely watched, and if the wine excite too much, it must no longer be given."

Were it consistent with our plan to enter into discussions concerning therapeutical principles and remedies, we should take issue with the author on the use of stimulants. So far from the great circumspection in their use which he enjoins being necessary, we are satisfied that, when sustaining measures are indicated, they may be administered more or less freely, according to the indications, so as to render the excitant remedies just referred to of subordinate importance, and even comparatively useless. We say this on the strength of considerable experience. As a rule, we think spirits are to be preferred to wine. The circumstances which denote the propriety of stimulants, and the extent to which their use is to be carried, are, of course, in a practical point of view, of great importance; but to consider them here would be a digression from our present object, which is simply to give a summary of the more important points pertaining to treatment which are contained in the work under reviewal.

Under the head of tonics, the author mentions only quinia. This holds, in his estimation, a low rank among the remedies indicated in typhus and typhoid fever. He has no confidence in the power which has been claimed for it of cutting short a continued fever as it does an intermittent or remittent. When this result follows, either the disease would have aborted without the remedy, or there has been an error of diagnosis. Continued through the whole career of the disease, as is the custom with some practitioners, he thinks it may act injuriously, especially in the second stage. The conditions under which it may be given with advantage are contained in the following extract:—

"When the excitantia have been given, and the symptoms against which these were prescribed are subdued, but the fever nevertheless continues, and the strength is very low, without any sign of approaching improvement; the pulse continues frequent and irritable, the skin either dry and rough, or covered with clammy perspiration, the spleen more or less swollen, but the tongue clean and moist, the quinine is in its place. Also, when, in consequence of the intestinal ulcerations, or suppurating ulcerations elsewhere, a state resembling pyæmia is developed, as well as in the cases where there exist marked remissions in the fever, which is not seldom seen in typhus cases occurring during a prevalent epidemic of intermittent." P. 155.

The following quotation contains all that is said under the head of dietetic rules:—

"The dietetic direction during the first stage being in conformity with the patient's own feelings, is limited to abstinence from food; the same proceeding is not quite so applicable during the second. My experience has shown that the patient then feels well from taking some food, although it must be of the simplest and mildest kind. For drink I allow warm milk from the beginning of this stage, mixed with carbonated water in equal parts, or soups of oats, sago, rice, also mixed with this water, and some wine, according to circumstances. Later in this stage, small quantities of chicken or veal broth are given—a tablespoonful several times a day. We must, however, carefully watch its effects, as should the broth seem to excite too much, its use must be suspended. Jellies, animal and vegetable, too expensive to be employed at hospitals, are in private practice very useful during this stage, if given in small quantities, and often repeated." P. 177.

The author evidently does not appreciate the importance attached, of late years, by some British and American writers (amongst whom the late Dr. Graves is especially to be mentioned), to alimentation in the treatment of fevers. For many years we have been satisfied that the administration of concentrated nutriment, in conjunction with stimulants, constitutes a branch of the management which, in general, ranks above all other measures. With the added experience of each year, we are the more convinced of the advantage of (to use Dr. Graves' expression) "feeding fevers." The practice of Prof. Huss in this respect is well as far as it goes, but it does not go far enough; and he interposes restraining cautions, which, in our opinion, are gratuitous. Alimentary analeptics are admissible earlier than he advises, and are useful by way of forestalling prostration. It is better to run the risk of entering on sustaining measures too soon than of deferring them too long, for it is easy to suspend their use if they are found to do harm, while lost time cannot be regained. So when they are indicated by existing prostration, the injury from an inadequate supply of stimulants and nutriment is vastly greater than from excess, provided the effect is watched, and the quantities thereby graduated.

The author devotes a distinct section to the treatment of special symptoms. We do not, however, find under this head aught which, from its novelty, interest, or importance, claims particular notice. The same remark is applicable to the management of convalescence, and of the *sequelæ*.

Although, in commencing to write this article, we did not intend to be hampered by a constant regard for brevity, we have occupied somewhat more space than we had contemplated; but we trust not more than, in the judgment of the reader, is due to the scientific interest and practical importance of the subjects, especially that to which the larger portion of our remarks has been devoted, viz., the non-identity of typhus and typhoid fever. In taking leave of the work by Prof. Huss, we must confess that it has disappointed our expectations, not because the author contends for the unity of continued fever, but in consequence of the manner in which he has treated this subject. Purporting to be a work devoted to statistics of typhus and typhoid fever, embodying the experience of several years at a large hospital, we had hoped to find the question of the identity or non-identity of these affections tested anew by a comparison of the results of the numerical analysis of a series of cases of each fever separately; and we were anxious to see whether the results of observations made in the capital of Sweden would correspond or differ from those obtained in France, England, and America. Instead of this, the work, so far as this question is concerned, only gives the opinions of the author, backed by whatever authority may be derived from the fact that he has seen and treated a large number of cases of both forms of fever. The force which belongs to such opinions different persons will undoubtedly estimate differently. We do not, however, hesitate to attach to them small importance when brought into antagonism with conclusions reached by the analytical investigation of recorded cases. The statistics relating to both typhus and typhoid fever indiscriminately possess a certain value, provided these affections are identical; otherwise they are comparatively valueless.

With the portion of the work devoted to treatment, we are less dissatisfied. Although there is here room for criticism, the therapeutical views which the author advances, and the pathological notions on which they are founded, are, we believe, in the main, in accordance with the opinions and practice of the most intelligent and judicious practitioners of the present time.

A. F.

ART. XII.—*Chimie Appliquée à la Physiologie et à la Thérapeutique.* Par M. le Docteur MIALHE, Pharmacien de l'Empereur, Professeur Agrégé à la Faculté de Médecine, &c. &c. Paris, 1856.

M. MIALHE's book is a reproduction, in great measure, of separate essays published by him at various intervals between 1840 and 1850; and it is remarkable to see how many of his physiological doctrines, whether adopted or original, which have been either modified or entirely superseded by the advance of the science since the date of their first appearance, are retained by the author, and re-stated with as much confidence as ever. After passing through, in the introductory pages, with some general considerations on the character of the chemical changes taking place in the healthy body, and the proper mode in which they are to be studied, he takes up, in the first chapter, the consideration of the phenomena of oxidation and nutrition—commencing with those of oxidation. He makes a division of all the alimentary substances according to Liebig's celebrated hypothesis, into *plastic* and *respiratory* elements. Of these, the former are mostly used in the nutrition of the tissues, and the latter—such as sugars and oils—almost completely destroyed by direct oxidation in the blood; terminating, therefore, soon after their ingestion, in the production of water and carbonic acid. The very important objections to this doctrine, which have recently been acknowledged by the leading physiologists, seem to have nearly or quite escaped the author's notice. He speaks constantly of those substances which, on being taken into the system, do not reappear in the excretions, as necessarily "burnt" in the circulation; and regards the natural heat of the body as the result of the same combustive process. These are all opinions which were adopted some time since, and are now modified or abandoned in consequence of their resting too evidently on insufficient data; several very important links in the proof being entirely wanting, or supplied only by inference. There is one theory, however, advanced by M. Mialhe, in this connection, which is, we think, a novelty, and at the same time a striking instance of the common, but very dangerous practice of inferring a chemical reaction to take place in the body without any direct proof, and simply because its materials exist there. It is in regard to the mode of action of various poisonous substances, and particularly of hydrocyanic acid. The author, after speaking of the constancy and rapidity with which the "intravascular oxidation" goes on in the body, and its importance to the continuance of life, goes on to remark, that any substance which should interfere with this oxidation, would, by that fact alone, become poisonous. Some substances actually do, as he thinks, have such an effect. Chloroform and sulphuric ether, for example, introduced into the blood, are thought to displace its oxygen in this manner, and to suspend life, during the continuance of their anæsthetic effect, by simply arresting the process of combustion. The volatile oils are considered as liable to exert the same influence by reason of their avidity for oxygen; and sulphuretted, seleniuretted, and arseniuretted hydrogen also act by depriving the blood of its oxygen, while they are at the same time converted into other compounds, poisonous by themselves.

"We can very easily understand, then," says M. Mialhe (p. 29), "how rapidly fatal would be the operation of any substance which should have the power of seizing at once upon all the oxygen contained in the blood, and destined for the supply of respiration and nutrition. Such would be the action of phosphorus, provided it were possible to administer this body in a gaseous condition. The same effect would be produced by any substance endowed with the property, without itself becoming oxidized, of suddenly putting an end to the process of intravascular combustion. Such a poison would act on the living body like a stroke of lightning. Now we know there is a poisonous substance, whose operation is in reality like that of a stroke of lightning, viz: hydrocyanic acid. It results from the researches of M. Millon that this acid has a remarkable tendency to interfere with certain phenomena of oxidation, or combustion; and that, even in very small quantity, it prevents entirely the powerful combustive action of iodic acid upon oxalic acid. Considering the relation which exists between the two phenomena of respiration and oxidation, we may conclude that the only effect of hydrocyanic acid, introduced into the organism, is to cut short the process of vital oxidation, and produce in that way an instantaneous death."

It would be difficult to imagine a physiological theory more destitute of direct evidence than this; or one which depended for its support upon remoter analogies.

In his chapter on the *digestion of starchy substances*, M. Mialhe reproduces almost entirely the opinions which he professed ten years ago with regard to the importance of "animal diastase," or the organic substance of the saliva, and its identity with vegetable diastase, as well as with the organic matter of the pancreatic juice. He was among the first to extract this substance from the saliva, and to recognize its power of transforming starch into sugar. He still continues to attribute to it a very important part in the chemical processes of digestion, though this opinion is now, and has been for some years, generally abandoned, for experimental reasons which do not seem to be regarded by the author as having the importance which is usually attributed to them

The question of the *origin of sugar* in the animal economy is disposed of in a still more loose and unsatisfactory manner. M. Mialhe contents himself with stating, in very concise terms, the important doctrine maintained by Bernard, that a certain quantity of sugar is constantly produced in the liver from metamorphosis of the elements of the organ itself; and then proceeds to express his dissent from it in the following brief terms:—

"For our part, we cannot share the opinions of M. Bernard. For us, the liver is not a secreting organ for the sugar, but only an apparatus of condensation, in which the sugar accumulates, after being taken with the food; in the same manner as the liver also condenses in its tissue certain metallic poisons introduced into the economy." (P. 61.)

The many experiments performed and reported by Bernard, in opposition to this very objection, and the long contest carried on, during the past year, before the French Academy on the whole question, in which Longet, Figuier, Bernard, and Lehmann all took a part, and during which a special committee investigated the matter and reported favourably to Bernard, are all passed over in silence; though they ought certainly to have some weight in deciding so very interesting a physiological question.

In his concluding paragraph of this section the author also misrepresents Bernard's doctrine in a very singular manner:—

"If the sugar be not derived," he says (p. 61), "exclusively from amylaceous elements of the food (since it is now demonstrated that muscular flesh and the white of egg contain a certain quantity of it), it is nevertheless an undeniable fact, admitted by M. Bernard himself, that the quantity of sugar existing in the organism is in direct proportion to the quantity of starchy matters absorbed from the digestive apparatus. So the liver, whether it be a secreting or simply a condensing organ, derives after all from the food the saccharine elements which it supplies to the circulation."

This is certainly unjust, both to Bernard and his doctrine; for one of the points upon which he most positively insists is, that the liver is *not* dependent for its saccharine supply upon starchy matters in the food; that as much sugar is produced by it under an animal as a vegetable diet; that even after several months' strict regimen on food carefully deprived of amylaceous matters, it is still as abundant as when the food was of a mixed character; and that, finally, the sugar of the liver, instead of being derived from any starchy elements, is produced in the tissue of the organ itself, by a transformation of its own substance. (Bernard, *Nouvelle Fonction du Foie*, Paris, 1853.)

In treating of the *destruction of sugar* in the animal economy, M. Mialhe describes first the usual reactions of a saccharine substance when treated, in solution, with acids, alkalies, and metallic salts, and particularly its power of reducing the salts of copper, when heated in an alkaline solution. Sugar alone, he observes, will not produce any reduction of the oxide of copper; but in order to produce this effect it must be accompanied with an alkali or alkaline carbonate. The body which becomes oxidized, therefore, at the expense of the copper, is not the sugar itself, but the new substances (ulmic, formic, and glycic acids) into which it has been previously converted by contact with the alkali. He regards the phenomenon of the reduction of metallic compounds which sometimes takes place in the body (as in the case of the salts of copper, red ferrocyanide of potassium, &c.) as owing to the presence of the formic and ulmic acids, &c. into which the sugar has been converted by the alkaline carbonates of the blood. It is in this way that he arrives at the following theory of the natural transformation of the sugars in the circulation:—

"On its arrival in the blood the glucose decomposes the alkaline carbonates, forming with their bases new compounds, *glycosates*, and setting free their carbonic acid; the glycosates, which are unstable compounds, are rapidly transformed into glycic, ulmic, and formic acids, or rather into glyciates, ulmiates, formiates, which combine with the oxygen of the blood, and undergo a veritable combustion, with the production of water and carbonic acid." (P. 67.)

The above theory of the destruction of sugar in the blood will be found, on examination, to rest on four successive propositions, each essential to its establishment, and all of them more or less hypothetical:—

1. In the reduction of copper from an alkaline saccharine solution, the alkali acts by first converting the sugar into ulmic, glycic, and formic acids.

2. When metallic salts, and particularly those of copper, are reduced in the animal economy to a lower state of oxidation, the agents of this reduction are the ulmic, glycic, and formic acids.

3. These acids are produced *from the sugar of the blood* by the action of the alkaline carbonates.

4. And finally, the water and carbonic acid, expelled from the system, are (partly) formed by direct oxidation of the above acids.

None of the above propositions are free from doubt. With regard to the first, though the presence of an alkali be certainly necessary to the operation of Trommer's test for glucose, we are not aware that its precise mode of action, as above described, rests on anything more than inferential grounds.

In the second place, the reduction of metallic salts, when it occurs in the animal economy, may certainly be owing to the action of other bodies beside formic acid, &c. The albuminoid substances themselves absorb oxygen with great readiness under every ordinary condition, and may even produce, by their presence, a partial reduction in the solution of copper, used as Trommer's test. Thirdly, formic acid has undoubtedly been found in the blood and various other fluids of the body; but its source is unknown. Even in the red ants, from which it was formerly obtained in the greatest abundance, it is yet quite uncertain whether it be produced in the body of the insect, or introduced with the food from some vegetable source. And, lastly, the direct oxidation of these acids, when present in the body, is itself a matter of doubt. Indeed, formic acid has been found (by Lehmann) in comparatively large quantity in the normal perspiration. If it were, therefore, so readily oxidizable in the system as to reduce the salts of copper, when these are present, it is not easy to understand how it should itself escape destruction by the free oxygen of the blood, and arrive unaltered at the surface of the skin.

The theory of the mode of disappearance of the animal sugars, adopted by M. Mialhe, conducts him very readily to an explanation of the morbid phenomena of diabetes. In health, the normal sugars of the blood are destroyed by the influence of its alkaline carbonates. Anything which diminishes the alkalescence of the blood will therefore tend to produce an accumulation of sugar in the system, and a consequent diabetic condition of the blood and all the secreted fluids. M. Mialhe does not hesitate, therefore, to attribute the condition of diabetes to a preponderance of acids in the system by which the alkalescence of the blood is neutralized, and the oxidation of the sugar prevented. This preponderance may be occasioned, he says, by an abuse of acidulated drinks, by an exclusively azotized diet, or by a suppression of the cutaneous transpiration. Animal food, containing principally compounds of sulphur and phosphorus, gives rise in the body, by oxidation, to sulphuric and phosphoric acids; while vegetable food contains salts of the organic acids (citrates, malates, &c.), which are destroyed by oxidation, leaving a residue of alkaline carbonates. A proper admixture of the two is thought to maintain the natural alkalescence of the blood, while a too great proportion of animal food diminishes or entirely neutralizes it. Finally, the cutaneous transpiration is one channel through which the free acids are eliminated from the system. There are, says M. Mialhe, five secretions with an alkaline reaction, viz., the tears, saliva, bile, and pancreatic and intestinal juices; and three which are acid, viz., the sweat, gastric juice, and urine, by whose constant activity the natural balance between acids and alkalies is preserved. If, however, the cutaneous transpiration be checked, its acid ingredients are retained in the system, the fluids lose their alkalescence, the sugar is not destroyed, and diabetes is the consequence. M. Mialhe therefore "maintains," in a formal manner, "that the cause of diabetes is the want of assimilation of glucose, through an insufficiency of the alkaline principles in the economy." (p. 77.)

We should anticipate at least, then, from so confident a statement, that this want of alkalinity in the blood, in cases of diabetes, had actually been observed; and that this fact served as a basis for the author's opinion. Far from it. M. Mialhe even acknowledges, with an admirable candor, the difficulty of the objection that, in point of fact, the blood of diabetic patients "is never acid or neutral; but always maintains an alkaline reaction;" and the singular manner in which so apparently stubborn a fact is disposed of, is not the least remarkable part of his theory. In the first place, he says it is "exceedingly difficult" to determine by experiment the precise degree of alkalinity of the blood; intimating, therefore, that it may be diminished in diabetes, without our having observed it. But the remaining part of his answer to the above objection is the more important, and its ingenuity deserves a quotation in the author's own words:—

"In the condition of health," he says (p. 76), "the alkalinity of the blood is determined mainly by the alkaline carbonates, but to a slight degree, also, by the alkaline phosphates; these last, notwithstanding their power of restoring the blue colour of reddened litmus, are not included by chemists in the list of alkaline substances proper; and, furthermore, they do not, as we have proved, give rise to the decomposition of glucose. Now it is our belief, that in diabetic patients the blood remains alkaline *because it is rich in phosphates and poor in carbonates*, so that the degree of alkalinity, produced by the presence of the phosphates, is entirely inefficient for the decomposition of the glucose; which can only be effected by the influence of the carbonates."

It is upon such grounds that M. Mialhe rests his theory of the pathology of diabetes.

The remainder of the first portion of the book is occupied with the consideration of the digestion of albuminoid and fatty matters, the endosmotic properties of albumen and albuminose, and the occasional passage of these substances into the excretions and exudations. It contains little that has not been already before the profession, or that is presented in such a way as to excite any great degree of interest.

The remaining chapters constitute by far the most interesting and important portions of the book. They are devoted to the *absorption and chemical transformation in the system of drugs and poisons.* But very little has yet been done in this field. Almost all we know with regard to the subject is, that such and such matters are, or are not, absorbed into the blood; or that they do, or do not, make their appearance in the secretions. The manner of their absorption, and the changes which they undergo before elimination, constitute an extremely important subject, the study of which may be said to be now first commenced in earnest by M. Mialhe. He commences by establishing the principles that no substance can have any action on the living body without being absorbed; and no substance can be absorbed without being liquefied and soluble; and then passes in review the actions of iodine, sulphur, phosphorus, metals and metallic salts, resins, volatile and fixed oils, and the vegetable alkaloids with their salts.

Notwithstanding the very slight solubility of *iodine* in water, when administered internally, or applied to a denuded surface, it rapidly undergoes changes which result in its absorption. A minute portion of it, according to M. Mialhe, is dissolved by the water of the fluids, and is then converted into iodides and iodates by the action of the alkaline carbonates; and, as the iodides of potassium and sodium themselves exert a powerful solvent action on free iodine, a large portion of this at once enters into solution, and, as the author believes, coagulates the animal matters of the fluids; the coagulum afterwards disappearing by the gradual conversion of the iodine into iodides and iodates by the alkaline chlorides and carbonates of the blood and their subsequent absorption. He lays it down, therefore, as a precept, that iodine should never be administered in substance or in alcoholic tincture, in any case where it is our object to produce merely a constitutional effect; since its coagulating tendency is productive of a troublesome local irritation, and interferes, at the same time, with the absorption of the drug. A much better form, under almost all circumstances, is the iodide of potassium, which is already soluble, and does not coagulate or irritate the tissues. Iodide of potassium, as it is usually administered, does, it is true, sometimes produce a considerable degree of gastric irritation; but this is owing, according to M. Mialhe, to the presence of iodate of potass, which not unfrequently, as he says, occurs as an accidental impurity in the iodide of potassium of the shops. This iodate of potass is decomposed by the acid of the gastric juice and its iodine, liberated from union with the potass, acts on the mucous membrane as a coagulating and irritating substance.

Sulphur is thought to be capable of absorption when administered internally, notwithstanding its insolubility in water. The fact seems to be sufficiently proved by its frequently producing a general constitutional excitement in addition to its laxative effect, by the sulphurous odour it communicates to the breath and excretions, and finally by the property which it communicates to the skin, after prolonged administration, of blackening certain metallic substances. This absorption is accomplished by the alkaline carbonates of the intestinal fluids, which transform the sulphur into alkaline sulphurets and hyposulphites, substances which are soluble, and, consequently, directly absorbed into the circulation. Arrived at the skin, these combinations are decomposed by the acid of the perspiration, and hydrosulphuric acid is disengaged if the excreted substance be a sulphuret, and sulphurous acid with free sulphur if it be a hyposulphite. Whether sulphur be administered by the stomach or by the endermic method, therefore, the author recommends that it be always associated with an alkali (potass, carbonate of magnesia, or soda), in sufficient quantity to neutralize the acid reaction of the gastric or cutaneous fluids, and in addition to form soluble sulphurets and hyposulphites with the drug.

Phosphorus, equally insoluble in water with sulphur, is thought to be absorbed by a very similar process, being converted by the alkaline intestinal juices into phosphoretted hydrogen and hypophosphites of soda and potass. It should therefore be given dissolved in oil or ether, in order that it may be thoroughly exposed to the contact of the intestinal fluids, and its transformation into soluble substances effectually secured.

Arsenic, in a metallic state, is regarded as entirely insoluble, incapable of absorption, and without action on the living tissues; but nevertheless as practically a very poisonous substance, because it readily becomes oxidized and converted into arsenious acid. M. Mialhe has convinced himself not only that metallic arsenic readily gives rise to arsenious acid when exposed to the contact of moist air, or water containing air in solution, but also that this oxidation is much facilitated by the presence of the chlorides of potassium or sodium; and as the greater part of the animal fluids contain both oxygen and the alkaline chlorides, powdered metallic arsenic must, when introduced into the body, always give rise to more or less arsenious acid, and become absorbed under that form.

In the treatment of arsenical poisoning, the antidote which has heretofore been regarded with most favour is the hydrated peroxide of iron. M. Mialhe proposes, as much more efficacious, the *hydrated sulphuret of iron*, which produces by decomposition an insoluble sulphuret of arsenic and a peroxide of iron. He says that a comparative experiment with these two substances and a solution of arsenious acid shows that the hydrated sulphuret of iron decomposes the poisonous substance much more rapidly than the hydrated oxide. The insoluble sulphuret of arsenic is, however, slowly reconvertible into arsenious acid by the chlorides of the intestinal juices; and the antidote should therefore be always administered in excess, in order to guard against such an accident. The great advantage, however, of the hydrated sulphuret of iron, and for which M. Mialhe particularly recommends it, is, that it is an antidote, not only for arsenic, *but also for all the metallic salts liable to be used as poisons, except cyanide of mercury*—reducing, in the same manner with arsenic, the salts of copper, lead, tin, antimony, bismuth, mercury, and silver; so that in any case of doubt as to the precise nature of the metallic poison which had been administered, it would be infinitely safer as an antidote than the hydrated peroxide.

In treating of the mode of action of the different preparations of *iron*, the author considers it as certain that nearly all of them are efficacious, to a certain extent, as remedies, and more particularly in the regeneration of the blood-globules in chlorotic patients. Those preparations which are insoluble in water, are mostly soluble in the acids of the gastric juice, and act afterward in the same manner as the soluble compounds. The mode in which he imagines the metallic preparation, however, to produce its final result, is a little complicated. He finds, in the first place, that all the soluble salts of iron, without exception, precipitate with the animal matters of the gastric juice. The insoluble preparations, including metallic iron, are first dissolved by the acid of the gastric fluids, and then precipitate at once, like the former, so soon as these fluids are in excess. A small portion of the iron, however, escapes precipitation, is taken up by the blood, and meets there with the alkaline carbonates, by which it is decomposed; the insoluble oxide of iron which is set free being appropriated by the blood-globules, and prevented by its insolubility from escaping by the secretions. It is in this way, according to the author, that it contributes to the regeneration of the blood-globules and the cure of chlorosis.

According to this theory, the only preparations of iron useful in the treatment of chlorosis, are those whose compounds, dissolved in the gastric juice, and absorbed into the blood, are decomposable by the alkalies, leaving an insoluble oxide to be retained in the system—such as metallic iron and its oxides, chlorides, bromides, iodides, and, without exception, all its oxysalts. On the other hand, those preparations, such as ferrocyanide of potassium, not decomposable by the alkalies of the blood, remain soluble, pass into the secretions, and merely traverse the body without producing any therapeutical effect. The preparation which the author regards as the most efficacious is the *double tartrate of iron and potass*, which he prefers for the following reason: All the other oxysalts, as has just been mentioned, after allowing a minute quantity to be absorbed from the stomach, precipitate with an excess of gastric juice, and pass into the intestine. Here they are decomposed by the alkaline fluids of the intestine, and the whole remaining iron set free in the form of an oxide, which passes through the intestine unaltered, and is discharged with the fæces. The only one of these preparations not decomposable by the alkalies is the tartrate of iron and potass. It therefore continues to be absorbed through the entire length of the intestine, and introduces into the blood a much larger quantity of iron, for the same dose, than can be the case with any of the other preparations. Once introduced into the blood, however, its tartaric acid is destroyed by oxidation, replaced by carbonic acid, and the carbonate of iron is then decomposed by the alkalies, and its oxide retained in the system, as already described.

How much of the above is the result of direct experiment, and how much inferential, it is not always easy to determine from the author's account. He starts, however, with some very grave errors, which detract considerably from the value of his conclusions. He regards, for instance, the two following facts as "incontestablement acquis à la science."

1. "The globules of the blood contain a combination of iron; *no other part of the living body contains iron.*" (P. 285.)

It should hardly have escaped the recollection of the author that, at the present day, iron has been demonstrated to exist, in the healthy condition, in the urine, the sweat, saliva, gastric juice, and bile, as well as in the blood-globules.

2. "The combination of iron contained in the globules presents the reactions of an *oxygenated compound* of the metal;" from which the conclusion is drawn that the iron is combined with the globules under the form of an oxide.

The grounds, however, upon which this opinion was first adopted, have been found to be quite insufficient; and it is now acknowledged by the first authorities in organic chemistry, that we are entirely ignorant as to the particular combination under which iron exists in the blood-globules. (Lehmann, Robin and Verdeil.)

Although these errors, however, may invalidate the author's theory with regard to the ultimate mode of action of the compounds of iron in the system, they do not necessarily impair his conclusions as to their mode of absorption, or the superiority which he claims for the tartrate of iron and potass over the other ferruginous preparations.

The researches of the author on the *preparations of lead* bring him to the conclusion that they are all, as well as metallic lead, when introduced into the digestive canal, acted on by the alkaline chlorides of the intestinal juices, and converted into chloride of lead; this again unites with the excess of chlorides remaining, so as to produce a double chloride of lead and potassium or sodium. This "alkaline chloro-plombate" is distinguished from the simple chloride of lead by being more soluble than it, and not forming any precipitate with an albuminous fluid. It is therefore much more readily absorbed, and enters freely into the circulation. When, therefore, any soluble and coagulating saturnine preparation—as, for example, the subacetate of lead—is taken into the stomach, its first effect is to precipitate with the albuminous matters of the digestive fluids. But it is afterward decomposed by the chlorides, and absorbed under the form of a double chloride into the circulation.

A very interesting series of experiments are reported by M. Mialhe, which he undertook with the view of ascertaining whether any of the compounds of lead could be given off as gaseous exhalations when mixed with spirits of turpentine. It has been thought that paints, having compounds of lead for their basis, when used with volatile oils, might give rise while drying to emanations containing lead, and become poisonous by inhalation. M. Mialhe has demonstrated, however, by a very ingenious and satisfactory contrivance, that this is not the case; and that any injurious effects produced by such emanations must be attributed to the spirits of turpentine, since they contain no lead that can be chemically demonstrated, even when examined in a very concentrated form.

One of the most important chapters in the book relates to the action of the *mercurial compounds*. According to the author's investigations, all the preparations of mercury in use as medicinal agents, are converted, to greater or less extent, by the chlorides of the animal juices, into corrosive sublimate; and that, whatever be the compound employed, the bichloride is the only active agent in the production of its constitutional effects. He finds that calomel, exposed to the action of a solution of chloride of sodium and sal ammoniac, produces, at the end of twenty-four hours, a quantity of corrosive sublimate, which varies according to the amount of alkaline chlorides present, and the elevation of the temperature at which the mixture is kept. Similar results were obtained with the other preparations of mercury. The addition of various organic matters—sugar, gelatine, albumen, &c. to the mixture, sometimes retarded, but never entirely prevented the reaction. It even took place when calomel was mixed with the serum of the blood; and finally, the author has reason to believe that he has detected bichloride of mercury in the urine, after calomel had been administered by the stomach. The bichloride itself, then, in minute doses, if managed with prudence, might replace all the other preparations of mercury. Still, calomel has some practical advantages, which will probably enable it always to retain its place as a therapeutical agent. Taken into the stomach in an insoluble form, it is very slowly and gradually tranformed into the bichloride, and constantly absorbed in successive minute doses during its entire passage through the intestinal canal. Its local action is, therefore, very mild, and an overdose is not liable to be attended with any serious results, since the amount of bichloride produced is not in proportion to the calomel ingested, but to the quantity of the chlorides which it meets with in the intestine; and these never occur in so concentrated a form as to produce dangerous results. The different preparations of mercury are, therefore, more or less active in proportion to the readiness with which they become converted into corrosive sublimate under the influence of the alkaline chlorides. M. Mialhe arranges them in the order of their activity, as follows: First, the bichloride itself; then the biniodide, the red oxide of mercury, calomel by precipitation, calomel by sublimation, the protiodide, and lastly metallic mercury. The protiodide is usually regarded as more active than it really is, because, according to the author, when prepared according to the method of the French Codex, it always contains, as an impurity, more or less of the biniodide, sometimes amounting to eight, or even ten per cent. of its weight.

The author directs the attention of the profession to two facts in this connection, which are very important in a medico-legal point of view: first, that corrosive sublimate may exist in the dead body, in cases of poisoning, and not be detected by the usual tests; and secondly, it may be detected in the body when it has not been administered during life.

"The method usually adopted by chemists," he says (p. 463), "to detect corrosive sublimate in an aqueous solution, is to extract it with ether. Now, we have ascertained that corrosive sublimate, when accompanied with a notable quantity of binoxide of mercury and an alkaline chloride, *will not dissolve in ether;* such is the mixture which is produced by the addition of a few drops of a fixed alkali to an alkaline chloro-hydrargyrate—that is to say, to a solution containing, at the same time, corrosive sublimate and an alkaline chloride."

The possible detection of corrosive sublimate in the body, when none has been taken by the stomach, results of course from what has already been said of the transformation of all the mercurial preparations by the alkaline chlorides of the intestinal fluids.

In the remaining chapters there are many interesting observations on the preparations of silver, the fixed oils, and vegetable alkaloids, the localization or stagnation of poisons, compatible and incompatible substances, pharmaceutical preparations, and the special mode of action of caustics, astringents, vesicants, purgatives, &c. The whole of this portion of the treatise is extremely suggestive; and though some of the author's conclusions may appear to be founded on too slight grounds—as, for example, what has been already quoted in regard to the preparations of iron—all of them are deserving of attention, and many will probably be more thoroughly established at some future time. The only danger, in this kind of study, lies in anticipating too confidently what reactions will take place in the animal fluids from what we know of their separate ingredients. It cannot be too constantly remembered, that it is impossible to foretell what will be the reaction of any chemical substance in an animal fluid. So many unexpected results have already been obtained from direct observation in this particular as to show the extremely uncertain character of inferential conclusions; and we cannot better express the present and future requisitions of the science, in this respect, than by quoting M. Mialhe's own words :—

"Chemical reactions do not take place with such simplicity and precision in the interior of organized bodies as in the experiments of the laboratory. The human body is not an inactive capsule, a simple test-tube, without influence upon the phenomena which take place in its interior. It is, on the contrary, an exceedingly complicated and movable organization, all of whose conditions and elements must be investigated, ascertained, and reunited, before we can properly appreciate their influence upon any new combinations which may arise; otherwise it is impossible to establish a single reliable conclusion. It is by too often forgetting these principles, and by misconceiving the composition of the animal solids and fluids, that we have sometimes retarded science rather than advanced it, while making a hasty application to physiology of incomplete chemical ideas." J. C. D.

BIBLIOGRAPHICAL NOTICES.

Art. XIII.—*Proceedings of American Medical Societies:—*

1. *Proceedings of the South Carolina Medical Association, at the Extra Meeting in Columbia, July* 5, 1854, *and of the Annual Meeting in Charleston, Feb.* 5, 1855. 8vo. pp. 104.
2. *Transactions of the South Carolina Medical Association, at the Extra Meeting in Greenwood, July* 18, 1855, *and at the Annual Meeting in Charleston, Feb.* 6, 1856. 8vo. pp. 54.
3. *Transactions of the Sixth Annual Meeting of the Medical Society of the State of North Carolina, held at Salisbury, N. C., May,* 1855. 8vo. pp. 40.
4. *Transactions of the State Medical Society of New York, at its Annual Meeting, Feb.,* 1856. 8vo. pp. 254.
5. *Proceedings of the Convention and of the Medical Society of California, held in Sacramento, March,* 1856. 8vo. pp. 36.

1. The proceedings of the Medical Association of South Carolina evince a laudable anxiety on the part of its members to cultivate assiduously the field of observation within their respective circles of practice, and to present the result of their labours as a contribution to the common fund of medical knowledge.

The communications presented at the several meetings of which the volumes before us comprise the *Transactions*, are replete with practical details of great interest and value. To a few of them, it may, perhaps, be objected, that too much space and prominence are given to disquisitions of a purely theoretical character. It is very certain that the chief value of the contributions made to the several State and County Medical Societies, throughout our country, will be in proportion as they present a faithful record of the personal experience and observations of the physicians of each locality, in reference to its prevalent diseases—their character, progress, terminations, and treatment, compared with the topographical peculiarities of the locality; the season at which the diseases were severally observed; the meteorological phenomena that preceded and attended their occurrence; the general character of the population—its pursuits, habits, and condition—and, especially, of that portion of it which appeared to be the most predisposed to suffer from the endemics of the place, or from any epidemic with which it may have been visited. It is only from a series of observations of this character, carefully recorded, year after year, that we are to derive the materials to serve as the basis for a correct natural history of diseases—embracing their etiology, characteristics, progress, and terminations—and from which may be constructed satisfactory views of their pathology, prophylaxis, and therapeutics.

The first communication comprised in the proceedings of the South Carolina Association is on *typhoid dysentery*, by Dr. R. W. Gibbes.

Dr. G. commences with the remark, which has also been made by other physicians, that typhoid disease has, of late, greatly increased in the State, though the mortality from it has been less than in the Northern States.

"Within twenty years," he remarks, "typhoid pneumonia has extended in all directions, and may now be found in all localities, and at all seasons. In the early part of my practice, I well remember, that for eight or ten years I never saw a case on a high land plantation, nor at any season than winter, while there has been a gradual extension from the swamps and creeks, where I had patients by hundreds, to the driest and most salubrious uplands, and to the town, in all sorts of weather, even in the midsummer heat, or the pleasant time of spring and autumn. We have yet to learn what is the cause of this and its kindred disorders. As so many different localities are affected, with every variety of soil and cultivation, the greater probability is that atmospheric influence is more concerned in their production and propagation, than an emanation from the soil. Possibly electrical changes in the air and the earth have a more important influence than is usually allowed, while diet and habits of life are also to be considered."

Dr. Gibbes gives the following as the characteristic symptoms of typhoid dysentery:—

"It comes on with symptoms of depression and debility, not accounted for by a looseness for a day or two, with small discharges of bloody mucus, and a substance resembling a mass of brain and blood beat together; florid at first, but soon acquiring, in bad cases, a bluish appearance, reminding one of a mass of placenta. There is but little fever, and, in the worst cases, none; that is, heat of skin and increase of force in the pulse; where this is the case, I consider the disease less dangerous; the pulse is quick but soft and relaxed, as in typhoid pneumonia, the breathing is but little disturbed. Usually, in the worst cases, the skin is soft and cool, often moist or damp, with a paleness or leaden aspect. The tongue is but slightly changed; in some cases covered with a whitish fur, generally broad and flat, and not more red than usual. In no case have I seen the sharp-pointed, acute, intensely red, raw beef-looking tongue, of acute inflammatory dysentery. The irritability of the rectum is very great, with distressing tenesmus, with twelve to twenty stools in twenty-four hours. In some cases there is persistent irritability of stomach during the whole course of the disease, in others, a soreness and pain in the iliac region, intense at times, but not always present. After a few days, tormina from flatus is a distressing symptom."

Nothing is said as to the average duration of the disease nor the mortality prodneed by it, and in regard to the treatment which was found most successful in its management, we are left to draw our conclusions from the history of three cases which are presented somewhat in detail. The principal remedies employed in these were opiates, astringents, and stimulants, with the oxide of silver and a milk diet. In children, Dr. G. states, that he has found the disease readily controlled by enemata of *nit. argent.* 10 grs. to one ounce of water, repeated every third or fourth hour, with the *oxid. argent.* and opium by the mouth. In some protracted cases he has given, with advantage, the tincture of cantharides, which is a favourite remedy with his friend, Dr. Trezvant, in cases attended with depressed nervous energy. In all his cases Dr. G. gave, freely, mint-toddy or port-wine negus, with solutions of gelatin, chicken-broth, or milk, for diet; articles, he remarks, presenting more nourishment in less compass than vegetable food, and of a kind more easily digested.

The three cases, the histories of which are given in the communication before us, were, we are told, the only fatal ones seen by Dr. G., but as no mention is made of the entire number of cases treated by him, the statement affords us no clue to the general mortality of the disease.

The next paper is entitled a "*monograph*" on *typhoid fever*, by Dr. J. McF. Gaston, of Columbia, S. C. As this monograph purports to present facts and deductions in reference to the particular form of disease of which it treats, derived from the personal experience of the writer, it is necessarily one replete with no trifling amount of interest. Disregarding the theoretical disquisitions to which so large a portion of the paper is devoted, we shall endeavour to give a brief account of such parts of it as have a direct practical bearing.

After noticing the tendency to an increased typhoid character in the diseases of his vicinity, Dr. Gaston remarks, that he recognizes typhoid fever as an essential or primary affection—the several local lesions occasionally found associated with it—whether of the intestines, brain, or lungs, etc., being viewed by him as purely secondary or symptomatic.

Premising a general history of the proper characteristic phenomena of typhoid fever, Dr. G. proceeds to describe several types of the disease, "not specially" coming under the general description, and, "perhaps, not included in the history of symptoms usually given in books of practice."

The first of these types is a fever of low grade, with hot and dry skin; without disturbance of the brain or bowels; with the peculiar typhoid pulse, of only moderate acceleration. The distinctive features of the pulse of typhoid fever, Dr. G. describes as a peculiar, quick, jerking movement of the artery when compressed by the finger. Without this peculiarity of pulse all the other symptoms, usually enumerated in connection with the disease, may be present, without, in the estimation of Dr. G., constituting a case of genuine typhoid fever; but, with this manifestation of irritability in the systolic and diastolic action of the heart, he would recognize the fever were all other traits undeveloped.

"It is, then," he adds, "with such a pulse as this—quickness, independent of frequency—a jerking propulsion of the blood with a perceptible cessation between the pulsations, however frequent, and, at the same time, a fixed uniformity, without much tension or force, that I associate the idea of typhoid fever. When a hot dry skin is associated with this description of pulse of moderate frequency, and *yet without any special local determination*, it must be classed as typhoid fever, and, accordingly, I include it, although differing from the ordinary acceptation of the books. This may progress, and the patient scarcely be confined to bed. A listless, languid, good-for-nothing impression is felt, or there may be a lively appreciation of surrounding scenes, and more than ordinary loquacity, connected with a restless activity of body, but inability to undergo much labour or exercise, without great fatigue and prostration. Both these conditions will be found associated with an abnormal state of the nervous system, and dependent on debility, or want of proper action in the cerebro-spinal centre."

This Dr. G. regards as the primary type of typhoid fever. The second type is one in which the surface of the body, and especially the extremities, is below the natural temperature, and dry; with a pulse decidedly small, feeble, and frequent; stupor; torpid bowels; dark brown, coated tongue, with red edges and tip. The disease apparently verging upon a malignant condition.

A third type is that in which bilious remittent fever, early in the attack, verges gradually into a continued form, and the tongue becomes red at its edges and tip, and covered on its upper surface with a dry brown fur. This form of fever, Dr. G. holds, must be regarded, both as to its pathology and treatment, as genuine typhoid fever; the difference in origin not necessarily constituting a difference in the nature of the pathological condition produced.

Dr. G. confesses his inability to throw any light on the etiology of typhoid fever. It occurs, he remarks, on the plains and in the valleys; amid the highest mountain settlements, and in the boggy marshes; in well-ventilated apartments, and in narrow confined cells; among well-fed luxurious men of leisure, and the robust plain living labouring classes; in males and females, whites and blacks. And yet, when once developed, we know that it is aggravated by certain conditions and mitigated by others, which is a circumstance of great practical importance in reference to its treatment. Dr. G. does not consider the disease contagious, though he believes it may become, in some instances, infectious, by the accumulation of morbid secretions and a vitiated atmosphere about the person of the patient.

The author's views of the pathology of typhoid fever are not very clearly or fully expressed. He would appear to consider the disease as the effect of some depressing influence, the primary action of which is upon the cerebro-spinal axis, from whence he traces the depression of nervous energy characteristic of the premonitory stage.

"We are thus enabled," he remarks, "to afford a rational explanation of the whole train of disturbances, and to apply a treatment which will obviate any serious result in most instances. This may be reckoned an hypothesis, but, if it be one which meets all the conceivable forms of the disease, and which proves itself in practical results, it must strengthen our belief in its correctness. I am aware that some abstruse allusions to the connection of this fever with the ganglionic system have been presented to the public. But, the symptoms presented at the outset of the disease are undoubtedly those of general nervous depression, afterwards of irritation, and subsequently prostration, and in referring them to the cerebro-spinal axis as a source, I am but pursuing a natural channel of association."

In proceeding to the treatment of typhoid fever, Dr. G. considers the remedial measures as they are adapted to, 1st, the premonitory stage; 2d, the stage of development; 3d, the progressive stage; 4th, the decline; and 5th, the convalescence.

In the first stage, he trusts mainly to a solution of bicarbonate of ammonia in gum-water, administered every hour or two during the day, with a Dover's powder at night to insure rest. Other stimulants, he remarks, may, doubtless, be used with advantage, but the carbonate of ammonia is the article he has relied upon in the premonitory stage, and it is with much confidence he recommends its use at this period of the disease.

In the second stage, when the disease has become fully developed, any attempt to arrest the course of the disease will be futile, but we must look for its continuance for a period of perhaps twenty-one days, or even longer. During this period, Dr. G. proscribes bloodletting, whatever may be the apparent indication for its employment; active purgatives, however torpid the bowels; all nauseating and relaxing remedies; the constitutional effects of mercury to the extent of producing salivation; the discharge from a blistered surface, even when counter-irritation may be demanded; and, in short, everything that can have a tendency to lower the vital energies of the patient.

The treatment recommended is careful and assiduous nursing: the abstraction of the patient from all depressing influences, moral and physical; the moderate and cautious administration of stimulants; and a farinaceous, well-regulated diet. When there is bilious complication, Dr. G. directs blue mass, with Dover's powder, assisted, if necessary, in its operation by a gentle enema given next day. When costiveness is present, he gives castor oil, combined with spirits of turpentine. Cooling applications are directed to the head. When there is abdominal distension, attended with tenderness on pressure over the right ilio-cæcal region, benefit will be derived from frictions to the part with camphorated spirits of turpentine. When the tongue is dry, red, and glazed, the best remedy will be spirits of turpentine, in small doses, internally, combined with camphorated tincture of opium and gum Arabic. When diarrhœa occurs, it is to be checked by the acetate of lead and opium by the mouth, and, as an enema, incorporated with starch. As a stimulant and tonic, Dr. G. employs quinia in this stage of the disease, giving it in the dose of from half a grain to a grain, two or three times in the day. In the abortive practice, by the employment of large doses of quinia, at short intervals, he has no confidence; he has tried it faithfully and courageously, but with only partial success in any case.

About the ninth day a crisis usually occurs, and the disease then assumes a milder or a more aggravated character. In the first case a gentle stimulus, such as cracker panada, with the addition of sound Madeira or Port wine, and the maintenance of the bowels in a regular condition by enemeta of corn-meal gruel, is the chief treatment that will be required. But if the disease augments in violence, more active stimulation will be demanded. "It is a matter of much consequence," Dr. G. remarks, "to be regular in the administration of stimulants at this stage of typhoid fever. The condition of the patient should determine the times and quantities, and the increase should be made as the prostration ensues, with the progress of the disease.

"If cerebral disturbance persists, in the progressive stages, a blister to the scalp, as a counter-irritant, will sometimes prove advantageous. But the indications of inflammation should be very positive to justify its application, as the mere functional disturbance will not be relieved by this mode of treatment, and may be aggravated. It is better to err on the safe side, and dispense with it in a doubtful case. I have seen uneasiness and jactitation, with a peculiar stare, and contracted state of the muscles of the face, giving an unnatural expression of countenance, entirely relieved by a free administration of brandy. These symptoms are frequently thought to be connected with inflammation of the brain, but they are really the result of nervous depression, the want of a due excitement of the brain; and when the equilibrium is restored by the influence of the stimulant, the patient becomes composed, and all the functions are performed with greater harmony."

The patient should be properly nourished. Dr. G. prefers, as a general rule, farinaceous articles, reduced to a fluid consistency. When the bowels are not disturbed, ripe fruits may be allowed, and mucilaginous drinks. Large draughts of water, iced or otherwise, have been invariably found to do harm.

"In the progress of typhoid fever, it is essential that the sick-room should be freely ventilated, and that everything about the bed and person of the patient be often changed for dry, fresh, and clean articles. The skin should be cleansed with soap and water every two days, and rubbed with a coarse towel afterwards, until a glow is established on the surface. All the changes of apparel, and the removals from bed, should be attended to by the nurse, with competent assistants, and the effort to do even slight things should be prevented, as the strength of the patient is more apparent than real."

"As the fever begins to decline, the husbanding of the strength is demanded by every means we can avail ourselves of. The patient must not be allowed to sit up too soon. Profuse sweating must be restrained by frictions with dry flannel, on which may be dusted a small quantity of powdered mustard and alum. Coolness of the extremities may be obviated by sinapisms to these parts, or to the spine. Moderate but adequate stimulation is still demanded, with a carefully regulated diet. Dr. G. prefers the use of farinaceous articles until the fever has nearly disappeared, and the appetite has become strong, when he gradually introduces the animal juices, and the more tender articles of a solid kind.

"At the close of the regular course of the fever, exacerbations sometimes occur in the afternoons, or perhaps without much uniformity as to time or frequency. We may give the quinia in the intervals to encourage this tendency, and continue it, in small portions, three or four times a day, as a tonic. Should night-sweats be present, the elixir vitriol may be added to the quinia, and given in conjunction with Port wine. The paroxysms will usually yield under this course, and the patient will forthwith enter upon the stage of convalescence." "A stimulant, with proper attention to diet, is important for a considerable period after the fever has disappeared. Brandy, Port-wine, or Madeira may be used, but Dr. G. has found good French brandy most reliable in this debilitated condition."

We have given, above, a brief outline of the views of Dr. Gaston in relation to the nature and treatment of typhoid fever. For details we must refer to the paper itself, which is well deserving of an attentive perusal. It is true, in many of his opinions, the author is very far from being orthodox, and employs the term typhoid fever in a much wider, though we think more correct sense, than that which has been given to it of late years. The typhoid fever of Dr. G. embraces a form of febrile disease, which, with various important modifications, has, within a short time past, rapidly increased in prevalence throughout the United States. Of this form of fever the monograph before us will be found to furnish a very interesting, though by no means complete account.

As a kind of appendix to the foregoing paper, Dr. Gaston presents some remarks on the criterion for the employment of stimulants.

The proper employment of stimulants as a therapeutic agent, the particular circumstances under which a resort to them is demanded, the extent to which they must be pushed, in any given case, in order that the favourable results they are adapted to produce may be obtained, and the indications for their discontinuance, are questions of no trifling importance, but in relation to which there is a great want of unanimity of opinion among medical practitioners. Even as to the indications for the fulfilment of which a resort to them is demanded, there is little or no agreement among our most authoritative therapeutists. Dr. G. believes that he has discovered a positive and unerring criterion by which the propriety or impropriety of the employment of stimulants in the treatment of disease may be decided. This criterion is the condition of the circulation in the capillaries of the surface, which he supposes to be an index of the condition of the capillary circulation throughout the body.

If the colour of the skin, at a point where pressure has been applied by the finger, is slow in returning, it indicates a want of tone in the capillaries of the surface, and, as Dr. G. infers, of the rest of the system, calling for a resort to stimulation, in proportion to the deficiency of tone thus indicated.

"It is not," he remarks, "when the general cutaneous surface presents the most florid appearance that the lancet is best practised; nor is it when the skin is wanting in colour that I would suggest stimulants. But, in either condition, there may be a debility, indicated by a torpor of the capillaries, when pressure is made by the end of the finger, and under such circumstances, I think, we will rarely be disappointed in resorting to a stimulant. Thus, we are not left to judge of the force, fulness, or frequency of the pulse, nor are we compelled to resort to tentative measures, of very doubtful propriety, but all may be satisfactorily determined, in the majority of cases, by a particular examination of the state of the capillary circulation."

Dr. G. wishes it to be distinctly understood that this criterion for the employment of stimulants has not been sufficiently established by observation to enable him to give any positive assurance as to its results. The subject is open for investigation, and he trusts that others will prove its importance in the treatment of all diseases to which stimulants are applicable.

"This test for the application of stimulants," he adds, "appears simple, but it will require much careful comparison of the healthy with the diseased, of the strong with the weak, and much discrimination between diseases themselves, and their tendencies, to render it useful as a diagnostic. It will require judgment to profit by it in the way proposed, and yet I trust that all these difficulties may be overcome, and that it may prove an adjuvant to other means of discrimination, if not a complete index to the condition of the vital forces."

On *typhoid pneumonia*, by Dr. R. S. Bailey, of Charleston. This paper is occupied, chiefly, by the history of two cases of the disease, to which are appended a few practical remarks.

The succeeding paper is an account of *epidemic dysentery*, as it appeared in the districts of Chester and Lancaster, S. C., during the years 1853–54, by Dr. Mobley, of Lancaster.

This communication is one of considerable interest and value. We regret, however, that the author has neglected to notice any of the circumstances observed during the epidemic of which he is the historian, calculated to throw light upon the etiology of dysentery, and that he has furnished no statistics showing the number of cases observed, the class, age, sex, and colour of the persons attacked, and the amount of mortality produced by the disease.

After very full details of the treatment pursued in the several types under which it presented itself in different cases, Dr. M. remarks:—

"But the most important agent in the treatment of this epidemic, the remedy *par excellence*, was opium, without which all our efforts to control the disease would have been fruitless. I am persuaded that others have confined themselves too much to the doses prescribed by custom, and have dreaded too much the poisonous effects to derive the full benefit of this drug in the management of dysentery. At any rate, the quantity which seems to have been given elsewhere would have fallen short of any visible effect on the disease as it appeared to us. It was an imperative necessity to check, or at least to moderate, the incessant purging, and, above all, to ameliorate the intolerable suffering from tormina and tenesmus, as the patient had been worn out and exhausted, and the vital powers had succumbed." "I have observed that small doses are more apt to excite the brain and nerves, while the larger seem to act as a sedative. Opium was also a grateful stimulant, particularly in the latter stages of the disease, maintaining the equilibrium of the circulation, and diffusing a general glow over the whole body. It thus enabled us to bleed, sometimes, in the early stage, where the pulse would not otherwise admit it. By subduing the erythism of the system, it secured us the chances of blistering, where otherwise it would not have been tolerated. But, above all, it gave us the stimulus of hope. In almost every stage of dysentery we have not so much the brain affected as great mental anxiety and despondency."

In the next paper, Dr. J. McF. Gaston gives the description of an "*abdominal spring pessary*," with drawings illustrative of its construction and application. This pessary is a combination of the stem pessary with the abdominal supporter; the two being united by a spring, which passes downwards from the front piece of the supporter, and curves backwards to be attached to the lower end of the stem pessary. The material of the pessary is silver, hollow within. Below it is a mere tubular stem, of ⅜ inch diameter, which gradually enlarges as it ascends, terminating in a hollow bulb, depressed above and anteriorly, so as to form an oblique concavity, with a rounded rim 6½ inches in circumference. In the depression above there is an opening, from which a tube passes downwards, and out at the lower extremity of the stem. The length of the pessary on its posterior face, from the rim of the bulb to the extremity of the stem, is 4½ inches, and on its anterior face 3⅜ inches. The difference of length on the two faces results from the obliquity of rim of the concave surface, and a slight curvature forwards of the upper portion of the instrument, corresponding with the axis of the pelvis. The largest diameter of the rim is from side to side; its front part is somewhat flattened and obtunded, to obviate collision with the rectum or bladder. An instrument of smaller dimensions may be used with good results when found better adapted to the condition of the parts. The upper portion has been also modified from the hollow bulb to a concavo-convex cup.

The experience of Dr. G. with this apparatus has satisfied him that better results are attainable with its use than from any other means which have been resorted to for the relief of prolapsus uteri and the relaxation of parts connected with it.

"When the apparatus is properly fitted to the person, and the pessary is introduced into the vagina, the neck of the womb rests in the concavity of the upper surface, and the organ is kept in its place by means of the spring attached to the stem, without any tension of the vaginal walls. In the use of all self-retaining pessaries, the vagina is so distended as to overcome its contractile powers, and increase the liability to prolapse after the removal of the instrument. Such a result does not attend this modification of the instrument; the stem is so reduced in size that it causes no dilatation of the rugous coats of the vagina, or of the sphincter. The tube, which affords an outlet to the secretions of the womb, admits, also, of the introduction of medicated injections, which come in contact with the os tineæ, and flowing over the rim of the pessary, are diffused over the entire lining membrane of the vagina. Thus the vaginal walls are contracted, and the broad and round ligaments are restored to their proper tone, and retain the womb in its normal position.

"The abdominal front piece takes off, to a great extent, the downward pressure of the intestines, and a radical cure is promoted, without the restraint and inconvenience which attend the ordinary treatment for prolapsus uteri. Instead of long confinement to the horizontal position, with its concomitant atonic condition of the physical organization, the patient may walk and take healthful exercise in the open air while the apparatus is worn."

The value of the apparatus just described must, of course, be decided by the results of experience. We should fear that more or less irritation will be produced, in the various movements of the patient by whom it is worn, by the stem of the pessary and the external spring at the point where they are connected in the upper commissure of the vulva. We should rather expect also a downward pressure, rather than an opposite effect upon the intestines, and of course upon the womb, by the action of what Dr. G. demonstrates "the abdominal front-piece."

Cases of pseudarthrosis, by Dr. R. W. Gibbes, of Columbia. Three cases are related. In the first, the ununited fracture was of the humerus, about three inches above the condyles. Perfect union was effected by friction of the fractured surfaces, at the end of six weeks. This case is replete with interest throughout. In the second case the ununited fracture was situated about the middle of the right femur. Union was brought about by inserting two steel needles into the unossified callus, and by them piercing and lacerating it freely, then allowing them to remain in for eighteen days. Union took place in about four months. In the third case there was an ununited fracture of both bones of the forearm; union was effected at the end of eight or nine weeks, by a seton introduced between the fractured surfaces.

In the first case phosphate of iron, and in the second, phosphate of lime were freely administered, and Dr. G. believes had a favourable influence in promoting the union of the fractured bones.

The volume closes with the *Address of the President of the Association*, delivered at the annual meeting in 1854.

The address contains some excellent remarks on the importance of medical organization, and the means best adapted to elevate the character and promote the efficiency of the medical profession.

There is one position assumed in the address to which, however, we cannot assent. It is, that the medical profession have no right to expect that any college should require every candidate for the degree of doctor in medicine be perfectly prepared to enter upon the practice of his profession, in all its various departments; inasmuch, as to demand such a proper action for graduation would drive the students from its classes to those of other schools where they can procure the doctorate with less difficulty. Hence all that we can ask of any medical college is, that they shall make their examinations as rigid as they can be made short of driving away the students.

The medical profession have interests which are paramount to the mere pecuniary interests of any or all of the medical schools. They have an unquestionable right to require of every college that those sent forth by it bearing its diploma should be precisely what that diploma declares them to be, individuals well instructed in the theory and practice of medicine. If, before conferring the diploma, they neglect to subject their graduates to an examination, sufficiently rigid to test their qualifications for its reception, they commit a fraud upon the medical profession and the public, and bring the doctorate into such contempt that it becomes no longer a distinction worth the trouble of acquiring. No school has a right to be governed by the will of its students, so far as to lower the grade of its examinations to adapt them to their incompetency; nor can the medical profession be turned aside from its demands for a full and thorough education of all who would desire to enter its ranks, by any fear that a compliance with those demands shall thin the classes and curtail the income of any set of medical teachers.

2. The *Transactions* of the South Carolina Medical Association, at its extra meetings in July, commence with a short but pertinent address by the President, Dr. J. P. Barratt, on the objects of the Association, and the duty of its members to zealously co-operate in their accomplishment.

Then follows a brief account of dysentery, as it has occurred, epidemically, during four consecutive years, in Orangeburg and the adjoining districts. The account was prepared by Dr. Salley.

The disease, we are told, did not seem to select low, damp situations, nor was it of a more intractable character when it did occur in such localities. In 1852, it began in the most elevated portion of Orangeburg.

The grave cases were always indicated by a foul tongue, high fever, frequency of pulse, great soreness over the abdomen, the urgency of the tenesmus, and the number of the evacuations, and if there were no other bad symptoms present, the rapidity of the pulse and rapid emaciation of the patient, were sufficient to excite anxiety for the result. Hiccup was not an unfrequent symptom, but of itself, was not regarded as a grave one; but when connected with a low delirium, and a relaxed state of the sphincter ani, it was the immediate precurser of death.

In the treatment of the epidemic general bleeding was inadmissible. Mercury Dr. S. found to aggravate the worst features of the disease.

The most successful treatment, in the hands of Dr. S. and the physicians of his neighbourhood, was by saline purgatives in very minute quantities. The sulph. sodæ was generally preferred, but not exclusively.

"In mild cases, sulph. sodæ, tinct. opii, each ʒj, in six ounces of water: a tablespoonful every third hour, is a very good prescription. The super tart. potass. in ten grain doses, with one drachm tinct. opii camph. is very much such a formula as the first, and equally efficacious. Dr. S. has used, more than anything else, a powder, made by substituting the sulph. sodæ for the sulph. pot.

in the Dover's powder, and adding two drachms of prepared chalk. The dose is from five to ten grains."

Dr. S. notices, also, a combination of bitart. potass., opium, and ipecac.; ten grains of the former to half a grain of each of the latter, as an admirable remedy, both for its efficacy and convenience. It may, he remarks, be safely relied on in the first stage of a large proportion of cases.

The pulv. nux vomica Dr. S. would not recommend when the stools are all blood, or serum, or blood suspended in serum, but has great confidence in it when the discharges are composed of blood and mucus intimately combined, or of mucus alone; discharges that are always attended with a great deal of tenesmus and pain.

The spirits of turpentine he considers to be a very efficacious remedy in cases attended by frequent discharges of fluid blood. Of the nitrate of silver he cannot speak favourably in the first stage of the disease.

In some bad cases he has known the patient suffer much from dysuria, for which distressing symptom he knows no better remedy than frequent large injections of cold water.

"The treatment of infants and children must be somewhat modified. They bear opiates so badly, that if care be not taken, the remedies will destroy more than they cure. Hyoscyamus should be substituted for opium in all these cases. From half to a grain of hyoscyamus, combined with from three to five grains of sup. tart. pot., I have found to be the best and safest prescription I have ever used. A child is often quieted by allowing him to sit in a tub of water, and by applying warm fomentations to the abdomen."

In the second stage of dysentery, when ulceration has probably occurred in the large intestine, there is great emaciation; very frequent pulse; sometimes cool extremities, with the rest of the surface hot and dry; a dry and often glazed tongue; the discharges are composed of blood and mucus, or they are of a purulent appearance or contain particles of pus. The best remedies in this stage Dr. S. has found to be the spts. of turpentine and nitrate of silver. Iodine, he has reason to believe might be advantageously administered.

Dr. Salley presents a description of a very simple, cheap, and convenient *fracture bed.* It is composed of two ordinary carpenter's trestles, upon which are nailed boards of the requisite length, to support a good wool mattress, covered with a blanket and sheet. A frame of scantling is then to be made, the sides of which are to project two feet beyond the bed. This frame is to be covered by a strong piece of cotton bagging, securely tacked to the side pieces. This is to be covered with a quilt and sheet, through which and the bagging, in a proper position, a hole is to be cut. The frame is to be laid upon the bed, and upon it, the patient. When the latter has a call to evacuate his bowels or bladder, or when it is desirable to cool the parts heated by contact with the bed, two assistants can remove the frame, with the patient on it, and place beneath its two ends a trestle two feet higher than the bed, by which it will be supported as long as is found convenient or necessary.

Dr. Bailey, of Charleston, read an entertaining essay on the want of medical faith and the evils thence resulting, whether the want of faith exist in the patient as to the efficacy of medicines generally, or those employed in his particular case, or as to the skill of his physician, or the want of faith be in the physician as to his competency, or his knowledge of the true nature of any case for which he may be called upon to prescribe. The essay, though it displays neither any great depth of reasoning nor aptness of illustration, is, nevertheless, replete with common sense and every day truths too apt to be overlooked by the members of our profession.

The annual meeting of the Association in 1856, was opened by some pertinent remarks on the condition, importance, and future action of the Association, and the propriety of the entire medical corps of the State lending their co-operation in the furtherance of its objects.

To this succeeds an oration by Dr. E. T. Miles. The theme of the orator is Medical Association, its scope and advantage—the benefits derived from it by the individual members of the profession, by the cause of scientific and practical medicine, and by the best interests of society at large in the augmentation of the means for the prevention and control of disease. Most ably is this interesting theme discussed and enforced, and most eloquently are the physicians of South Carolina urged to render it, by their acts, the efficient instrument for obviating the enfeebling separation of mind from mind, and for enabling our profession to stand forth, with dignified strength, among the formative elements of society, and prevent the intelligence, philosophical bias, and noble aspirations engendered by the pursuits and objects of the true physician to struggle, with divided energy and object, against the forward presumption of the deceitful and secret arts of ignorance and imposture—to make it the means of marshalling the ranks of those enlisted in the cause of legitimate medicine, with renewed vigour, to the work of enlightenment and amelioration.

Two interesting cases are detailed by Dr. Robert Lebby. The first is a case of rupture of the bladder, on its posterior surface, a little below the fundus. The patient was a strong, healthy man, in the vigour of life. On descending a flight of six steps, the heel of his right shoe caught on the edge of the first step and precipitated him forwards; he made a violent exertion to save himself by which he was hurried, without falling, to the bottom of the flight of steps. No inconvenience was experienced for some ten or fifteen minutes, when the patient was seized with a violent pain in the epigastrium, extending to the umbilicus, and attended with swelling of the abdomen. In the course of the ensuing night, he voided per urethram about a gill or more of pure arterial blood. The next day his countenance was pallid and anxiously distressed, surface cold and clammy; great tumefaction of abdomen, hard and unresisting; pulse thread-like, feeble, and frequent; voice husky and hollow; intellect clear; great restlessness. The patient survived the accident nearly five days. On examination after death the rupture of the bladder was detected; the cavity of the abdomen was filled with urine and extravasated blood; no mention is made of peritoneal inflammation.

The second case is one of tubal pregnancy, with rupture of the right Fallopian tube. The sac, entire, about the size of a walnut, and filled with a limpid fluid in which floated a fœtus, of between three and four months' development, had escaped into the cavity of the abdomen, where it was surrounded by a coagulum of blood of large size.

Dr. L. details, also, the history of three other cases of the accident that have occurred in Charleston within the last thirty years.

"It will be observed," the Dr. remarks, "that there is a striking similarity of symptoms in all of the four cases; and the reference hereafter, may enable the practitioner to form somewhat of a clear diagnosis of so terrible a calamity. While our art could afford no relief, yet the progress in medical research and advancement may determine positively the character of the accident."

He informs us that the symptoms of the case seen by him led him to believe it to be an attack of cholera, for which it was treated.

"The cramp in the abdomen and extremities; the serous fluid thrown up, with the alvine dejections of a simliar character, sustained such a diagnosis. These symptoms agree, in part, with Dr. Simon's case. There was, likewise, no tympanitis, and very little tenderness over the stomach; the abdomen was not swelled. In both Dr. Simon's and Holbeck's cases, there was no tympanitis, but excruciating pain when the abdominal parietes were touched. In Dr. L.'s case there were no positive symptoms, except the pallid lip that indicated hemorrhage, and this not more so than he has frequently seen in cholera patients. In Dr. Simon's case, the tube, between the place of rupture and where it enters the uterus, was nearly obliterated. This was not so in Dr. L.'s case, and, he concludes, was not so in Drs. Holbeck or Mitchell's, although they are silent on the subject."

A report of the committee on registration follows, with the draft of a bill to be presented for enactment to the legislature of South Carolina. The objects of this bill are thus concisely and accurately stated.

"1st. To ascertain the relative number and proportion of births, deaths, and marriages, in order to ascertain the progress and increase of the population.

"2d. The causes of death; so as to be able to trace the operations of natural and physical causes on the health of the inhabitants.

"3d. The season of the year, and duration of illness, and locality, where certain diseases prevail, so as to suggest means for abating them.

"4th. The age, sex, condition, colour, nativity, and occupation; in order to know how these various circumstances influence marriages, births, and deaths.

"5th. With a proper and complete record of these events in human life, are involved great public and private rights, such as claims to property, etc. etc."

The physicians of nearly every State appear to be impressed with the immense importance of securing a regular and continuous registration of the births, deaths and marriages which occur within its borders; and are moving with energy and zeal to secure its accomplishment. When will the profession in Pennsylvania awake from their apathy in relation to this matter, and be willing for their own and the public good, to give the slight amount of labour required at their hands for carrying it into effect. When the public shall become fully aware of how materially their interests will be promoted by a registration law, physicians will be compelled to do what they ought to be the first voluntarily to perform as an act of duty they owe to themselves and to the public.

A unique case of dislocation of the patella is reported by Dr. Wragg. It occurred in a negro, who, while engaged in loading lumber upon a boat, was caught by a loaded car, whilst in motion, and jammed against the cross-sticks on which the piles of lumber rested. A complete revolution of the patella on its longitudinal axis had taken place, so that its outer edge corresponded, nearly, to the inner edge of the articulating surface of the femur; its anterior face was turned backwards, and rested on the articulating surface of the femur; its inner edge looked outwards and a little forwards, forming a projecting edge in front and on the outside of the joint; and its posterior or articulating face was under the skin, looking forwards, with a slight inclination backwards.

Having ascertained that, in coming to its new position, the inner edge had been forced forwards and then outwards, the reduction was readily effected, by the thumbs of both hands being placed on the outer and under edge of the projecting border of the patella, while the index and middle fingers were pressed against the other border, in a direction outwards and backwards, and force being applied with the view to roll the bone over into its place. The first effort failing, a bystander was directed to pass his hands under the knee-joint, and make forcible and intermittent flexion of the leg. In a moment, the bone performed an evolution, slipped into its place, and the man rose up and walked. He experienced no further inconvenience; the ligaments, cartilages, and investing membranes of the joint having received no injury from the extensive displacement of the patella.

3. The *Transactions* of the sixth annual meeting of the Medical Society of the State of North Carolina present, first, a report on surgery by Dr. N. J. Pittman. It comprises a series of interesting cases, that occurred in the practice of the reporter. Among these we would notice, especially, a case of vesico-vaginal fistula, of eight months' standing, operated upon according to the method of M. Jobert, with very promising success. A case of compound fracture of the left scapula, from a violent blow on the shoulder, treated by Desault's apparatus for fractured clavicle. A perfect union of the fracture ensued, without deformity or any impediment to the motions of the arm remaining, and a case of perineal fistula, of five years' standing, operated on by freely laying open the sinuses, and removing as much of the integuments as seemed advisable. Dressings of lint and cold water were applied, and perfect rest enjoined. The case is still under treatment, and, so far, doing well.

This report is followed by an address, delivered by the same gentleman, on the "Nature of Auscultation and Percussion as a Means of Diagnosis in Disease." The subject is treated with great ability and clearness. The advantages to be derived from these means, for the physical investigation of disease, are strongly insisted on, and the necessity of every practitioner becoming familiar with their mode of application pointed out. With great propriety, Dr. P. points to the necessity of the introduction into our language of a plain nomenclature of auscultation. It would, certainly, greatly facilitate a more general resort to it in the investigation of the diseases of the chest and its viscera.

The next report is by Dr. W. H. McKee. It comprises a case of confluent smallpox, of a very bad character, in which Dr. M. was induced to employ the muriated tincture of iron, from having seen it used with so much success in erysipelas.

"The patient," he remarks, "may have recovered without anything, but as his case was a bad one, and he recovered so promptly, I thought it not amiss to mention it here. Neither the pain in the head nor the delirium should deter the physician from giving the iron, either in smallpox or erysipelas, as I can safely say it is by far the best remedy I have ever used in phlegmonous erysipelas." "If, on further trial, the muriated tincture of iron should be found to possess as much therapeutical virtue in the treatment of smallpox as it does in the management of erysipelas, it will relieve the profession, as well as the community, of some of its terrors."

Dr. M. also reports three cases of puerperal convulsions, in which injections of spirits of turpentine appeared to have the effect of suspending the convulsions, and, at the same time, in producing labor when the functions of the uterus were apparently suspended.

In reference to the dysentery that prevailed, with the ordinary symptoms, more or less, in Raleigh, and the surrounding country, throughout the year 1854, Dr. M. remarks, that the treatment most successful in his hands was the saline and opiate. He used very little calomel, or mercurials of any kind, as they appeared rather to irritate than soothe the disease. In all cases of long standing, he found the nitrate of silver, in grain doses, with a half to a grain of opium, every four or six hours, to give prompt relief.

The scarlet fever and measles, which prevailed during the same period, were, in some instances, so hybrid in their appearance, that it was difficult, in the early stage of the attack, to discriminate between the two, and it was only in the sequel that the real character of the disease was developed. In some cases, the scarlet fever assumed, in its initiatory stage, a congestive type, resembling a chill, accompanied by gastric fever. The patient, instead of presenting a scarlet appearance, would be pale, labour anxiously for breath, and vomit; in a short time, the bowels would become relaxed; cold, clammy perspiration, and death, soon closed the scene. Dr. M. saw some few cases of a putrid or malignant character.

"The winter of 1854," Dr. M. informs us, "was the driest and coldest known for years, and yet, pneumonia prevailed to a much more alarming degree than it had for some time. About the middle of January, 1855, it first appeared as an epidemic. It was not confined to any particular class of citizens, but prevailed generally, attacking, in some instances, nearly all in a family, and, in others, only one. In many cases, the patient would be taken suddenly, and complain of violent pain in the head, which would be followed by stupor, cold extremities, hot head, leaden appearance of the skin; pulse small, quick, 120 to 140; breathing quick and short, bowels as often loose as bound. If nothing was done for the patient at this stage of the attack, he would gradually rouse up in twelve hours, and often express himself as feeling much better, and ask for something to eat, and, if allowed to do it, would eat a hearty meal; but soon after, fever would set in, with delirium, and, in some instances, raving. Most of the cases Dr. M. saw in the country, were at this stage of the disease. The treatment consisted in giving a dose of Epsom salt in some warm, red pepper tea. This, in a short time, would vomit freely, unloading the stomach, and operating several times on the bowels. Afterwards, a decoction of seneka and liquorice-root was given, in tablespoonful doses, every two hours; flaxseed tea, acidulated with lemon-juice, being allowed freely as a drink, with, occasionally, a teaspoonful of equal proportions of oxymel and compound syrup of squills, to aid expectoration, and, at night, a dose of morphia, to procure sleep. If the pain in the side was very acute, cups were applied. The head was only relieved by shaving the top, and applying a blister. Some other cases Dr. H. treated with quinine and hive syrup, as an alterant and expectorant. In every instance, he had to use stimulants at some stage of the disease. In not a single instance was he able to employ the lancet. If the patients survived the ninth and eleventh day, they invariably recovered. The deaths took place, generally, on the fifth, sixth, or ninth day of the disease."

Speaking of chronic intermittent fever, usually accompanied with a chloro-anemic condition, and indications of dropsy, and enlarged spleen, Dr. M. states that quinine and muriated tincture of iron will, in most cases, effect a cure, if given three times a day for two or three weeks. The combination will sometimes be rejected by the stomach, especially in children. When this is the case, he has found the following equally successful: grains 60 of quinine, and grains 180 of phosphate of iron, intimately combined, and divided in 36 parts, of which one is to be given to an adult, in syrup or water, three times a day, and to children, in doses adapted to their age, until the whole is taken.

These *Transactions* close with the valedictory address of the President, Dr. J. H. Dickson. Its subject is the dignity, scope, and importance of the profession of medicine; a theme which the writer enforces with commendable zeal, and no little force and eloquence.

4. The *Transactions* of the State Medical Society of New York open with an able eulogium on the life and character, and professional labours, of Dr. Theodric Romeyn Beck, by Dr. F. H. Hamilton. It presents a very interesting memorial of one distinguished by his indomitable perseverance, his ardent devotion, his honesty of purpose, and excellent talents, who, during his lifetime, occupied a high rank in the scientific world, and whose name will be handed down to posterity, if by no other of his publications, by, at least, his *Elements of Jurisprudence.*

The second paper is a report on "Tuberculosis and Tubercular Pneumonia," by Dr. C. B. Coventry. Though short, compared with the vast importance of the subjects embraced in it, it is, nevertheless, replete with valuable hints and suggestions, and presents a nearer approach to a correct pathology of what have been denominated tuberculous diseases—or those associated with tuberculous depositions—than that which has heretofore been taught in the generally received practical treatises.

We prefer the denomination of tubercular pneumonia, applied by Dr. C., to the disease of the lungs known as tubercular phthisis, consumption of the lungs, pulmonary tuberculosis, etc., inasmuch as it more clearly expresses the true character of the affection, which is, in fact, pneumonia modified in its phenomena and progress by its occurrence in subjects labouring under pulmonary tuberculosis. It is very certain that tubercles may exist in the lungs for a long time without the occurrence of inflammation, and without undergoing the process of softening.

"We usually find consumptive patients refer the commencement of the disease to some definite period when they have suffered from some unusual exposure, or when, as they term it, they have taken cold. Perhaps they are more correct than is generally imagined. When tubercles exist in the lungs, any of the ordinary causes of pneumonia are sufficient to excite inflammatory action. We have no proof that tubercles produce inflammation in the lungs; but when inflammation is excited by other causes, they aggravate the difficulty, and increase the danger, in the same manner that meningitis, in children, is rendered more dangerous and fatal by the existence of tubercular deposits. The presence of tubercles may be properly considered as constituting a predisposition, and then slight causes, which would not be injurious were the lungs in a healthy condition, may be sufficient to excite disease."

It is, we are persuaded, by the study of pulmonary consumption in this light, that satisfactory results can alone be arrived at, in reference to its prophylaxis and proper treatment.

"The history of phthisis is sufficient to demonstrate the importance of a correct diagnosis of tuberculosis of the lungs. We find not only many different affections have been confounded under the general name of consumption, but that many of the ablest writers have differed as to what actual pathological conditions should be embraced under this general term. The term phthisis pulmonalis signifies simply a general wasting and exhaustion, consequent on pulmonary disease, and may embrace chronic bronchitis, chronic pneumonia, or pleuritic effusions, as well as pulmo-tuberculosis. In point of fact, the two first are almost invariable concomitants of the latter when it proceeds to a fatal termination, and even pleuritic effusions are not unfrequent in the advanced stage of pulmo-tuberculosis. The danger from these different affections is very much increased from their connection with tuberculosis. To distinguish tuberculosis from other affections, and to determine how much is to be attributed to the one, and how much to the other—to be able to say whether the disease is simply chronic bronchitis, which has so often been mistaken for pulmo-tuberculosis—whether it is simply condensation of the lungs in consequence of congestion or inflammation—whether it is suppuration as a consequence of simple inflammation—whether there is pleuritic effusion, and, if so, whether it is the consequence of simple pleuritic inflammation, or complicated with diseased structure of the lungs, are questions of vital importance in forming a diagnosis and prognosis in this disease. It is, however, sufficient for all practical purposes to divide it into three stages; the first, embracing the period of simple tuberculosis, without any evidence of inflammatory action; the second, after inflammation has supervened—as true tubercular pneumonia; and the third, after softening and suppuration have taken place, with expectoration of purulent and tuberculous matter."

Of the several signs or symptoms by which the diagnosis of these different conditions is to be determined—the physical and the rational, Dr. C. has presented a concise, but clear and instructive outline.

The sketch of the treatment demanded, as well for the arrest of the tuberculous dyscrasy of the pulmonary tissues, as for the cure of the inflammation occurring in lungs affected with tuberculosis, presented by Dr. C., is based exclusively upon the results of his own personal experience. The treatment laid down by him is, we are convinced, rational and judicious. It corresponds, in its general outlines, with the plan we have ourselves pursued for many years, and with such results as justify our unshaken confidence in it. If we hope to lessen the mortality—alleviate the sufferings, or prolong the lives of our consumptive patients, it must be by a careful study of the pathology of the disease so as to acquire correct views as to its character and causes, and by a system of treatment based upon the teachings of general therapeutics, with an entire abandonment of all reputed specifics, and of all plans of medication founded in a gross misconception of the morbid conditions it is our duty to remove.

The third article is a report, by Dr. Thomas W. Blachford, on rest, and the abolition of pain in the treatment of disease.

The importance of rest in the treatment of all acute diseases, has long been recognized by every observing and skilful physician, and strongly enforced in the leading medical works of a recent date. In the various acute affections of the head, thorax, abdomen, pelvis and limbs, and in nearly all fever, our remedial measures must be aided by perfect rest, or we shall fail in procuring from them their desired results. The same holds also in respect to dysentery, diarrhœa, hemorrhage, and many other diseases. It is true, as is properly remarked by Dr. Blachford, that there are a numerous class of ailments, having their origin in long-continued sedentary habits, confinement within doors, and deficient or unnutritious food, in which regular out-door exercise, active or passive, according to the condition of the patient, and graduated in its kind and extent by his capability of undergoing it, constitutes an important therapeutical agent, without which a cure can scarcely be anticipated.

To abolish pain is one of the important missions of the healing art. It in many cases can be accomplished only by the cure of the disease by which it is produced, and with which it is as intimately connected as the effect with its cause; so long as the latter exists must the former continue. Pain is not always, however, to be abjured. In many affections, especially those of internal parts, it is the voice of nature's sentinel, disclosing the condition within, and could we succeed in abolishing it, we should place ourselves in the condition of one in a labyrinth, extinguishing his lights that he may grope his way in the dark. If, however, the physician may not always aim at the sole object of abolishing pain, it is his duty always to use every proper means for its abatement. This he often affects by placing his patient or the organ chiefly affected in a state of perfect rest; by encouraging, by prudent and admissible means, sleep at proper intervals, and, generally, by the employment of the remedies adapted to remove the pathologieal condition of which the pain is a consequence. In very many cases he has it in his power to alleviate pain by the opportune and judicious employment of opiates, narcotics, or other anæsthetic agents internally, or locally to the external parts which are the seat of pain.

The entire subject of rest, and the abolition of pain in the treatment of disease is one of great importance. The report of Dr. Blachford presents a series of interesting hints in reference to it. The subject is not, however, discussed as fully and satisfactorily as we should have desired.

The fourth article is on the treatment of pneumonia, by Dr. Saunders. This is a very short paper. Dr. S. has seen but three cases of the disease during the last two years, which, in his judgment, were of so grave a character as to require bleeding.

"My usual treatment," he reports, "is solution of tart. ant. et potass., with some form of anodyne, in mucilage and sugar. I as often use the tinct. of opii and camphor, with antimony, as any other preparation for adults, and the ext. belladonna for children, combining them in sufficient quantity merely to allay irritation. I scarcely have a severe case of this disease, and were it not for the opportunity I have of knowing cases treated homœopathically, I should be inclined to think that the severe cases did not belong, as a general thing, to the region in which I live. I occasionally use calomel, and sometimes blisters, with apparent good effect."

The fifth article is on malignant pustule, and scrofulous gangrene, by Dr. Howard Townsend, of Albany. Two cases of what the writer denominates scrofulous gangrene, are detailed. They both occurred in children, females, both under three years of age; inmates of the Orphan Asylum of Albany. The first case strongly resembled gangrenopsis; in the second, the disease, in place of being located in the centre of the cheek, was at the outer angle of the left eyebrow. It commenced with a red pimple, from which was developed an ulcer of a dusky, almost purplish red hue, with a dry, hard, gangrenous spot in the centre; with thirst, loss of appetite, diarrhœa, and fever; but without any gangrenous affection of the gums or mouth. Both cases terminated fatally. This disease seems to Dr. T. to be a peculiar form of inflammation and ulceration, superinduced by the strumous diathesis of the patient, and which could scarcely be developed in an individual of full, robust health, and free from all scrofulous taint.

The sixth article is the history of fœtation, from coition to parturition, by Dr. Thomas Goodsell. The paper is an interesting one—conjectural, as must necessarily be the case, in treating of a vital process, or series of vital processes, from the careful observation of which we are completely shut out. We cannot spare sufficient space on the present occasion to present an analysis of it, and feel no inclination to attempt a criticism of the views advanced by the author.

The seventh article is an able account of encysted osseous tumours, or those consisting of a thin secreting membranous cyst, developed in a cancellous structure, and surrounded by a thin bony wall; by Dr. Alden March. This, like all the contributions of Dr. March, is of a strictly practical character. The account he presents of the peculiar and rather unfrequent form of disease which is the subject of the paper, is from personal observation, and the writings of Baron Dupuytren. It will be read by the surgeon with equal interest and profit.

A short paper by Dr. J. L. Phelps, follows, intended to show that the mode of reducing dislocations of the femur backwards and upwards on the dorsum of the ilium, by a peculiar movement of the limb, which has recently attracted attention in consequence of the paper read by Dr. Reid, of Rochester, at the session of 1852, and subsequently claimed as having originated with Dr. Nathan Smith, who demonstrated it before the class in Yale College, in the course of 1815-16, was performed by Dr. Physick as early as January, 1811, in the Pennsylvania Hospital.

The ninth paper is the history of a case of chronic nephritis, resulting in disorganization and entire absorption of the substance of the left kidney, communicated by Dr. G. J. Fisher, of Westchester County. Few details could be collected of the previous history of the case of a satisfactory character. In the place of the left kidney was a sac filled with fluid, slightly turbid, resembling urine that had been voided several hours. The sac was of the same general outlines as, but much larger than, the kidney, with a cord extending from it to the bladder, being the obliterated ureter. The right kidney was slightly softened. The liver and spleen hypertrophied and enlarged. The patient was a convict, of intemperate habits, 56 years of age. He was subject to frequent attacks of pain in the lumbar region; his extremities were œdematous; and he had for years been affected with a degree of nervousness, which, for some time previous to his death, amounted to complete chorea.

The closing article is a biographical sketch of Dr. Thomas Brodhead, an old and respectable physician of Columbia County, N. Y., communicated by Dr. P. Van Buren.

5. Pursuant to an invitation addressed to the members of the medical profession throughout the State of California, a convention, composed of a numerous delegation from the various sections of that commonwealth, assembled in Sacramento City, on the 12th of March, 1856, and organized the State Medical Society of California, with auxiliary societies in each town or county. The proceedings of that convention and of the first meeting of the State Society are before us. They show that a right spirit animates the body of the profession there, to secure to themselves an entire coöperation, and the cultivation of that friendly intercourse which should ever be manifested between those engaged in common pursuits having for their objects the alleviation of suffering, the development of the physical energies, and the prolongation of the lives of their fellow men—laying thus the foundation upon which must be based, in the first instance, the means for the amelioration of the condition of every community, and their advance in civilization, refinement and happiness. Without which coöperation and fraternal feeling the proper standing, and the true and legitimate interests of the medical profession can never be attained, while its individual members, isolated from each other, and regardless of the rights and interests of other physicians—striving to promote their own popularity and pecuniary success without reference to what is due, in an ethical point of view, to their fellow practitioners, bring themselves into merited contempt, and lower the entire profession in the estimation of the public. The physicians of California have taken the proper steps, and in a proper direction, to advance their common good, and to place themselves, as a body, in their true position in society; and at the same time, by a combined effort, each member within his field of observation, doing his share of the work, to present, in the investigation of the etiology, character, progress, treatment, and results of the endemic and epidemic maladies of California, a valuable contribution to the common stock of medical knowledge. D. F. C.

Art. XIV.—*Reports of American Institutions for the Insane.*

1. *Of the Maine Insane Hospital, for the years* 1854 and 1855.
2. *Of the New Hampshire Asylum for the Insane, for the years* 1854 and 1855.
3. *Of the Vermont Asylum for the Insane, for the years* 1854 and 1855.
4. *Of the Massachusetts Lunatic Hospital, Worcester, for the years* 1854 and 1855.
5. *Of the Boston Lunatic Asylum, for the year* 1852.
6. *Of the New York City Lunatic Asylum, for the years* 1854 and 1855.
7. *Of the Maryland Hospital for the Insane, for the years* 1853, 1854, and 1855.
8. *Of the Mount Hope Institution, for the years* 1854 and 1855.
9. *Of the Western Lunatic Asylum, Virginia, for the years* 1854 and 1855.
10. *Of the South Carolina Lunatic Asylum, for the years* 1853 and 1855.

1. By the report of Dr. Harlow, of the *Maine State Asylum*, it appears that the number of patients at that institution, on the 30th of Nov. 1853,

	Men.	Women.	Total.
Was	61	58	119
Admitted in course of the year . .	57	53	110
Whole number	118	111	229
Discharged, including deaths . . .	56	58	114
Remaining Nov. 30, 1854 . . .	62	53	115
Of those discharged, there were cured .	26	23	49
Died	16	16	32

Causes of Death.—Dysentery 16; general paralysis 5; consumption 2; old age 2; marasmus 2; serous apoplexy 1; congestion of brain 1; typhoid fever 1; gangrene 1; epilepsy 1.

"About the first of August," says the report, "an *epidemic diarrhœal dysentery* broke out in our wards, and for three months little else than the sick and dying occupied our attention. There was scarcely an individual connected with the hospital family who escaped the ravages of the disease. Officers, attendants, nurses and assistants shared alike with the patients in the attack. Just in the midst of the epidemic, when it would seem the services of the superintendent and steward were most needed, we were prostrated and unable to perform our duties. Having no medical assistant, we were obliged to call in a neighboring physician to attend the patients. Fortunately, the trustees were able to procure the valuable services of Ex-Governor Hubbard, who was formerly, for several years, a member of their board, and who has always felt and taken a deep interest in the hospital. He visited us daily for four weeks, and attended upon all the sick in the house till we were able to attend to our duties." Of ninety persons attacked by this epidemic, seventeen, of whom sixteen were patients, and one a female attendant, died.

The number of patients admitted, since the first opening of the hospital for their reception, is 1430. Discharged, 1316, of whom 590 had recovered. Died 175.

To avoid the labour and the inconveniences attendant upon the return of patients who, on the supposition of recovery, have left the hospital with the formalities of a regular discharge, but who, after a few days, either suffer a relapse or give evidence of imperfect restoration, Dr. Harlow has adopted the plan pursued at some of the European hospitals, of discharging all in regard to whom he has "doubts of their fitness, on trial, for a period of two weeks."

Of 1200 *patients* who have been in the hospital, 586 had insane relatives. It is not stated whether these 1200 were so many *persons*, or merely so many *cases*, including a considerable number of re-admissions of the same person—conditions which materially affect the percentage.

In some remarks upon the deleterious effects of a forced, early *intellectual* education, Dr. H. remarks that he "was most forcibly struck, in reading an account of a class of students who graduated at one of our New England Colleges, in 1827. It was found that of this class, numbering twenty-three, all but two had survived the lapse of quarter of a century; and it was also found that nearly every member of the class had arrived at adult age before entering college, thus escaping that premature excitement and development of the intellect which paves the way to mental disease, and furnishes tenants for many an early grave."

At the date of this report an additional wing for females was in course of construction.

In the report for 1855, we are informed that the new wing is completed, and occupied. The original design is thus finished, and the hospital can now accommodate two hundred and fifty patients.

	Men.	Women.	Total.
Patients in the Hospital, Nov. 30, 1854 .	64	51	115[1]
Admitted in course of the year . .	66	62	128
Whole number	130	113	243

[1] The number assigned to each sex, does not correspond with that of the report of the preceding year.

	Men.	Women.	Total.
Discharged, including deaths . . .	44	44	88
Remaining, November 30, 1855 . .	86	69	155
Of those discharged, there were cured .			41
Died			19

Deaths from general paralysis 5, epilepsy 3, chronic diarrhœa 3, tubercular consumption 2, congestion of the brain 3, old age, nephritis, and typhoid fever, 1 each.

"The propensity," says Dr. Harlow, "that exists in the minds of many of the friends of our patients, to remove them from the hospital too soon after they have been admitted, continues to be an evil which we should be glad to see eradicated. We are happy to say, however, that the evil appears to be growing less from year to year."

Patients admitted since the hospital was opened	1559
Discharged recovered	631
Died	193

"Owing to the two epidemics, and the great calamity by fire, with which the hospital has been visited since its existence, the bill of mortality is larger than (that of) some similar institutions."

Basing his calculation upon the results obtained by the commission which took the census of the insane and the idiots in Massachusetts, in 1854, Dr. Harlow concludes that, in Maine, there are 1365 lunatics and 560 idiots. "The question arises," he remarks, "where are all these 1365 lunatics, and what is their condition? Some are cared for at home, by their friends, either chained or caged, if unmanageable, and some 150 are in the hospital, while by far the largest proportion of them are at the various Almshouses in the State, many of them caged and chained, because they can be kept a few cents less per week than it costs at the hospital." Where is that *other* "Maine Law?"

2. At the New Hampshire Asylum for the Insane, on the 31st of May, 1853, the number of

	Men.	Women.	Total.
Patients was	70	73	143
Admitted in the course of the year . .	72	69	141
Whole number	142	142	284
Discharged, including deaths . . .	67	56[1]	123
Remaining May 31st, 1854 . . .	77	84	161
Of those discharged, there were cured .	34	29	63
Died	7	7	14

"During the whole year our household has enjoyed remarkable physical health. We have been entirely exempt from epidemics of all sorts, and acute disease has been almost unknown. Cleanliness, regularity of life, and a most healthful location have been the chief causes of this desirable state of things. The deaths which have occurred, with a single exception, were of those who for a long time were considered incurably insane, and who at last were literally worn out by the continued and unremitting force of their malady.

"Through the whole year our female halls have been full, and often crowded, and our male halls at all times crowded." This condition "prevents a proper classification of patients, and seriously interferes with all curative measures." Dr. Tyler therefore recommends that an additional wing be erected.

"We can in almost no case infallibly pronounce a person incurably insane; certainly the records of the asylum for the year show the recovery of some whose improvement seemed impossible, and whose present condition, among their friends and in perfect health and soundness of mind, seems a miracle."

"The house is now lighted with gas, and we not only find its use more con-

[1] These numbers are quoted from the report. But if 67 men and 56 women were discharged, the number remaining would be 75 and 86, instead of 77 and 84.

venient, comfortable and cleanly than oil, but its brilliant light a curative means, in making our previously half-lighted halls cheerful and pleasant."

Report for 1855.

	Men.	Women.	Total.
Patients on the 31st of May, 1854 . .	77	84	161
Admitted in course of the year . . .	45	40	85
Whole number	122	124	246
Discharged, including deaths . . .	50	41	91
Remaining May 31, 1855	72	83	155

Among the patients who were discharged recovered, Dr. Tyler says there was "a man of intelligence and education who was for nearly eleven years an inmate of this institution."

The asylum is rapidly becoming filled with incurables. But about one-half of the applicants for admission can be received. The Doctor recommends that an additional wing be erected. A building for the violent patients is in progress.

From the answers to circulars sent to every city and town in New Hampshire, and from other sources, Dr. Tyler ascertains that there are 35 insane persons belonging to the State who "are supported by their friends or guardians in hospitals in other States; and that there are now resident in the State more than 550 insane persons, only 155 of whom are in this asylum. Of the remainder, many are kindly and comfortably taken care of at home, or with friends, or at almshouses; but others are chained, and caged, and sadly neglected; in filth, and exposure to the inclemencies of the weather. Some instances of cruelty and neglect have lately come to our knowledge, that, if known, would startle the neighbourhoods in which they have occurred."

Whole number of patients from the opening of the Asylum .	1284
Discharged cured	547
Died	118

3. At the Vermont Asylum for the Insane, on the 1st of August, 1853, the number of

	Men.	Women.	Total.
Patients was	183	189	372
Admitted in course of the year . . .	77	86	163
Whole number	260	275	535
Discharged, including deaths . . .	72	74	146
Of whom there were recovered . . .			80
Died			40

It appears that a large number of the patients at this Asylum are employed on the farm, in the garden, and in the workshop. Dr. Rockwell also encourages them to join in "all amusements which require exercise of the body as well as diversion of the mind, and especially riding, walking, playing billiards, ten-pins, quoits, and the like." He would "rather they would play chess, draughts, cards, and such like games than do nothing."

	Men.	Women.	Total.
Patients, August 1st, 1854	188	201	389
Admitted in course of the year . . .	78	86	164
Whole number	266	287	553
Discharged, including deaths . . .			159
Remaining, August 1st, 1855 . . .			394
Of those discharged, there were recovered			79
Died			52
Whole number of patients since the opening of the Asylum			2393
Discharged, recovered			1127

The unusually large number of deaths during the last year, is accounted for, in part, by the prevalence of a severe and fatal form of dysentery which appeared among the patients in the early part of summer, and continued with unabated severity throughout that season. The number of attacks is not mentioned, neither is that of the cases in which it proved fatal. Warned by the two epidemics which have been mentioned, the directing authorities of the institution have ordered the construction of two infirmaries, one for either sex, wherewith, in the event of a future similar invasion of disease, the invalid patients can be isolated from the others. These apartments have been commenced.

4. The State Lunatic Hospital of Massachusetts, at Worcester, has for several years been greatly, almost unjustifiably crowded with inmates. It, its officers, and its patients have at length obtained some relief. The inconvenient and unwholesome condition of things has been changed for the better. Another State Hospital has been erected at Taunton. To this, on the seventh of April, 1854, "and on each of the five succeeding Fridays, a *car load* of patients" were transferred from the hospital at Worcester. The number thus removed was 210. No accident occurred in this rarely-paralleled migration. "The patients were mostly of a very orderly class, and they were gratified with the ride." Notwithstanding this great abstraction from its wards, the hospital was left "quite full, but not crowded," and it became possible to abandon the use of a number of cells and improperly-contrived rooms which had long been tenanted by patients.

	Men.	Women.	Total.
Patients in the Hospital, Dec. 1, 1853 .	266	254	520
Admitted in course of the year . . .	125	174	299
Whole number	391	428	819
Discharged, including deaths . . .	198	240	438
Remaining Nov. 30, 1854	193	188	381
Of those discharged, there were cured .	45	77	122
Died	15	19	34

Causes of Death.—Marasmus 5; consumption 4; lung fever 4; maniacal exhaustion 7; apoplexy and palsy 3; epilepsy 2; erysipelas 2; suicide, dropsy, chronic dysentery, diarrhœa, congestive fever, asthma, and jaundice, 1 each.

In connection with the causes of insanity, Dr. Chandler makes the following remarks: "Probably in no part of the world are the causes of insanity more numerous and more active than among the population of Massachusetts. Here the mind, and body too, are often worked to the extreme point of endurance. Here wealth and station are the results of well directed efforts; and the general diffusion of intelligence among the people stimulates a vast many of them to compete successfully for these prizes. But in the contest, where so many strive, not a few break down. The results on their minds may not, perhaps, be any less disastrous, whether wealth and station are obtained, or not. The true balance of the mind is disturbed by prosperity as well as by adversity. It is only in a sound body that the manifestations of the mind are sane and entirely healthy. As a people, we cannot boast of the highest standard of physical health, although we may of general intelligence, enterprise, and hard work."

In the course of the year 1855, very important improvements were made in this establishment. Not the least of these was the introduction of the apparatus for heating by steam, and that for ventilating by mechanical power. Relieved, by the hospital at Taunton, of its great excess of patients, and brought, by improvements, more nearly into conformity with the idea of the times, this institution may still, for a long number of years, continue its career of usefulness. Indeed, it seems that Dr. Chandler is unwilling to acknowledge that it has ever merited the impression which has been made upon the public mind in regard to it. "Whatever," he remarks, "may have been said against this hospital—and most of what has been said about its defects, has been so said as an excuse to make it still better—it has always afforded, and does now, with all the progress made in others, a residence as comfortable and as cheering, and as healthful to the patient, as any similar institution in this country."

In this expression we believe Dr. C. is mainly correct. The only exception suggested relates to the hygienic condition of the building. It can hardly be assumed that, with its comparatively low ceilings, and its imperfect ventilation, it can be so healthful, other things being equal, as some of the similar edifices more recently erected. For the impression which has gone abroad in regard to it, the Board of Trustees who have the control of it are chiefly responsible. They drew the picture of its defects; and if their painted grapes bear such a semblance to reality that the birds have pecked at them, truly it is not the birds that should bear the blame. All who have visited the hospital are well aware that the picture was a sketch of the shady side alone, and that another, drawn from the sunny side, might be made as attractive as the first was repulsive.

From its earliest years we have been a not unfrequent visitor to this hospital, and in this place we feel bound to acknowledge our belief that, from its origin, it has been not only *well*, but *very* well managed. We would shun invidious distinctions—we shall make none; yet justice demands from us the expression, that there is no institution in the country at which we could, at any time, have placed a friend with greater confidence that all his necessities would be supplied; that his comforts would be carefully ministered to; that he would be shielded from abuse; and that his restoration would be wrought for with watchful care, with constant assiduity, and with that skill which is the result of a good professional knowledge, combined with practical experience.

"We avail ourselves of this occasion," write the trustees, in their report, "to bear testimony to the fidelity and signal ability with which Dr. Chandler has discharged the duties of his position, and to the great success which has attended his labours during the whole period of his superintendence."

Dr. Chandler has resigned his office, and Dr. Merrick Bemis, for some years one of the assistant physicians of the hospital, has been appointed as his successor:—

	Men.	Women.	Total.
Patients in the hospital Dec. 1, 1854	193	188	381
Admitted in the course of the year	86	113	199
Whole number admitted in the course of the year	279	301	580
Discharged, including deaths	111	133	244
Remaining, Nov. 30, 1855	168	168	336
Of those discharged, there were cured	50	59	109
Died	13	14	27
Admitted from Jan. 18, 1833, to Nov. 30, 1855	2,451	2,505	4,956
Discharged, recovered	1,089	1,195	2,284
Died	281	272	553

Of this aggregate number of deaths, 87 are attributed to marasmus; to "consumption 67; apoplexy and palsy 59; maniacal exhaustion 59; epilepsy 50; suicide 22; lung fever 22; disease of the brain 21; disease of the heart 20; diarrhœa 19; erysipelas 17; old age 14; typhus fever 11; dysenteric fever 10; dropsy 10; inflammation of the bowels 8; hemorrhage 6; cholera morbus 5; chronic dysentery 5; gastric fever 5; cholera 4; mortification of the limbs 3; from intemperance 3; bronchitis 3; congestive fever 3; hydrothorax 3; convulsions 2; asthma 2; disease of the bladder 2; cancer 2; jaundice 2; land scurvy 1; concussion of the brain 1; fright 1; rupture 1; pleurisy 1; chorea 1."

In reference to the salubrity of the hospital, this schedule of the mortality among almost five thousand patients, in the course of a period but little less than twenty-three years, is well worthy of a careful perusal. Its testimony is more reliable than that of individual opinion; more forcible than arguments deduced from theories of architectural construction. The almost entire exemption from fatal epidemics, from severe endemic fevers, and from other acute diseases, to which it bears record, will find but few parallels in any other institution of the kind in any quarter of the globe.

Under the table of causes we find the following remarks:—

"Spiritualism of the present day is of the last (moral) class of causes. This singular mental phenomenon has, for some years, engaged a part of the minds in this vicinity, and some few cases have been brought to us the past, as well as p e s years, arising, it was supposed, from investigating its phenomena, and from believing in its supposed truthful revelations of the future state of existence. If it was true that this process of investigation did really open to the mind any knowledge of the world to come, not revealed to us by the Scriptures—which many of its votaries assert and believe—then it would be a cause calculated in the highest degree to engage, excite, and disturb the mind. But it has been said by those best prepared to investigate closely, that the responses through the mediums contain no ideas of this or the next world, that were not then, or had not previously been, in the mind of some one present. It may be a new faculty of the mind, but its field of operation lies this side of the grave."

In regard to moral treatment, Dr. Chandler writes as follows: "We recognize the principle of giving the largest liberty, and the greatest freedom from restraint, in each case, consistent with the security of the individual and safety of the community. * * * About one-half of our patients perform some kind of labour, more or less useful. For plain work, the patients are ready and very efficient. One day this autumn the patients, with one hired man, dug, took off the tops, and put into the cart, four hundred and eighty bushels of carrots. Some are ingenious mechanics. Two have assisted the carpenters most of the season. One gentleman has made all the soft soap—three hundred and fifty barrels a year—and some of the bar soap, for five or six years. He has gathered the materials, made and distributed, and attended to the economical use of it. No one can make better soap than he. Two have made our baskets for years, and have supplied themselves, in part, with clothing. One female has made pantaloons and vests to supply the demand in our family. The females make the shirts, and knit the stockings; they wash and mend; they cook, and they help about all our domestic affairs. * * * Whip-lash braiding * * * is the best employment I can think of to introduce among our patients in-doors."

5. The report for the fiscal year ending with the month of November, 1852, is the latest which we have seen from the Boston Lunatic Asylum:—

	Men.	Women.	Total.
Patients at the beginning of the year	100	141	241
Admitted in course of the year	41	11	52
Whole number	141	152	293
Discharged, including deaths	34	15	49
Remaining at end of year	107	137	244
Of s discharged, were cured	17	5	22
Died ha e	14	8	22

Causes of Death.—Consumption 8; debility 3; general paralysis 3; epilepsy 2; chronic mania 2; smallpox 1; "Asiatic diarrhœa" 1; old age 1; marasmus 1.

"It is a noticeable fact," writes Dr. Walker, "that no death from dysentery has occurred. This disease has prevailed extensively among us for several successive years, always bringing with it great suffering, and ceaseless anxiety. Early in August it appeared in a very violent form, bringing several of our household rapidly to the verge of the grave. Fires were immediately lighted in the furnaces morning and evening, so that when the patients were rising and retiring, a current of warm air should be passing through the halls and bedrooms. * * * The most unpromising cases speedily began to amend, and at the time when the disease usually raged the most fiercely, not a case was under treatment."

The report for 1851 from this institution, contained a brief but interesting account of the case of an Irish boy, among the patients. This account was in whole or in part transferred to our notices. The report before us states that the boy has left the institution "giving promise of future usefulness."

6. *New York City Lunatic Asylum,* on Blackwell's Island.

	Men.	Women.	Total.
Number of patients on the 1st of January, 1854	232	310	542
Admitted in course of the year	224	262	486
Whole number	456	572	1,028
Discharged, including deaths	211	262	473
Remaining, Dec. 31, 1854	245	310	555
Of those discharged, there were cured			186
Died			190

Among the cases cured, there were four of delirium tremens. Of the cases admitted, nine were improper subjects for the institution.

Causes of Death.—Cholera 83; consumption 34; paralysie générale 19; typhomania 9; "debilitas" 9; epilepsy 8; congestion of brain 7; dysentery 3; chronic diarrhœa 3; old age 2; typhus fever, pneumonia, erysipelas, hydrocephalus, albuminuria, suicide by suspension, injuries of head, injuries from fall, "submersion," peritonitis, gastroscirrhus, pericarditis, ascites, 1 each.

Dr. Ranney gives the following account of the cholera, by which, as will have been perceived, nearly one-half of the mortality was occasioned:—

"The epidemic commenced on the 22d of July, and terminated on the 22d of August. An attendant, however, was attacked on the 11th of September, and died in twelve hours. Four of the other attendants had cholera of a severe form, but all recovered. It seemed more violent, and proved more fatal than in 1849, and nearly the same class was affected, viz: those in whom the constitution was greatly impaired from chronic disease, and the mind reduced to the most hopeless state. Frequently, the first warning was complete collapse, characterized by blueness of the skin, coldness of the surface, and loss of pulse. Cramps were less common than in 1849. If diarrhœa occurred, as a premonitory symptom, it was readily checked by medicine."

"Chronic diarrhœa has become much less frequently a cause (of death) since the introduction of Croton water on the island."

Of the 486 patients admitted in the course of the year, only 97 were natives of the United States. Of the foreigners, 241 were from Ireland; 91 from Germany; 21 from England; and 9 from Scotland. The remainder were from various countries. One hundred were supported by the Commission of Emigration, and all these were immigrants of the preceding five years.

"A large proportion of the recent immigrants recover; the derangement of mind being generally produced by privations on ship-board, and the changes necessarily incident on arriving in a strange land. Their exposures and sufferings are occasionally very great in crossing the Atlantic, and, in a few, the aberration of intellect has seemed to depend entirely on the want of sufficient nourishment. A poor German boy was admitted last March, who had just arrived in New York. His suffering from starvation had been so great as to obliterate from his memory all knowledge of having crossed the ocean, and he fancied himself in his father-land! He would implore me, in the strongest terms, to allow him to go on his journey, as in a few hours he would meet his father and mother, who were anxiously awaiting his return. Then a change would come over him, and he would imagine that he was detained as a culprit. He would plead his innocence with feeling eloquence, and in the most melting terms. These delusions were so firmly fixed that he would listen to no explanation, and the only effectual quietus was the liberal and constant supply of nutriment. His thirst fully equally his appetite for food. I subsequently learned that he was a native of the Grand Dukedom of Baden, and that he had been seventy days in making the voyage from Bremen to New York. In two weeks the delusion disappeared, and he became fully conscious of his condition. In two months his mind was perfectly restored, when he left the asylum, as noted for excessive fatness as he had previously been for his emaciated and meagre appearance."

We rejoice to learn, as we do from the report for 1855, that one of the foulest blots which has rested upon the practical psychiatry of our country, has at length been effaced. "The most decided improvement ever made in this asylum," remarks Dr. Ranney, "has been consummated the past year. I refer to the entire removal of prisoners, not only from their immediate connection with the insane, but from the institution.

"From 1826 to 1847, the work of the asylum was performed, and the principal charge of its inmates taken, by persons transferred from the different penal institutions on the island. At the commencement of the year last named, six of that class were employed in each of the halls, and between fifty and sixty engaged as domestics about the building. One-fourth of the whole number at the asylum being convicts, the institution differed little, in its *morale*, from a prison. It was urged upon the common council, 'that the same individuals who were committed in the city as criminals, and required an armed keeper in the penitentiary, were sent here to take charge of a class who require the most mild and soothing treatment.' But the memorials sent, soliciting a change in the system, produced no effect."

And be it remembered that no action was taken upon the subject until after the asylum had ceased to be one of the footballs of partisan politics, by that worthy act of the State Legislature, which wrested the government of the Almshouse Department of the City of New York from the municipal authorities, and vested it in a Board of Governors selected in equal, or nearly equal numbers, from the two most prominent political parties of the day. The change commenced in 1850, when prisoners were removed from three of the halls for patients, and has gradually progressed to its final completion.

	Men.	Women.	Total.
Patients in the asylum Dec. 31, 1854	245	310	555
Admitted in course of the year	163	208	371
Whole number	408	518	926
Discharged, including deaths,	170	183	353
Remaining, Dec. 31, 1855	238	335	573
Of those discharged, there were cured			200
Died			100

The disease of six patients, recorded among the cured, was *delirium tremens*.

Deaths from consumption 29; paralysie générale 18; epilepsy 7; chronic diarrhœa 7; typhomania 6; old age 5; congestion of brain 5; hemiplegia 3; anasarca 3; inflammation of brain 2; apoplexy 2; typhus fever 2; hypertrophy of heart 2; pneumonia 2; bronchitis, pleurisy, hydrothorax, ascites, erysipelas, scorbutus, and accidental drowning, 1 each.

So long as the circumstances controlling the population of this institution shall continue such as they are at the present time, so long must its annual records present a large bill of mortality. It is, in fact, the receptacle of the offscourings of the civilized world. Of the 371 patients received in 1855, only 78 were natives of the United States, while 293 were foreigners. Of the latter, 288 were Europeans. Ireland was represented by 178; the German states, including Austria and Prussia, by 68; England by 19, and eight of the other nations by smaller numbers. Some of these came with broken constitutions, many of them under the depressing influence of disappointed hopes, many with the typhoid effects of the voyage by sea still upon them, and some labouring under a combination of two or more of these vultures to vitality. There are also other causes, perhaps of minor importance, but still of sufficient magnitude to swell the sum of forces tending to a fatal issue.

The moral treatment at this institution is gradually becoming broader, more systematic, and more effective. Musical concerts, or parties, have been held from two to three times in each week. "New Year's day, the Fourth of July, Thanksgiving, and Christmas were appropriately observed. The oration delivered by one of the inmates, on the Fourth, is a creditable production. The reading of the Declaration of Independence, the music, and the original ode, would compare favourably with the usual ceremonies on similar occasions. About three hundred and fifty patients joined in the celebration.

"One of the most pleasant and interesting of our amusements has been the holding of 'Moot Courts.' Many could directly participate in these, either as plaintiff, defendant, counsel, judge, or juryman. The minor offences alone were tried by this supreme court of Blackwell's Island. The judge, noted for benevolence and wealth, and preferring to pay the damages rather than have any one suffer from the uncertainty of the law, gave decisions—unlike those of the city courts—satisfactory to both parties."

7. The reports by Dr. Fonerden, of the Maryland Hospital for the Insane, are very brief, limited almost exclusively to a short account of the changes in the patients resident, and to such subjects appertaining to the management of the hospital as are of merely local interest. The statistics of those now under review, are condensed into the subjoined table:—

	1853.			1854.			1855.			AGGREGATE.		
	M.	W.	Tot.	M.	W.	Tot.	M.	W.	Tot.	M.	W.	Tot.
Patients on the 1st of January .	68	62	130	57	60	117	56	63	119	68	62	130
Admitted in course of the year .	29	21	50	23	23	46	42	28	70	94	72	166
Whole number	97	83	180	80	83	163	98	91	189	162	134	296
Discharged, including deaths .	40	23	63	24	20	44	39	29	68	103	72	175
Remaining, December 31 . .	57	60	117	56	63	119	59	62	121	...	...	...
Recovered	8	3	11	10	7	17	13	13	26	31	23	54
Died	7	2	9	5	3	8	13	4	17	25	9	34

Previously to the year 1855, some cases of *mania à potu* were received at this institution; but we are informed by the report for 1850, that such cases are not enumerated in the tabular accounts of the insane.

8. From the report of Dr. Stokes, Physician to the Mount Hope Institution, near Baltimore, we extract the subjoined numerical results for 1854:—

	Men.	Women.	Total.
Patients on the 1st of January, 1854 .	45	87	132
Admitted in course of the year . . .	54	51	105
Whole number in course of the year .	98	139	237
Discharged, including deaths . . .	41	48	89
Remaining, Jan. 1, 1855	56	91	147[1]
Of those discharged, there were cured .	19	18	37
Died	7	8	15

Causes of Death.—Acute mania 2; apoplexy 1; Bright's disease 2; epileptic convulsions 2; puerperal mania 2; exhaustive mania 3; phthisis 2; "gradual senile decline" 1.

"Erysipelas and dysentery prevailed to a considerable extent during the summer, but in no case did they prove fatal.

[1] All these figures are given as they are in the report, without an attempt to harmonize them. Of men, there were 45 at the beginning of the year, and 54 admitted; yet the total is made 98. Of the women, the two items and the aggregate similarly disagree. It is stated, in general, that 41 males and 48 females were discharged; yet, immediately afterwards, in giving the details of cures, improvement, deaths, &c., the number of males is made 42, and that of females 47.

"During the entire year the institution has been rather more than comfortably filled."

From the remarks upon "premature removals," we make the following extract: "Those practically familiar with the habitudes of the insane, and the motives and influences under which they act, know full well that many, who are violent, noisy, and outrageous whilst under the care of their friends, become calm and docile when subjected to the mild but firm discipline and moral treatment of an asylum. Such a change does not indicate a cessation, or even (in some instances) the mitigation of disease; it merely shows that it is held under control by the varied influences brought to bear on it. * * * * Many of our inmates who are peaceful and contented, cheerfully occupied throughout the day, entering with pleasure into the amusements and recreations afforded them, or rambling at will in the grounds of the asylum, would become unhappy and unmanageable if restored to the exciting cause of their malady."

We proceed to the report for the year 1855:—

	Men.	Women.	Total.
Patients on the 1st of January . . .	56	91	147
Admitted in the course of the year . .	49	46	95
Whole number in the course of the year .	105	137	242
Discharged, including deaths . . .	59	61	120
Remaining, Jan. 1, 1856	46	76	122
Of those discharged, there were cured .	19	7	26
Died	7	7	14

Of the patients who were discharged improved, or unimproved, forty-six belonged to the District of Columbia, and, being supported by the national government, were transferred to the Government Hospital for the Insane, near Washington.

Upon the subject of injudicious visits to patients, by their friends, Dr. Stokes says: "It is astonishing with what a reckless and criminal disregard of the most earnest representations of the injury likely to be inflicted, this course is persisted in. Thus it is that the patients' mental health and future happiness are often jeoparded by the indiscreet action of those most interested in their recovery. Strange to relate, after informing them that such a step is calculated to entail chronic insanity upon the patient for life; that its certain effect will be to protract the disorder, and thus increase and prolong the trouble and expense of his maintenance, many instances have occurred during the past year wherein they have obstinately persisted in their insane course."

The following case is related in the observations upon epileptic mania: "In a case now under treatment the person, whose attacks seldom amount to spasms, or even a distortion of the features, but in whom the loss of concioneness is complete for the time, would really seem to possess two natures. His life presents two decidedly distinct phases; the one embracing a period of a week preceding or following the attacks, during which he is suspicious, timid, apprehensive of plots to destroy him, malicious and vindictive. He is then irritable and imperious, violent and gloomy. In the other phase, in a manner normal, his character manifests itself under an entirely different aspect, exhibiting the capacities of a man in possession of good sense, and free from all extravagance."

In four cases, the abuse of opiates is alleged as the cause of the mental aberration. "Opium," remarks Dr. S., "is much more used by females than by males, and there exists abundant proof that the vicious habit of this indulgence prevails much more extensively than is supposed. From two to four ounces of laudanum a day is by no means an unfrequent allowance."

Among the facilities, and the adopted plans for moral treatment mentioned in this report, are books, music, embroidery, excursions, a saddle-pony, musical reunions, dancing, books, games, and newspapers. In the report for 1844, it is mentioned that the anniversaries of the Fourth of July and Christmas are appropriately observed.

9. The report by Dr. Stribling, of the Western Lunatic Asylum, Virginia, extends over two fiscal years:—

	Men.	Women.	Total.
Patients in the Asylum, Oct. 1, 1853 .	217	160	377
Admitted in the course of two years .	90	63	153
Whole number	307	223	530
Discharged, including deaths . . .	81	61	142
Remaining, September 30th, 1855 . .	226	162	388
Of those discharged, there were cured .	32	30	62
Died	36	22	58
Whole number of patients admitted from July 1, 1836	801	537	1338
Discharged, cured	302	214	516
Died	186	109	295

Since the last preceding report the Asylum has been so much crowded with patients that 141 applicants were rejected. Hence Dr. Stribling requests the Board of Directors to "again invoke the attention of the general assembly to the subject of founding another asylum for the insane," and expresses his confirmed opinion that if another institution of the kind be determined upon, it should be placed in that part of the State which is west of the Alleghany Mountains.

Dr. Stribling has frequently been called from his hospital duties, by subpœna, to act as an expert in courts of law. "The Board of Directors, perceiving the evil likely to result therefrom to the interests of the asylum, presented the subject, in their report for 1843, to the legislature, and asked 'that this officer be released from obligation of obeying such mandates, and that he be allowed, as some other officers of the Commonwealth, to give his testimony or opinion in the usual form of deposition.' The suggestion was promptly acted upon, and a law passed to that effect." Subsequently, upon receiving a subpœna in a criminal case, he refused, under this law, to obey it. The question of the constitutionality of the law, so far as relates to criminal trials, was thereupon discussed before Judge Fulton, and he, in the language of Dr. Stribling, "sent his officer with an attachment to *coerce* my attendance. The attachment was not executed, only because, under the advice of learned and able counsel, I became satisfied that, in this case, at least, 'prudence was the better part of valour.'"

Now, in our humble opinion, Dr. Stribling and his Board of Directors were wrong in the premises. We think that no superintendent of an institution should be exempt from obedience to a subpœna, in any case, either criminal or civil, in which his opinion as an expert is important to the issue. We have few experts of the kind. They are, almost without exception, connected with the institutions for the insane. Those institutions have, or ought to have competent assistant physicians. Thus, we believe that a law releasing the superintendents from duty before legal tribunals, would be more seriously detrimental to the cause of justice, and to the welfare of society, than useful to the inmates of the institutions over which they preside.

10. From the few statistics of the reports of the State Lunatic Asylum of South Carolina, we select the following:—

	1853.			1855.		
	Men.	Women.	Total.	Men.	Women.	Total.
Patients at the beginning of the year			135			174
Admitted in the course of the year .	40	35	75			62
Whole number in the course of the year			210			236
Discharged, including deaths . .			38			65
Remaining at the end of the year .	91	81	172	86	85	171
Discharged cured			22			18
Died			9			31

In regard to the mortality in 1855, Dr. Trezevant says: "We have lost 31 patients: 15 of these, from their enfeebled state, would have died under any circumstances, but their death was hurried on by the improper accommodations of the house, and the unwholesome condition of the yard. The rest suffered from bowel complaint, then prevailing, and were the victims of our want of proper ventilation and arrangements. * * * In dry seasons the mortality is about five per cent., but in wet it has been equal to about one in three. In the present year the bowel affections commenced with the rainy season, continued whilst it lasted, and ceased when the earth was no longer saturated with moisture."

We have carefully perused the reports before us, and find therein but little which comes within the scope of our notices, while that little is upon subjects already fully laid before our readers. The chief burthen of the reports from this institution, for several years past, consists of an exposition of the imperfections of the Asylum, and the necessity of a new one. The building is old, and imperfect in its architectural construction and arrangements. Its grounds are too limited, and are immediately surrounded by dwelling-houses of citizens of Columbia. It appears that one or more of its wards are so damp as seriously to affect the health of the inmates. The whole is so much crowded that, as stated in one of the reports, there are fifty patients more than can be properly accommodated. The heating and ventilation are bad. There are no proper arrangements of baths and water-closets. In short, judging from the reports, the whole establishment stands but as a representative of the past. It is acknowledged as such by the Regents, the Physician, and the Superintendent. This has been granted for years. The question, therefore, has been, What shall be done? We have exposition after exposition of the defects. We have suggestions for erecting additional buildings to those which now exist. We have propositions to erect an entirely new establishment upon the lands now occupied. We have argument upon argument to prove that a new structure should be erected more remote from the town. And yet the question is—What shall be done? There is a liberal appropriation yet unexpended. Different models have been presented for the new edifice. One of these is preferred and highly extolled by one party, but rejected and condemned in the strongest terms by another. And still, alas! still the question is—What shall be done? And the relic of the past, with "all its imperfections on its head," continues unmolested, and its inmates rejoice in the comforts of antiquity, because the powers that be cannot agree upon a substitute.

ART. XV.—*Deux Mémoires sur la Physiologie de la Moelle Épinière, lus à l'Académie des Sciences*, le 27 Août et le 24 Septembre, 1855. Par le Docteur E. BROWN-SÉQUARD. Lauréat de l'Académie des Sciences, etc. etc. 8vo. pp. 42. Paris, 1855.

Recherches Expérimentales sur la transmission croisée des Impressions Sensitives dans la Moelle Épinière. Par le Docteur E. BROWN-SÉQUARD, etc. etc. 8vo. pp. 19. Paris, 1855.

Propriétés et Fonctions de la Moelle Épinière: Rapport sur quelques Experiences de M. BROWN-SÉQUARD. Lu à la Société de Biologie, le 21 Juillet, 1855. Par M. PAUL BROCA, Professeur Agrégé à la Faculté de Médecine, etc. 8vo. pp. 35. Paris, 1855.

Two Memoirs on the Physiology of the Spinal Cord, read to the Academy of Sciences, August 27 and September 24, 1855. By E. BROWN-SÉQUARD, M. D.

Experimental Researches into the Decussation which takes place in the Transmission of Sensitive Impressions through the Spinal Cord. By E. BROWN-SÉQUARD, M. D.

Properties and Functions of the Spinal Cord: A Report on some Experiments of M. BROWN-SÉQUARD. Read to the Biological Society, July 21, 1855. By M. PAUL BROCA.

THE recent investigations of Dr. Brown-Séquard have thrown very important light on the physiology of the spinal cord, especially on the manner in which sensitive impressions received by the different portions of the body are transmitted, through it, to the brain.

While the fact is now, apparently, well established, that the posterior roots of the spinal nerves are the sole route for the transmission of sensitive impressions to the sensorium, there still continues to exist much diversity of opinion as to the portion of the spinal cord through which these impressions are conveyed to the brain. According to Backer, Kuerschner, and Longet, it is solely by the posterior fasciculi of the cord. Bellingeri refers the transmission to the central and Stilling to the posterior portion of the gray substance alone, while Ludwig Türck refers it to the lateral fasciculi. Eigenbrodt, while he describes the posterior fasciculi as the principal medium of transmission, believes that it may also take place through the gray substance, probably by the white fibres contained in this portion of the cord. According to Schiff, both the gray substance and the posterior fasciculi are the media of transmission, and one of these portions of the cord may supply the action of the other. Rolando and Calmeil suppose that every portion of the spinal cord is capable of transmitting sensitive impressions to the brain.

This diversity of opinion in reference to a subject that would appear, at first sight, so easy to determine by experiment, Dr. Brown-Séquard supposes to have arisen from ignorance on the part of the experimenters of one or other, or several of the following circumstances:—

1st. The existence of reflex movements.

2d. The decussation which occurs in the transmission through the spinal cord of sensitive impressions.

3d. The possibility of this transmission being made by parts devoid themselves of sensibility; and,

4th. The possibility of exposing the spinal cord, without causing an excessive loss of blood, and without exhausting the sensibility of the animal.

By a series of well devised and skilfully executed vivisections, Dr. Brown-Séquard has very clearly demonstrated that, it is not by the posterior fasciculi of the spinal cord that ultimately takes place the transmission to the brain of the sensitive impressions made upon the trunk and limbs, but by the gray substance of the cord, and especially by its central portion.

Dr. Brown-Séquard has endeavoured to show, by a number of ingenious and very striking experiments, carefully made by him upon the living animal, and varied so as to avoid, as much as possible, all sources of error, that the transmission of sensitive impressions through the spinal cord is made, in great part, if not entirely, in a decussative manner; that is to say, the impressions that come from the right side of the body are transmitted to the brain by the left half of the cord, and *vice versa.*

The general conclusions deduced from these experiments, and verified by numerous pathological facts, are as follow:—

1st. The decussation of the elements by which sensitive impressions are conveyed to the brain, does not take place, as it has been asserted, at the anterior extremity of the spinal protuberance.

2d. The gray substance of the cord does not possess the property, as some physiologists pretend, of transmitting sensitive impressions in every direction.

3d. The most part, if not all the elements by which sensitive impressions are transmitted, decussate in the spinal cord; that is to say, those coming from the right half of the body pass into the left half of the cord, and *vice versa.*

4th. The decussation of these elements occurs, in part, almost immediately after their entrance into the spinal cord; a few of them decussate at a certain distance above the place of entrance, while others, on the contrary, and much the greatest number, descend into the cord and decussate a certain distance below the point of entrance.

5th. If there be some of the elements by which sensitive impressions are transmitted that ascend from the limbs or trunks along the entire course of the spinal cord to make their decussation in the brain, their number must be very inconsiderable.

6th. The lesions capable of producing a paralysis of sensibility, seated at any point of a lateral half of the cerebro-spinal centre, produce always the paralysis of sensibility in the opposite side of the body. There is no difference, in this respect, between the brain and spinal cord, as has heretofore been supposed.

In a more recent memoir, Dr. Brown-Séquard describes a series of further vivisections, which, besides confirming the correctness of the general conclusions in reference to the functions of the spinal cord deduced by him from his former experiments, have conducted to results, in reference to the organization and physiology of that important organ, of a character at once novel and highly interesting.

In previous experiments, Dr. B. S. demonstrated that when the two posterior fasciculi of the cord are divided transversely, both the divided surfaces remain sensible. This fact would appear to prove, contrary to what physiologists have universally admitted, that the transmission of sensitive impressions may take place, in the posterior fasciculi of the cord, in two opposite directions. The following experiment performed by Dr. B. S., leads, on this question, to results much more positive:—

"In a dog, cat, or full grown rabbit, we divide transversely the two posterior fasiculi of the spinal cord, at the inferior portion of the dorsal region; we then dissect these fasciculi from the divided edges, longitudinally, for the distance of two or three centimètres, so as to separate from the surface of the cord that distance, two laminæ, continuous, the one by its superior, and the other by its inferior extremity, with the rest of the cord. The sensibility persists, but weakened, in both of the separated laminæ, and we have verified the fact a great number of times, since 1852 when we first announced it, that the inferior lamina appears to be more sensitive than the superior."

Subsequently, Dr. B. S. has varied this experiment, by taking two animals of the same species, and in each separating a single lamina from the surface of the posterior fasciculi, leaving it continuous with the cord at its upper extremity in the one, and at its lower extremity in the other. In comparing the sensibility of the laminæ in the two animals, it was found, as in the preceding experiment, that the one which remained attached to the cord by its lower end, exhibited a greater degree of sensibility than the other.

If, remarks the Doctor, we dissect up laminæ comprising not only the posterior fasciculi, but also a part of the lateral fasciculi of the posterior gray cornua, we find the sensibility to be much more acute in the two laminæ than when they are composed only of the posterior fasciculi. The length of the flaps has also a considerable influence upon the degree of their sensibility. The shorter they are the greater their sensibility. When over four or five centimètres in length, they have scarce any sensibility near their free extremity.

It is evident that the impressions made upon the free extremity of a flap detached from the posterior fasciculi of the cord, excepting at its lower end, must be centrifugal, and as, in those fasciculi, the only nervous element we can detect for the transmission of sensations are fibres, it therefore results, according to Dr. B. S., that fibres, capable of transmitting sensitive impressions in a centrifugal direction, exist in the posterior fasciculi of the spinal chord. By the following experiments, he shows that these fibres merely pass in the posterior fasciculi, and after a short course pass out again and penetrate the gray matter.

We divide, transversely, the posterior fasciculi on a level with the tenth dorsal vertebra, and from the surface of these fasciculi, below the section, we separate a flap of about two or three centimètres in length, and leave it attached to the cord by its inferior extremity. Having assured ourselves that this flap retains its sensibility, we then divide transversely the two posterior fasciculi, at the distance of one centimètre below the spot where the flap is connected with the cord, and we find that the flap is deprived of all or nearly all its sensibility.

"If, in place of making the second section at only one, we make it at five or more centimètres below the spot at which the flap remains continuous with the cord, we find that the sensibility of the flap continues unimpaired. In this case, the fibres for centrifugal transmission have quitted the posterior fasciculi to pass into another portion of the cord, because the second incision did not reach them, as it did in the first case, where they were all or nearly all divided."

The fibres referred to it is evident, therefore, quit, after passing a short distance, the posterior fasciculi; whence go they? The following facts show that they pass into the central gray substance.

"If in three animals, after having separated a flap from the posterior fasciculi of the cord, adherent by its inferior extremity, we divide transversely, at about four or five centimètres anteriorly to the flap, in one of the animals, the lateral fasciculi, in a second, the anterior fasciculi, and in the third, the gray substance, we find that, in the last animal, the sensibility of the flap is destroyed, while it still continues in the other two. But if we divide in these the central gray substance, on a level with the spot at which the flap is continuous with the cord, the flap is deprived of its sensibility."

It is therefore in the central gray substance that pass the descending fibres of the posterior fasciculi, or those for centrifugal transmission. Analogous experiments show that in the flaps of the posterior fasciculi that adhere by their superior extremity, the ascending fibres, or those for centripetal transmission quit, also, very soon the posterior fasciculi to penetrate into the central gray substance of the cord.

"The foregoing experiments," remarks the Doctor, "would seem to authorize the following conclusions:—

"1st. That there are two species of sensitive fibres in the posterior fasciculi of the cord: the one ascending, or for centripetal transmission; the other descending, or for centrifugal transmission.

"2d. That in the posterior fasciculi, either the descending fibres are more numerous than the ascending, or they are capable, under certain circumstances, of inducing a greater amount of pain than the ascending fibres.

"3d. That the ascending as well as the descending fibres merely pass into the posterior fasciculi, and after running along them for a short distance, come out again to penetrate into the central gray matter of the cord."

Dr. B. S. has shown, by direct experiment, that a considerable number of the ascending and descending fibres are derived from the posterior spinal nerves; or, in other words, immediately upon their arrival in the cord, these nerves send fibres into the posterior fasciculi, of which a portion pass towards the brain, while another portion take an opposite direction. But all of these fibres quit soon the posterior fasciculi to penetrate into the central gray substance of the cord. The following experiment shows that they pass from the right posterior fasciculus to the left portion of the gray matter.

"In a rabbit we divide a lateral half of the cord, transversely, on a level with the first lumbar vertebra, and then cut longitudinally the cord to the extent of two centimètres in the direction of its antero-posterior plane, downwards from the transverse section, and at a right angle with it. A small portion of the cord is thus separated at every part excepting its inferior extremity. In another rabbit we in the same way separate a small portion of the cord at every part excepting its superior extremity. Thus, in the first rabbit the impression, when the posterior nerves that are inserted in the partially separated portion of the cord, will be transmitted by the descending and in the second by the ascending fibres. If it is on the right side of the cord that the incisions have been made, and we divide, on the left side, the posterior fasciculus, at the distance of five centimètres above the part at which the first incision has been made, in irritating the posterior nerves which are inserted in the partially separated portion of the cord, we find them to be still sensible, but if, at the part where the left posterior fasciculus is divided, we cut through, transversely, the left lateral half of the central gray substance, the nerves referred to lose their sensibility."

Experiments detailed by Dr. B. S., in which, after two transverse sections of the posterior fasciculi, made at a short distance from each other, sensibility has been diminished or lost in the posterior nervous roots included between the incisions, seem to prove that a considerable number of the fibres of these roots pass to the posterior fasciculi. Other experiments, in which, after two transverse sections of the posterior fasciculi, the posterior roots, included between the incisions, retain in a striking degree their sensibility, would seem to show that the fibres of the nervous roots which pass by the posterior fasciculi, come out again after running a certain course.

"The cut surfaces of the section of a segment of the posterior fasciculi, resulting from two transverse divisions of these fasciculi, appear," remarks Dr. B. S., "always to differ, the one from the other, in their degree of sensibility; the greatest amount appearing to exist in the uppermost.

"In the experiment performed by dividing transversely the posterior fasciculi in two places, very near to each other, we obtain a very curious result. We refer to the hyperæsthesia which exists everywhere below the inferior section. Of the three segments which result from a division, at two points, of the posterior fasciculi, the upper or cephalic has a normal sensibility, the middle, a very feeble sensibility, and the posterior or caudal, an exaggerated sensibility. This exalted sensibility of the lower segment is always observed, excepting when the division has been made near to the caudal extremity of the cord, and it is, I may add, the greater in direct proportion to the size of the segment.

"The state of sensibility in a segment of the posterior fasciculi, included between two transverse sections, has a direct relation with that of the nervous roots inserted in the segment, and of those portions of the body which derive their sensitive fibres from these roots. That is to say, when the sensibility of the fasciculi is diminished or augmented in a certain proportion, there is a corresponding diminution or augmentation in the nervous roots and all the parts of the body to which these send fibres.

"If, as we have attempted to show, the fibres of the posterior nervous roots pass, in part, into the posterior fasciculi, we should find, after having divided transversely the entire cord, excepting the posterior cords, that sensibility persists, to a certain extent, in the posterior fasciculi and nervous roots, behind the section; and such is actually the case, as we have shown in a preceding memoir. In this experiment, the posterior roots of the two or three pair of nerves that are immediately behind the point where the cord is divided, retain their sensibility through those of their fibres that pass by the posterior fasciculi. This is not the case, however, with the nervous roots situated at a greater distance behind the point of division; their sensibility is lost, because, such of their fibres as pass by the posterior fasciculi have already quitted the posterior fasciculi and penetrated into the gray substance beyond the point of division.

"The following experiment shows that the fibres of the posterior nervous roots which pass by the posterior fasciculi a short distance behind where the latter have been divided, again leave these fasciculi a short distance in front of the division.

"In a cat or dog, after a transverse section of all the cord, save the posterior fasciculi, on a level with the tenth dorsal vertebra, we assure ourselves that sensibility persists in the posterior fasciculi, for the extent of some centimètres behind the point of division, as well as in the posterior roots of the two or three pair of nerves that are immediately behind this point. Then, upon one animal, at the distance of one centimètre, and in another, at the distance of five or six centimètres, in front of the first described section, we divide transversely the posterior fasciculi; in the first animal we find that sensibility is destroyed, while, in the second, it continues behind the part at which the first described section had been made. If, however, we divide, in this latter, transversely, the central gray matter, at the point where the posterior fasciculi had been divided, we shall find that the sensibility is lost."

"It is probable," Dr. B. S., remarks, "that certain fibres of the posterior nervous roots pursue a similar course in the gray cornua with those which go to the posterior cords, that is to say, after penetrating into the cornua, the fibres separate into ascending and descending, and after a short course penetrate the central gray substance. It is at least what may be rationally concluded from the following experiments:—

"Before and behind the posterior roots of a pair of nerves, we thrust into the posterior gray cornua, in a direction perpendicular to the longitudinal axis of the cord, a flat needle with a double cutting-edge, so as to cut the cornua transversely. We find subsequently that the posterior nervous roots between the four punctures made in the cornua have lost a considerable portion of their sensibility."

"We divide, transversely, on a level with and anterior to the last pair of dorsal nerves, the greater portion of the fibres of the posterior fasciculi, saving, as much as possible, the surrounding gray substance. We afterwards perform the same operation behind the second pair of lumbar nerves; so as to comprehend three pair of nerves between the two divisions. The sensibility we find still persists sufficiently acute in the posterior nervous roots intermediate to the points of division. If now the two sections are enlarged laterally, so as to divide the remaining fibres of the posterior fasciculi as well as the posterior gray cornua, the sensibility is diminished in a manifest degree in the nervous roots referred to. If, in addition to the sections already made, we also divide a considerable portion of the lateral chords, we find that these roots lose, still more, their sensibility."

From these experiments, it would appear that the posterior gray cornua as well as the lateral fasciculi, at least their posterior portion, are the parts for the passage of a certain number of the fibres of the posterior nervous roots. In regard to the lateral fasciculi, this conclusion is rendered still more probable by the following experiment:—

"At two places, immediately before and behind the posterior roots of three pair of nerves, we divide, transversely, the posterior portion of the lateral fasciculi, taking care to avoid, as much as possible, the central gray substance and the posterior cornua, and we find that an evident, though not very considerable diminution, occurs in the sensibility of the posterior roots of the three pair of nerves included between the divisions. The diminution of sensibility is much more evident when the two, or rather four sections, are so performed as to include only a single pair of nerves between them."

The fibres of the posterior nervous roots that pass into the lateral fasciculi, as well as those which proceed to the gray cornua, are ascending or descending like those which go to the posterior fasciculi. Besides, the fibres of the nervous roots which pass a certain distance along the lateral fasciculi and the posterior cornua, quit soon these parts to penetrate into the central gray substance. These facts are demonstrated, in regard to the posterior cornua and lateral fasciculi, in the same manner as in reference to the posterior fasciculi.

It would appear, then, that in the spinal cord, the posterior spinal roots are arranged very similar to the ganglionar root of the trigeminus nerve, which, as we are aware, is divided in the spinal protuberance and bulb, into three portions, of which two, of little size, are the one ascending, and the other transverse, while the third, the bulbar root, is very large, and descending.

From the facts and reasoning Dr. B. S. has adduced, he believes that he is able to draw two series of conclusions, as follows:—

"I. *Conclusions relative to the distribution of the Fibres of the Posterior Nervous Roots in the Spinal Cord.*—1. The fibres of the posterior nervous roots appear to pass in part to the posterior fasciculi, and probably also, but in a very small number, to the lateral fasciculi.

"2. The fibres of the posterior roots which pass to the posterior fasciculi, appear to proceed, in part, towards the brain, and, in part, in the opposite direction; so the one portion are ascending, and the other descending.

"3. The fibres of the posterior roots which pass to the lateral fasciculi, seem also to be composed of two series, the one ascending the other desending.

"4. In the posterior gray cornua, there appears to be, also, ascending and descending fibres derived from the posterior roots.

"5. In the posterior and lateral fasciculi, as well as in the posterior gray cornua, the descending fibres appear to be more numerous than the ascending.

"6. The ascending and descending fibres derived from the posterior nervous roots appear, after passing for a short distance, to leave the posterior and lateral fasciculi, as well as the posterior gray cornua, to penetrate the central gray substance.

"II. *Conclusions relative to the transmission of Sensitive Impressions in the*

Spinal Cord.—1. On their arrival at the spinal cord the sensitive impressions pass by the posterior fasciculi, the posterior gray cornua, and probably, also, by the lateral fasciculi.

"2. In these different portions of the cord, the sensitive impressions mount or descend, and, after a short course, towards the brain or in the opposite direction, they quit these portions of the cord to enter the central gray substance, in which, or by which they are finally transmitted to the brain."

The fifth conclusion of the first series is one which, according to Dr. B. S., is the least positively established of the six. In saying that descending fibres appear to be more numerous than the ascending, he wishes only to be understood as offering the probable explanation of the hyperæsthesia of those portions of the body which are behind the point at which the posterior fasciculi of the cord have been divided transversely. He is aware that there are two other explanations that may be given of this phenomenon which possess perhaps equal probability. Thus, it is possible that it is a property of the descending fibres to possess a greater amount of sensibility than the ascending, if so it is not necessary to explain the fact referred to by supposing that there should be more descending than ascending fibres. It is very certain that there is a special cause of the hyperæsthesia experienced, after a division of the posterior fasciculi, in the parts below that division, and consequently the descending fibres should cause more pain than the ascending in the experiments of Dr. B. S., because the properties of the descending fibres cannot be tested until after the posterior fasciculi, or one of them have been divided.

"It is possible, then, that even though inferior in number, the descending fibres may cause a greater amount of pain than the ascending. Let the question be settled as it may in reference to the relative number of the different fibres, an important anatomical and physiological fact results from the facts reported in this memoir, it is that the posterior nervous roots of the cord, in the same manner as the great root of the trigeminus in the bulb, send into the cord sensitive descending fibres, or those for centrifugal transmission. Anatomy must decide as to the *number*—with respect to the question of the *existence* of these fibres, anatomy has already confirmed what vivisections so positively teach. We have seen, and the most skilful microscopists have likewise seen descending fibres proceeding from the posterior nervous roots."

D. F. C.

Art. XVI.—*Clinical Lectures on Surgery.* By M. Nélaton. *From Notes taken by* Walter F. Atlee, M. D. Philadelphia: J. B. Lippincott & Co., 1855. 8vo. pp. 755.

This volume, according to the preface, "contains the publication of notes taken, during a period of three years, 1851–52–53–54, from the remarks made upon cases to which attention was particularly directed. The course adopted in their arrangement has been, as a general rule, to class under the same head those in which the same pathological lesion existed, though in some few instances, when the great interest of the case lies in the diagnosis, this plan has been departed from, and the case has been classed with others, from the fact that it was *not* one of them."

The preface further informs us that the additions of the editor "are so placed as to be at once distinguished. This has been done very rarely, in fact almost solely, in order to make the work as respects surgical pathology more complete, by stating the results of microscopical investigations. These results have been taken from the works of M. Charles Robin, and of M. Lebert."

The title of the work, although not altogether in accordance with the statements of the preface and the actual contents, must insure for it an amount of attention, which we are glad to say there is much to gratify in the notes of which it is composed. Clinical lectures are always interesting; and the name of Nélaton as the lecturer is at present so attractive, that almost any report of his hospital teachings would be eagerly sought after by a numerous crowd of admirers in this country. We remember him ten years ago in the very same field of labour, which he has since rendered so pre-eminent, as even then one of the best and most popular lecturers on his branch, although Berard and Blandin, Lisfranc and Roux, as well as the now veteran Velpeau, were still in full vigour and activity. We have read the notes of Dr. Atlee, therefore, with unusual interest. They do great credit to his industry and enterprise; and we are satisfied that they are unusually full and faithful, and may afford an excellent idea of the distinguished clinical professor's mode of teaching, as well as of much of his theory and practice.

We regret, however, that they have been left to work their way without the guarantee of authenticity, if not of special authority, which is naturally looked for in a production of such extent and character. The very high reputation of the author of the lessons which they are understood to represent, and the consequent importance of the doctrines and experience which they exhibit, obviously increase the necessity for accompanying their publication with some kind of token, on the part of M. Nélaton, of assent to their appearance, and of affirmation of the facts and opinions which they impute to him.

We understand that the desired approval was obtained by Dr. Atlee, and that accident alone has hitherto prevented its announcement. A voucher to this effect would certainly very much enhance the value of the work, and give, in many eyes which now view it with distrust, an entirely different aspect to an offering which has been too handsomely produced, and has cost too much valuable time and labour, to be presented under any but the most favourable auspices. It is to be hoped, therefore, that the objection may be removed in the next edition. This seems to be all the more needful, because new or peculiar modes of practice in treatment and operations, and independent views of pathology and therapeutics, may be met with here and there, which must prove rather startling to the previous notions of many readers. A few of these might be dwelt upon to more or less advantage in our notice; and we might be tempted to risk a doubt or two, so far as this country is concerned, in relation to some others, did they come before us more directly from their author.

Several of the cases which suggested peculiarities of practice or pathology, are unfortunately inconclusive, because, owing to various impediments, no results were ascertained. The value of a number of the observations is seriously impaired, in this way; many cases of interest—not a few decidedly important—being abruptly terminated through the disappearance of the patient, or the withdrawal of the lecturer or reporter. Others may be noted also, which, although natural enough in the course of an every-day clinique, and proper enough, perhaps, in an elementary text-book, seem hardly to be entitled to the space they occupy in a collection of selected cases. They were certainly not required to establish either the interest or completeness of the series. We do not say this in a fault-finding spirit; we are not the first to make these remarks, and we repeat them as a matter of duty, especially in behalf of that influential class of readers who regard a big book as a great evil. In our practical day and generation the worst of troubles in a book intended to be much and widely read, is too often in its own specific gravity: the deadliest foe to popular interest in the *nature* of the matter of an author's pages, is its extra *amount* in bulk. As bulk, then, is one of the difficulties which is barely escaped in Dr. Atlee's volume, although doubtless fully overcome in its successful circulation, he will excuse us if, with a sincere desire to avoid disparagement, we express the belief that the matter which is added to the clinical notes for the purpose of pathological illustration might have been advantageously compressed into the form of foot-notes or appendices in smaller type. This appears to us especially desirable in the portions relating to the microscopical conclusions of the authorities cited in the preface, since these conclusions are not those of M. Nélaton himself; nor do the recent investigations and discussions, in the French Academy and elsewhere, appear to aid in settling mooted points or in sustaining the weight of these authorities against him and his fellow-surgeons. We cannot help doubting the utility of such additions in a work which, as the *Clinical Lectures* of the Professor of Clinical Surgery in the Medical School of Paris, from notes taken in the wards or amphitheatre of the Clinical Hospital of that school, might be regarded, notwithstanding the qualifications of the preface, as intended to exhibit the precepts and practice of that Professor, and of him alone. In adding to the commentaries of M. Nélaton the editor runs the risk of a confusion, if not of conflict of opinions, which might materially change the character of his book.

Still no one can fail to become deeply interested in its pages, or to be decidedly benefited by the many admirable hints on diagnosis and treatment afforded by the cases and comments which occur in the greatest profusion and variety, and are repeatedly presented in graphic and vivid colours. We take pleasure, therefore, notwithstanding some, perhaps immaterial, objections to one or two features of the publication, in recommending it to the careful study of advanced students and practitioners. To the latter, especially, it must prove not only very interesting but in the highest degree instructive, as we should be glad to show by a few extracts, had we space for them, and by a hasty glance at the headings of the principal chapters.

Among the almost bewildering array of surgical diseases and injuries which are often forcibly and always usefully illustrated, in the twenty-three chapters, may be mentioned burns, contusions, wounds, and local disorders of different kinds, affections of the bloodvessels, cancerous and other tumours, abscesses, fractures, and luxations, diseases of the joints and of the bones, injuries of the head, affections of the eye and of the nose, affections of the soft parts of the face, of the neck, of the mammary gland, tumours of the abdomen, diseases of the anus, rectum, and intestines, of the male genital organs, of the bladder, of the female genital organs, affections of the foot.

Under these separate heads almost the whole range of ordinary practice, together with much that is by no means of every-day occurrence, even in hospital experience, is presented in an agreeable and familiar and, as already intimated, often particularly clear and striking manner. M. Nélaton's happy faculty of teaching principles, as well as his lucid modes of demonstration, are well retained by Dr. Atlee in his notes. Indeed, in spite of frequent Gallicisms and occasional obscurities of language, the extreme literalness of the translation increases its genuineness to us, and affords the strongest evidence of the fidelity of the reporter. The very Gallicisms in words and phrases are full of associations with the lecture-room in which they were originally taken down, and recall to our mind the language of the lecturer more forcibly than the purest English that could be written. Let us not be understood to be the apologist for errors of revision, which we doubt not will be fully atoned for in a future effort. These are minor blemishes, although annoying to many readers and injurious to the reputation of a translation, but they are not serious enough to interfere with the legitimate uses of a scientific work intended solely for professional men who ought to be familiar with the language from which they are derived.

Our thanks are due to the publishers for the handsome style in which the volume is produced. It would be gratifying to see their example on this occasiou more frequently followed. E. H.

Art. XVII.—*Human Physiology.* By Robley Dunglison, M. D., LL. D., Professor of the Institutes of Medicine in Jefferson Medical College, Philadelphia, etc.: "Vastissimi studii primas lineas circumscripsi." Haller. With five hundred and thirty-two illustrations. Eighth edition, revised, modified, and enlarged. Two volumes, 8vo. pp. 729–755. Philadelphia, 1856: Blanchard and Lea.

In the notice of a scientific work, which, in the midst of a host of contemporaries of high reputation, has already reached to its eighth edition, it would be a work of supererogation to enter into a formal criticism of either its matter or its plan. It has, unquestionably, been found to answer, in a good degree at least, the purposes for which it was originally prepared, and to keep pace with the progress of discovery and elucidation in its particular department, or the call for edition after edition would not have been made. A very inferior treatise on physiology, or one behind the knowledge of the day, would not have been tolerated, when so many others of acknowledged value were at hand to supply its place.

In a work which, like the one before us, is chiefly valuable as a correct and satisfactory exponent of the actual state of physiology, deduced from the observations and experiments of preceding and contemporary investigators, we are not to look so much for originality of matter as for fulness, accuracy, and impartiality, in the exposition of the labours of the most reliable cultivators of the science, and for clearness and system in the arrangement and treatment of the subjects embraced in it; so that it shall present a faithful and useful reflection of received facts and doctrines, with, of course, the views of its author on all those questions that still remain problematical, or, in regard to which a difference or opposition of opinion is entertained by authorities of equal weight.

In this latter point of view, the treatise of Dr. Dunglison is one admirably calculated to meet the wants of the student of human physiology. The author has, with commendable industry, noted the new facts, as well as the modifications of those previously recorded, that are due to the labours of the more recent physiologists, and the changes that, in consequence, the before received explanations of vital phenomena have undergone; these, with its clear exposition of the established truths and doctrines, render the present edition as fair an expression as can be desired of the physiology of the day—such as it has been rendered by the labours of a host of energetic and discriminating luvestigators.

We may, it is true, in a careful analysis of the work, find ourselves obliged to differ from the author as to the validity of one or two of the opinions he has drawn from established facts, and, occasionally, to accuse him of having given undue importance to certain series of observations and experiments, and the doctrines based upon them; as a whole, however, we can candidly say, that we know of no treatise better adapted for the use of the medical student, or of those who, although they are not preparing themselves for admission into the ranks of our profession, may desire, nevertheless, to become acquainted with the vital laws and phenomena of the human organism.

The work is well and richly illustrated; for several of the illustrations contained in former editions, others of a superior quality have been substituted, while about sixty entirely new ones have been added. D. F. C.

Art. XVIII.—*A Practical Treatise on the Diseases of the Testis, and of the Spermatic Cord and Scrotum.* With numerous wood engravings. By T. B. Curling, F. R. S., &c. &c. Second American, from the second revised and enlarged English edition. Philadelphia: Blanchard & Lea, 1856. 8vo. pp. 419.

Mr. Curling's admirable monograph has been the standard authority on its subject ever since it first appeared some twelve or thirteen years ago. The new edition may be safely recommended as not only sustaining, but decidedly surpassing the reputation of the old one in all the characteristics of a classical treatise, and in none more than in its practical tendencies. The peculiarly happy qualifications of the author for the preparation of such an essay, have evidently been at work in enabling him to make the utmost of the unusual opportunities afforded by the long interval between the two editions, and by the immense field of observation and research within his reach. Those who are familiar with the original work, superior as it was to all of its predecessors, cannot fail to be satisfied that the evidence of progress presented by the volume before us is fully in proportion to the advance of practical science generally, if not greater than there was reason to expect in a work already so complete in most respects and confined to the disorders of a single organ.

This is the impression which a careful comparison of the first and second issues, of which both English and American copies are now upon our table, has made upon ourselves. The whole book has been subjected to a laborious revision by its able author; and has been correspondingly improved in style and arrangement, as well as in the addition of a large amount of valuable matter. In the course of this improvement new chapters have been added, many have been rewritten, and as the preface very modestly ventures to hepe, nearly all of them contain additional facts of practical interest and importance. In order to accommodate the fresh matter and additional wood-cuts without increase of bulk, the introductory part on the anatomy of the testis is omitted in the London and New York copy. A smaller type and larger page have enabled the Philadelphia publishers to retain this section in their edition, without making their volume as large as the other, at the same time that some notes and several extra illustrations have been introduced by Dr. W. H. Gobrecht, who was called upon to incorporate the cases of the author's appendix in the text, and to supervise the passage of the latter through the press.

We find upon examination, that notwithstanding the retention of nearly twenty pages on the anatomy, including seven wood engravings, together with three brief notes and eight new wood engravings in the remaining chapters, the American reprint occupies just one hundred pages less than the London and New York original. It should be said also that the paper and printing of the American edition are as good as usual, and the execution of the wood-cuts is all that need be desired—quite equal to that of their prototypes from the hands of the English artists.

It is difficult to make selections where there is so much to engage the professional reader. Nor is it much easier to point out the portions of the volume which, either on account of novelty or practical interest, may seem to demand especial notice. Without attempting such distinctions, we may say that in glancing over the pages our attention has been arrested by Chapter I., On Congenital Imperfections and Malformations—particularly Sect. III., On Imperfect Transition of the Testicle; Chaper IV., On Hydrocele; Chapter VI., On Orchitis, and particularly Sect. II., On Chronic Orchitis; Chapter VII., On Tubercular Disease of the Testicle; Chapter VIII., On Carcinoma of the Testicle; Chapter XIX., On Castration; Chapter I. of the part on Diseases of the Spermatic Cord, On Hydrocele: Chapters IX., X., XI., of the Third Part, On Diseases of the Scrotum, occupied with adipose, fibrous, and cystic Tumours of the Scrotum. The chapters just enumerated are but a few of the thirty-four which are worthy of study as containing much that is not to be found in the pages of the former edition. They may serve in some degree to show the nature of the advance made by the author in his twelve years' inquiries and records in relation to the subject of his elaborate and most instructive work. In addition to his own valuable accumulations, Mr. Curling was enabled to avail himself of the manuscript copy of a prize essay on the diseases of the testis, by Mr. Harvey Ludlow, a young and promising surgeon, recently a victim of the Eastern war at Scutari. Valuable tables and cases of interest well observed and recorded in this essay, are quoted and handsomely acknowledged by our author.

We conclude our notice with two or three extracts which appeared to be sufficiently interesting to reward a perusal here; at the same time that they will afford a very fair idea of the general tone and style of the book.

His remarks upon the use of the seton in the treatment of hydrocele were especially acceptable to us, inasmuch as they speak well and to the purpose of a remedy for which we have been taught to entertain more respect than is generally accorded to it:—

"The seton is a better mode of treating hydrocele than the other plans which I have described; but though a remedy less severe than these, it is not free from the same objection, of being very liable to produce more inflammation than is requisite for the cure of the complaint. It is, however, a very useful remedy in certain forms of the disease, and in vaginal hydrocele under certain circumstances. The plan I adopt is to pass an ordinary curved needle, armed with a single or double silk ligature, through the skin and sac in front, leaving a space of an inch or an inch and a half between the ends of the ligature, which may be tied loosely together to prevent the seton escaping. The two or four threads should be sufficient to fill up the apertures made by the needle, and thus prevent the admission of air and escape of blood. The fluid in the sac then drains away along the threads. Inflammation of the sac soon arises, and causes fibrinous exudation. This is known by the greater solidity of the tumour, and it is then necessary to remove the threads, usually from the second to the third or fourth day after the operation. The inflammation and swelling afterwards subside, and the hydrocele is permanently cured by adhesion. In this way of employing the seton, the sac is disturbed much less than in the ordinary method, and the inflammation excited is usually mild. I have resorted to it in many cases of encysted hydrocele of the cord and testicle; and as the tumour in these cases is usually small in size, the seton proves the best means of cure. In cases of simple hydrocele, after the failure of injections by others, I have also used the seton with success, and I have tried it too in cases where no other treatment has been adopted. The great objection to its use in simple hydrocele is the uncertainty of its operation. I have generally found it both a sure and gentle remedy, though occasionally I have been disappointed by its producing high inflammation, which it was impossible to control, and which speedily ran on to suppuration." (p. 132.)

As appendix to the foregoing, it will be useful to add the following summary view:—

"A careful inquiry into the merits of the various modes of effecting the radical cure of hydrocele fully establishes the superiority of the treatment by injections, especially iodine. The older surgeons committed a great error by endeavouring to excite too high a degree of inflammation; for, not perceiving that the disease could be arrested by altering the action of the vessels of the part, they sought to obtain the closure of the natural cavity, which, moreover, they endeavoured to effect by producing suppurative inflammation and granulation, instead of by the gentler process of adhesion. The improvement in treatment consists in reducing the amount of inflammation to the lowest possible standard, the chief risk incurred arising from the plans employed proving too mild to be efficacious and sure. Injection has now been largely tried in this and other countries; and experience warrants us in asserting that, though it is not an infallible remedy, of all the plans hitherto practised it combines the greatest number of advantages. The pain attending it is slight; its effects are mild, and at the same time tolerably sure; if properly performed, it is free from danger; and it frequently succeeds without altering the natural condition of the parts. I know it is a question whether the cure by adhesion, though less perfect than that in which the disposition merely of the vessels is changed, is not upon the whole preferable. In the latter there is a possibility, if not a probability, of a relapse at some future period, the causes conducing to hydrocele still remaining; whilst the inconvenience produced by an impediment to the free movements of the testicle, in cases cured by adhesion, is regarded as too trivial to be any disadvantage. But, in the absence of data showing the degree to which the disease is liable to return after the cure without adhesion, I feel perfectly satisfied with such a result, and much prefer leaving a patient exposed to the doubtful chance of a relapse, than subjecting him to severer treatment in order to make sure of exciting sufficient inflammation to secure adhesion and obliteration of the sac. Injections, however, are not capable of effecting a cure in every case, nor are they adapted for every constitution. The judicious surgeon, therefore, whilst resorting to them as his ordinary remedy, will be prepared to avail himself, in particular and difficult cases, of other means more certain in their effects, such as the seton and incision." (pp. 141, 142.)

Next we present a long but curious and instructive account of spermatozoa in encysted hydrocele.

"In investigating the history of the cases of encysted hydrocele containing spermatozoa which came under my notice, I found in a majority of instances that the swelling had gradually formed after an injury to the testicle; and in two cases it was clear that a small cystic swelling had long existed in a stationary state, but after a slight blow had enlarged. So that it was most probable that a duct had been ruptured by the contusion, and that the irritation consequent on the injury, and perhaps on the addition of the spermatozoa to the fluid contents of the cyst, had led to its further growth. After several attempts to establish by anatomical examination the existence of a communication between the duct and the cyst of the hydrocele, which failed owing to the difficulty of injecting the tubes in the head of the epididymis, I have recently, with the assistance of Mr. John Quekett, succeeded in detecting a communication in two instances. A man, aged fifty-three, died in the London Hospital in July, 1854. His testicles being enlarged, were removed. On laying open the tunica vaginalis, I found a cyst containing about four drachms of milky fluid attached to the head of the epididymis in both testicles. At my request Mr. Quekett inserted a tube into the vas deferens, and injected the glands with mercury. The metal passed into the epididymis, and escaped freely into the cyst attached to it in both organs. The ducts of the epididymis, loaded with mercury, were found ramifying over the walls of the cyst, having been drawn out and expanded by the growth of the hydrocele. On examination of the interior of the cysts, the open mouth of the duct from which the mercury had escaped was distinctly visible. There was an oval opening in the membrane of the cyst, the edges of which were even and rounded, and at a point in the centre of this opening globules were seen escaping from a minute aperture in one of the ducts. The open mouth of the duct, into which a bristle has been passed, may be distinctly seen in the preparation.

"The examination of these two testicles affords the true solution of the diffi-

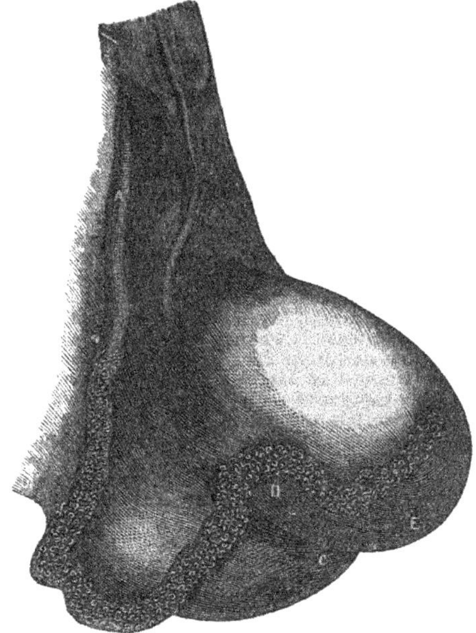

A. Vas deferens. C. Testicle. D. Epididymis, with the ducts expanded over the cyst. E. Cyst.

culty which has hitherto existed in satisfactorily accounting for the presence of spermatozoa in encysted hydroceles. It appears that as the hydrocele increases in size, the delicate tubes are drawn out and extended over the cyst, a position in which they are peculiarly exposed to accidental rupture. That the opening was of old standing, and not produced by the pressure of the column of mercury, is shown by the character of the aperture. It may be objected that if such a patent opening existed, the hydrocele should go on steadily increasing from the ingress of the spermatic fluid, and not remain stationary, as we often witness in these cases. We can readily conceive, however, that in the full distension of the cyst, the ducts would be so compressed and obstructed as to cause the seminal fluid to flow through the other efferent tubes. If the hydrocele were emptied by puncture, the channel would again become free, and fresh spermatozoa would then enter the cyst. In some instances the opening of the duct appears to become permanently closed, so that after the puncture of the cyst there is no return of the hydrocele, as in the following case. An old man consulted me on account of a large hydrocele which extended up to the abdominal ring, the testicle being situated at the bottom of the scrotum. It was on the right side, had been forming for eight years, and had never been tapped. I introduced a trocar, and drew off thirty-two ounces of a milky fluid, which contained myriads of spermatozoa. I saw him two months afterwards, and found a fulness on the right side of the scrotum from the collapsed sac, but there was no return of the hydrocele.[1]

"The ducts of the epididymis, when extended over the cyst, must not only be liable to rupture from a slight contusion, but also to be punctured in the operation of tapping; and no doubt they are occasionally wounded in this way. This appears to have happened in the following case: A man, aged fifty-one, had an encysted hydrocele, which was tapped by one of my colleagues, and about an ounce of limpid fluid was removed from two distinct cysts. He was again tapped by the same surgeon a month afterwards, and on neither occasion were any spermatozoa detected in the fluid removed. In a few weeks afterwards he applied to me in consequence of a return of the swelling, attended with a good deal of uneasiness. I performed acupuncture in three places, and in the drops of fluid which escaped, spermatozoa were found.

"Spermatozoa are stated to have been found in some two or three instances in fluid removed from the tunica vaginalis. It is not improbable that these cases may have been encysted hydroceles mistaken for simple. The diagnosis is sometimes very difficult, and in the case of the cyst examined by Mr. Paget, this error was made before death by a hospital surgeon. I have, however, found spermatozoa in the sac of the tunica vaginalis, and the following case will account for their presence. A man, aged fifty-four, died in the London Hospital of disease of the kidneys, of one of the ureters, and of the bladder, which appeared to be consequent on a severe blow on the loins about six weeks before. The tunica vaginalis of one of the testicles contained two ounces and a half of slightly opaque fluid, in which a few spermatozoa were found. There were three small cysts containing fluid, immediately connected with the epididymis, and also at one spot an irregular ragged membranous appearance, evidently caused by the rupture of a cyst. It is most p that the spermatozoa had escaped from this cyst, which may indeed robablbeen burst at the time of the injury. I have examined the fluid from the tunica vaginalis in a

[1] "The above explanation of the occurrence of spermatozoa in hydrocele is in complete accordance with the interesting observations of Professor H. Luschka in a Paper on the 'Appendicular Structures of the Testis' (*Virchow's Archiv. f. Path. Anat. u. Physiol.*, vol. vi. p. 310, 1854), with which I have only recently been made acquainted by Mr. Busk in a note in his recently published translation of *Wedl's Pathological Histology*, p. 465 (Syd. Soc.) Luschka states that the cavity in many cases communicates so openly with the seminiferous canal that the hydatid may be taken to represent a vesicular dilatation of the extremity of the latter, projecting beneath the epididymis. The communication with the seminal tube when narrower can, however, always be demonstrated by the introduction of a bristle, or by mercurial injection. But not unfrequently no communication can be discerned, and in these cases the cysts contain no seminal elements. Professor Luschka seems to have found less difficulty in detecting the communication with a seminal tube than I experienced.

large number of instances without finding these bodies, and I believe their occurrence in vaginal hydrocele to be extremely rare." (pp. 152–155.)

"From these observations, it will appear that I consider the treatment by pressure to be applicable either for the cure or relief of the majority of cases of varicocele occurring in practice. Certainly, in all those cases in which tolerably firm pressure with the fingers, at the abdominal ring, removes the sense of weight and uneasiness along the cord, this plan may be resorted to with every prospect of a beneficial result; and its simplicity, freedom from all risk, and efficiency, render it preferable to all operative modes of treatment. The truss should be applied whilst the patient is recumbent, so as to make rather firm pressure at the external ring. It sometimes happens that the truss, though worn with comfort after being adjusted in the morning, begins to produce uneasiness towards the after part of the day. When this is the case, the pressure should be diminished by loosening the thigh-strap. In general, the truss should be worn only during the day, though in some instances I have thought it advisable to recommend its use during the night also. Thus, in one case the patient suffered uneasiness in lying on the side affected, and was able to pass a better night on wearing the truss. When the scrotum is unusually pendulous, or when the veins are very long and form a plexus of any size, I advise the addition of the silk net suspender, which may be readily adapted to the truss." (pp. 373.)

Lastly, a short extract in regard to the treatment, radical as well as palliative, of varicocele, by pressure with a truss—in which Mr. Curling has had much experieuce and has met with great success.

The truss which is above referred to is delineated and described on p. 366, and several cases in illustration are given on the succeeding pages in order to explain its method of application and beneficial operation. This plan of treatment and its rationale have been known to the profession through Mr. Curling for several years, but we suspect that they have not attracted the attention they deserve. We remember listening with great interest to a lecture on the subject, read by Mr. Curling ten years ago, at a meeting of the Medico-Chirurgical Society of London. The report of this paper and the discussion on it were subsequently published and very generally quoted. His recommendation of the employment of the truss as he directs it for the removal of this common and vexatious infirmity, was no more decided then than it is now after a ten years' further trial.

E. H.

Art. XIX.—*Manual of Materia Medica and Therapeutics.* Sixth edition, revised and enlarged. By Prof. Fr. Oesterlen: published by Haupp & Siebeck, Tübingen, 1856.

The author of the above manual has been long favourably known to the literary and scientific world, not only by this *Materia Medica*, but also by his work on *Hygiene*, one on *Medical Logic*[1] (a work alike important to physician and naturalist), and various other productions. His manual of materia medica having in the course of a few years passed through so many editions, we may be allowed the conclusion that it must possess more than ordinary merits to commend it, for, considering the vast number of similar works, it could not otherwise have passed into the hands of so many thousands of readers in nearly every part of the world.

We are all aware that there is scarcely a department of medicine, for the development of which we need the aid and co-operation of so many various collateral sciences (more especially chemistry, pharmacy, physiological and chemical medicine, natural history and the like), as in that of materia medica and therapeutics. Such difficulties can alone be surmounted by a mind possessed of qualities, resources, and talents, such as are found united in the au-

[1] Published in English by the Sydenham Society.

thor of the book before us. Nor has there come under our eye a work on materia medica, in which the doctrines derived from these auxiliary sciences have been brought into so intimate a relation and connection with the infinite mass of remedies, and with all the practical details, as in Oesterlen's manual; in fact, in every chapter to which we turn, we discover that the author is as familiar with the natural sciences and physiology as with nosology and clinical medicine.

From the great number of compendiums that have been published on this branch of medicine, it may not be irrelevant in the first place to inform the reader of what he will find in Oesterlen's work—in other words, what he may and may not expect; for this reason we here annex a brief survey of its contents.

In his Introduction, after considering definition, properties, and qualities, physiological and therapeutic actions of the various medicines and poisons, their manner of application and their classification, our author treats of the single substances in the following order:—

1. Metals.
2. Alkaline and earthy bases and their salts.
3. Metalloids, such as sulphur, iodine, chlorine, and others.
4. Acids.
5. Bitter and astringent substances: iron and manganese.
6. Volatile excitantia and stimulantia, such as æther, camphor, æthereal oils, balsams, &c.
7. Vegetable acria.
8. Narcotic substances and such as produce asphyxia.
9. Indifferent nutritive substances (emollientia diætetica), such as fats, starch, and substances containing albumen and gum.
10. Water.
11. Mineral waters.
12. Physical agents (imponderabilia), as heat, cold, cold water cure (hydropathy), electricity, galvanism, magnetism, electro-magnetism.

A special appendix treats of dietetics, climates, gymnastics, and the like, and the work finally concludes with a large number of well chosen formulas, a toxicological table, and a collection of chemical tests for all of the most important substances.

Besides its being so complete and comprehensive, what, in our opinion, more particularly distinguishes the work in question is, that the description of all these subjects, of themselves often so dry and tedious, appear in this book less tinctured with their dulness than is usual in manuals of this kind, and that his manner of elucidating his subject bespeaks a mind of the highest order, well stored with universal literary attainments, and endowed with a most penerating judgment.

The botanic and pharmaceutic qualities of medicines, in a word their natural history, we find throughout the work, to be well though briefly described, but his chief stress the author lays on the *modus operandi* and the therapeutic application of all these substances, and in doing so, he has taken the science of materia medica in the sense and acceptation in which it should certainly be regarded by the physician and student, unless we intend to sacrifice it to the interest of the pharmaceutist. In this respect particularly, Oesterlen's *Materia Medica* differs from Pereira's, and from all other English works known to us on this subject; these have laid the chief weight on the natural history and pharmacy of substances. On the other hand, we find in Oesterlen's work, a more detailed and complete description of the actions and applications of medicines (so essential to the practitioner at the sick-bed), than is to be met with in any work on materia medica in the English language.

To show that Oesterlen has at least partially traced out the right course, we may mention the fact, that in the short space of eight years his *Materia Medica* has passed through six editions (each including upwards of two thousand copies), and that it has now become at all the universities in Germany and among practising physicians a *standard work.*

In every part of the book we find moreover a more careful and circumspect use of English and American, as well as of German and French and other foreign literature, than is generally met with; a literary and scientific apparatus so complete must prove indeed a welcome treasure to every reader. In confirmation of the above we have for instance only to refer to the chapters on mercury, iron, iodine, ætherization, cod-liver oil, cold-water cure (hydrotherapeutics), mineral springs, and so on; a mere cursory perusal of these will lead him to the conviction that the chapters above referred to may well lay claim to the title of concise monographies—all, nevertheless, concentrated in *one* volume.

In studying this work, the reader will become convinced sooner than from the study of any other similar work, that materia medica (therapeutics), like all other branches intimately connected with the natural sciences, has, in the course of time, undergone an almost entire revolution in respect to its foundations, principles, and scientific tendencies. The materia medica of the present day is not that of some twenty or even ten years' date; the physicians, too, must *nolens volens*, follow the current of the age, the more surely as this but leads onwards and nearer to truth, the highest aim of medical science and art. Taking this view of the subject, Oesterlen appears to us the chief representative, if not in many respects, even the author and originator of this system, or so to say, of this school; in no other work on materia medica have we seen so many an illusion and delusion, so many a superstition of the old school of therapeutics subjected to so consistent and so critical a scrutiny, and yet in nowise running into the opposite extreme of therapeutic nihilism, of mere negation and rejection.

The notice we have thus taken of Oesterlen's work, brief as it is, will suffice to explain why it was, that during our sojourn in Europe, we have heard expressed by competent judges, English, French, Russian, and German, but *one* opinion, and that the *most favourable* as to the merits of his *Manual of Materia Medica and Therapeutics*, an opinion corroborated by many German reviewers of the recent edition. It is also for this reason that we have felt ourselves induced to commend the work so highly to the attention of physicians, and to students of medicine at home. J. C. T.

Art. XX.—*New Remedies; with Formulæ for their Preparation and Administration.* By Robley Dunglison, M. D., Professor of the Institutes of Medicine, etc. in the Jefferson Medical College. Seventh edition. Philadelphia: Blanchard & Lea, 1856. 8vo. pp. 769.

Although the *New Remedies* of Prof. Dunglison has been before the medical public for a long time, and therefore its general scope and character are well understood, yet the announcement of a new and seventh edition not only warrants, but seems to require a brief notice; more especially, as it has not been particularly described in this journal for a few years past.

The remedial means, which are introduced into this edition for the first time, either from their recent discovery, or from new applications of old remedies, are twenty-eight in number; some of them being of a very important character.

Among others, we notice the chloride of bromine; of which, the mode of preparing and the manner of using are described. This is the article employed by Dr. Landolfi, Surgeon of the Sicilian Army, in the treatment of cancer, and, as it is affirmed, with an unusual amount of success. His experiments are now attracting considerable attention in Europe.

Santonin, the active principle of the European wormseed—semen contra—obtained from the various species of artemisia, is another of the articles newly introduced. This is now manufactured in Philadelphia, and the experiments made with it here coincide with those given in the work; namely, that it is peculiarly destructive to the long round worm. Its comparative tastelessness and small dose afford great advantages over the ordinary vermifuges.

In the article on *Cauterization and Catheterism of the Larynx and Trachea,* is to be found a *résumé* of our present knowledge on this subject. The instruments employed, the mode of introducing, the solutions for medication, and the diseases, in which the supposed introduction has been tried, are noticed in detail. The author says, "There can be no doubt, that injections can be thrown into the bronchial tubes; but it is difficult to suppose, that they can often reach tuberculous excavations in such quantity as to exert any direct action on the diseased surface. In many cases of bronchitis, however, they may prove beneficial."

Quinidia, the new alkaloid obtained from Peruvian bark, or rather from the cheaper barks of the northern coast, is described; and the experiments to determine its therapeutical value are succinctly referred to, which prove it to be an efficient substitute for the sulphate of quinia. The other remedies, used for the same purpose and now introduced for the first time, are Cedron seeds, Cinchonicine, and Apiol.

The latter is a yellow, oily liquid, obtained from the common parsley, and is given in the dose of fifteen grains. "In the intermittents of Europe, apiol has succeeded in 86 cases out of 100. It has not been so fortunate in the fevers of hot countries: and MM. Joret and Homolle conclude, as the result of all observations, that it cannot be employed with the same advantage as the sulphate of quinia, in the intermittents of torrid regions; but may very well be substituted for it in those of Europe."

From the mineral kingdom, the metals—cerium, nickel, and tellurium, and the salts—chloride of iron, chloride of sodium, hyposulphite of soda and silver, iodide of sodium, permanganate of potassa, phosphate of lime, and the saccharine carbonate of iron and manganese; together with caffein, carbazotic acid, cod-liver olein, Eau de Pagliari, galvanic cautery, hydriodic ether, pumpkin seeds, rennet, and traumaticine, are introduced either as "new remedies," or as old articles with new uses.

The foregoing, however, does not convey a correct idea of the additions in the present volume, for a careful comparison of the leading and more important articles of the previous edition, shows that much care and attention have been bestowed upon their history. So that a full and fair exhibit of the present knowledge of the profession of their therapeutical properties is given.

We might allude to aconitia, atropia, extract of hemp, cinchonia, colchicum, &c. &c., but it is unnecessary to enter into further detail. On the subject of anæsthetics, much valuable information is to be found in the articles on congelation, chloroform, and ether.

There is one feature in this work which is particularly valuable, as the remedies it treats of are new either in introduction or in application. It is the precise reference for the asserted facts, to the authors and works by whom they are announced and from which they are taken. So that the student can refer to the original sources for more ample illustration.

Another equally valuable feature is the subscription of formulæ to most of the articles, for the administration of the remedies described.

Upon the whole, therefore, we are disposed to consider this edition as not only sustaining the high reputation of the work which has carried it through six previous ones, but as being entitled to the favourable consideration of the profession as a faithful summary of the leading facts known, whether it be in the modes of preparation, the manner of using, or the effects of new remedies.

R. P. T.

ART. XXI.—*The Principles of Surgery.* By JAMES MILLER, F. R. S. E., F. R. C. S. E., Professor of Surgery in the University of Edinburgh, &c. &c. &c. Fourth American, from the third and revised English edition. Illustrated by two hundred engravings on wood. Philadelphia: Blanchard & Lea, 1856. 8vo. pp. 696.

THE publication of three Edinburgh and four Philadelphia editions, within not more than twelve years, decidedly indicates the high standing and sustained popularity of Professor Miller's treatise. Our readers are doubtless familiar with its merits as a favourite text-book. These are so generally known and have been already so repeatedly pointed out in previous notices, that we need scarcely do more on this occasion than announce the new edition.

On account of the absence in Europe of Dr. Sargent, the present volume has been passed through the press without his editorial supervision. The aim of the publishers, as the advertisement informs us, has been "to render the work an exact transcript of the author's last and revised edition," in which such use had been made of the American annotations as the Professor himself had deemed advisable. In this desirable object we think the publishers have very happily succeeded. The result is certainly a book as handsome as their former issue, and one of more convenient dimensions, although amply furnished with useful matter, and bearing evidence of the usual progress in proportion to its date.

We have looked it over with particular attention, and have compared its pages, throughout, with those of its immediate predecessor in this country. Our examination has satisfied us that it has been carefully revised by its accomplished author, and that, notwithstanding considerable accessions to the old contents, he has so managed by condensation and alteration as to reduce rather than augment the size of the whole. Much space has been gained for instance in the article on anæsthetics, in which a few brief paragraphs have been advantageously substituted for the long appendix on chloroform which formed an unduly prominent feature of the last edition. The additions are so incorporated into the context of the different chapters as to make no change in the good order and precision of arrangement and fluency of style which have always characterized the work. Although introduced with marked discrimination, they are yet sufficiently full to justify the long-established reputation of the author as a conscientious teacher of the actual state of surgical pathology and therapeutics; while they show him to be eminently free from the tendency to beguile the student with displays of reading or ingenious speculations in regard to unsettled questions or points of minor practical importance.

On these accounts, especially, apart from the well known elegance and clearness of language, as well as comprehensive range of topics and elevated scientific tone of Professor Miller's treatise, we are glad to believe that its high position as one of the acknowleged exemplars of the *Principles of Surgery*—perhaps the best of its class—is abundantly maintained. We heartily commend it to the attention of pupils and practitioners as a valuable elementary preceptor. They may safely resort to it and, within the limits of a text-book, depend upon it as a reliable monitor and guide in their earlier studies; while they will be apt to find it, along with works of greater compass and pretension, no mean instructor in any stage of a professional career.

E. H.

Art. XXII.—*The Dissector's Manual of Practical and Surgical Anatomy.* By Erasmus Wilson, F. R. S., author of "A System of Human Anatomy," &c. Third American, from the last revised London edition. Illustrated with one hundred and fifty-four wood engravings. Edited by William Hunt, M. D., Demonstrator of Anatomy in the University of Pennsylvania. Philadelphia: Blanchard & Lea.

We have here the third American edition of this useful and popular work. Not claiming to be a complete "System of Human Anatomy," but a manual for dissectors; it will, we think, be found fully to meet the wants of those for whom it is intended, while its convenient size and arrangement will make it of more practical value in the dissecting-room than a more elaborate work could be.

The edition before us, "besides being much enlarged and modified," has evidently been prepared with care; and it would seem to have been the aim of the editor rather to correct inaccuracies which had escaped observation in former editions than to add new matter of his own. Where additions have been made, they are of practical value and deserving the student's attention; thus, on page 29, he writes:—

"The attention of the dissector should also be directed to some general facts in regard to the position of certain structures and their relative importance in the economy. Thus, he should remember that the great bloodvessels are placed upon the line of flexion, and as near as possible towards the inner side, and that this line includes all of the anterior aspect of the body with the exception of the legs. By this arrangement these essential parts are most effectually protected from injury, and least exposed to disturbance from the movements of the body. He should also not lose sight of the ordinary laws of physics and mechanics, in his study of the human frame, for by an intelligent application of these, he will frequently be enabled to comprehend and give a purpose to a part (as of a muscle, for example) even before he has an exact idea of its position and relations. * * * When the subject is injected with chloride of zinc, a plan generally adopted in this country, care should be taken not to remove too much of the integument at once, as the parts when exposed will dry and become hardened very rapidly," &c.

We scarcely need add our belief that the reputation acquired by former editions will be fully sustained by this.

Art. XXIII.—*Atlas of Cutaneous Diseases.* By J. Moore Neligan, M. D., Edin., M. R. I. A., &c. &c. Philadelphia: Blanchard & Lea, 1856. 4to. Pl. XVI.

The object of the author in the publication of this book of Plates, "is to supply the student and junior practitioner with a work moderate in size, and cheap in price, which can be readily referred to in the study of what is admittedly an obscure class of diseases;" and he has "endeavoured to combine faithfulness in representation with accuracy of finish, without which it could not prove a faithful guide."

It is entirely beyond the power of language to convey, in many cases, accurate ideas of external characters, and hence the difficulty of learning to discriminate the various diseases of the skin, is insurmountable without the opportunity of studying them in a hospital appropriated to their treatment, or by the aid of accurate representations.

The latter have been supplied by Dr. Neligan, and we can safely recommend his Atlas to students, and especially to country practitioners, as affording them a safe and reliable guide in the diagnosis of an obscure and important class of diseases. The American edition possesses all the accuracy of the original, and, in point of artistic execution, is very superior.

QUARTERLY SUMMARY

OF THE

IMPROVEMENTS AND DISCOVERIES

IN THE

MEDICAL SCIENCES.

ANATOMY AND PHYSIOLOGY.

1. *On the Animal Starch and Cellulose Question.*—VIRCHOW (*Archiv.*, vol. III. heft. 1) has given the results of further investigations on this subject. He divides the substance into true and false corpora amylacea, relying on the reaction of iodine and sulphuric acid, and on the fact that the true corpora amylacea are not soluble in hot alcohol, ether, &c., and are destroyed by concentrated acids and alkalies. Among the false bodies he classes: 1st. The brain-sand, probably the same which Busk described as being found in the corpus callosum, and which was coloured externally of a yellowish-red hue by iodine. 2d. Various gelatinous and albuminous grains spoken of as colloid-grains in certain tumours. 3d. The concentric epidermal globules often found in the thymus gland and cancroid tumours. 4th. The bodies found in coagulated blood described by Gulliver, Gerber, and Hassall. 5th. The medullary matter described by Virchow himself on a previous occasion. 6th. The leucine grains obtained from extract of milk.

According to Virchow the following are the places wherein true amyloid degeneration is certainly to be found. They are—1st. The nervous system. Besides the fore-mentioned parts, the spinal ligament of the cochlea, and many parts of atrophied brain and spinal marrow, show it. He had found it in the gelatinous and cellular softening of these structures, and he mentions its discovery by Busk in one case almost throughout the brain and the choroid plexus; by Willigk in cicatrices of brain; and by Rokitansky in atrophied parts of brain and other structures. 2d. In the spleen. In the follicular cells and pulp, the thickened walls of arteries, especially circular fibres, and in the trabeculæ. 3d. In the liver. In the waxy degeneration, chiefly in the cells, but also in intervening tissue. 4th. In the kidneys, which are pre-eminently the subject of the degeneration. The Malpighian bodies and the arteries leading to them become first affected; then the areolar tissue in the neighbourhood of urinary tubes of papillæ; and then the other parts. Virchow says, that in most organs where they are found we have undoubted changes of the tissue elements, and that probably there is a "conversion into vegetable matter."

These starch bodies, chemically as well as morphologically, are very allied to starch bodies of plants. Busk says he has often seen in the smaller ones a dark cross by polarized light, whose arms intersect each other in the middle of the grains at an angle of 45°, the majority only showing a simple dark line. It seems necessary to guard against error by the remembrance that in several false amylaceous bodies a yellowish-red colour, called by Meckel iodine-red, is found by addition of iodine; and this is the case also with all blood-holding parts. The later addition of sulphuric acid will be requisite to determine the presence of true amyloid substance. This yellow or iodine-red appearance is compared by Busk to the appearance produced in unripe cellulose, such as is wont to occur in the lower plants. But in plants we have quantities of cellulose mixed with gelatinous substances, so that in the treatment with iodine and sulphuric acid we have all sorts of immature colours, indicating a mixture of blue and red, brown and yellow. Such a play of colours takes place in the spleen, especially in the amyloid substance from the pulp and follicles, but in no case does the blue or blue-red come forward with such clearness as in the Malpighian bodies and afferent arteries of the parenchyma of the kidney. Our author concludes that sooner or later the albuminous substance of the tissues disappears, and is replaced by amyloid substance. In those instances where the substance differed still more from starch proper it becomes more like cellulose proper; and the organs affected show that peculiar look called waxy or lardaceous. The same idea is acknowledged by Virchow to have arisen also at Edinburgh independently of himself. Generally the indurated organs are enlarged, leaving no doubt of the deposit of new matter. The co-existence of the same alteration in the spleen, liver, and kidneys leads naturally to the recognition of a common cause, a constitutional disturbance.

Since the above was written by Virchow in the *Archiv*, he has made another communication on the same subject; but before speaking of this, we will mention a communication made[1] by Mr. Carter, entitled the "Extensive Diffusion and Frequency of Starch Corpuscles in the Tissues of the Human Body." In this, it will be seen, a different view is maintained on certain points. This observer saw the starch bodies in a tumour involving the optic nerve, and also the pineal gland of man and sheep; and, since then, made extensive experiments, examining in succession thirteen human bodies out of the clinical wards of Professor Bennett, of Edinburgh. He met with two kinds of starch, one resembling wheat, the other potato starch; and he found them in the liver, spleen, kidneys, brain, pancreas, mesenteric glands, suprarenal capsules, Pacchionian bodies, mesentery, lungs, ovaries, scrofulous matter, pus, urine, epidermis, blood, and other places, in organs as well healthy as diseased. In one case he found them around an apoplectic clot, but could not find them in any other part of the brain. In a case of diabetes, the other organs presented an unusual amount, but the liver was free from any. He never seems to have found them in the muscular structure of the heart. In the sheep, oxen, and lower animals, they were found in the same indiscriminate way; and the author says that they have hitherto been mistaken for fatty oil globules, to which, from form and refractile powers, they have much resemblance. He considers them as of physiological, not of pathological interest, being ordinary constituents of the body, and, as he calls them, "the thermogenic magazines," analogous to fatty substance, and capable, possibly, of conversion into grape sugar and carbonic acid, or into the lactic acid of the gastric juice.

In the second paper by Virchow (*Archiv*, p. 364), to which we have alluded, the author thinks he has made considerable advances on the subject. In all the cases in which he found the cellulose, chronic and extensive disease of the osseous system existed; and he thinks these diseases exercise a determinate influence on the production of the waxy "degeneration"—the disease, especially caries and necrosis, inducing a deficit of nutrition and cachexy, thus robbing the spleen, kidneys, &c., of their natural elements, and disposing them to take on the degeneration. He has never met with the amyloid substance in the bones, but has so done in the cartilage of the joints of an old person with senile arthritis.—*Brit. and For. Med.-Chirurg. Rev.*, April, 1856.

—

2. *The Earthy Phosphates in Urine.*—NEUBAUER, who has conducted a very laborious and precise investigation respecting the quantities of earthy phosphates present in urine under various conditions, has arrived at the following results:—

1. In the normal state, a growing man of 20–25 years old, partaking of a mixed diet, voids in twenty-four hours, as the mean of fifty-two observations, from .9441 to 1.012 grammes of earthy phosphates. The maximum voided in

[1] Edinburgh Medical Journal. August, 1855.

twenty-four hours amounted, upon an average, from 1.138 to 1.263 grm., and once only to 1.554 grm. The minimum amounted, upon an average, to .8 grm., and once only to .328 grm.

2. The phosphate of lime, as a mean of fifty-two observations, amounted to from .31 to .37 grm. The mean maximum was from .39 to .37 grm.; the mean minimum was nearly constant, .25 grm., and only once amounted to .15 grm.

3. The phosphate of magnesia amounted to .64 grm., as the mean of fifty-two observations. The maximum was, upon an average, .77 grm.; only once were .938 grm. voided. The mean minimum amounted to .5 grm., but once sank to .178 grm.

4. In the normal condition, upon an average, three equivalents of 2 Mg O, $P O_5$ were voided to one equivalent of 3 Ca O, $P O_5$. As a mean the entire phosphates consisted of 67 per cent. of phosphate of lime, and 33 per cent. of phosphate of magnesia in 100 parts.

5. Salts of lime, when taken, pass over, either not at all or in very small quantity, into the urine. The entire quantity of normal phosphates passing into the urine undergoes, in consequence, no important increase.

6. In disease, the absolute quantity of earthy phosphates, as well as the relative proportion between the lime and magnesia phosphates, appear to depart considerably from the normal condition.—*Lancet*, April 26, 1856.

MATERIA MEDICA AND PHARMACY.

3. *Quinated Cod-Liver Oil.* By M. Donovan.—A preparation of cod-liver oil, called *oleum aselli cum quina*, has been lately introduced into medical practice, and is favourably noticed by some practitioners. It is probable that the tonic effects of quinine, conjoined with the restorative powers of the oil, may afford a combination of greater efficacy than is possessed by either separately. To many persons, the mawkish taste of the oil modified into the decided bitter of the quinine is an improvement. I have been informed that the combination of sulphate of quinine with cod-liver oil is effected by exposing them in a state of mixture to a certain temperature: if the heat be too high or too low, the combination, it is said, will either not take place or it will be subverted. I have made some trials with very unsatisfactory results, the quantity of sulphate which dissolved being very small, as might be expected from the character of sulphates in general.

Aware that the alkaline basis of sulphate of quinine possesses some of the properties of a resin, it seemed probable that it might dissolve in oil; and, on making the experiment, I found that this is actually the case.

The alkaloid quinine is known to possess little efficacy as a medicine on account of its insolubility in aqueous liquids; hence, it is always administered in the state of acidulated disulphate, or, in other words, in the state of sulphate. Oil, by rendering quinine soluble, develops the medicinal virtues of that alkaloid, and thus, for every useful purpose, acts the part of sulphuric acid.

A few trials convinced me that quinine may be dissolved in cold cod-liver oil in even greater ratio than is ever necessary for the purposes of the physician. A solution of eight grains to the ounce is intensely and persistently bitter. When the mixture is first made, a very disagreeable and peculiar smell is developed; but by exposure to the air for an hour or two, or better by filtering, the smell exhales and is dissipated. The colour of the oil is deepened by the combination.

This compound, which may be briefly named *oleum aselli quinatum*, has this advantage, that two active medicines, of coinciding effects, may be thus administered at one dose. To some, it is a severe trial to swallow either of them; and to such persons it would be a relief, instead of taking two separate disagreeable doses at different times, to swallow both at once, and have done with them.

There are constitutions which will not tolerate the free exhibition of cod-liver oil, and patients of this class are precluded from availing themselves of advantages which might have been of the utmost value to them. Perhaps the quinated oil would agree better with such stomachs.—*Dublin Medical Press*, March 26, 1856.

MEDICAL PATHOLOGY AND THERAPEUTICS, AND PRACTICAL MEDICINE.

4. *Asphyxia, its Rationale and its Remedy.*—By MARSHALL HALL, M. D. The term Asphyxia, which ought to be exchanged for apnœa, designates that condition of the animal system which results from the suspension of respiration.

Respiration involves two processes—the inhalation of oxygen, and the exhalation of carbonic acid.

The remedy for the suspension of respiration is, on every principle of common sense, the restoration of respiration. This view might be considered, irrespective of physiological inquiry and proof, as self-evident; but that proof is amply supplied by physiology.

Of the two functions suspended, it is certain, from physiological inquiry, that the retention of the carbonic acid is by far the more fatal, and that, in a word, asphyxia is the result of carbonic acid retained in the blood, which becomes, in its excess, a blood-poison.

If this view be correct, it is evident that restored respiration is to the blood-poison in asphyxia what the stomach-pump is to poison in the stomach; and that it is *the* special remedy, the *sine quâ non*, in asphyxia.

But this blood-poison is formed with a rapidity proportionate to the circulation, which is, in its turn, proportionate to the temperature. To elevate the temperature, or to accelerate the circulation, *without* having *first* secured the return of respiration, is therefore *not to save*, but in reality *to destroy life!*

Now, let me draw my reader's attention to the *Rules* for treating asphyxia, proposed and practised by the Royal Humane Society. They are as follow:—

"1. Convey the body carefully, with the head and shoulders supported in a raised position, to the nearest house.

"2. Strip the body, and rub it dry; then wrap it in hot blankets, and then place it in a warm bed in a warm chamber free from smoke.

"3. Wipe and cleanse the mouth and nostrils.

"4. In order to restore the natural warmth of the body:—

Move a heated covered warming-pan over the back and spine.

Put bladders or bottles of hot water, or heated bricks, to the pit of the stomach, the arm-pits, between the thighs, and to the soles of the feet.

Foment the body with hot flannels.

Rub the body briskly with the hand; do not, however, suspend the use of the other means at the same time; but, if possible, immerse the body in a warm bath at blood heat, or 100 deg. of the thermometer, as this is preferable to the other means for restoring warmth.

"5. Volatile salts or hartshorn to be passed occasionally to and fro under the nostrils.

"6. No more persons to be admitted into the room than is absolutely necessary."

My first remark on these rules for treating asphyxia is, that "to convey the body to the nearest house," is doubly wrong. In the first place, *the loss of time* necessary for this purpose is—*loss of life!* on the contrary, not a moment should be lost; the patient should be treated instantly, on the spot, therefore. In the second place, except in very inclement weather, the exposure of the face and thorax to the breeze is an important auxiliary to the special treatment of asphyxia.

But most of all, the various modes of restoring the temperature of the patient, the warm-bath especially, are objectionable, or more than objectionable; they are at once inappropriate, unphysiological, and deleterious.

If there be a fact well established in physiology, it is that an animal bears the suspension of respiration in proportion, not to the warmth, but, within physiological limits, to the lowness of the temperature, the lower limit being about 60° Fahr. A warm-bath of 100° Fahr. must be injurious.

All other modes of inducing warmth are also injurious, if they divert the attention from *the one remedy* in asphyxia—artificial respiration,—or otherwise interfere with the measures to be adopted with the object of restoring this lost function.

Such, then, are the views which the scientific physician *must* take in regard o the late rules for treating asphyxia promulgated by the Royal Humane Society.

I now proceed to state the measures by which those rules must be replaced.

I revert to a proposition already made: as asphyxia is the result of suspended respiration, the one remedy for the condition so induced is, self-evidently and experimentally, the restoration of respiration.

But there is an impediment to artificial respiration never before pointed out. It is the obstruction of the glottis or the entrance into the windpipe, in the supine position, by the tongue falling backwards, and carrying with it the epiglottis—an event which can only be effectually remedied by adopting *the prone position*.

In this position the tongue falls forward, drawing with it the epiglottis, and leaving the ingress into the windpipe *free*.

But even when the *way* is patent, there remains the question, how is respiration to be effected? The syringe or the bellows may not be at hand, and if they were, the violence used by them is apt to *tear* the delicate tissue of the lungs. The mode proposed by Leroy, of compressing the thorax by means of a bandage, and allowing its expansion by the resilience of the costal cartilages, is proved by experiment to be futile, chiefly, no doubt, from its being attempted in the supine position, with the glottis obstructed.

The one effectual mode of proceeding is this: let the patient be placed in the prone position, the head and neck being preserved in their proper place. The tongue will fall forward, and leave the entrance into the windpipe free. But this is not all, the thorax and abdomen will be *compressed* with a force equal to the weight of the body, and *ex*piration will take place. Let the body be now *turned* gently on the side (through rather more than the quarter of a circle), and the pressure on the thorax and abdomen will be removed, and *in*spiration—effectual *in*spiration—will take place! The expiration and inspiration are augmented by timeously applying and removing alternately pressure on the spine and ribs.

Nothing can be more beautiful than this life-giving—(if life *can* be given)—this breathing process.

In one series of experiments, twenty cubic inches of air were *ex*pelled on placing a corpse in the prone position, and ten cubic inches more by making pressure on the thorax and ribs, the *same* quantities being *in*haled on removing that pressure, and on rotating the body on its side. But I must give the experiments in detail:—

A subject was laid on the table, and pressure made on the thorax and ribs, so as to imitate the procedure of Leroy. There was no result; a little gurgling was heard in the throat, but *no inspiration* followed. The tongue had fallen backwards, and closed the glottis or aperture into the windpipe! All inspiration was prevented.

Another subject was placed in the *prone* position. The tongue having fallen *forwards*, and the glottis being free, there was the *ex*piration of twenty cubic inches of air, a quantity increased by ten cubic inches more on making pressure along the posterior part of the thorax and on the ribs. On removing this pressure, and turning the body through a quarter of a circle or rather more, on the side, the whole of the thirty cubic inches of air were *ins*pired!

These manœuvres being repeated, ample respiration was performed!

Nay, there may be a question whether such considerable acts of respiration may not be too much.

It is to be observed, however, that, in this mode of artificial respiration, *no force* is used; the lung therefore is not injured; and that, as the air in the trachea and bronchial tubes undergoes little or no change in quantity, the whole inspired air passes into the air-cells, where the function of respiration is alone performed.

It deserves to be noticed, that in the beginning of this experiment in the prone position, the head had been allowed to hang over the edge of the table: all respiration was frustrated! *Such is the importance of position.*

Reserving the full exposition of this method of *postural respiration*, this theseopnœa (from θεσις, position), for another occasion, I will conclude by reducing these views into the simplest *Rules* for the treatment of asphyxia.

New Rules for the Treatment of Asphyxia.

I. Send with all speed for medical aid, for articles of clothing, blankets, &c.

II. Treat the patient on the spot, in the open air, exposing the face and chest freely to the breeze, except in too cold weather.

I. *To excite Respiration,*

III. Place the patient gently on the face (to allow any fluids to flow from the mouth).

IV. Then raise the patient into the sitting posture, and endeavour to *excite* respiration,

1. By snuff, hartshorn, &c., applied to the nostrils;
2. By irritating the throat by a feather or the finger;
3. By dashing hot and cold water *alternately* on the face and chest.

If there be no success, lose no time, but

II. *To imitate Respiration,*

V. Replace the patient on his face, his arms under his head, that the tongue may fall *forward*, and leave the entrance into the windpipe free, and that any fluids may flow out of the mouth; then

1. Turn the body gradually but completely on the *side, and a little more*, and then again on the face, alternately (to induce *in*spiration and *ex*piration);
2. When replaced, apply pressure along the back and ribs, and then remove it (to induce further *ex*piration and *in*spiration), and proceed as before;
3. Let these measures be repeated gently, deliberately, but efficiently and perseveringly, *sixteen times* in the minute *only;*

III. *To induce Circulation and Warmth,*

1. *Continuing* these measures, rub all the limbs and the trunk *upwards* with the warm hands, making *firm pressure* energetically;
2. Replace the wet clothes by such other covering, &c., as can be procured.

VI. *Omit the warm-bath until respiration be re-established.*

To recapitulate, I observe that—

1. If there be one fact more self-evident than another, it is that artificial respiration is the *sine quâ non* in the treatment of asphyxia, apnœa, or suspended respiration.

2. If there be one fact more established in physiology than another, it is that within just limits, a *low* temperature conduces to the protraction of life, in cases of suspended respiration, and that a more elevated temperature destroys life. This is the result of the admirable, the incomparable, work of Edwards.

3. Now the *only* mode of inducing efficient *respiration* artificially, at all times and under all circumstances, by the hands alone, is that of the postural manœuvres described in this paper.

This measure *must* be adopted.

4. The *next* measure is, I have stated, to restore the *circulation* and *warmth* by means of pressure firmly and simultaneously applied *in the course of the veins*, therefore *upwards.*

5. And the measure *not to be adopted*, because it tends to extinguish life, is *the warm bath, without* artificial respiration.

This measure *must* be relinquished.

These conclusions are at once the conclusions of common sense and of physiological experiment. On these views human life may, nay, must, sometimes depend.—*Lancet*, April 12, 1856.

5. *On Jugular Venesection in Asphyxia, Anatomically and Experimentally Considered.*—A paper on this subject was read before the Medico-Chirurgical Society of Edinburgh (March 19th, 1856), by Dr. Struthers. The object of the paper, which was illustrated by preparations and drawings of the valves in the cervical veins of the human subject, was to ascertain whether distension of the right side of the heart could be relieved by opening the external jugular vein in the human subject. The experiments of Drs. John Reid, Cormack, and Lonsdale, had satisfactorily shown that, in the lower animals (dogs, cats, and rabbits), the right side of the heart could be thus disgorged so as to restore its action, which had been arrested by a simple mechanical cause, over distension. He considered that the indication of restoring the heart's action by jugular regurgitation, had not received that attention which Dr. Reid's suggestive paper demanded for it. Dr. Struthers described the anatomy of valves which he had found in the cervical veins, as well as those usually alluded to as present in the external jugular. A pair of valves at or within the mouth of the internal jugular vein; a pair in the subclavian vein immediately external to the point of union with the external jugular; a pair at or within the mouth of the external jugular; a second pair in the course of the external jugular, at the upper end of its sinus, or large portion, about 1½ inch above the clavicle, and various lesser valves at the mouths or within the tributaries of the external jugular. The varieties, and relative position of the two portions of each pair of valves was described, as he had found them in numerous careful examinations. With the view of ascertaining whether regurgitation could take place notwithstanding these valves, Dr. S. performed a series of experiments on the dead subject. A pipe was fixed in the femoral vein, and tepid water thrown freely upwards. The general result was, that the external and other jugular veins very soon became distended, and that when the lancet opening was made, at about an inch above the clavicle, the fluid regurgitated freely. At first a jet came, emptying the distended sinus, and then it continued to flow, never in a jet, but in an active stream across the neck, escaping by the wound with a wriggling motion, evidently due to the obstruction offered by the valve which it had overcome. Care was taken to ascertain that the fluid came by regurgitation, not from above; but, if allowed, it also came freely from above, having ascended by the internal jugular. The introduction of a probe so as to hold aside the guardian valve of the external jugular did not much accelerate the regurgitating flow. When the catheter was introduced, however, the fluid came very freely by it—as freely as from a distended bladder. It is easy to introduce a common male catheter to the vena cava or right auricle, by directing it backwards and inwards, as well as downwards, from the point of venesection. But as soon as the catheter has entered the subclavian vein, the fluid comes as freely as when it is pushed farther. As soon as the point of the catheter is withdrawn into the external jugular, the fluid ceases to come by it. In one subject the fluid could not be made to regurgitate. This was at the time attributed to the circumstance that the cranium had been opened for the removal of the brain, the fluid pouring out by the cranial sinuses; but, on dissection, two pairs of valves were found in the external jugular below the lancet opening, besides the pair above it, as usual.* Regurgitation seems to be prevented by two pairs of valves, though one pair may be overcome. In these experiments the veins of the arm did not become distended, and no regurgitation took place from a lancet-opening in the axillary vein, although afterwards it was seen that only two pair of valves had stood in the way, between the heart and the opening. By "pair," Dr. S. meant the two separate portions which act together as one valve. He (Dr. S.) drew the following conclusions: 1. No venesection can be of any use in asphyxia, except in the neck, on the principle of regurgitation; which, how-

ever, may also relieve congestion of the head. 2. That, besides warmth and friction, and (the most simple and effectual of all means) continued artificial respiration by alternate compression and relaxation of the sides of the chest, jugular venesection should be tried. 3. With reference to Dr. M. Hall's recent recommendation of the prone position, to prevent the tongue falling back and closing the glottis, the question occurred—Does the tongue fall back, under passive circumstances, in the supine position? Is not the closing of the superior glottis, under all circumstances, a muscular act—both the carrying down and back of the tongue and epiglottis, and the lifting upwards and forwards of the larynx? The mouth, however, should be cleared of frothy mucus. 4. That to obviate the evident risk of entrance of air into the veins, the wound should be closed as soon as regurgitation is about to cease, and artificial respiration be then commenced; the jugular venesection having been performed as early as possible.—*Edinburgh Medical Journal*, May, 1856.

---

6. *Syncope Senilis, arising from Gastric Irritation.*—Mr. John Higginbottom has given the name of syncope senilis to an affection common, he says, to all ages, but which occurs in a more aggravated form in infancy and old age. The symptom of syncope is not very apparent in the former period of life, but is so in old age, and is the first symptom requiring prompt attention, for if remedies are neglected, convulsions and death follow.

"It is," Mr. H. observes, "about thirty years since I first noticed partienlarly the syncope senilis. The subject was about seventy years of age. I thought at that time it was a precursor of an attack of apoplexy, the patient having had a slight paralysis when about twenty-three years of age, which affected him slightly through life. I was glad to find, on his recovery, that there was no increase of his paralytic symptoms. Since that time, I have often observed the same syncope, unattended by any permanent ill effects.

"My patients have been from sixty-eight to eighty-six years of age; the youngest sixty-eight, the oldest eighty-six. I am not aware that they have laboured under any organic disease whatever; but we all know, that at an advanced age the brain and heart, the nervous and vascular system, are frequently more inactive, and in an impaired condition.

"In the cases I have attended of syncope senilis, gastric irritation appears to have been the sole cause of the attack. At that advanced age, mastication of the food is very imperfectly or not at all performed, for want of teeth; solid animal food has been eaten when the stomach has been in an unfit state to assimilate it, usually after having had a longer walk than the patient has been accustomed to, or had more muscular exertion than usual, so as to produce fatigue, and sometimes after exposure to cold; all which tend to weaken the power of the stomach. On this account the food remains an indigestible mass in the stomach, and gives rise to gastric irritation, producing syncope and convulsion, which sometimes follows, often slight at first, but becoming more formidable, or even fatal, if proper remedies are not promptly used.

"I was called to a patient about three o'clock in the morning, his wife having been awoke by his hard breathing and noise in his throat. She found her husband was in a fit. I was directly sent for. When I arrived he had partially recovered, but very soon after he had a second fit, which had the appearance of a slight attack of epilepsy, attended with convulsion, but had no bitten tongue, as is usual in severe attacks of epilepsy. As soon as he was sufficiently recovered from the attack, so that he could swallow, I gave him half a drachm of the powder of ipecacuanha with fifteen grains of the bicarbonate of potass, which was followed by full vomiting; he ejected lumps of solid beef, which appeared to have been swallowed, or rather bolted, without having been masticated at all; one of the pieces, I observed, was about an inch long and three quarters of an inch in thickness. Although the food had been taken into the stomach about sixteen hours, the acute corners and edges of the beef appeared as if just cut with a sharp knife, not the least digested. No further remedy was required after the emetic, but attention to the bowels, which he reluctantly submitted to, saying he was quite well.

"In a month afterwards he had another fit of a similar nature. He fell down in a moment on the floor, and remained in the same state as in the former case for half an hour; the same remedies were resorted to as before, and he recovered quickly. I expect the patient will have a return of the syncope, as he is very wilful, and will not attend to any means of prevention. This patient was the youngest, being sixty-eight years of age. Previous to the first fit he had been using much muscular exertion, still being active in business.

"Another case is that of an old patient of eighty-six years, who at intervals of a few weeks had several similar attacks of syncope. After the last fit, attended with slight convulsion, I was induced to think it had been occasioned by taking solid food, which was swallowed after imperfect mastication; on that account I forbade him the use of animal food altogether. This regimen he has now strictly adhered to for some months, except a few times having taken a small quantity of tripe. He has had no return of his fainting fit, a much longer time having now elapsed than the interval after which he had several of the previous attacks. I would make an observation here, as a contrast to the former case I have related in the younger man, that at a more advanced age the patient does not recover so quickly from the attack, but requires particular attention to the digestive organs for some days, with gentle aperients, and saline medicine in a state of effervescence.

"It is not unusual for even young men to have similar attacks from indigestion, when sudden syncope for a short period comes on, recovery taking place in a few moments. The same attack at an advanced age, I presume, would be attended with aggravated symptoms, such as those I have witnessed."

Mr. H. considers the last illness of the Duke of Wellington to have been syncope senilis, and believes with Dr. M. Hall that if efficient vomiting had been induced, the Duke's life might have been saved.

Mr. H. says that he knows "no emetic equal in such a case to half a drachm of the powder of ipecacuanha, with the addition of ten or fifteen grains of the bicarbonate of potass, as it corrects any acidity in the stomach, and produces full vomiting both safely and quickly; it has also the power of raising the system to its normal condition, without producing any unnatural excitement, and promotes the healthy secretions of the various organs of the body. The nausea and inefficient vomiting arising from natural efforts to empty the stomach, I have no doubt produces debility and exhaustion, when a full vomiting from ipecacuanha has the contrary effect. Should the first half-drachm of ipecacuanha not operate, a second such dose may be given with the greatest safety, it only having the effect of a more speedy operation. If vomiting still should not follow, the fauces might be irritated with a feather, to excite it. I have for the last forty years given ipecacuanha emetics with the same freedom as I have purgatives, and never saw any bad result.

"It might be thought by some individuals that abstaining from animal food at the period of old age might be attended with the loss of health and strength. I had an instance in a relation of my own family, who, at seventy years of age, quite abstained from animal food, and also from wine. After the lapse of ten years, when at the age of eighty, he was requested by his relatives to resume his animal food and wine, he excused himself from taking either of them by saying he did not want them, for he was very healthy, and in good spirits, although very thin in body. He lived till he was nearly ninety years of age. This old gentleman, I apprehend, would have been a likely subject for the syncope senilis had he been in the habit of taking solid animal food, which he could not masticate, and would most probably have shortened his days.

"At an advanced age, when the physical powers of the body are declining, and second childhood approaching, and at that period when comparatively little exercise only can be taken, the body does not require the same solid food. Nature points out the use of milk and light farinaceous matter as an aliment, as being more natural, and adapted to that period of life; such food alone is sufficient to keep the body in a healthy, cheerful, and happy state. It has been erroneously stated that "wine is the milk of old age;" I believe the truth is, that milk is the wine of old age, for both the first and second childhood, the most natural and the most nutritious. Dr. Erasmus Darwin used to say,

"Milk is white blood." The oldest individuals I have known, have lived principally upon milk diet. Second childhood may be treated much in the way as directed by the late Dr. James Hamilton, Professor of Midwifery in the University of Edinburgh: "Plenty of milk, plenty of flannel, and plenty of sleep or rest."—*Lancet*, April 26, 1856.

7. *On Treatment of Fever by Large and Frequently Repeated Doses of Quinine.*—Contradictory reports have been made by different practitioners as to the success attending Dr. Dundas's mode of employing quinine in the treatment of fever, and with a view of contributing to the establishment of the truth Dr. Thomas B. Peacock has reported (*Med. Times and Gaz.*, Jan. 12 and 19, 1856) the results which he has obtained from the quinine treatment as employed in St. Thomas's Hospital, and compared the average mortality and duration of the cases in which it was administered, with the similar facts as to those in which the more ordinary treatment was had recourse to.

"On referring," he states, "to the hospital records, I find that during the present year, from January to October inclusive, there were treated in St. Thomas's, 139 cases of fever of all kinds, excluding the cases entered as febricula and ephemera. Of the 139 cases, 20 were subjected to the quinine treatment. In one case, 4 grains of the drug were given every two hours; in a second, 5 grains were exhibited three times daily; in a third, 5 grains were administered every three hours; in four others, 5 grains every four hours; in two, 6 grains every three and every six hours; in two, 8 grains every four hours; in two, 10 grains every two hours; in three, 10 grains every six hours; and in one, 15 grains every six hours. In three cases (one male and two females), the remedy was only given in doses of 2 grains three times daily. In six of the cases, the exhibition of the quinine was commenced on the day of the patient's admission into the hospital; in eight, on the following day; in one, on the third day; and in one, on the fifth day from admission. In one case, in which the patient took fever in the hospital, the precise period of the disease at which the quinine treatment was commenced, is not stated, but it may be inferred not to have been later than the third or fourth day. In all the cases, stimulants and support were had recourse to, as required. Of the twenty patients, fifteen were males, and five females; the respective proportions of the sexes being 75 and 25 per cent.

"The mean age was in males, 24.1; the extremes, 17 and 35
" " females, 20; " 14 and 29
" " both sexes, 23.4.

"The mean period of admission was in males, 9 days.
" " " females, 10 "
" " " both sexes, 9.1.

"Deducting the three cases in which small doses only were given, the mortality was—

In males, 2; in females, 1; or,

In males	14.2 per cent.
females	33.3 "
both sexes	17.6 "

"The mean period of residence of the cases cured, excluding those in which small doses only were given, and one case detained in hospital eighty-four days, from accidental circumstances, was—

In males	28.7 days.
females	20.5 "
both sexes	29 "

"During the same period of nine months there were, as before stated, 119 other cases of fever treated in the hospital. In some of these cases, little else was given than soda water, and suitable support and stimulus. In others, the treatment consisted in the exhibition of chlorate of potash, dissolved in water or decoction or infusion of bark, with or without hydrochloric acid, in doses of 8 or 10 grains, every two or three hours. In yet other cases, the sesquicarbonate of ammonia, in doses of 5 to 8 grains, was given in infusion of serpentary or decoction of bark at intervals of 2 to 4 hours; this treatment being commenced either at an early period of the disease, or towards its termination. In both these sets of cases, diffusible stimulus and support were also given, according to the amount of prostration.

"Of the 119 cases, 73 were males, and 46 were females, being respectively 61.3 and 38.6 per cent.

"The mean age of the patients was—

In males,	24.5;	extremes, 4 and 72
females,	24;	" 5 and 58
both sexes,	24.4	

"The mean period of admission was—

In males	10.4 days.
females	9.5 "
both sexes	10.2 "

"The mortality was in males, 10; in females, 5; or,

In males	13.6 per cent.
females	10.8 "
both sexes	12.6 "

"The mean period of residence of the cases cured (deducting those detained in the hospital from accidental causes), was—

In males	27.2 days.
females	29.8 "
both sexes	28.1 "

"It will be seen, on comparing these two series of observations, that they bear a very close general resemblance, as regards the circumstances which most materially affect the results of the treatment pursued; as the age and sex of the patients, and the period of the disease at which they were admitted into the hospital; indeed, in the last two particulars, the advantage was rather in favour of the cases treated by quinine. The two series may, therefore, be admitted as affording some test of the respective merits of the systems of treatment pursued; and it will be seen, that in the quinine cases the rate of mortality is considerably higher, and the durations of residence longer, than in others.

"It may, however, be objected that a calculation founded upon the respective duration of residence of the cases in hospital, does not afford a satisfactory standard of comparison, as being liable to be affected by accidental causes; and there can be no doubt of the truth of this remark. The period during which a patient is detained in bed, would, exceptional cases being omitted, afford more exact results; but the comparison of the periods at which the patients are regarded as free from fever, as adopted by Dr. Gee and Mr. Eddowes, or the period of convalescence, would be a still less satisfactory standard, because liable to greater variation from the views of different observers. In the calculations above given, I have endeavoured to guard against incorrect results, by excluding all cases detained for a longer period than usual, from casual circumstances.

"It may also be contended, that the number of cases in which the quinine treatment was had recourse to, was so small, that the inferences deduced from them cannot be depended upon. Admitting the force of this objection, I have collected all the cases in which the quinine treatment was employed in the Hospital during the year 1854. These I find amount to twenty in number, of which twelve were males and eight females; but two, one male and one female, took the remedy only in small doses. Deducting these, there remain eighteen cases in which the quinine was exhibited, in doses varying from 2 and 4 grains every four hours and three times daily, in boys of 8, 10, and 15 years of age, to 5, 8, and 10 grains every two, four, six, and eight hours, in adults. The remedy was commenced on the day of the patient's admission into the hospital in seven cases; on the following day, in five cases; on the third day, in three; the fourth, in one; and on the seventh, eighth, and ninth days from admission, also in one case each. The general circumstances of the cases were also more favourable for treatment than either of the other two sets, the mean age of the patients being only 19.3, and the extremes 10 and 45; and the mean period of admission the sixth day of illness. The results were also more favourable both as regards the mortality, and the duration of the cases cured; the deaths being only two males; and the period of residence in the cases which recovered, only twenty-six days; deducting the three cases in which the quinine was not given till the seventh, eighth, and ninth days from the admission of the patients into the hospital, and in which the period of residence was twenty-seven, sixty-three, and sixty-nine days.

"Adding these two series of cases together, and deducting those in which the remedy was only given in small doses, we get a total of thirty-five cases treated by quinine; of these, twenty-five were males, of whom four died; giving an average mortality of 16.0 per cent.; and ten were females, of whom one died, or ten per cent.; or in the thirty-five patients of both sexes, the mortality was five, or 14.2 per cent.

"The mean period of residence of the cases cured, was, in twenty males (excluding the one detained eighty-four days), 27.9 days; and in six females (excluding the three in which the patients did not commence the remedy till the seventh, eighth, and ninth days from their admission into the hospital), 25.3 days; or, taking the two sexes together, the mean period of residence of the patients was 27.3 days.

"It will thus be seen, on comparing these results as to the thirty-five cases treated by quinine with those obtained in the other 119 cases, that while the mortality in the quinine cases was considerably greater than in the others (1.6 per cent.), the mean period of residence of the cases cured under that treatment was very nearly the same as in the other cases (.8 less).

"This statement, embracing, as it does, so large a number of cases, including all those treated in the hospital by quinine during a period of nineteen months, and that, too, in the practice of different medical men, must, I think, be regarded as affording a fair indication of the results of the quinine treatment, and a legitimate comparison with that of the other methods. There do not appear any circumstances which should affect disadvantageously the results in the quinine cases; indeed, the general characters of the cases so treated are rather more favourable for treatment than those in which the more ordinary plans were pursued. If, therefore, quinine really possessed the power of cutting short an attack of fever, without reference to its particular type or form—and such is distinctly the assertion of Dr. Dundas—the average duration of the cases cured under that treatment, and their mean mortality, should be less than those under the ordinary plans; and if such does not prove to be the case, the fair inference is, that the remedy does not possess the asserted power.

"It is, however, quite possible that, though the quinine treatment may fail to exhibit satisfactory results, when applied to all the cases which occur, taken indiscriminately, without reference to their peculiar character; when applied to a more select set of cases, it may prove to be capable of arresting some of them, or, at least, of materially mitigating their severity."

Dr. Peacock gives the details of seven cases of fever in which he made use of the remedy with a view of ascertaining by direct observation, how far it possesses the asserted power of arresting fever, or of proving, when exhibited in large and frequently repeated doses, a useful auxiliary to the employment of other means.

"In all these cases the most marked effect produced by the large doses of quinine was the depression of the power and frequency of the pulse. In one case the beats were only 48 in the minute on the fourth day after the commencement of the remedy, and when sixteen 10-grain doses had been exhibited; and, in this instance, the only other effect produced by the drug was slight frontal headache, and singing in the ears, and the patient steadily improved during its employment. In two cases the torpor and depression of strength increased under the use of the remedy; but, as these symptoms subsided, while it was still persevered in, it is not clear whether they should be ascribed to the action of the quinine or to the natural progress of the disease. In one case only was there more than transient headache or vertigo from the use of the remedy; and this was also the only case in which there was very marked tinnitus aurium. In one case there was decided deafness, but, in this instance, the hearing was impaired from the time of the patient's admission. In one of the only two cases in which vomiting occurred, an emetic had been given at the commencement of the treatment. In one case the diarrhœa, previously present, was considerably aggravated under the use of the quinine."

The general results of the treatment may be stated as follows:—

"1. In one of the cases of typhus, the quinine was certainly not productive of any benefit, and probably added to the torpor and depression of strength. In the other case of typhus it produced the most marked depression, and the patient was only saved by its discontinuance and the liberal exhibition of stimulants. In both cases, though the patients recovered, the disease seemed to follow its natural course, and to be in no degree curtailed in duration by the exhibition of the remedy.

"2. In one case of typhoid, the depression of power and torpor increased under the use of the quinine, but the notes are too imperfect to allow me to speak confidently as to its effects. The patient recovered after an illness of average duration.

"3. In two other cases of typhoid, the remedy appeared to exert neither beneficial nor injurious effects; the disease followed its usual course, and the patients recovered.

"4. In another case of typhoid, it certainly added to the torpor and depression. The remedy was only exhibited in small doses, and for a short period, and was entirely discontinued after six doses had been given, in the course of a day and a half, and stimulants and other means were then freely had recourse to; the prostration and torpor, however, increased, and the patient died comatose.

"5. In the fifth case of typhoid, in which the affection was combined with bilious complication, the quinine was decidedly beneficial, the patient steadily improving under its use. The attack was certainly of shorter duration and less severity than might have been expected from the urgency of the symptoms when the treatment was commenced; but, in this case, the amendment was gradual, and no sudden improvement in the symptoms at any time occurred.

"In all the cases the patients had stimulus and support as required, and other accessory treatment, such as astringents, aperients, and anodynes, etc. While also the quinine was exhibited in the various cases in different doses and at various intervals, the different results bore no relation to any of these circumstances.

"The facts and observations which I have now related must only be regarded as a contribution towards the solution of the question of the usefulness of large and repeated doses of quinine in the treatment of the continued fevers of this country. So far, however, as they go, they are opposed to the views of Dr. Dundas, that quinine possesses the power of cutting short the attack; on the other hand, they indicate that the remedy is, in some cases, beneficial; but only as an auxiliary to other measures. It remains to decide, by more extended observations, in what forms of fever, and under what peculiar circumstances, local and individual, the remedy may be advantageously employed; and whether the quinine is more useful in moderate doses at distant intervals, or in the large and frequently repeated doses which have been recommended."

—

8. *Bronzed Skin and Disease of the Supra-Renal Capsules.*—In our last number (p. 489 *et seq.*), we noticed the connection which has recently been pointed out as existing between bronzed skin and disease of the supra-renal capsules. Mr. Jonathan Hutchinson has given (*Med. Times and Gaz.*, March 8, 1856), in a tabular form, the prominent characters observed in twenty-seven cases, and which tend very conclusively to support the opinion that the peculiar bronzing of the skin is really indicative of a fatal cachexia, and of organic disease of the supra-renal capsules:—

No.	Reference.	Sex.	Age.	Occupation, etc.	Previous health, etc.	First symptoms.	Degree of bronzing.
1	Dr. Addison's Work, p. 9.	M.	32	Baker.	No history given, excepting that the skin was white when in health.	Troublesome cough, followed very shortly by debility and bronzing of skin.	Colour of a mulatto; scrotum and penis darkest. (See Plate I.)
2	Dr. Addison's Work, p. 12.	M.	35	Tidewaiter, married; exposed to weather, and often living on salt provisions.	Rheumatism eight years ago; of bilious temperament but generally in good health.	An acute illness, with vomiting, constipation, headache, and delirium; much debility was left by this, and the bronzing of the skin soon followed.	Dark olive brown; pigmentary deposits in lining of lips. (See Plate II.)
3	Dr. Addison's Work, p. 15.	M.	26	Carpenter; married; intemperate.	Very good until 3 months before the change in colour was noticed.	Pain in the back and right leg, followed by debility, wasting, and attacks of giddiness.	Dark olive brown,—deepened in patches. (See Plate III.)
4	Dr. Addison's Work, p. 19.	M.	22	Stonemason.	No history. He died the day after admission into Hospital.	Liability to pain in stomach, and vomiting; tic douloureux.	Face, axillæ and hands of a dingy bronzed colour.
5	Dr. Addison's Work, p. 23, from Doctor Bright's Reports.	F.	Ad't	Not stated.	No history.	No history.	"Complexion very dark."
6	Dr. Addison's Work, p. 25.	M.	—	A barrister of middle age.	No history.	No history.	Surface generally dark and dingy; face, neck and arms covered with patches of deep chestnut-brown;—patches of white skin interspersed. (Plate XI.)
7	Dr. Addison's Work, p. 30.	F.	60	Not stated.	No history. The cancer of the S. R. C. was secondary to cancer of the breast.	Cancer of the breast.	The colour of the skin of the arms, chest and face was of a peculiar light-brown, swarthy hue.
8	Dr. Addison's Work, p. 32.	F.	53	A servant; single.	Always thin, but of good health.	An eruption on the skin four months before, which being cured, stomach symptoms began.	Skin generally very dark; axillæ and areola of umbilicus remarkably dark;—patches darker than surrounding skin.—(Plates IX and X.)
9	Dr. Addison's Work, p. 35.	M.	53	Sailor; married; sober.	Very good; a muscular, strong-built man.	About two months before admission began to lose appetite and feel generally unwell.	The face of yellow bronzed tint, and grew darker while under observation. (See Pl. VI.)
10	Dr. Addison's Work, p. 33.	F.	28	Not stated.	Died of cancer of uterus; the disease of S. R. C. being secondary.	Those of cancer of the uterus.	"A peculiar dingy appearance."

General symptoms, complications, etc.	Whole duration of disease.	Mode of death.	Autopsy.	Remarks.
Excessive weakness; some emaciation; of puerile demeanor; urine healthy; pain in left lumbar region; cough; sense of soreness about epigastrium.	3 years.	Acute pericarditis and pneumonia.	S. R. C. both as hard as stones, as large as eggs, and quite destroyed. Evidences of recent pericarditis and pneumonia; no tubercle; no other visceral disease.	A very well marked case; no chronic disease found at autopsy excepting in the S. R. C.
Pinched, anxious expression; tendency to vomiting; pulse of usual frequency, but extremely feeble; liable to occasions of alarming depression; constipation of bowels; tenderness at epigastrium; numbness of fingers, legs, and tip of tongue occurred early, but passed off.	6 months.	Not stated.	S. R. C. both contained compact fibrinous concretions. Inflamed gastric mucous membrane; no tubercle; no other visceral disease.	The deposits in the S. R. C. resembled tubercle, but there was no tubercle in other organs.
Thin, pale, and very feeble; liable to fainting on rising from bed; sickness and hiccough; pain in back; partial loss of consciousness at times; *angular curvature of spine; leucocythemia.*	7 months.	Gradually sank into a torpid or typhoid state.	S. R. C. each completely destroyed and converted into a mass of strumous deposit; psoas abscess, and caries of lumbar vertebræ; tubercle in lungs; spleen rather large.	The blood was examined both before and after death, and contained a large excess of white corpuscles.
Sickness, vomiting, and pain in stomach; great debility, and some emaciation. The prostration preceding death was so peculiar as to suggest that some poison had been taken.	Several months.	Died from collapse, without apparent cause.	S. R. C. wasted and destroyed, weighing together only 49 grains. No other important disease.	The disease of the S. R. C. was an atrophy, apparently consequent on inflammation.
Extreme debility; bilious vomiting; emaciation considerable; abscess in the breast, and swelling of the right parotid. "There was no indication but to support her strength." —Dr. Bright.	Not stated.	Gradually sank; before death became drowsy; had pain in forehead, and was liable to "wander" occasionally.	"The only marked disease was in the S. R. C., both of which were enlarged, lobulated, and the seat of morbid deposits, apparently of scrofulous character." They were four times the natural size; the left had suppurated.	The account of this case was recorded by Dr. Bright long before any suspicion was entertained as to the importance of disease of the S. R. C.
Emaciated, but not to an extreme degree; great anæmia; extreme languor; stomach exceedingly irritable, and vomiting urgent and distressing; pulse of good size, but exquisitely soft and compressible.	1 year.	"The patient speedily sank." No details given.	The S. R. C. both greatly enlarged, of irregular surface, and much indurated; natural structure lost; microscope could find no nucleated cells; no important disease of other organs.	In this case the vomiting had been so urgent that the idea of malignant disease of the stomach had been suggested.
No history. The woman died of ulcerated cancer of the breast, and the diagnosis of diseased S. R. C. was only formed when, in the post-mortem theatre, the bronzing of the skin was first noticed.	Not stated.	Not stated.	"Both S. R. C. contained a considerable amount of cancerous deposit, invading their entire structure."—Dr. Lloyd.	.. ..
Emaciated and very feeble; much irritability of stomach.	4 months.	Died "of exhaustion" three days after admission.	Cancer of the pylorus; left S. R. C destroyed by cancer.	In this case the extent of change of colour in skin was proportioned to that of the disease of S. R. C., one of them being yet sound.
Sensation of sickness, but no actual vomiting; complained only of weakness and loss of appetite; rigors every five or six hours; no pain; pulse 80, rather feeble; bowels irritable.	3 months.	He became gradually weaker and weaker, and so died.	Tubercular deposit was found in one S. R. C.; tubercular matter was also in the spleen, and the kidneys were degenerate; lungs not examined; deposit of black pigment in omentum, mesentery, and cellular tissue of abdomen.	In this case only one S. R. C. was disorganized, and the degree of bronzing appears to have been only proportionate.
Until the body was in the post-mortem theatre, the discoloration of the skin was not noticed; it was then remarked, and disease of the S. R. C. foretold. No history of symptoms had been preserved.	Not stated.	Died of exhaustion from cancer.	The right S.R.C. healthy; the vein emerging from the left was obstructed by a malignant tubercle, and the organ itself occupied by a recent extravasation of blood, its structure being otherwise healthy.	In this case the degree of bronzing was but slight, the disease affecting but one capsule, and being of but recent occurrence.

No.	Reference.	Sex.	Age.	Occupation, etc.	Previous health, etc.	First symptoms.	Degree of bronzing.
11	Dr. Addison's Work, p. 39.	M.	Ad't	Not stated.	Died of cancer of lungs, etc.	Those of cancer in the thorax.	"The patient's face presented a dingy hue." Freckles about the face, and brown discoloration at root of nose and angles of mouth.
12	*Med. Times & Gaz.*, Dec. 15, 1855, p. 593. (Dr. Burrows)	M.	24	Hawker; single.	Had lumbar abscess in childhood.	Pain across the back, followed by emaciation and bronzing of skin.	Of a dark copper-bronzed tint generally; patches of lighter skin on chest and belly; skin of penis and scrotum almost black,
13	*Med. Times & Gaz.*, Jan. 19, 1856, p. 60. (Dr. Gull.)	M.	24	Carpenter; temperate.	Robust.	Debility; breathlessness on exertion; nausea; "biliousness."	Skin generally of a sallow olive brown. The dark colour most marked about the knees; inside of lips mottled with black pigmentary deposit.
14	*Medical Times and Gazette*, Jan. 19, 1856, p. 62. (Mr. Bakewell.)	M.	28	Labourer.	Not known.	Not known.	Skin generally of deep brown or bronzed appearance, the tint being darkest over the thighs.
15	*Med. Times & Gaz.*, Feb. 20, p. 189. (Dr. Thompson; Mr. Sibley.)	M.	20	Baker; sober.	Good.	Bronzing of the skin.	Skin generally of a peculiar, dark, dirty-brown colour.
16	*Med. Times & Gaz.*, Feb. 23, 1856, p. 190. (Dr. Rowe.)	M.	29	Not stated.	Delicate.	Delicate health, and bronzing of skin.	Skin generally brown, with some darker spots.
17	*Med. Times & Gaz.*, Mar. 8, 1856, p. 233. (Dr. Farre.)	M.	37	A publican; intemperate.	A year before had suffered from pain in the lumbar region, which subsided under simple measures.	He was admitted for delirium tremens.	Skin generally of a peculiar yellowish-brown.
18	Dr. Addison's Work, p. 29.	M.	60	Not stated.	No history.	No details.	Skin generally dark and bronzed, with patches blanched and white. (Plate XI.)
19	*Med. Times & Gaz.*, p. 233. (Dr. Stocker.)	M.	56	Physician.	Dyspeptic, but not otherwise in bad health.	General malaise and irritability of stomach; increasing debility and emaciation.	Patches of dark brown discoloration first appeared about the neck, hands, and abdomen. These increased, but the face remained, except some small patches, of natural colour.
20	*Med. Times & Gaz.*, Dec. 15, 1855, p. 594. (Mr. Startin.)	M.	12	At school; Irish.	Had suffered from abscesses in the neck and slight cough, but was, on the whole, strong and robust.	Loss of flesh and gradually increasing languor; fanciful appetite.	Copper brown in all parts, the face and neck being tinged deepest.

General symptoms, complications, etc.	Whole duration of disease.	Mode of death.	Autopsy.	Remarks.
No history preserved, the nature of the disease not having been suspected during life.	Not stated.	Died of cancer.	One S. R. C. entirely disorganized by cancer, the other healthy.	In this case but one capsule was affected, and the bronzing was proportionately slight. A note as to the discoloration of skin had been taken during life, and without any suspicion of diseased S. R. C.
Irritability of stomach, with Vomiting; pain across the back; great debility; emaciation; partial loss of appetite; urine natural.	8 months.	Died from exhaustion consequent on the action of an aperient dose.	Both S. R. C. contained pus, and some concrete bodies resembling hardened tubercle; there was no active disease of the Vertebræ, nor any important lesion of other viscera.	In this case the chain of morbid phenomena was Very complete.
Nausea; vomiting; great *malaise* and exhaustion; emaciation; urine healthy; blood loaded with white corpuscles.	5 months.	Died rather suddenly, from exhaustion.	Both S. R. C. atrophied and destroyed, the left contained cysts, the right some solid concretions; no other organs examined.	.. ..
He was known to have been for some weeks in a low weak state; no further history; not materially emaciated.	Unknown.	Died from the exhaustion consequent on a short journey.	Both S. R. C. completely atrophied, and containing calcareous concretions; emphysema of the lungs, and fatty degeneration of the heart.	.. ..
Became suddenly languid, then sank into collapse, and died after a three days' illness; no rigors had preceded it; his friends had for six weeks noticed the change in tint of the skin, but there had been no other symptom.	6 weeks.	Died in collapse.	Each S. R. C. enlarged to the size of half a kidney; their structure was quite destroyed, being converted into a firm tubercular-like material, and in parts softened down.	This appears to haVe been idiopathic disease of the S. R. C.; no tubercle was found in other organs.
Had also disease of the knee-joint; general health rather improved, until within three days of the fatal seizure; he remained muscular and fat.	8 months.	Diarrhœa, followed by an epileptic fit; a succession of fits, attended by incessant vomiting and occasional delirium; ended in death on the fourth day.	Both S. R. C. destroyed, and containing cheesy, gritty, and semi-purulent deposit; a complete examination was made, and no other visceral disease of importance was discoVered.	In this, as in case 23, a peculiarly disagreeable odour was obserVed to exhale from the patient's body for three or four weeks before death.
He died after a fortnight's illness from delirium tremens.	3 weeks or more.	Sank into a typhoid state with low delirium, for some days before death.	Both S. R. C. were converted into abscesses, but their cortical structure was not wholly destroyed; circumscribed abscess in the liver.	In this case the suppurative inflammation of the S. R. C. had probably been acute and quite recent.
Anæmia; extreme feebleness of heart's action; uneasiness and irritability of stomach; slight œdema of upper extremities.	Not stated.	Died of debility; cancer in the mediastinum was suspected.	No autopsy.	This case, Dr. Addison states, bore the closest resemblance to case No. 6. The cachexia was precisely that of diseased capsules,—cancer in the mediastinum was suspected from the œdema of the upper extremities.
Great debility and wasting; no organic disease excepting that of the S. R. C. being indicated.	About 6 months.	Sank from exhaustion.	No autopsy.	In this case the presence of the bronze patches enabled Dr. Addison to predict the patient's speedy death at a period when there were no other alarming symptoms.
Some emaciation; great and increasing debility; heavy oppressed aspect; urine healthy.	9 months.	Sank under an attack of diarrhœa, and just before death had a succession of convulsive spasms, (epileptic?)	No autopsy.	For four months before death, the boy had been getting gradually weaker and weaker.

No.	Reference.	Sex.	Age.	Occupation, etc.	Previous health, etc.	First symptoms.	Degree of bronzing.
21	*Med. Times & Gaz.*, Dec. 29, 1855, p. 648. *Ibid.*, May 24, 1856, p. 519. (Dr. Peacock)	F.	14	At school.	Healthy.	Lassitude; muddy complexion, and slight cough.	Of a brown muddy tint, deepest on face, arms, and shoulders. No mottling.
22	*Med. Times & Gaz.*, Jan. 19, 1856, p. 61. (Dr. Burrows)	F.	28	Married; temperate.	Delicate.	Menorrhagia and subsequent debility 2 years before the change of colour.	A tawny or yellowish brown tint, most deeply marked on the face, arms, thighs, and legs. Patchy discoloration in parts.
23	*Med. Times & Gaz.*, Feb. 23, p. 191. (Dr. Rowe.)	M.	45	Carter; married; temperate.	Robust.	Spots of dark tints in various regions of the body. At first there was no illness or discomfort.	Skin generally of dusky brown, not unlike a Mulatto; darker in some parts than in others.
24	*The Association Journal*, Jan. 19, p. 42. (Dr. Budd.)	F.	42	Married.	Good.	A brown tinge of skin, followed by a three weeks' illness (typhus fever), after which the bronzing became more marked.	Tint of skin generally like that of a North American Indian; certain parts darker than others.
25	*The Association Journal*, Jan. 19, p. 43. (Dr. Budd.)	F.	40	Not stated.	Not stated.	.. ..	Very dark, general discoloration, large black patches in mouth.
26	*Med. Times & Gaz.*, Feb. 23, 1856, p. 189. (Dr. Thompson.)	M.	33	Married.	Good.	Paroxysmal pain in the abdomen; loss of strength; amenorrhea.	The skin generally became suddenly of a peculiar dirty brown tinge.
27	*Med. Times & Gaz.*, Dec. 22, 1855, p. 629. (Dr. Rankin.)	F.	68	Married.	Formerly very stout and of large frame.	Loss of strength and flesh.	Face and hands dark brown; "as brown as a Japanese;" other parts not seen.

9. *Starch as an External Application in Cases of Smallpox and other Skin Diseases of an Inflammatory Nature.*—Dr. Thos. W. Belcher extols (*Dublin Hospital Gazette*, April 1, 1856,) the efficiency of starch used externally, in skin diseases generally, and more particularly in smallpox. He relates several cases of smallpox in which he used the starch. This article is made thick, and frequently applied. The entire surface of the body was sponged with tepid water at least once daily, after which the mucilage of starch was immediately laid on. It allays the itching, and completely prevented pitting.

SURGICAL PATHOLOGY AND THERAPEUTICS, AND OPERATIVE SURGERY.

10. *Amputations.*—Dr. Menzies read a very interesting paper on this subject before the Military Medical and Surgical Society (Feb. 28, 1856).

Although, he remarked, the works of our most distinguished civil and military surgeons would appear to embrace and elucidate every point of the question or difficulty connected with the subject, the matter he had selected for the Society was one of interest at the present time, and, without venturing to suggest any novelty or theory of practice, he felt it a duty to elicit every possible information which might hereafter tend to preserve either life or limb. Three

General symptoms, complications, etc.	Whole duration of disease.	Mode of death.	Autopsy.	Remarks.
Countenance expressive of extreme languor; some emaciation; great debility; liability to faintings, and to short "seizures."	18 mont's.	Died suddenly in an epileptic fit; had been progressively losing strength up to the time of death.	A chalky concretion found in the medulla oblongata; supra-renal capsules were not examined.	.. ..
Appetite very bad, some thirst; great debility; pains in the loins; menorrhagia; expression languid and anxious.	7 months.	Not known.	No autopsy.	.. ..
No material loss of general health until within a few weeks of death; debility then supervened, and loss of appetite; great irritability of stomach; failure of memory for some months; urine normal.	3 years.	He sank under incessant vomiting; delirium preceded death.	At the autopsy, the chief condition noted was the presence of tubercle in the lungs. The S. R. C. were not examined.	A peculiar and disgusting odour was noticed to exhale from the body a few days before death. See case 16.
About eight months after the first bronzing was noticed, she began to lose flesh and strength: a harassing cough now occurred; irritability of stomach; extreme anæmia and debility.	16 mont's.	Gradually sank from exhaustion.	No autopsy.	Eight months after the change in colour began, the patient was confined of a healthy infant, which did well.
Anæmic, and extremely feeble; sickness and vomiting.	Not stated.	Gradually sank from exhaustion.	No autopsy.	This case is very imperfectly reported, but is stated to have resembled very closely the preceding one.
Previous to the change in colour of skin, she had been anæmic and very feeble. Coincident with that change, she fell into a peculiar collapse, and continued for several days much prostrated.	5 weeks.	Recovered under the use of tonics, and the skin resumed its condition of simple pallor.	Recovered.	In this case the disease of the S. R. C. might be conjectured to be merely inflammatory, and, therefore, susceptible of cure.
Sinking at pit of stomach; nausea; complete loss of appetite; great and increasing loss of strength. Heart's action very feeble; secretions healthy.	.. ..	Still living.	Living at the time of Report.	In this case the symptoms all combine to indicate the renal-capsular cachexia.

questions suggested themselves: 1st. In any given case, why should we amputate? 2d. When should we amputate? and 3d. How, or in what manner should the amputation be performed? The first and second questions involved the nature and extent of the injury, the condition of the patient, and the circumstances of locality, both present and eventual. They comprised what was called Conservative Surgery, and, if he might use the expression, the antagonistic radicalism of Surgery. He would therefore ask in the first place, What extent of lesion of soft parts without detriment to a principal artery or fracture of bone can justify amputation? Most of us have seen a fatal shock to the system by a large shot or fragment of shell traversing the axis of a limb, or passing through its soft parts. He remembered a soldier of the 79th Highlanders wounded in the trenches by a large fragment of a shell passing transversely through the muscles of both thighs, but without injuring the bone, which case terminated fatally in four hours. This case proved fatal, in consequence of not applying a tourniquet, as the track of the large vessels of the limb was not injured. He would, therefore, caution his younger brethren against neglecting so simple a precaution, as many causes may tend to produce hemorrhage during the transit of the patient to the hospital. In such cases he considered our duty was to assist nature in the subsequent extensive suppuration, for it is astonishing to what an extent injury of the soft parts may be repaired. He then mentioned a case in which the arm and leg were both extensively injured: The arm was amputated on the field, but in the leg the foremost artery had been laid bare, just below Poupart's ligament; two inches of the thumb had been exposed; still it gradually covered over. Everything was against this man, from the nature and extent of the injury, the prostration from his wounds and the amputation, and the circumstances which precluded his being treated in the Crimea. He imagined, therefore, from this and similar cases, that in the majority of uncomplicated lesions of soft parts, if the system rallies from the first shock, the chances are in favour of recovery without amputation. He then referred to the valuable properties of the compound tincture of benzoin, or friar's balsam, in extensive lacerated wounds; it would be of advantage more especially in a long passage by sea to the hospital, after an action, as had already occurred in the Crimea. Where sloughing had actually occurred, the application of pure nitric acid (but not beyond the dead surface as in hospital gangrene) speedily converts an offensive source of irritation and fever into an innoxious, inodorous healthy substance, and greatly expedites its removal. The infliction of a wound on the principal artery of a limb, or even one of its large branches, forms a most serious complication in the lesions of the soft parts received in action; happily it is not frequent, as arteries, from their elasticity and peculiar structure, often escape; still it does occur, and the question is, what influence it should have on our practice. A man of the 93d Highlanders was wounded by a ball in the popliteal space, and the artery opened. The vessel was skilfully tied by Dr. Logan, above and below. Mortification ensued, and amputation was performed as a *dernier ressort*, and the man died. Now, although there can be little doubt that, had amputation been performed in the first instance, this man's life would have been saved, it does not follow that this would have been the correct practice. He trusted that we might hear some results of the experience of Alma, Balaklava, and Inkerman on this point. His own opinion was, that, unless under very peculiar circumstances, the primary consideration should be the immediate security of the patient's life by deligation of the artery, leaving amputation to follow as a possible but not probable consequence. Our next consideration was regarding fractures of bone received in battle as connected with amputation. The solution of continuity will of course depend much on the missile, etc. Limbs have not much chance in the track of a round shot or shell, and leave us little choice of action. He believed that as regarded the upper extremity and below the knee an ordinary bullet will waver, and a Minie seldom causes such extensive comminution as to justify amputation. The old bullet was easily turned in its course, but the Minie produced longitudinal fracture and sometimes comminuted it in an extraordinary manner; still the reparative process of fracture was often equally extraordinary. He then mentioned a case in point. The success that had attended the operation of resection of joints proved that it was not absolutely necessary to amputate because a ball had not penetrated any articulation of the upper extremity, or a fracture extended into it. Wounds of the carpus and tarsus were also amenable to the principles of conservative surgery, of which he had seen several admirable results. He would now refer to compound fractures of the thigh—though last, the most important, and embracing the first question, Why should we amputate? It was a most serious and sacred duty of the surgeon to weigh well this question. All personal feelings of *éclat* or vanity must be spurned. At the cavalry charge of Balaklava General Canrobert exclaimed, "Mais ce n'est pas la guerre;" and although it may be equally magnificent to a professional eye to see Weiss's bright steel flashing through wounded limbs in graceful curves, it was not always surgery. There was no operation that he would not have an honest pride in performing; but he maintained that it was not always necesary to amputate in compound fracture of the femur. Can life be insured when amputation of the thigh was performed? certainly not. Must it be sacrificed without a hope of saving the limb? certainly not. There is a living proof to the contrary this moment in the camp. Under what more unfavourable circumstances could the wounded have been placed than after Alma, Balaklava, and Inkerman? Still the cases proved remarkably successful. He then referred to the modes of protecting the limbs from motion during very rough transit, to which military men, under such circumstances, were subject, and recommended the gutta percha splint, and also observed on the best mode of applying it. The French surgeons said they now never attempted to save a compound fracture of the femur; no doubt many English surgeons held the same opinion. He was aware that those cases required extreme vigilance; but what had happened might happen again, and he trusted that attempts would be made to preserve the limb in such cases, should we have another campaign. The rifle bullet generally split the femur in the direction of its fibres. His experience of wounds of large joints led him to the conviction that either amputation or resection must be performed to give the patient a chance of his life. He was in favor of the resection of joints. The next question was, When is it to be performed? Is it to be primary or secondary? Primary operations he considered to be within thirty-six hours, or before adhesive inflammation had fairly set in. The consequences of secondary operations during that period were very fatal when the operations were delayed to the true secondary period. When the constitution had become in some degree accustomed to the drain on the system, the results became very favourable. He then gave some tables of the re-results of secondary operations at Scutari, but the returns were not very complete; however, the conclusion naturally was, that if amputation were to be performed, the sooner it was done the better after the receipt of the injury; and if delayed, no operation should be performed until local and constitutional circumstances were favourable. He would continue the subject on another day.

Dr. Williams said that as the practice of some was very different from what had been so ably stated by Dr. Menzies, he hoped that those who were there from the commencement of the war would give their experience. With reference to the tincture of benzoin for wounds, he had not used it himself, but had found copaiba of the greatest use in lacerated wounds.

Mr. Blenkins felt sure the author must have had considerable experience in gunshot wounds. He could bear his testimony to the admirable effects of the tincture of benzoin. He thought it a valuable remedy, and had used it in cases of hemorrhage from the surface of scorbutic sores with the greatest benefit.

Dr. Crawford differed somewhat from Dr. Menzies, but agreed with him in cases of wounds of the humerus. He considered wounds of the large joints as cases for resection; however, they were not always hopeless cases, and he mentioned the case of an officer of the 18th Regiment who was wounded in the knee-joint, treated by Dr. Ryan, 18th Regiment, by rest, and whose limb was saved without an operation. Compound fractures of the femur were also not without such success as to leave hope of saving the limb. He also mentioned some cases of compound fracture of the tibia that afterwards required operations; still he in general agreed with Dr. Menzies, that many cases would still require operations.

Dr. Trotten mentioned a case at Scutari of a wound of the knee-joint, where an attempt was made to save the limb, but amputation was subsequently required.

Dr. Crawford, in reply to Mr. Blenkins, said the synovia escaped from the wound of the knee-joint.

Dr. Robinson could not corroborate Dr. Menzies' statement of the advisability of preserving the limb, where the injury was below the knee; the amount of injury almost always required amputation, and if not done primarily, would require to be subsequently performed with more risk to the patient.

Dr. Gordon, after a long experience here and elsewhere, never had reason to regret not having saved the limb when the joint had been injured; he had never seen a case in which the head of the tibia was injured that had recovered without an operation.

Dr. O'Leary read his successful case of excision of the head of the femur.

Dr. Shelton mentioned a case of compound fracture of the middle of the humerus which recovered without operation; he was an advocate for conservative surgery.

Mr. Blenkins thought that Dr. O'Leary's case was a favourable one for excision, and he had an opportunity of seeing the man while under treatment in the 68th Regiment Hospital, and was struck with the simplicity of the apparatus employed.

Dr. O'Leary said, that as allusion had been made to the resection of the hip-joint, he had read the case that had proved so eminently successful.

Dr. Robinson had a case of gunshot wound of the knee-joint; there was no splintering of the bone, and it was considered an apt case for an attempt at conservative surgery. The patient, however, subsequently died.

Dr. Gibant had seen two excisions of the elbow and two of the knee both successful.

Dr. Burke said his experience during the Sutlej campaign was in favour of primary amputations.

Mr. Rodgers mentioned a case of wound of the knee-joint that proved fatal.

Dr. Williams considered the same amount of mortality would not have occurred had the ease happened under different circumstances. In hot climates he considered that primary amputations should generally be preferred.

Dr. Gordon corroborated Dr. Burke, and said that he, out of twenty-two operations on the upper extremity, had only lost one.

Mr. Thornton was greatly in favour of early operations after injuries, and mentioned a case of a soldier whose arm he had amputated at the neck of the humerus, who was walking about the fifth day.

Dr. Burke in reply to Dr. Williams said, with reference to the heat of climate, it was in the northwest provinces of India, where the climate is occasionally colder than it is here. The heat of India had nothing to do with the fatal results in the cases he had mentioned.

Dr. Crawford thought, as far as he could gather the opinion of the members, that amputation was considered necessary in cases of perforating wounds of the knee-joint. Inflammation of the synovial membrane appeared to have been the cause of dread; but he hoped that he might live to see the day when amputation would not be considered altogether necessary in those cases.

Dr. O'Leary mentioned a case of wound of the knee-joint in which he could introduce his little finger; there could be no mistake that the joint was injured, as the synovia was escaping from the wound. He was going to amputate, but was ordered not by the principal medical officer; the man died in a few days of pyæmia. In another case the knee was wounded by a piece of glass, the synovia escaped from the wound; ice was constantly applied, and tartar emetic administered; on the seventh day inflammation set in and mercury was given; the joint gradually improved, the wound became chronic, and is now progressing favourably. He was of opinion that synovia may come out of a wound and yet the limb may be saved. This was not a clean wound.

Mr. Wyatt considered that we should not trust too much to the absence of any sanguineous effusion immediately after an accident. He had no experience of the tincture of benzoin, but he did not approve of the tincture of matico. He imagined that neither of them could be applied except in cases where hemorrhage occurred only from the surface of sores and wounds. The author of the paper, in speaking of the French practice here, in reference to the wounds of the middle and upper thirds of the thigh, had been somewhat in error, the fact being that they scarcely ever operate in such cases, but leave the patient to nature; and they find it as successful as in cases where for similar injuries they had previously operated. He could bear testimony to the extraordinary course a Minie ball would sometimes take, and mentioned a case that occurred at Inkerman.

Mr. Bowen thought the question raised respecting the employment of primary or secondary amputations a most important one. He could speak most favourably of the employment of aconite as an antiphlogistic remedy instead of tartar emetic. He did not approve of the gutta percha splints recommended by Dr. Menzies, but preferred those made of thin wire, which are light and cleanly.

Mr. Wyatt had seen the splints mentioned by Mr. Bowen; they were constantly employed in the French ambulances, and were found very useful.

Dr. Sclaveroni said the wire splints had been used in the Sardinian army in a few instances, and were highly approved of.

Mr. Blenkins had been edified by the discussion, and he proposed a vote of thanks to Dr. Menzies.

---

11. *Analysis of Cases of Amputation of the Limbs in the Radcliffe Infirmary, Oxford.*—Edward L. Hussey, Esq. communicated to the Royal Medical and Chirurgical Society (April 8, 1856) the following statement:—

"The capital operations in the Radcliffe Infirmary are recorded in a register kept for the purpose, the entries being made from notes taken at the time of the operation. In this register and in the admission-books are noted 164 cases of amputation from all causes, which are arranged in the paper in separate tables. Among the cases of disease, 91 were for diseases of joints; 55 of these were in the thigh, of which 10 were fatal; 6 died from the immediate effects of the operation, and 4 did not recover sufficiently to be sent home. The mortality varied in the practice of the different surgeons. Of 20 cases in the leg, only 1 died; of 6 cases in the upper arm, and 10 in the forearm, all recovered. Among those who recovered from the operation, 17 never permanently regained their former health; 3 died from accidental illness; in 1 the cause of death was not ascertained; 16 others died with phthisis, at various periods after the operation; the subsequent history of 5 was not known; the rest are all now in good health. The mortality was not affected by the duration of the disease, or the extent of disorganization of the joint. The proportion of men who undergo amputation in early stages of disease is greater than that of women; in later stages the proportion of women is greatest. The operations for diseased joints in boys and girls under puberty are not successful; a larger proportion than in adults die from the effects of the operation, or do not recover their health after amputation. In 5 cases of malignant diseases, 2 died after operation; in 1 the disease returned within a year; the other 2 are living. In other diseases, necrosis, caries, gangrene, elephantiasis, old ulcerations, and inconvenient limbs, all the patients recovered. Of 6 cases of primary amputation of the thigh, only 1 recovered, and in that case the injuries were confined to the leg, below the knee. In all the fatal cases, the operation was performed after very severe injury. All the operations on the leg (12 in number) succeeded. Of 15 on the upper arm, 3 died; and of 14 on the forearm, I died. Among the secondary operations, only 1 died, after amputation at the shoulder-joint for a burn. The operations were mostly done by circular incision. The chief veins of the limb were tied whenever they bled, without any bad consequences. The stumps were generally tied at the time of the operation. In several cases, where the stump was left open after the operation, there was secondary hemorrhage, and in all of them union was very slow. The healing of the wound, or the discharge of the patient, was retarded by so many accidental causes, that it was not easy to make a fair estimate of the time occupied in the recovery. The forearm generally healed rather sooner than the upper arm, and the upper arm rather sooner than the leg, the thigh being much the latest. After amputation for diseased joints, the stumps healed sooner than in other diseases. The greatest delay was after primary operations for accidents.

"Mr. Erichsen asked how it was that the rate of mortality varied so greatly in the practice of different surgeons in the Radcliffe Infirmary; whether the variation was accidental, or due to the adoption of different methods of treatment. The paper appeared to indicate that (as, indeed, might be expected) amputations and excisions for disease were on the whole more successful in the country than in London. Skill, he believed, had little to do with success in such cases. In the country the surgeon had not to deal with persons who were broken down by debility as in London, and he could place his patients in far better hygienic circumstances. The mortality at the Radcliffe Hospital did not appear to arise from pyæmia, secondary abscesses, and the like, which so frequently occasioned death in London. The mortality, however, in cases of primary amputation of the thigh, appeared to be as great there as elsewhere. This was, perhaps, the most fatal operation in surgery. In many institutions not one patient in ten had recovered. Such a result would almost lead one to adopt the plan of the French surgeons, who had given up the operation entirely. He believed that not a single case had proved successful either in the French or British camp.

"Mr. Hussey said, the six deaths after amputation of the thigh resulted from pyæmia. He had no doubt that operations were more successful in the country than in London, the constitutions of the patients being better. In London he never saw a wound after amputation heal by the first intention. In the case of recovery after primary amputation of the thigh, the thigh-bone was not injured. When the bone was injured he had never known a patient to recover. He should be glad to know the result in London of operations for diseased joints in children. His own impression was, that amputation for diseased joints was never required before puberty. Such cases, he found, recovered in the country; and if they did not, amputation, he believed, would be of no service.

"Dr. Barker said, he knew two officers who had recovered after primary amputation of the thigh; and, he believed, without a bad symptom.

"Mr. Paget mentioned two recent successful operations for gunshot wounds; one by Mr. Hewett, at St. George's Hospital, where there was an extensive fracture of the lower part of the femur; and the other by himself, at St. Bartholomew's, where the gunshot went through the condyles of the femur. In both cases, he said, recovery was perfect.

"Mr. Curling thought Mr. Erichsen had taken a more gloomy view of the operation than facts warranted. He had seen many cases recover.

"Mr. Erichsen said, he had in view 12 cases at Edinburgh, all of which died; 10 in the Royal Infirmary, Glasgow, and the same number in St. Thomas's Hospital, not one of which recovered. In the hospital with which he was connected, nearly half the cases had been saved; so that as to personal experience he did not take so gloomy a view as was supposed; he simply referred to the statistics which had been published.

"Mr. Arnott said, that in regard to the operation in question, the experience of the Peninsula was similar to that of the Crimean campaign—that it should not be attempted except in cases of absolute necessity."—*Med. Times and Gaz.*, April 26, 1856.

---

12. *Excision of Elbow-joint.*—Mr. SYME states (*Lancet*, April 19th, 1856), that he has recently adopted the following method of excising the elbow-joint, and found it to wonderfully facilitate the process.

Having made the ordinary incisions be exposed the convex osseous surface, held the ulnar nerve to the side by a hook, and sawed through the bones about the middle of the olecranon. Nothing, he says, could be easier after this, than insulating first one and then the other extremity, and sawing them off to the requisite extent.

---

13. *Excision of the Knee-Joint.*—By PETER BROTHERSTON, Esq. In 1854, when visiting Edinburgh, I had frequent opportunities of seeing two cases, in which the operation of excision of the knee-joint had been successfully performed by my friend, the late Dr. Richard Mackenzie, of Edinburgh, in the Royal Infirmary; and, being struck by the appearance, strength, and usefulness of the limbs operated upon, I determined, whenever a suitable case presented itself, to give the operation a trial.

Robert Strang, æt. 10, son of a collier residing in Clackmannan, has had strumous disease of the left knee-joint for two years. The leg is slightly flexed, the joint very much enlarged, and an ulcerated opening, about half an inch in diameter, over the inside of the joint. A probe, introduced into this opening, and pushed backwards, enters the joint. He has continual pain, aggravated on motion, and the discharge is very considerable. The boy is pale and emaciated, and has a quick pulse, of about 120. Having stated to the parents that an effort should be made to save the leg, and explaining to them the nature of the operation for excision of the knee-joint, they at once consented to have the operation performed without delay. I wrote to my friend, Dr. James Gillespie, of Edinburgh, requesting his assistance in this case, he having assisted the late Dr. Richard Mackenzie in his previous cases at the Royal Infirmary; and, accordingly, on the 19th May, 1854, I performed the operation as follows: The boy being put under the influence of chloroform, I made a free incision across the front of the knee-joint, below the patella, from a little above the posterior edge of the inner tuberosity of the tibia, across to the posterior edge of the outer tuberosity; and having divided the lateral and crucial ligaments, I proceeded to separate the connection round the condyles of the femur, which being done, about three quarters of an inch of the condyles were sawn off. A slice of about one-third of an inch in thickness was then taken from the head of the tibia, and the cartilage was removed from the inner surface of the patella by means of a gouge. Four arteries required ligature. The ends of the bones were then placed in accurate apposition, and the wound was closed with seven sutures. A splint, covered with lint, was applied to the ham, and the whole secured with a bandage.

It is needless to give a detailed account of this case; but I may remark, that in seven months, complete anchylosis of the bones had taken place, and the boy could walk with freedom. There were two or three sores in the neighbourhood of the incision; but they were superficial and unconnected with the bone.

Second Case.—The progress and cure of the case just related was anxiously watched by a gentleman in Alloa, whose son, eleven years of age, was labouring under acute synovitis and ulceration of the cartilages of the right knee. From seeing the case of the boy Strang progress so favourably, he asked me if a similar operation might not save his son's limb; and on being told that the case was a remarkably favourable one for the operation, he at once consented to have it done. I may state there was urgent necessity for this operation, or amputation being immediately performed. The extreme paroxysms of pain which came on whenever the boy attempted to sleep, caused by the ulceration of the cartilage being brought in contact with the opposing bone during sleep, when the natural control of the limb was lost, and his state of nervous debility, showed that he could not have borne up longer under the source of irritation. There was no other external ulceration, except a sinous opening in the ham, which discharged a quantity of matter. I was assisted again by my friend, Dr. James Gillespie, and the operation was performed on the 12th January, 1855, in every way similar to the former case.

There was a considerable quantity of pus in the joint, and distinct ulceration of the cartilage on the condyles of the femur and head of the tibia. The incision nearly all healed by the first intention, and everything went on favourably till about the beginning of March, when an abscess began to form on the outside of the thigh, a little above the seat of the operation. This I opened on the 28th of March, and shortly afterwards the abscess gradually closed, and finally healed altogether. It is now eleven months since the operation was performed, and the limb is fairly anchylosed. All swelling has disappeared, and the limb is as straight as its fellow, and only an inch shorter. The patella is found slightly movable, a little above its former seat, and he can walk with a firm decided step, without a crutch, although he uses one at present, by my orders, to save the limb.

I may mention here the great benefit I found from the use of sand bags, recommended me by Dr. Richard Mackenzie, laid on each side of the leg, along the sides of the joint, and fastened with two bits of tape, one above and another below the knee. They served admirably to keep the bones in accurate apposition, and from their weight, kept the leg *in situ*, especially preventing its movement during sleep.—*Edinburgh Med. Journ.*, April, 1856.

---

14. *Tic Douloureux cured by Excision of a Mass of Phosphate of Lime, adhering to the Supra-orbital Nerve.*—By Hugh Sharp, Esq. On the 17th of December, 1855, a man, G. F., æt. about 50 years, residing in Cullen, had a very severe attack of tic-douloureux in his left brow, which continued, without intermission, for several hours; it again returned on the 18th, at the same hour as on 17th, but with greater violence, when I was called on for advice, etc. Seeing at once the nature of the case, and without examining minutely the seat of the severe pain, I prescribed for him some croton oil and calomel pills, to be taken at proper intervals. This had the desired effect, until the 20th, when the pain returned with the same violence as formerly, when I was again called in, when, on pointing out to the man the course of the supra-orbital nerve, which would have to be divided, or rather a small part of it removed altogether, in order to give relief, even for a limited time, I detected a small hard tumour, about the bulk of a pea, somewhat flattened, firmly adhering to, and immediately over, the supra-orbital nerve, as it emerged from the notch, and concealed by the eyebrow. I inquired if he knew how long the small tumour had been there,

when he stated that it had been there about thirty years, but had never felt any pain in it, or near it, and did not think it had any connection whatever with the pain; but on my stating my firm belief that the small tumour was the sole cause of the acute suffering, he agreed to my proposal of removing it immediately, which I proceeded to do. I thought the small tumour was a firm encysted one, but soon found out my mistake, for, on attempting to transfix it, my small bistoury was stopped. I then laid open the skin over the tumour, and grasped it firmly in a common dressing forceps, but found I could not dislodge it from its adhesions without the aid of a small scoop. This small tumour was in reality a small piece of phosphate of lime, which I transmitted to Professor Syme, along with the details of the case.

I have further to add that the Tic was completely cured by the removal of the tumour, and has not again returned, even in the most modified degree, to the very great satisfaction of the patient. In many cases, I am of opinion that tic is produced by the presence of a tumour, of one kind or other, on the nerve, though situated so deep as to elude detection. I may here add, that the patient has suffered, every week almost during the past thirty years, from severe headaches, but since the removal of the little tumour he has had no return of headache whatever.—*Edinburgh Med. Journ.*, April, 1856.

15. *Gunshot Wounds.*—Dr. G. H. B. Macleod, in some "Notes on the Surgery of the War" (*Edinburgh Medical Journal*, May, 1856), makes the following interesting remarks on gunshot wounds:—

"Of the 'peculiarities' of gunshot wounds, none strikes one earlier than the results which flow from the fact, that their being essentially of a contused character, their tract must suppurate before it closes. Superficial wounds through muscles, sometimes, though rarely, form exceptions, as they have been seen to adhere by the first intention. Thus I have seen one case, in which a superficial wound of the belly of the gastrocnemius by a ball, was said to have healed by the fifth day. The separation of the sloughs from the tract of a ball have, in the case I have had under my charge, taken place at different periods between the sixth and twenty-seventh days, according to the depths of the parts traversed. This separation gives rise to another feature in these wounds, the occurrence of secondary hemorrhage, as well as the fact, that if the orifices of the tract become clean and adhere while suppuration is going on within, most troublesome accumulations of pus and burrowing abscesses will result. The greater contusion at the orifice of entrance causes it, in general, though by no means universally, to be longer of taking on the adhesive process than the orifice of exit.

"The eccentric course often pursued by balls, has frequently been remarked upon in former wars, and though we have had many most striking instances of this peculiarity, still I suspect we have had less of it than occurred in the experience of former campaigns. The Minie ball is seldom content to dally with a limb, or run round a cavity. Its force, on the contrary, suffices not only to carry it through any of the great cavities, but has been seen to lodge in the body of a third man, after perforating that of his two front rank comrades. The old ball is still sometimes used, and most curious is its occasional wandering. Thus I have known it enter above the elbow, and be cut out from the posterior wall of the axilla of the opposite side, while in another instance it entered the right hip, and was found embedded in the left popliteal space. This circumstance often makes the search for balls exceedingly difficult, more particularly as the feelings of the patient frequently give one but little assistance. That such a search should be instituted at the very earliest possible moment before inflammation and swelling have come on, is a most imperative maxim; and unless greater injury be inflicted by its removal than is likely to follow its retention, the necessity of extracting the ball and all foreign matters it may have introduced along with it, is of the utmost importance, both immediately and remotely. Two instances may be mentioned as illustrating the necessity for an early and careful search—though such an obvious point hardly requires elucidation. One case occurred to myself. A soldier, wounded on the 18th of June, was brought under my care in the General Hospital in camp. He had sustained a compound fracture of the right arm, which was much swollen on admission. I was told, and accepted the story, that the accident had been caused by a piece of shell, to which species of injury the wound bore every resemblance, and that a surgeon who had seen him in one of the trenches, had removed it. At the earnest solicitation of the patient, I contented myself with applying the necessary apparatus to try and save the limb, without minutely examining the wound. The injury turned out to be much masked and to be more severe than was at first supposed—the shaft of the humerus having been split into the capsule—and when removing the limb at the shoulder, some days after, a large grape-shot dropped out from among the muscles. I once saw a piece of shell weighing nearly three pounds, extracted from the hip of a man at Scutari, after the battle of the Alma, which had been overlooked for a couple of months, and to which a very small sinus alone led. This latter case, too, illustrates another curious circumstance in gunshot wounds, viz., the way in which the elasticity of the soft parts often permits bodies to pass in behind, which they close, so as to make it a matter of wonder how such masses could have got admission.

"The sensation caused by a ball striking a limb appears to be of the most trivial and transient nature, and is commonly likened to a smart blow from a cane. If a cavity be entered, the collapse and mental trepidation are often, however, very appalling.

"Shell wounds are more destructive to the soft textures than those caused by rifle balls, being frequently followed by wide-spread sloughing; but the hard parts often suffer less. The bone may be fractured, but it is frequently not much comminuted. The shell falling vertically, gives rise sometimes to most wonderful escapes.

"The constitutional fever which follows gunshot wounds is, in general, proportioned to the importance of the part implicated, though most curious exceptions to this not unfrequently arise. That old soldiers, if sober, are much less affected by this constitutional disturbance than others, is, I think, very observable. The mitigation of this, and of the local inflammation, the prevention of all accumulations of matter, by the making of judicious dependent openings, the relaxation of several muscular fibres, the application of light unirritating dressings, rest, and attention to the general principles of surgery, comprise all the treatment which gunshot wounds usually demand. In the profuse suppurations which so often follow these injuries, the use of cod-liver oil has been markedly advantageous. The extreme simplicity of the appliances and dressing employed during this war, and the nearly total absence of poultices and such like 'cover-sluts,' would, I think, merit the approbation of even Mr. Guthrie. The era when the 'Oleum catellorum' and the tenting of wounds was in vogue, has entirely passed away forever; and, though wondrous virtues are ascribed to water, it is not on account of any 'magical or unchristian' power which it is supposed to possess. Water dressing and the lightest possible bandaging is in universal repute in this army, though not seemingly so popular with our allies the French, with whom grease, divers coloured washes, heavy pledgets of charpie and much cloth, still hold their place. There is, however, one application to profusely suppurating wounds, which I have seen the French employ with more manifest advantage than many of the astringents we use, viz., a solution composed of the perchloride of iron in the preportion of one to three of water.

"Splints, too, of the simplest pattern are now employed, and the straight position universally preferred in the treatment of fractures. Bandaging is reduced to the fulfilment of the most necessary essentials, and all complications studiously avoided. Endless rollers, multiplied splints, and various contrivances are still too often seen in the French ambulances. Stiff bandages have been but little used by us, though one felt much tempted to apply them after their recorded success in the Schleswic-Holstein war. The 'appareil amovo-inamovible' is said to be popular with our enemies, and an illustrated book on its employment, published in 1851, for the use of the army, was found by a friend who was with me in the hospital library of Fort Kinburn.

"The long believed and much feared effects of the wind of balls, has so completely passed away into the mythology of surgery, that if it were not that one of my own wards, at this moment, contains two most excellent instances proving its utter nonsense, I would not at all refer to it. The haversack of one man was struck by a round shot on the 8th September, and though his back was slightly discolored, he was not knocked down; and the other suffered a trivial abrasion of the thigh by a like cause. I had lately two under my notice—a sergeant who was struck on the chin by a 9 lb. ball, and though it fractured his jaw severely, in no way affected his brain; and another soldier had a piece of flesh, about the size of the fist, cleanly nipped out of his hip in the same way."

16. *Hemorrhage following Gunshot Wounds.* By G. H. B. Macleod.—Hemorrhage following gunshot wounds is not now so dreaded as it used to be, because it is known to be by no means so frequent in occurrence as it was formerly believed to be. I have heard surgeons declare that tourniquets might have been left at home, so far as any use they were of at the battles of the Alma and Inkerman, but I suspect, though cases did not often require them when seen by the medical man, that hemorrhage is in reality the chief immediate cause of death in the case of the majority of men killed in the field. It would be a dangerous experiment to make, but withal a very interesting one, to go over a field of battle immediately after a fight, and record the apparent causes of death in each case.

The returns fail to inform us of the numbers of cases in which secondary hemorrhage succeeded gunshot wounds in the course of this war, and though I have no figures to which I might refer in corroboration of the statement, I am inclined to think that the proportion is higher than that set down by Mr. Guthrie. The period of its occurrence has appeared to range, on an average, between the fifth and the twenty-fifth day, without drawing any minute distinction, as is done by Dr. John Thomson, between hemorrhage due to sloughing, ulceration, or simply excited arterial action at different stages of the process of cure. The fifteenth day has, curiously enough, been that on which it has taken place in the vast majority of the cases of which I have retained notes. One instance, the particulars of which I failed to learn, was said to have occurred as late as the seventh week, when the wound—a gunshot wound of the thigh—was nearly cicatrized. Hemorrhage occurring early has been almost universally treated on the principle laid down by Bell, and so well supported and elucidated by Guthrie, of tying both ends of the wounded vessel; but when the limb is much swollen, the parts infiltrated matted together and disorganized, it is all very well to say the same principles must be carried out notwithstanding the additional risk that the coats of the vessel may be diseased, but any one who has tried it a few times will know that to do so is no easy task. With a vessel like the posterior tibial, which has repeatedly bled and infiltrated the tissues of a large muscular calf, changing their appearance and matting them together, and with a large irregular wound, into which the blood from the vessel does not seem to be poured in a collected form, but to well out from a large sloughing surface, so as to afford no guide to its exact position, the undertaking is one of the most difficult that can be imagined. The rules and precepts laid down in books about passing probes from the surface towards the seat of the bleeding, the appearance assumed by the vessel, and the dissecting-room directions to find it, are all utterly useless in actual practice; and the knowledge of them is often more a hindrance than an assistance. Watchful eyes and careful cutting, are the only reliable guides.

I believe that pressure so carefully applied over a long tract of the main vessel above, as will diminish, without arresting, the stream passing through it, will, in many cases, be sufficient to allow such coagulation to take place in the open mouths of the vessels as will prevent any future annoyance—that is always supposing a very large extent of an artery be not ripped open, as it were, and as I have seen it, by a rifle ball. The French do not, seemingly, act so unreservedly on the principle of putting a ligature on both ends of a bleeding vessel, as we do. They perform Anel's operation in not a few cases. The interesting and instructive nature of the following case is evident: A Russian boy, wounded at Inkerman, was received into the French hospital at Pera. He had sustained a compound fracture of the leg from gunshot. On the fifteenth day after injury, profuse hemorrhage took place from both openings. Pressure failed to arrest it. The popliteal was tied the same day according to the method of deligation recommended by M. Jobert, viz., on the inner side of the limb, between the vastus and hamstring muscles. The foot remained very cold for four days, and then violent reaction set in, and on the eighth day from the ligature of the main vessel hemorrhage recurred both from the original wound and the incision of ligature. Pressure was tried in vain. The superficial femoral was then ligatured on the tenth day from the deligation of the popliteal. Four days afterwards the bleeding returned from the wound, and pressure then seemed to check it. The ligature separated from the femoral on the twelfth day after its being tied, and the third day after, *i. e.*, the twenty-fifth day from the first occurrence of hemorrhage bleeding again set in from the wound, the limb was amputated in the thigh, and the unfortunate patient ultimately recovered. Would Mr. Guthrie not have saved this man's limb and the surgeons much trouble? It was a matter of common conversation in the hospitals at Constantinople, that when the weather was close and sultry, with little wind, there was certain to be a large number of cases of secondary hemorrhage.

A soldier, resting his right hand on his musket, was struck by a ball on the web between the thumb and forefinger. The wound seemed trivial, but the whole hand swelled exceedingly. On the fourteenth day arterial hemorrhage occurred, and pressure was applied. The bleeding repeatedly recurred, and still pressure was persevered in. Finally the radial, and then the ulnar, was ligatured before the hemorrhage was commanded. An early search in the wound, and a thread appled to the orifices of the vessel, would have saved much annoyance and risk. The following occurred under my own notice:—

M'Garthland, a soldier of the 38th regiment, an unhealthy man, who still suffered from the effects of scurvy, which had been followed by fever, was shot through the left leg from behind, and externally forwards and inwards, on the 18th of June. The fibula was broken, and the edge of the tibia was injured. He walked to the rear without assistance. On admission the limb was greatly swollen. This swelling very much diminished in a few days. On the fifth day, arterial bleeding, to a limited extent, took place from both openings. Recalling a case put on record by Mr. Butcher, of Dublin, the wound of the post-tibial, I determined on trying the effects of well-applied pressure along the course of the popliteal and in the wound, and employed cold, while the limb was raised and fixed on a splint. The object of the pressure on the main vessel was to diminish, not arrest, the flow of blood through it. On the eighth day there was again some oozing. Pus had accumulated among the muscles of the calf (one great objection to using pressure on the orifices of gunshot wounds), and required incision for its evacuation. On the ninth day a pulsating tumour was observed on the external aspect of the leg, and next day the bleeding returned from both wounds.

I wished then to cut down and tie the vessel in the wound, but a consultation decided on waiting a little longer, in the hope that the bleeding might not return. On the night of the eleventh day most profuse hemorrhage recurred. The attendant, though strictly enjoined, failed to tighten the tourniquet, but the necessary steps to arrest the bleeding were taken by the officer on duty. Next morning, when I first heard of the occurrence, I found the patient blanched, cold, and nearly pulseless. A consultation decided that the state of the parts made the securing of the vessel in the wound very problematical, and that as the limb would not recover if the main artery was taken up, amputation must be performed so soon as he had sufficiently rallied. When reaction had fairly taken place, I amputated the limb. The removed parts were much engorged, sloughed, and disorganized. The anterior tibial was found to have been opened for about an inch shortly after its origin, and on it was formed the aneurism, which had a communication with both orifices of the wound. The artery should have been tied in the wound on the occurrence of the second bleeding. I say the second bleeding, as it very often happens that even when hemorrhage has taken place, to a considerable extent, and evidently from a vessel of large calibre, it never recurs. Many most striking instances of this have come under my notice. But though more than even this is true, and that frequently blood thrown out repeatedly is spontaneously arrested, still the great preponderance of cases in which it recurs in dangerous repetitions and quantities, as in the above instance, should cause us, I believe, to interfere on its second appearance, if it be in any quantity more particularly, and that we should not delay, so as to run the risk of such a return as will cause exhaustion. Not to interfere unless the vessel is bleeding, must not always be understood too literally, or we will often be prevented from performing a necessary operation till our patient is beyond our help. The hemorrhage recurs over and over again, and the surgeon, though as near as is practicable, arrives only in time to see the bed drenched, and the patient and attendant intensely alarmed. There is at the moment no bleeding, and he vainly hopes there will be no return; and so on goes the game between ebbing life and approaching death, the loss not great at each time, but mighty in its sum, till all assistance is useless.

The use of acetate of lead, or gallie acid, though often trusted to in these hemorrhages, are surgical farces—mesmeric passes along the vessels would be of infinitely more service.—*Edinburgh Medical Journal*, May, 1856.

17. *Escape of Great Vessels by their Elasticity, from Balls.* By G. H. B. Macleod.—There is no circumstance in gunshot wounds which is more striking than the wonderful way in which the great vessels, by their elasticity, escape from the ball in its transit. Thus bullets innocuously traversed parts where one would suppose a pin's head could not be placed, without wounding a vessel. True, the fact that such cases remain to be seen, results from the vessel not having been opened, and we do not know in how many cases the result was not so fortunate, but still, viewed merely as happy escapes, they are curious and interesting. In the course of the femoral vessels, this phenomenon is particularly common. Through the axilla, through the neck, out and in behind the angles of the jaw, between the bones of the forearm and leg, balls of every size often take their passage without harm to the vessels. Take the following cases as examples: A soldier was wounded at Inkerman, by a ball which entered through the right cheek and escaped behind the angle of the left jaw, so tearing the parts that the great vessels were plainly visible in the wound. Three weeks after he was discharged without having had a bad symptom. A soldier of the Buffs was struck in June last, when in the trenches, by a rifle ball, in the nape of the neck. It passed forwards round the right side of the neck, up under the angle of the inferior maxilla, fractured the superior maxillary and malar bones, destroyed the eye, and, escaping, killed another man who was sitting beside him. This man made a recovery without a bad symptom.

A French soldier at the Alma was struck obliquely by a rifle ball, near, but external to the right nipple; the ball passed seemingly right through the vessels and nerves in the axilla, and escaped behind. His cure was rapid and uninterrupted. Endless numbers of similar cases may be seen in any military hospital.—*Ibid.*

18. *The Warm Bath in the Treatment of Wounds, Especially those made in Amputation.*—M. Langenbeck, of Berlin, has published in the *Deutsche Klinik* for September 15th, 1855, an account of a process by which wounds, especially those made in amputation, can be constantly subjected to the influence of a warm bath. He first examines the modes of application of cold and warm water, and concludes that, in many cases, these are insufficient. He relates the advantages which he has obtained from the use of large warm baths after capital operation, such as disarticulation of the shoulder-joint, excision of the scapula, lithotomy, etc. These baths have been employed from half an hour to an hour once or twice daily, not being contraiudicated by traumatic fever and inflammation of the edges of the wound; at a temperature of 97° Fahrenheit, they maintain warmth, diminish fever, heat, and the frequency of the pulse, calm pain, and keep the wound clear. Topical warm baths have often been

employed by MM. Langenbeck and Stromeyer, in gunshot wounds of the extremities, with or without injury of the bones, before and during suppuration. Stromeyer first recommended the use of the permanent warm bath after the operation for vesico-vaginal fistula.

The following is a description of the apparatus employed by M. Langenbeck:—

The apparatus intended for the upper extremities consists of two oblong basins, of various sizes; they are placed in a hollow of the mattress near the edge of the bed, so that, as the patient lies on his back, the arm may rest comfortably in them. The reservoir for the leg is triangular; the base is directed upwards, and the apex is fixed on a board, and moves on a hinge. By means of a wooden structure, which works into the supporting board, and is fixed at the upper end, the latter can be raised or depressed at convenience. The whole apparatus forms a double inclined plane, on which the leg, bent at an angle of about 120°, rests in the water. The basin has a cover fastened down, with an opening at the upper part to admit the leg. The opening has a projecting border, on which is fixed one end of a sleeve of vulcanized cacutchouc, the other end embracing the thigh and leg; in this way, the evaporation and cooling of the water are prevented. In the interior of the reservoir, three straps are fixed to hooks, so as to sustain the limb; while two other straps pass over the limb and keep it in position. At the bottom of the bath is a short tube, with a stopcock, for removing the water. Two openings, with movable coverings, are made in the cover of the apparatus; one being for introducing water and the other for receiving the thermometer.

Injuries of the knee, and the stump after amputations of the thigh, require the horizontal position, and consequently another form of apparatus. This consists of a square zinc box, from half a yard to a yard in length, fourteen inches wide, and arranged internally in the same manner as the apparatus already described. For stumps, the wall which looks towards the thigh has a large hole, with a projecting border, to which, by means of an iron ring, a caoutchouc tube passes and embraces the thigh. For injuries of the knee, the India-rubber tube is first applied to the thigh; then the leg is passed through the openings in the box and the lower caoutchouc tube; the lower border of the tube fixed on the thigh is then fastened by an iron ring, which is brought together by screws, to the projecting rim of the opening in the basin; and the apparatus, being thus adjusted, is filled with water.

M. Langenbeck, as a rule, leaves large wounds without dressings. But when they are the result of recent opperations, attended with loss of substance, he applies charpie and a bandage to obviate secondary hemorrhage. These applications, however, are removed the next day, without disturbing the limb. In amputations, resections, etc., sutures are employed, an aperture being left at one corner of the wound for the escape of secretions.

In general it is best not to employ the apparatus until the risk of secondary hemorrhage has ceased; for instance, in amputation, not within eighteen or twenty-four hours. In several cases, however, M. Langenbeck has applied the bath immediately after operation, before the patient had recovered from the effects of chloroform. This proceeding has the advantage of not being troubled by dressings, and the pain in the wound is rendered very trifling. If consecutive hemorrhage arise, the limb must be removed from the apparatus.

Great attention must be paid to the caoutchouc bands, so that they may neither compress the limb too tightly, nor allow the escape of water. Notwithstanding these precautions, œdema and gangrene may be produced, even by the slightest constriction, in some cases; especially over such parts as the crest of the tibia, where the bone is immediately under the skin. These inconveniencies may possibly be removed by further improvements; but it is well to examine the wounds carefully twice a day, when the water is renewed, and to shift the position of the caoutchouc sleeves, which should be sufficiently long.

The temperature of the water must vary according to the indications, whether it be desired to relieve pain, to prevent consecutive hemorrhage or inflammation, or to favour granulation. Further observations will probably point out the modifications required by the kind of lesion, and by the strength, age, and temperament of the patient. When the apparatus is used immediately after operation, the temperature employed at first is from 50° to 55° Fahrenheit; if the water be not renewed, the temperature rises, in from three to twelve hours, up to 59°, 68°, or 88. After the first day, this temperature is the most agreeable to the patient; at a later period when the wound begins to suppurate, water at 93° or 95° is used. In general, the feelings of the patient are the best guide on this point. It is easy to keep the temperature almost constant, by covering the apparatus more or less, and by adding warm or cold water. In summer, at a temperature of from 72° to 77° in the room, the heat of the bath rose, in twelve hours, from 93° to 95° or 100°. On the other hand, in winter, the temperature of the room being 63.5°, the water fell nearly constantly to 86° or 88° in the same period.

In general, it is sufficient to renew the water twice a day. If there be a large wound, or abundant suppuration, the apparatus must be carefully cleaned every day, by drawing off the water, and wiping the walls of the bath with sponges dipped in a chlorinated solution, taking care not to disturb the wound. When, however, the wound is large and not dependent, it is advisable to pass a stream of water into it to remove the secretions.

The advantages of this procedure are thus pointed out by M. Langenbeck:—

1. *Diminution of the Pain following Operation.*—However large the wound may be, pain is not complained of. In two cases, after injuries of the extremities, pain was produced in the sound foot and hand which were placed in the water, probably by distension of the thick epidermis. This pain, however, soon disappeared. When the water is being changed, and the injured part is exposed to the air, a cold sensation is experienced, attended with pain, which is removed as soon as the water is again poured in. If the wound remains exposed for a quarter of an hour, rigors are produced. M. Langenbeck has never seen rigors follow important operations, when the patient has been placed in a bath during anæsthesia.

By the use of the bath, the necessity for bandages, plaster, etc., is removed. The sutures can be removed without disturbing the limb, and cleanliness is maintained. Unfortunately, in amputation of the thigh, the apparatus is likely to produce œdema. This objection, however, may be removed by further improvement.

2. *Diminution of Fever.*—The traumatic fever, and that attending suppuration, lose their intensity. The pulse is usually from 88 to 90; at first, it is commonly as high as 120, but sinks as soon as suppuration commences. When the water is removed, the pulsation increases from 10 to 24, and again decreases when the water is added. If there be violent inflammation of the wound, or phlegmon of cellular tissue, the pulse may rise to 120 or 150, with corresponding general heat. During suppuration, Langenbeck once only observed rigors, indicating the formation of a large purulent deposit.

3. *Removal of the Secretions.*—So long as the water has free access to the wound, the stagnation and decomposition of its secretions are impossible, in proportion to the fluidity of these, and the dependent position of the limb. In deep and sinuous wounds, as after resection of the knee-joint, injections must be used. Complicated wounds, as those attending fracture of the thigh, with injury of the knee-joint, must be carefully watched; for, even though the surface of the wound be clean, there may be deposits in the subcutaneous cellular tissue, and when the wound is small, or when phlegmonous inflammation has set in. Incisions must then be employed, as in the ordinary treatment.

4. *Promotion of the Healing Process.*—M. Langenbeck has not yet been able to determine how far the use of the bath promotes union by the first intention. In one case, however, of circular amputation of the leg immediately below the knee, the wound healed by the first intention in the course of the sutures. In an open wound, subjected to the influence of the bath, the layers of coagulated blood, adherent to the wound, lose their colour; the fibrin remains, until, on the third or fourth day, it is removed by the granulations. The surface of the wound, in five or eight hours after operation, assumes a yellowish-gray colour, somewhat white, resulting from the decoloration of the superficial parts, and from the layer of exudation, which adheres to the wound. The limb, especially

in the vicinity of the wound, swells from the imbibition of water, and regains its natural dimensions on the removal of the water. This absorption must have a beneficial influence in promoting removal of the secretions, and preventing disorders in the capillary circulation. M. Langenbeck has observed inflammation of the edges of the wound and phlegmonous redness only in cases where purulent deposits were formed, or where the sutures were too tight.

In three or four days, the dead layer is removed in portions by the water, and granulation commences. In a very hort time, the deeper parts become filled up, the ends of the bones are covered, and the granulations from the medullary canal unite with the others. In the bath, the granulations attain a development, which is not observed with other modes of dressing. Their semi-transparent appearance shows that this depends in part on the absorption of the water. When the wound is covered with granulations, cicatrization commences. This is probably somewhat retarded by the bath; hence at this stage M. Langenbeck has recourse to the ordinary dressings.

To ascertain whether wounds heal more rapidly under water than when exposed to air, a large number of comparative experiments would be required; and even then we must remember that the period of healing varies even for the same operation. In three cases of subcutaneous resection of the tibia and fibula, healing took place in five, seven, and twelve weeks; while in two cases of subcutaneous excision of ankylosed elbow-joints, the wounds healed in the water bath in four weeks. A case of excision of the knee-joint, performed at Kiel, required fourteen weeks; while another case, under the influence of the bath, required only eight weeks. It must be remembered, however, that operation wounds sometimes heal very rapidly under the ordinary treatment, Nevertheless, M. Langenbeck is inclined to believe that the use of the bath promotes cicatrization.

Will the employment of the bath obviate the danger of pyæmia? This question cannot yet be decidedly answered; but M. Langenbeck has never seen pyæmia attend this treatment, although it occurred at the same time in other patients under his care. Chilling of the wound, retention and decomposition of the secretions, and miasmata, are the causes of pyæmia. These are obviated by the use of the bath; although the possibility of the occurrence of pyæmia cannot be denied.

M. Langenbeck relates several cases in which he has employed the treatment described, viz:—

1. Compound comminuted fracture of the right leg: 2. Osteosarcoma of the right tibia; amputation immediately below the knee: 3. Carcinoma of the foot; amputation by Lisfranc's method: 4 and 5. Ankylosis of the right elbow; subcutaneous resection: 6. Medullary cancer of the patella; removal of the patella, and excision of the ends of the bones: 7. Large fibrous tumour on the outer side of the knee; extirpation; joint opened; extensive gangrene and sanious suppuration. Recovery took place in all the cases except the last.

In the *Deutsche Klinik* for October 13, 1855, Dr. Fock publishes some further observations. The following are the cases in which the use of the bath is indicated: 1. All large wounds of the soft parts, whether it be desired to heal them by the first intention or not. 2. Penetrating wounds of the joints. 3. Compound fractures, as soon as inflammation and suppuration of the skin and cellular tissue set in. 4. Lacerations of the soft parts of the hands and feet, with or without injury of the bones. 5. After lithotomy, urethrotomy, operation for hernia, removal of uterine tumours, extirpation of the ovary. 6. Caries. 7. Whitlow, diffuse phlegmon, and acute suppurative œdema. 8. Gangrene. 9. Burns. 10. Acute and chronic inflammation of the joints. 11. Operations for ankylosis and contracted joints, whether by rupture or osteology. [12. The Cæsarean section?]—*Association Med. Journ.*, March 8, 1856.

---

19. *Surgical Uses of Glycerine.*—In our preceding No. (p. 518), we noticed some observations made by M. Demarquay on the surgical applications of glycerine. Since M. Demarquay published his remarks, further experiments have been made on the subject, the result of which has been published (*Gazette*

Médicale de Paris, January 26, 1856) by M. Lutton. He describes first the physical, and then the therapeutic effects of glycerine.

1. *Physical Effects.*—Being of an oily appearance, while it is of the consistence of syrup, it prevents the dressings from adhering to the wound; and by its solubility in water, it allows the wounds to be readily cleaned. Glycerine evidently moderates suppuration; and on the other hand, being very hygrometric, it keeps the parts constantly moist, and prevents the products of exudation from concreting. To obtain this result, it is necessary to apply the glycerine in abundance, and to impregnate the charpie and linen well with it. It protects the parts from the action of the air, and maintains them at a sufficiently high temperature. In these respects, glycerine is superior to fatty matters for surgical dressings.

2. *Therapeutic Uses.*—The first effect of the application of glycerine is to produce a slight prickling sensation, which, however, is soon calmed, and is never very distressing.

Simple Wounds.—In ordinary wounds, whether accidental or surgical, and free from complication, glycerine has no very manifest action. Under its application, wounds heal at least as soon as under most neutral local applications, and almost the only circumstance of any note is the small amount of suppuration. Besides this, there is scarcely ever an exuberance of granulations.

Burns.—In different degrees of burns, glycerine is a very convenient and efficacious application. Patients who have been treated by the transcurrent cautery, on account of white swelling, sciata, etc., have objected to be dressed with glycerine, on the ground that the burn healed too quickly, and did not "draw" enough. The happy effect of glycerine has been remarkably observed in a case of burn in the second degree, produced by an explosion in a mine.

Diphtheritis of Wounds.—In the Hospital of St. Louis, wounds, during the first days of their production, present a grayish, almost diphtheritic appearance, and become clean slowly. Under the influence of glycerine, this condition, more troublesome than serious, is arrested; the wound assumes a rosy aspect, without any exuberance of granulations.

Hospital Gangrene.—It was for this affection that glycerine was first employed in the Hospital of St. Louis. The disease in the first case was very extensive, and had been unsuccessfully treated by lemon-juice, quinine, and even by strong nitric acid and the actual cautery. In this, as in two other cases, glycerine was completely successful.

Abscesses and Purulent Deposits.—In deep wounds and sinuous ulcers, glycerine has been used, either by being introduced on a piece of charpie, or as an injection. The amount of suppuration has been remarkably diminished, and the period of cicatrization has been smaller. M. Demarquay has also injected glycerine into cold and congestive abcesses, and those in connection with inflamed bones, with complete success.

Ulcers.—Chronic, varicose, gangrenous, and other ulcers, have become rapidly clean under the influence of glycerine. The surface throws out granulations, and cicatrization soon takes place. Rest is a powerful and necessary aid.

Chancres.—Glycerine though it has no specific action on chancres, rapidly cleans the surface, and causes them to assume a healthy appearance.

Diseases of the Neck of the Uterus.—MM. Trousseau and Aran have already employed glycerine, but with little satisfaction, in uterine affections. M. Demarquay, however, has found it useful in simple or granular ulceration of the cervix. When the ulceration has been chronic, or when the cervix was rather enlarged and tumefied, caustic applications were also made. Glycerine was then applied by means of wadding: after the separation of the eschar, the secretions, commonly so abundant and fetid, were remarkably moderate in quantity.

In vaginitis, also, glycerine has been applied; but here, as in diseases of the cervix uteri, nothing conclusive can as yet be arrived at regarding its efficacy.

The editor of the *Med. Times and Gaz.* states (April 22, 1856) that he has lately had an opportunity of watching a trial of the remedy by Mr. Skey, in St. Bartholomew's Hospital. The first few cases in which it was resorted to appeared greatly benefited, and Mr. Skey was induced by their result to direct its general use. His final conclusion, however, as stated in clinical remarks, has been, that the remedy possesses no peculiar virtues whatever. A considerable number of sores heal rapidly during its use, as, indeed they would do under that of any non-irritating application which would exclude the air and prevent drying; in those, however, which have assumed an unhealthy state, and which resist the influence of other like remedies, it effects nothing whatever. A smaller series of trials by Mr. Hutchinson on patients at the Metropolitan Free Hospital, have led him to the same conclusion with Mr. Skey. Unhealthy sores dressed with it for periods of three weeks have remained precisely *in statu quo.* It is an agreeable application, causes no smarting, excludes the air, keeps the sore moist, and does not adhere to its edges; but beyond these it appears to possess no recommendations. While more expensive, it seems little, if at all, superior to olive or almond oil. It may seem difficult to reconcile the great discrepancy between foreign and English experience which these conclusions show. It might, perhaps, scarcely be deemed fair to insinuate, that on the Continent the employment of dressings which simply exclude air, and are themselves non-irritating, is not so well understood as among ourselves, and that, consequently, credit has been given to a single remedy which belongs rather to the whole class. Such, however, we suspect is, to some extent, the case. In one case, recorded by M. Petel, the source of fallacy is transparent. A woman came under his care for phagedænic stomatitis. Glycerine was applied, and *chlorate of potash given.* A very rapid cure, of course, occurred. The narration reminds one of Voltaire's assertion, that he could easily kill a flock of sheep by spells of witchcraft, provided, at the same time, he might mix a little arsenic with their food.

—

20. *New Method of Treating Phagedæna.*—Mr. Cock has recently been trying, in Guy's Hospital, a plan of treating phagedænic ulcers by constant irrigation. The method is, to have the sore well exposed, and the affected limb placed on some waterproof material; a reservoir above the bed is then filled with lukewarm water, and, by means of an elastic tube, a stream is kept continually flowing over the surface of the sore. By this means all particles of discharge, etc., are washed away as soon as formed, and the ulcer assumes the clean, pale appearance of a piece of meat which has been long soaked. In all the cases in which it has been practicable to employ the irrigation efficiently, a speedy arrest of morbid action has been secured, and the number has included several in which the disease was extensive and severe. The theory of the treatment is, that phagedænic action is a precess of local contagion—the *materies morbi* by which the ulcer spreads being its own pus. Admitting this supposition—which there is every reason for doing—to be true, the object to be kept in view in curative measures is either to decompose or to remove the local virus. This end is accomplished somewhat clumsily by such remedies as the nitric acid, which, unless so freely used as not only to char up all the fluid matters, but to destroy the whole surface of the ulcer to some depth, fails to prevent a recurrence. Mr. Cock's plan of subjecting the ulcer to a perpetual washing attempts the accomplishment of the same end by a more simple and direct method. It involves no pain to the patient, and does not destroy any healthy tissues. Its one disadvantage seems to be, that, excepting on the extremities, its use would be attended with some inconvenience, from the difficulty of preventing the water from running into the patient's bed. Should, however, further trials confirm the very favourable opinion which has been formed at Guy's as to its value, these difficulties might, no doubt, be surmounted by the contrivance of suitable apparatus. The directions as to temperature of the water are that it should be as warm as comfortable to the feelings of the patient; and, as preventive of smell, Mr. Cock advises the addition of a small quantity of the chloride of lime or of soda.—*Med. Times and Gaz.*, April 12, 1856.

—

21. *Is it always necessary to resort to Amputation when a Limb is attacked with Sphacelus?*—Prof. Bardinet, of Limoges, has brought this important question before the Academy of Medicine of la Haute Vienne, and has answered it in the negative.

We are too ardent partisans of conservative surgery, having ourselves sufficiently often protested against the excessive tendency to operate everywhere and at all times, not to hasten to submit to our readers the reasons adduced by M. Bardinet in support of his opinion.

The following is the *résumé* of his memoir:—

1st. In this memoir I report eight new cases of sphacelus (two of the finger, three of the forearm, and three of the leg), in none of which amputation was performed. The task of eliminating the dead parts was intrusted to Nature, except that her operations have been actively aided by the employment of the ordinary disinfectants, and especially by the early resection of the dead parts near the eliminatory circle.

In these eight cases recovery took place.

Had amputation been performed, it is, on the one hand, extremely probable that a certain number of patients would have died; on the other, several of them would have been deprived, in consequence of the necessity of amputating above the eliminatory circle, of a portion of their limbs (the knee, for example, or the upper part of the forearm), which they are fortunate in having been able to preserve.

It is, therefore, not always necessary to amputate in cases of sphacelus.

2d. We should, above all, be extremely cautious in having recourse to amputation in cases of spontaneous gangrene—first, because in such cases, whatever we do, and even after the establishment of the eliminatory circle, we can never be sure that the gangrene will not reappear, and that we shall not thus needlessly add the pain and dangers of a serious operation to those of the original disease.

3d. Because the fear of amputating in parts whose vessels are diseased, obliges us to carry the section up to a considerable height, and thus involves, sometimes very uselessly, the sacrifices of parts which might have been preserved, and the loss of which is to be lamented.

4th. Because the gangrene may attack several limbs in succession, and even all the limbs, of which I have quoted two examples, and we should then find ourselves compelled to perform a series of sad mutilations.

5th. Because, on the contrary, in confining ourselves to cutting away the dead parts near the circle of elimination, we perform an operation which is always practicable and always useful, as it liberates the patient from a focus of infection.

6th. Because we avoid the risk of performing an amputation, all the benefits of which will be lost if the gangrene makes fresh advances.

7th. Because, in adopting the new mode, we do not unnecessarily remove parts which the patient is much interested in preserving.

8th. Because we have still the power of performing amputation, if it should become necessary.—*Dublin Med. Press*, April 9th, 1856, from *Presse Médicale Belge*, March 23, 1856.

---

22. *Practical Deductions from a Clinical Record of Twenty-six Cases of Strangulated Femoral Hernia.*—Mr. Birkett, in a paper read before the Medical Society of London (April 26th, 1856), commenced by stating that the object of the paper was, first, to bring prominently into the foreground the causes of death; 2d, The circumstances by which those causes are brought about; and, 3d, The means by which they may be avoided. It was shown, by means of a table of the cases, that a certain number of unfavourable circumstances occurred in each case, and that, in proportion to the aggregate, as a general rule, the case was cured, or terminated fatally. But in some of the cases only two, three, or four unfavourable circumstances existed, and yet the patients died; and in these, as well as others with a larger number, the causes of death were sought for and demonstrated. Of the twenty-six cases, all of which were operated upon by the author, one-half terminated fatally. In the fatal cases, death resulted from causes over which the operation could have but little influence; and it was undertaken only with the view to place the patient in a condition more favourable to recovery. The causes inducing the fatal result may be thus enumerated:—

1. The consequences of a journey performed while the patient was suffering with strangulated femoral hernia.

2. The defective constitutional nutrition of the patients generally.

3. Irrecoverable prostration, the result of long-continued vomiting and strangulation of the bowel in aged women.

4. Violence inflicted on the hernia. To this cause, the death of not less than five out of the thirteen is to be attributed.

5. The administration of purgatives before the operation.

The author unhesitatingly preferred to reduce the hernia without opening the peritoneal sac in those cases in which the surgeon would be justified in returning the protrusion by the taxis, if it could be accomplished.

In the twenty-six cases, the peritoneal sac was opened in twelve, and the causes which prevented the reduction of the hernia without so operating were the three following:—

1. The contents of the sac.

2. The morbid condition of the contents of the sac.

3. The dimensions of the neck of the sac, and the unyielding state of its tissues.

Six cases were related in which the author had reduced the hernia by a simple division of the fibrous tissues about the neck of the sac, and external to that covering of the hernia known as the fascia propria. To this simple method of relieving the constriction around the bowel the author gave the name of "The Minimum Operation." The causes of death in the fatal cases were shown, by *post-mortem* examination, to be referable to peritonitis, injury of the bowel inflicted in the taxis, exhaustion after fecal fistula, phlegmonous inflammation, collapse, acute bronchitis, and perforation of the bowel. Of the cured cases, the minimum of hours during which the bowel was strangulated was three hours; the maximum was seventy-seven hours. Of the fatal cases, the minimum period of strangulation of the bowel was eleven hours, the maximum seventy-nine hours. Of the cured cases, the average number of hours during which the bowel was strangulated amounted to twenty-three. Of the fatal cases, the average period of strangulation of the bowel was forty-six hours. The causes of death were primary and secondary: 1. Prostration; peritonitis; gangrene of the intestine; perforation. 2. Bronchitis; abscess behind the peritoneum; phlegmonous inflammation and suppuration. The circumstances by which they were brought about: Age; a journey; the defective constitutional nutrition of the patient; the morbid state of the canal above the strangulated piece of bowel; injury of the hernia caused by the constriction of the ring, and by manual violence inflicted on it; the duration of the sufferings; the intensity of the constitutional sympathies; fecal fistula; neglect of the tumour; the administration of purgatives; the warm bath. The means by which they may be avoided are: By care in manipulation; the early relief on the bowel from constriction; the reduction of the hernia without opening the peritoneal sac; the exhibition of opium, and the avoidance of all causes likely to induce exhaustion.—*Med. Times and Gaz.*, May 3, 1856.

---

23. *Mode of Reducing Strangulated Hernia, after Failure of the Taxis, by a Bloodless Operation.*—M. Seutin, the eminent surgeon of Brussels, is endeavouring to establish, in a Belgian Medical journal, the superiority of *tearing* either the inguinal or crural ring, over incising the same, for the reduction of strangulated hernia. He quotes experiments on the dead body, and several successful cases; and is confident that his method will soon supersede the operative measures generally resorted to. He places, first, great reliance on graduated taxis continued with due precautions for a considerable period; and when this fails, he endeavours to hook his index-finger round the margin of the ring, by passing it between the tumour and the abdomen; and by using a certain force, he causes the fibres of the external oblique to give way and crack to an extent sufficient for the reduction of the hernia. M. Seutin defends his practice with considerable ability, and hopes trials will be made.—*Lancet*, April 26, 1866.

24. *Radical Cure of Hydrocele.*—A man, aged 31, has recently been under Mr. Lloyd's care, in St. Bartholomew's, on account of a hydrocele, which had been several times tapped, and on one occasion treated by the injection of iodine, with the hope of permanent cure. The latter expedient, however, had failed, the sac having refilled. Mr. Lloyd adopted a plan, which has long been a favourite with him, of introducing a little of the red precipitate into the sac. The fluid having been drawn off by a canula, large enough to allow a director to enter it, the latter instrument, oiled, and then dipped in the powder so as to carry a few grains adhering to it, was introduced and moved about in the cavity. The introduction was repeated two or three times; some inflammation followed, and a perfect cure ensued. The practice has the advantage over that by injection of not requiring any special apparatus. Mr. Lloyd believes it also to be more uniformly successful.—*Med. Times and Gaz.*, April 12, 1856.

OPHTHALMOLOGY.

25. *Anemic Protrusion of Eyeball.*—Robt. Taylor, Esq., Surgeon to the Central London Ophthalmic Hospital, relates (*Med. Times and Gaz.*, May 24th, 1856) the following cases, illustrative of a disease which has only within a recent period attracted attention, and the true pathological explanation of which is yet a desideratum.

"*Case* 1.—Mrs. T., aged 26, has been married eight years, but has never been pregnant. Her menstrual periods have been regular; but the discharge has always been in excess, and she has had several attacks of menorrhagia, losing much blood on each occasion. She has long been subject to leucorrhœa, which, six months ago, became very profuse, and shortly after this she was attacked with palpitation of the heart. About the same time she observed a swelling in her throat, and her eyes became so prominent as to attract the attention of her friends. These symptoms, which appeared as nearly as possible simultaneously, have gone on increasing slowly but steadily. Leeches and tincture of iodine have been applied to the throat, but without producing any diminution in the swelling.

Present State.—She is very pale and feeble. She suffers from spinal tenderness, intercostal neuralgia, ringing in the ears, œdema of the ankles, and other symptoms of anæmia. She is exceedingly nervous, starting and trembling violently when suddenly addressed; she has occasional hysteric fits. The pulsations of the heart average 134 per minute, and are very distressing; the carotid arteries also throb violently. The thyroid gland is enlarged to about three times its natural size, its surface being smooth and regular; several of its enlarged arteries can be felt pulsating near the surface. The eyeballs protrude so as to expose a broad rim of the sclerotica around the margin of the cornea, giving her a wild and staring appearance, which attracts attention and exposes her to annoyance in the streets. The amount of protrusion varies, within certain limits, with the degree of nervous excitement, being always much greater when she is agitated. The eyeballs can be readily replaced by gentle pressure, but they speedily resume their prominence when the pressure is remitted. There is some congestion of the conjunctival vessels, and slight increase of the Meibomian and mucous secretions; in other respects the eyes have a healthy appearance; their movements are perfect in every direction, and the sight is unimpaired. The eyelids, which are of a dusky colour, cannot be closed without a slight muscular effort.

The treatment, which extended over a period of three months, consisted in the administration of iron in several forms; astringent injections, per vaginam, to check the leucorrhœa; and belladonna plasters over the region of the heart, which afforded great relief by diminishing the violence of the palpitation. As her general health improved, the heart's action approached more and more to the natural standard, and the prominence of the eyeballs was reduced, until they ultimately resumed their proper position; but no change took place in the size of the thyroid gland, so long as she remained under observation. She subsequently had a slight relapse, brought on apparently by mental agitation, but a similar plan of treatment again proved successful in a few weeks.

Case 2.—Mrs. C., aged 40, has had eight children, the last two of whom were twins, and were born four years ago. One of these she suckled for twelve, and the other for sixteen months; during which time, as on previous similar occasions, she menstruated regularly and abundantly. When she had suckled both infants for a year, she first observed an enlargement of her throat, and the swelling increased slowly for about two years, since which it has remained stationary. Some months after she first observed this enlargement her eyes began to protrude, so as to attract the attention of her friends. She then applied to a surgeon, who told her that she had disease of the heart—a fact which she then learned for the first time, as she had never felt the slightest uneasiness in that region; how long the palpitation may have existed it is impossible to say, as even now, although it is very violent, she is quite unconscious of it, unless when much excited.

Present State.—Pale, anemic, and highly excitable. The eyeballs protrude so as to expose a narrow rim of sclerotica around the cornea. They can be readily replaced by gentle pressure; their movements are perfect in every direction, and the vision is unimpaired. The protrusion varies with the amount of nervous excitement. The conjunctivæ are slightly injected, but in other respects the eyes appear to be perfectly healthy. The heart beats violently and rapidly, the pulsations being 142 per minute; but it is probable that this exceeds the usual standard, and is partly due to excitement, consequent on a stethoscopic examination. The carotid arteries pulsate strongly and visibly. The thyroid gland is enlarged, chiefly in a lateral direction, to more than thrice its natural size; its surface is smooth and regular.

The treatment was conducted upon the same general plan as in the preceding case, and extended, with one or two interruptions, over a period of five months. The general health was restored, and the eyes resumed their natural position; but there was not any diminution in the size of the goitre.

Case 3.—Mrs. R., aged 26, has been married nine years, but has never been pregnant. For many years she has been subject to profuse leucorrhœa, and her health has been still further impaired by insufficient nourishment, and by close application to needlework. Two years ago, she began to suffer from palpitation of the heart, and soon after this her throat became enlarged, and her eyeballs unnaturally prominent.

Present State.—Pale, thin, and excessively nervous and excitable, trembling almost convulsively when suddenly spoken to, or even when looked at. The eyes protrude to such an extent that she cannot, by any effort close the eyelids, and she complains much of the discomfort caused by their remaining half-open during sleep. The eyeballs can be replaced by gentle pressure; their movements are perfect, and the sight unimpaired. The protrusion varies considerably, with the amount of nervous excitement. The conjunctivæ are somewhat congested; in other respects the eyes appear perfectly healthy. The thyroid gland is enlarged to about four times its natural size, and numerous dilated arteries can be felt near its surface, which is smooth and regular. The heart, under the agitation of being examined, beats violently, the pulsations being 144 per minute. The carotid arteries also throb visibly.

This patient remained under treatment for two months, the remedies employed being iron, astringent injections per vaginam, and belladonna plasters over the region of the heart. She had improved considerably in health, and her eyes had receded so far that she could close the eyelids without any effort, when she left town, and remained without medical treatment of any kind for some months. A short time since, she again made her appearance at the hospital, in nearly the same condition as at her first visit. The treatment has been resumed, and she is again progressing favourably.

In each of the above cases, a careful stethoscopic examination of the chest was made by my friend Dr. Hare, who has kindly permitted me to condense and make use of his report.

In the first there was some hypertrophy, with a little dilatation of the heart, but no valvular disease. In the second, the condition of the heart was almost exactly similar, but there was a doubtful murmur with the first sound, the exact nature of which could not be clearly ascertained, on account of the excited state of the circulation at the time. In the third, there were slight hypertrophy and dilatation, with a distinct, though not loud systolic murmur at the base, 'which,' Dr. Hare says, '*may* be anemic.'

Case 4.—I have reserved this case for the last, although it is the first entered in my case-book, as I am desirous of calling attention to a very striking peculiarity which it presented, in the sudden appearance of the exophthalmia.

Letitia M., aged 21, was subject to fits, probably epileptic, in childhood. These gradually ceased as she attained the period of puberty, but she remained excessively nervous and hysterical, and has long suffered from spinal tenderness, intercostal neuralgia, coldness of the extremities, and other symptoms of nervous debility. Three years ago, after a fall by which she severely bruised her right side, she began to suffer from palpitation of the heart; this has continued ever since, being constant and annoying, interrupting her sleep, and greatly aggravated by the slightest agitation or exertion. One year after this, the thyroid gland began to enlarge, and gradually increased until it attained its present volume, about four times that of the healthy gland. She was for some time under hospital treatment for this, as well for the palpitation, but without receiving any benefit. About a week before I first saw her, she felt an unusual sensation in the brows one morning on awaking, and on looking in the mirror, she found that her eyes, which had been perfectly natural in appearance when she retired to rest, were protruded to such an extent that she could scarcely close the eyelids.

Present State.—The eyeballs protrude, as above described: their movements are perfect; the sight is not impaired, and they appear to be perfectly healthy. They can be readily replaced by gentle pressure, but resume their abnormal position when the hand is removed. She says that the prominence varies very much, and that at times it is scarcely perceptible. The action of the heart is very violent; the pulsations, under the excitement of being examined, are 140 per minute. There is a slight blowing murmur with the first sound; on percussion, the dulness over the heart is rather more extensive than natural. The carotid arteries throb violently. The enlarged thyroid gland is smooth and regular, and several of its dilated arteries can be felt near the surface.

Under treatment of a similar character to that adopted in the preceding cases, and extending over rather more than two months, the eyes had very nearly resumed their normal position, and the general health was very much improved, but there was no diminution in the size of the thyroid gland. She then left town, and I have not had an opportunity of seeing her since.

In addition to the above, I have collected from the various medical journals twenty-one cases, which have been given sufficiently in detail to render them free from doubt; others are alluded to as having occurred, but without any particulars being given. Of the twenty-five reported cases, twenty occurred in females, and four in males; in one the sex is not mentioned, but, from the context, the patient appears to have been a male. Three deaths have occurred, in each instance in males. In two there was a post-mortem examination. In the first, related by Sir Henry Marsh, the patient had long suffered from extensive organic disease; there was considerable dilatation, with hypertrophy, chiefly of the left side of the heart, and some amount of valvular disease, chiefly of the right; the right internal jugular vein was very much dilated; the patient died of general anasarca, followed by erysipelas and gangrene. In the second, detailed by Dr. Begbie, the patient suffered from organic disease of the heart, enlargement of the liver, general dropsy, and jaundice; of which complication of disorders he died. The heart was found to be large, soft, and flaccid; all the cavities, but especially the ventricles, were dilated; the valves were larger than usual, having accommodated themselves to the increased size of the cavities; but they were otherwise normal. The aorta, in comparison with the pulmonary artery, was small. The internal jugular veins were much dilated. The blood in the heart and great vessels was very fluid. In none of the other cases has stethoscopic examination detected any very serious amount of cardiac disease; in some there has been slight dilatation with thinning of the walls, but without valvular disease; in others there does not appear to have been any structural alteration.

With one exception, the enlargement of the thyroid gland has appeared to be due to simple hypertrophy of its normal structures, with a great increase in the activity of its circulation and size of its bloodvessels. In the exceptional case recorded by Mr. MacDonnell, the goitre was of the cystic variety, and had attained a considerable size.

In no instance has there been any disease of the eyeball. It is true that in a few cases it is described as having been enlarged; but this is evidently a mistake, as the vision was unimpaired. The eyeball is not subject to enlargement, except as a consequence of long-continued inflammatory disease, destructive of vision, by which the tough, unyielding tissue of the sclerotica is softened, and gives way to the pressure from within, bulging, generally, in a very irregular manner. The protrusion must be due to some other cause, the nature of which, in connection with the general pathology of the disease, we have now to consider.

It must be borne in mind that the protrusion may, as in *Case* 4, come on suddenly; that it varies in degree according as the patient is agitated or tranquil; and that the eyeballs can be replaced in their natural position by gentle pressure. It cannot, therefore, be due to any solid tumour, or fluid effusion in the orbit; nor can it be ascribed to paralysis of the recti muscles, for the eye can be moved in every direction as readily as in health. The cause to which it is most commonly ascribed is, congestion of the deep-seated veins of the orbit; and this seems to afford a more probable explanation than any other, both from its being quite reconcilable with the variable amount of exophthalmia, and from the well-known effect of impeded return of blood from the head in causing prominence of the eyes, as witnessed, for example, in strangulation. But how are we to account for this congestion; and how are we to explain its association with the peculiar condition of the heart and the thyroid gland? for the cases already on record are too numerous to permit us to suppose that these are merely coincident symptoms; together they evidently constitute a distinct disease, and there must be some common cause capable of producing each, and of rendering them mutually dependent upon each other.

It has appeared to me, that a key to the true solution of this question has been given by Dr. Marshall Hall, in his valuable writings on the subject of convulsive and paroxysmal diseases. He has shown that, in such diseases, there is a tendency to spasm of the muscles of the neck; and that the seizures are the direct result of impeded return of blood from the head, the deep-seated veins being compressed by the irregular muscular action. Now, the subjects of anemic protrusion of the eyeball are eminently of the class to which Dr. Hall's remarks apply. Some of them are subject to fits, hysterical or epileptic; in all the nervous system is in a state of extreme excitability, so that the slightest agitation produces starting and trembling, sometimes so violent as almost to resemble convulsion in a minor degree. Is it not probable that, as in the confirmed epileptics, there may, in these cases also, be an impediment to the free return of blood from the head, only to a less amount, and, perhaps, more continuously? In the only two post-mortem examinations that have been made, the internal jugular veins were found to be greatly dilated, as though they had long been subject to distention by some obstructing cause towards the lower part of their course; and, as in neither case was there any solid growth by which they could have been compressed, it does not seem unreasonable to suppose that the obstacle was due to muscular spasm. The same explanation would account for the enlargement of the thyroid gland, which, as has been already stated, is due to simple hypertrophy of its normal structures, and would be a probable result of long-continued hyperæmia. The palpitation of the heart does not require any explanation here, as it is common to all cases of anæmia, whether accompanied or not with protrusion of the eyes.

The different stages of the disease, then, may be stated as follow: First. Some debilitating disease, or exhausting discharge, producing—secondly, anæmia; thirdly, that peculiar state of the nervous system, in which there is a tendency to spasm of the muscles of the neck; fourthly, as the result of such spasm, and consequent impeded return of blood from the head, hyperæmia, and hypertrophy of the thyroid gland, and dilatation of the veins of the orbit, causing exophthalmia.

This explanation I offer merely suggestively. I am well aware that it is open to many objections; but none have as yet occurred to me which appear insuperable. It is supported by the histories of all the carefully described cases, and by the necroscopical appearances in the only two post-mortem examinations that have been made; and it accounts for the association of three symptoms, the connection of which it seems otherwise impossible to divine. If it fail to stand the test of rigid investigation, it may still have the good effect of attracting the attention of those who are able to expose its errors, and to substitute a perfect one in its place.

It is unnecessary to dwell at any length upon the treatment, which is essentially that of anæmia. A few cases have occurred in which patients have been attacked who were already the victims of extensive diseases of the thoracic and abdominal viscera, and in such the treatment must be merged in that of the more serious disorder. But in the great majority of instances, any structural changes that have been detected have been comparatively slight, and amenable to remedial measures. The patient should, therefore, be encouraged to look forward with confidence to a successful issue. In the words of Dr. Begbie, whose valuable paper contains the latest and most complete *résumé* of the subject, 'it is of great consequence to impress those suffering from this affection with the belief of its curable nature, and to urge upon them the persistent employment of the means of restoring the red particles of the impoverished blood, and improving the general health.' The *starting point* of the disease must first be ascertained, and in females this is almost always some form of exhausting discharge in connection with the uterine organs, which must be checked by appropriate remedies. The various preparations of iron, nutritious and unstimulating diet, pure air, and absence of excitement; the treatment, in short, which is found successful in cases of anæmia not thus complicated, are the further means to be adopted. No local applications are necessary, either to the eyes or to the thyroid gland; but as some patients are dissatisfied without them, they may be directed to use the eye-douche, or to bathe the eyes with cold water from time to time. The only local application which I have found really serviceable, has been a belladonna plaster over the region of the heart, which, in some instances, has had a marked effect in diminishing the violence of the palpitation. The progress towards recovery is generally slow, and the treatment may require to be prolonged over many months; but if judiciously selected and carefully persevered in, we may look forward with confidence to the restoration of the general health, and the complete disappearance of the deformity caused by the unnatural prominence of the eyes.

In many of the recorded cases, the swelling of the thyroid gland has also subsided, but this has by no means uniformly followed; it has occurred, so far as I am able to judge, more frequently in private patients, who are more under control, and have the means of carrying out more fully the prescribed medicinal and dietetic regulations, than in the less regular and less favourably situated class to which the out-patients of hospitals belong. But as the enlargement is rarely to any extent, and as a certain amount of diminution invariably takes place, the persistence of a slight and scarcely perceptible fulness is not a matter of any importance."

---

26. *Observations on Cataract.*—In commenting on a case of cataract recently operated, Mr. Wharton Jones made some excellent clinical remarks on the subject of cataract generally, as the result of his experience in University College Hospital. The opinions expressed by the operator are corroborated also by the scientific observations of Mr. Bowman and Mr. Critchett at the Ophthalmic Hospital in Moorfields, so that they may be taken as a fair representation of London ophthalmic practice on the subject of cataract.

As to the use of atropine to dilate the pupil, though this was used in the present case, Mr. Wharton Jones, like Mr. Dixon, does not think atropine or belladonna necessary. If the patient be in the recumbent position, and can be induced to remain without making any muscular effort, that is all that is required.

Next, as to the direction in which the section of the cornea should be made, whether upwards or downwards, though a "great deal has been said on both sides," Mr. W. Jones believes that one mode of operating is as good as the other; and for himself, he sometimes operates in the downward direction, sometimes in the upward direction. The advantages of the section of the cornea, in an upward direction, he is inclined to believe, after some experience of it, are only imaginary. Something, no doubt, is due to the peculiarities of each case; if the patient be excessively nervous, and, from some reflex or excite-motor influence, turns the eye up, it is difficult to operate in either direction. (Mr. Wharton Jones here showed the different steps of the operation for cataract, by sections of the cornea in both directions, on some fresh eyes from the lower animals, bringing out the lens in each case with remarkable facility.) A great deal depends on the treatment of cases of cataract after they have been operated on; it is necessary for the patient to rest with the eye closed up for at least three days. In the case of the man operated on in the present instance, it appeared that the iris, or pupil, was dragged to the side from loss of vitreous humour, but this did not siguify; in a fortnight he could see very well; seventeen days was the earliest convalescence the operator had met in a case of operation by the upper section, but five or six weeks is not an uncommon average for convalescence. Hemorrhage into the vitreous humour is one of the accidents to be avoided, as it is a disastrous complication of every mode of operative proceeding.

Mr. Wharton Jones next referred to the two other operations, depression, and division of the lens, which the surgeon is sometimes called on to perform; division of the lens is quite a different operation, he remarked, from depression or couching, so that no correct or fair comparison can be instituted between them. Extraction and depression, on the other hand, can be compared; after extraction, as familiarly known, the best eye is procured. Yet by depression, though the eyesight is not so good, and we have more inflammation to guard against, as the depressed lens acts something like a foreign body, yet, in persons of the age of fifty years, or above that period, very great success is found to obtain from this operation. It must not be forgotten, however, that, especially in gouty and rheumatic subjects, we must calculate on the dangers of the inflammation caused by the displaced lens attacking the retina and iris. Sometimes, even from other considerations, it may be advisable to have recourse to the operation of couching. A case was here cited by Mr. Wharton Jones, where he recently tried couching, for the reason that the opposite eye had been operated on previously in the City for extraction, but it had failed. He did not know the reason why—perhaps something in the patient's constitution; yet depression had succeeded very fairly in the opposite organ. The operator next made some practical observations on the character of the cataract glasses the surgeon should order for his patient. A four and a half focus is about the best; a five may, in rare instances, be required; but for reading, a two and a half glass will be necessary.—*Association Medical Journal*, March 29th, 1856.

---

27. *Traumatic Cataract and its Treatment by Operation.*—Mr. J. V. SOLOMON, in a paper read before the Birmingham and Midland Counties Branch of the Prov. Med. and Surg. Association, after giving an outline of the physiological anatomy of the lens and its capsule, which, he said, was of interest, by throwing light upon some of the nutritional changes of which the lens is the subject, and as affording a *rationale* of certain operations which are performed for their cure, defined traumatic cataract as an opacity of the lens or its capsule, in consequence of a blow upon, or penetrating wound of the eyeball. Mr. Solomon then considered the subject under three heads.

a. In cases of traumatic cataract, attended by little or no inflammation, and where the capsule having been ruptured accidentally the lens is undergoing absorption, his practice is to break it up ten or fourteen days after the accident, and clear the pupil of capsule, and so prevent the formation of a capsular cataract within the area of the pupil. The operation is performed by penetrating the cornea with a fine needle, etc. (Keratonyxis). Where the case is complicated by an ununited wound of the cornea, his first care is to obtain union by closing the eyelids with strips of plaster, and enjoining rest of the organ. Prior to which, any portion of recently protruding iris is returned within the anterior chamber by gently pressing upon it with the spoon end of the "curette," whilst the patient is under the influence of chloroform: but when that drug is contraindicated, or lymph covers the irident tumour, it must be snipped off, unless it should happen to be very small, with a pair of sharp-cutting eye scissors. When the wound is central, belladonna is to be immediately applied to the brow, and a drop of atropine to the conjunctiva; but when such is not the case, the application must be delayed until cicatrization has taken place.

b. In cases where the cataract is dislocated against the back of the iris, or is pushing its way through the pupil, and is attended by severe ocular pain and inflammation, Mr. Solomon's invariable practice is to extract the lens by Gibson's operation, which, by removing a cause of irritation, alleviates suffering, and accelerates recovery. In the event of these cases being treated only by the ordinary means applicable to internal inflammation of the eyeball, all the symptoms are protracted, and the pupil remains small, and obstructed by thickened opaque capsule, or organized lymph. Moreover, the deep seated structures are prone to be affected by inflammatory disorganization. In a word, the eye is left, on the subsidence of the ophthalmia, in a very unfavourable condition for any operation that may be at any time undertaken with the intention of clearing the pupillary aperture; unless the canula scissors can be made of use. It is in this class of cases that chalky or bony material forms withing the capsule.

c. With regard to cases of single traumatic cataract, occurring in an organ in other respects, as far as can be judged, healthy, the author advocates the operation of solution (Keratonyxis), on the grounds that it (1) removes a deformity which, to many persons, is a serious obstacle to their comfort and well-being in life, and that (2) it tends, if the patient occasionally exercise the eye by wearing a suitable cataract spectacle, to preserve a healthy condition of the retina. Deprive an organ, he said, of its natural stimulus, and its nutrition will become either feeble or perverted; in illustration of which, might be cited those cases where amblyopia or amaurosis is persistent after the removal of a congenital cataract from an adult.

The primary effect of the removal of a single cataract, as respects vision, is in many instances to render it double or confused; the patient, however, soon ceases to regard the impressions conveyed through the retina of the eye which has lost its lens, and recovers single and clear vision. In illustration of this, the cases recorded by Dr. Andrew Smith in the *Edinburgh Medical and Surgical Journal*, No. 74, are most apposite and conclusive. Three saw objects double when the bandage was first removed, and for nearly twenty-four hours, and then singly. Two saw double about three hours; and one of them, two days afterwards, upon being surprised, and opening his eyelids suddenly, experienced, for a few seconds, the same imperfection. A sixth saw constantly double for four days, and after that, as distinctly as ever he did; and the other three cases, as above remarked, always single.

Mr. Cheshire.—The able paper read by Mr. Solomon had evidently been written with great care; he, however, could not agree with the practice which it advocated. Though the author said that double vision subsided, he had omittted to state that the vision was forever after the operation confused; indeed, it must be palpable to every one, that the loss of the lens must induce confusion of vision. Whereas, if the cataract was not interfered with, the fellow eye became as good as two. Clear sight must be better than confused vision.

Mr. L. Parker (the Preisdent) considered the paper they had heard read a very valuable one; he regretted that the author had not illustrated it by a series of cases from his own practice. The question of the propriety of an operation was purely a question of fact; if one successful case could be adduced, that would be an answer to the objection that had been made.

Mr. Solomon said, in reply, that the objection which had been raised to the removal of a single cataract by the operation of solution, on the plea that the difference thereby produced in the adjusting power of the two eyes must give rise to permanently confused vision, was a theoretical one, and was nullified by cases recorded by Dr. Andrew Smith, R. Carmichael, Stevenson, and others, also by his own experience in the last seven years at the Birmingham Eye Infirmary; during that period no single instance of permanently confused vision, as a result of the operation in question, had come before him. He had not kept records of this class of cases, never anticipating that the propriety of the operation would have been made, in another place, the subject of a hostile attack; this deficiency in his paper he would, however, supply at the next meeting of the Branch, by producing some patients who had lost the lens from one eye, and from whom the members of the Society could elicit full particulars bearing upon the point in discussion. In his experience, he had met with several persons in whom the power of adjustment was different in the two eyes, and yet the vision was single and clear; the patients having only discovered the defect by accidentally closing the perfect eye. He might observe, in conclusion, that from inquiries he had made, he found that some of the most distinguished ophthalmic operators, metropolitan and provincial, in this country, and on the Continent, operated on cases of single traumatic cataract by solution. —*Association Med. Journ.*, March 15th, 1856.

MIDWIFERY.

28. *Spontaneous Version of the Child.*—Dr. Benda relates an interesting case of this. A woman was found with an arm-presentation, the waters having escaped. The right arm, as far as the half of the humerus, was outside the vagina, little swollen. Dr. Benda diagnosed on careful examination the second shoulder-presentation. In spite of attempts by himself and his colleague, Dr. Lehfeldt, it was impossible to pass the hand into the uterus to seize the foot. While waiting for chloroform, the following process, which took place very rapidly, was minutely observed. The hitherto relaxed perineum was suddenly distended, and the presenting right arm was drawn back into the genital organs; at the same time that the pelvic end of the child rose, the right side of the abdomen came first against the perineum, then the pubic end, and during a half-revolution upon the long axis the back was directed against the symphysis, the left hip was evolved over the perineum, whereupon quickly and in one pain, the legs folded upon the abdomen, and the head bent upon the breast followed. Thus, out of the second shoulder-presentation, and by strong uterine contractions alone, working in a capacious pelvis, the first breech-presentation had been developed; a half-turn upon the transverse axis taking place, as well as a half-turn upon the long axis. The child, at first asphyxiated, recovered perfectly.—*Brit. and For. Med.-Chirurg. Rev.*, April, 1856, from *Verhandl. d. Ges. für Geb.*, 1855.

---

29. *Complete Inversion of the Uterus, at the Time of Labour, with remarkable Absence of the Ordinary Symptoms of that Accident.* By F. W. Montgomery, M. D., Professor of Midwifery in the King and Queen's College of Physicians.—On the 10th of Sept., 1854, Mr. M. called on me to request that I would immediately visit his wife, whom he stated to be dangerously ill after her confinement. I accompanied him at once, and on my arrival at the patient's house, at 9 o'clock, A. M., found a physician accoucheur, of experience and discretion, in attendance, who subsequently gave me the following account of what had occurred before my arrival:—

"He had been sent for to see Mrs. M. about eleven o'clock, P. M., of the evening before, when he found her in labour of her fourth child, with the head presenting. She was twenty-eight years of age, healthy, and her former labours had been quite favourable. The liquor amnii had been discharged about twenty-four hours previously, without pain; for some time after the doctor's seeing her, the pains, which had recently set in, were pretty active, and as the pelvis was a roomy one, he expected that the labour would terminate in two or three hours. It was not, however, till about half-past seven o'clock that the child, a female, was born. During the night, two half drachm doses of ergot had been given, with little apparent effect, and it was not till after a pretty large dose of laudanum and peppermint was administered that the pains became really efficient. There was no hemorrhage, but as the placenta did not seem likely to come away speedily, the womb being sluggish, and not disposed to contract, the nurse-tender was directed to make pressure over the uterus, while the doctor drew down the cord. In about ten or fifteen minutes, the placenta came away, followed, on the instant, by a *large round tumour, which passed completely out of the vagina,* and was, for an instant, supposed to be the head of a second child, which it equalled in size.

"It was, however, soon ascertained to be the uterus completely inverted, no os being to be felt. The tumour was at once returned within the vagina without much difficulty, but pressure on the fundus failed to effect its restoration to its proper place. There was some hemorrhage, both on the sudden descent of the uterus and after its return, *but not much.* The patient felt a pressing desire to make water, and a distressing sense of pressure on the bladder, and becoming anxious, it was deemed advisable to have further advice. Although alarmed, from the knowledge that there was something wrong, she presented little change in countenance or pulse, no faintness, and but little hemorrhage. Her recovery, after the replacement of the uterus, went on most favourably, and at the end of a month she was as well as after any previous confinement." "Feb., 1856: she has been in good health ever since, and now considers herself two or three months pregnant."

Such are the accounts I received of this case at the time of the accident and since, and I am now to state what I was myself present at. I was at the patient's bedside at nine o'clock, delivery having taken place at half-past seven o'clock. I found her looking tranquil, her pulse good, firm, and quiet, and although she was anxious about herself, believing that there was some cause of alarm, there was not the least approach to that kind of overwhelming nervous distress which so often accompanies so serious an accident. She complained of nothing except the sense of pressure on the bladder; there were very smart periodical pains, which, however, she rather made light of, as she regarded them only as after-pains, such as she had had after former labours, which, indeed, they perfectly resembled; there was very little hemorrhage.

On examining the abdomen, there was to be felt *a considerable tumour in the supra-pubic region,* and taking this fact with the other conditions above mentioned, I confess I felt almost certain that it could not be a case of inversion, the symptoms were so widely different from those which almost universal experience would lead us to expect. An examination *per vaginam,* however, soon removed all doubt. I found that passage, indeed I may say the whole pelvic cavity, filled up with a firm fleshy tumour, *which was perfectly insensible;* and on passing the finger along it upwards, it was found to terminate in a *cul de sac* all around, and about an inch within the margin of the os uteri; so that the inversion, or perhaps, more properly, the eversion of the organ was as complete as I believe it ever is *in the first instance.*[1]

In proceeding to effect the reduction, I, in the first place, put the patient fully under the influence of chloroform; I then introduced my hand, and grasping the tumour, I compressed it as strongly as I could from the lateral circumference towards the centre, and at the same time pushed it upwards and forwards

[1] When the displacement has been for some weeks or months in existence, the tissue of the organ having gradually contracted and greatly diminished in bulk, the *cul de-sac* vanishes.

towards the umbilicus; for several minutes, this proceeding seemed quite without effect; but at length, I felt the tumour begin to yield, receding and gliding, as it were, by a spontaneous movement *of the whole tumour* upwards, and not of the lowest part of the fundus re-entering itself; and then, all at once, it suddenly almost sprung away from my hand, and was restored to its proper place. I pressed my hand into its cavity, up to the fundus, and kept it there for a few minutes, and before withdrawing it, I took the precaution of making sure that there was no dimpling in, or cupping of the fundus, by feeling the hand so retained with my other hand through the parietes of the abdomen. The resistance to the replacement of the inverted organ was so great, that I do not think I should ever have succeeded had I not put the patient to sleep, and subdued its contractile efforts by the administration of chloroform. I cannot but consider myself very fortunate, indeed, in having succeeded in restoring this uterus fully an hour and a half after its complete inversion, during which interval, moreover, active contractions had not ceased to occur. Dr. Merriman says that under such circumstances, unless the inversion be reduced in a few minutes after the accident has happened, all attempts to return it will be ineffectual. And Denman tells us that although present at the moment when the accident occurred in a patient of his own, and only waiting until he had separated the placenta, he could not possibly effect the replacement of the organ.

Inversion of the uterus at the time of delivery is, like the spontaneous evolution of the child, an accident of such rare occurrence, especially in private practice, that few, even of those most extensively engaged in practice, have ever seen a case of it; and still fewer have been actually present at the moment it took place. I have spoken with several practitioners on this subject, and, like myself until lately, none of them had ever met with it in private practice; one gentleman said that, in forty years, he had been called in once to a case of the kind, but found the lady dead when he arrived; another gentleman had seen it once in thirty years. The late Dr. Douglass told me, within a year or two before his death, that he had, just then, met with it for the first time, in private; and he assured me that it had taken place after he had left the lady apparently safe and well. Denman says expressly (Introduction, p. 566, 5th edit.), that it was an accident of very rare occurrence during the whole of his life; and Dr. Ramsbotham, whose practice and experience were equally extended, says he never saw a case immediately after inversion.

The production of this accident is, I think, too generally ascribed to injudicious traction of the cord to bring down the placenta; and the inevitable consequence of this presumption is, that whenever it is found to have occurred, it is taken for granted, that the attendant practitioner must be to blame as having thus caused it, when, in truth, all that depended on him may have been done with all proper care and skill, and the accident have arisen from causes over which he had no control; at the same time, undue pressure over the fundus uteri, and strong traction by the cord, are likely to be productive of so many untoward, or even fatal consequences, that no prohibition of their adoption can be too strongly enforced; and, I may add, that the last two cases of inversion, of which I am aware, as having happened in this city, were, I believe, justly attributed to the combined action of these agencies; but, if this displacement were easily produced by the mismanagement alluded to, instead of being, as it confessedly is, very rare, it would assuredly be of very frequent occurrence indeed, considering that the objectionable plan of interference is so constantly that of midwives, and too often of better educated practitioners.

I think we have quite sufficient grounds for believing, with Merriman,[1] that "there can be no doubt that a spontaneous inversion has sometimes occurred;" or, to use the words of Dr. Blundell,[2] that "the whole uterus may be pushed down, and this independently of anything done by the obstetrician." Ruysch states that the accident may happen, and did so in his own practice, when no undue force was used; and after animadverting on the impropriety of forcible extraction of the placenta as the general cause of this accident, he adds, "aliquando tamen, ortum ducit a conatibus post partum remanentibus."

[1] Synopsis, &c., p. 1857. [2] Principles and Practice of Obstetricy, p. 688.

Rokitansky[1] describes a condition of the uterus immediately after delivery, which might readily lead to inversion: it consists in a paralysis of the placental portion of the uterus, occurring at the same time that the surrounding parts go through the ordinary processes of reduction; the part alluded to is thus, he says, "forced into the cavity of the uterus by the contraction of the surrounding tissue, so as to project in the shape of a conical tumour, and a slight indentation is noticed at the corresponding point of the external surface. And he adds an observation, the truth of which I had occasion to verify, I may say anticipate, several years ago. "The close resemblance of the paralyzed segment of the uterus to a fibrous polypus may easily induce a mistake in the diagnosis, and nothing but a minute examination of the tissue can solve the question. The affection always causes hemorrhage, which lasts for several weeks after childbirth, and proves fatal by the consequent exhaustion."

The following case was an instance of this occurrence. In July, 1831, I was summoned, at four o'clock in the morning, to see a lady who had been delivered at 10 o'clock the previous night. The placenta was still retained, although she had had, all through the night, rather severe expulsive pains; she had lost a good deal of blood. On examination, I found the serous surface of the placenta lying upon, and pressed against, the internal surface of the os uteri; but, although the uterine contraction continued, I could not get it down by traction of the cord. On passing my hand into the uterus, I found the placenta was adhering to a globular tumour, which seemed to be as large as a good sized orange, and which, at the moment, I had no doubt was a fibrous tumour projecting from the inner surface of the uterus. To this tumour the placenta was morbidly adherent, and was only separated therefrom with difficulty. Having, however, accomplished this, and turned my hand freely in the uterus, to secure its complete contraction, the tumour, which was evidently the "placental portion" of the uterus partially inverted, completely disappeared, and the lady afterwards recovered well. Denman relates a case very much resembling this.[2]

With regard to those cases, in which inversion has been supposed to have occurred *spontaneously*, after the departure of the medical attendant, I think we may take for granted that in not a few of them the displacement had *commenced* while he was present, though without his knowledge; perhaps with very slight manifestations of its occurrence; or it may have remained unnoticed from want of sufficient observation and proper examination on his part. In the *Gazette des Hôpitaux*, for 7th Feb. last, there is a case reported in which partial inversion of the uterus was only discovered on the 6th December, in a patient who is stated to have been *safely delivered* on the 13th November; but from the whole details of the case, it appears almost evident that the inversion occurred at the time of labour, but was not then noticed.

There is obviously this danger in supposing, as so many do, that this accident is always attended and announced by a particular train of urgent symptoms; that if such symptoms are not observed, the attendant may be induced to conclude, what he would naturally so much desire, that no such accident could have happened, and so the patient is left to die, or linger out a life of misery. The instances in which this has happened are numerous indeed; one such is above referred to, and another we may quote from Dr. Merriman,[3] in which it is stated that "the placenta came away without any difficulty, and certainly without any suspicion of injury to the uterus;" but, between six and seven months afterwards, it was discovered that the uterus was inverted.

Now, when we succeed in effecting the replacement of a completely inverted uterus, how is its restoration really accomplished? Is it, as is generally stated in books, by re-inverting first the dependent fundus, or, in the words of Sir C. M. Clarke, "by making pressure on the lower part only of the tumour, so as to cause this part to be received into that above it,"[4] and so on, gradually up to the angle where the cervix is flexed on itself? Judging from what happened in this case of Mrs. M., and from the accounts given by others of what hap-

[1] Pathological Anatomy, vol. ii. p. 304.
[2] Op. jam. cit. p. 564.
[3] Synopsis, p. 299.
[4] Diseases of Females, Part i. p. 151.

pened in their cases, I think the above is not the mode of reduction; but that, as we compress the bulk of the tumour, and try to press the fundus back into itself, and push it upwards, *the flexure at the cervix* yields, and presently the fundus seems to escape upwards by springing as it were from our hand; so that the part which was last inverted is the first restored. This springing away from the hand is expressly mentioned by more than one writer of authority,[1] and is, I presume, produced by the contraction of the orbicular fibres of the partially restored cervix lifting up quickly the globe of the fundus.

I have now only to observe that, however small is the number of cases of inverted uterus met with in practice, it would be still smaller, if it were the universal rule carefully to examine every recently delivered woman, both through the abdominal parietes, to ascertain the size and form of the uterus, and also *per vaginam*, to be satisfied that there was no tumour protruding into that canal; nothing can excuse the neglect of this simple proceeding, and if it were *invariably* adopted, I think, with Mr. Newnham,[2] that "chronic inversion of the uterus would be known only by description."—*Dublin Hospital Gazette*, April 1, 1856.

---

30. *Placenta Prævia.*—In our previous number (p. 523, *et seq.*), we gave some interesting cases of placenta prævia, by Dr. Thos. Radford, and now continue them:—

Case X.—Jan. 2, 1823, Mrs. Fildes, midwife, sent for me to visit a hospital patient residing in Cock Gates, in labour and flooding. She was at the end of pregnancy, and in going up stairs had fallen, and immediately felt sick and faintish. In about an hour afterwards, she had a discharge of blood, followed by pains, which continued to increase in frequency and strength. The hemorrhage was now great; her countenance was very pale; her pulse was frequent and feeble. On an examination *per vaginam*, I found the os uteri opened to about the size of a shilling; but it was firm. On passing the finger through it, I detected the placenta. I plugged the vagina, and had the abdominal bandage put on, with the uterine compress placed under it, and then tightened, so as to effectually support the womb; the retaining bandage was also applied. She was carefully watched for some time; and as there was no external bleeding, or indication of any internal loss, I left her in the care of her midwife, strictly directing her to send again for me if there were any grounds for alarm.

In about four hours I called, and found the pains recurring more frequently and stronger. There had been no bleeding, and she seemed much better. I now withdrew the plug, and ascertained that the os uteri was considerably dilated, and softer, and the loosened placenta lying within it. There was some bleeding during the pains. After having placed on the regulating bandage, I passed the hand, and further detached the placenta to such an extent as I thought would allow the head of the child to pass, and then ruptured the membranes, directing the midwife at the same time to tighten the bandage. The water freely escaped; and in a short time the head of the child began to press on the os uteri, which soon yielded. The loosened portion of the placenta fell to one side, and the child passed by it, and in about three hours it was born alive. The placenta followed in about half an hour. There was no further hemorrhage, and her recovery was uninterrupted. A drachm of laudanum was given.

Remarks.—This case is another example of the value of the plug. A very short time elapsed between the accident and the occurrence of labour pain. The location of the placenta on the cervix and os uteri tended to produce these effects sooner than if this organ had been situated elsewhere. The irritation which the os sustained by the mechanical separation of the placenta was soon felt by the fundus and body of the uterus. The hemorrhage was brought on by the fall; but sooner or later flooding would doubtless have occurred, if no such accident had happened.

Case XI.—May 5, 1827, I visited a hospital patient residing in Cook Street, Salford, under Mrs. Booth's care, who was stated to be in labour, and in danger

[1] Merriman, Synopsis, p. 229.

[2] Essay, p. 8.

from flooding. She was in the last month of her seventh pregnancy. The pains were frequent and sharp; she felt faintish; looked pale; and her pulse was feeble. The discharge of blood had continued for three hours, and was now excessive, and increased on the accession of each pain. She had a slight attack a month before, which was soon suppressed by rest, cool air, and cold external applications. The os uteri was now dilated to the size of a shilling, but extremely rigid; it had the feel of a cartilaginous ring. I passed my finger through it, and I thought I perceived the placenta. Under these circumstances, I determined to effectually plug the vagina, to place on the abdominal bandage, and under it the uterine compress, and to fix the retaining bandage. She was carefully watched for some time, and feeling assured she was safe, I left her, having directed the midwife to send for me if any unfavourable symptom occurred.

In about six hours I was sent for, as the pains were now very frequent and strong. She was much improved in appearance, and her pulse was firmer. There had not been the slightest bleeding. On withdrawing the sponge, some small coagula followed, and immediately afterwards there was a fresh flow of blood. The os uteri was now opened fully to the size of a crown-piece, and felt considerably softer, and, as I thought, dilatable. A portion of the placenta with the membranes were found, in the absence of the pain, within it; and above I could feel the head of the child. As the uterus was now acting well, after having had placed on the regulating bandage, I passed my hand onward to the side where the membranes offered, and having first freely detached a sufficient extent of the placenta to allow the head to pass, I then ruptured them. The bandage was kept so tight as constantly to compress the uterus, as it changed in size by the escape of the waters. The pains were very strong; and the head of the child soon engaged within the os uteri, pushing the placenta aside as it descended into the pelvis. The child was born alive. The placenta was found lying loose in the vagina, and withdrawn. A drachm of tinctura opii was administered; and the circular bandage and uterine compress were applied.

Remarks.—No other means would have answered in this case so well as the plug; blood was saved and time obtained for the os uteri to soften and dilate; in fact, no other plan could have been safely adopted. If the membranes had been ruptured (which might assuredly have been done by means of a stilette), the hazards of protraction would have been very great with the os uteri so hard; and the child to a certainty would have been destroyed by the contusion and the laceration which the placenta must sustain from the pressure of its head on so unyielding a tissue. To prevent such an injurious effect on the placental structure, is one object in my practice of detaching a considerable portion of it from the uterus before rupturing the membranes is adopted.

Case XII.—On October 25, 1832, at 11 o'clock P. M., I was desired to see a hospital patient residing in Oldfield Lane, Salford, by Mrs. Blomeley. She was at the latter part of the sixth month of her fifth pregnancy. She had suffered from slight hemorrhages at different times for several weeks. During the afternoon and evening (of this day, 25th Oct.), she had copious discharges of blood, which recurred with each pain. When I arrived, she was very much exhausted; the pulse was feeble and indistinct; her lips were pale, and her face was deadly white; her forehead was bedewed with cold sweat; and her hands and arms (uncovered) were very cold; her feet felt warmer; her voice was very weak. Upon gently turning her on her side, to examine her, she fainted, and remained in an apparently lifeless state for some time, from which she slowly recovered, and was very much exhausted. The vagina was found full of coagulated blood; the os uteri was high in the pelvis, and was felt (with considerable difficulty) to be firm and undilated. Although I suspected that the placenta was placed here, I was quite unable to verify my suspicion. The hemorrhage continued, but it was rather less violent.

Her exhausted state demanded that some plan should be adopted, which would immediately suppress the bleeding. The undeveloped cervix, and the hard undilated os uteri, were unfavourable for any but that of effectually plugging the vagina. After the abdominal bandage was put on, and the uterine compress placed under it, the vagina was completely filled with pieces of sponge: the first piece I carried up forcibly against the os uteri; the retaining bandage was afterwards fixed. She was ordered absolute quietude; and as the surface of her body felt cold, she was warmly covered. Some brandy was administered with gruel, and repeated from time to time.

Although the vital power was so depressed, the pains increased in frequency and power, and in the course of five hours the plug was pushed further outwards; and on removing the bandage placed to retain it, the sponges were forcibly expelled. On examination, I found the placenta advanced to the os externum; and this organ, in connection with the entire ovum, was immediately forced away. The discharge ceased from the moment the plug was passed, and never returned; only a little coagulated blood came along with the ovum. The bandage was tightened over the compress. A drachm of tinctura opii was given.

On examining the placenta, a portion of its edge appeared to have been first separated; its surface was dark-coloured, and its tissue was loaded with coagulated blood. This poor woman was well nursed, and after some time she recovered, having been kept perfectly quiet, well supported, and her bowels regulated.

Remarks.—The value of the plug is eminently conspicuous in this case; it effectually arrested the bleeding at a time when perhaps the loss of very little more blood would have been fatal. The existence of uterine pain led me to conclude that some dilatation was going on at the upper portion of the cervix, and therefore I pushed the first piece of sponge more forcibly against the os uteri than I should have done whilst it was so high, under other circumstances.

The fallacy of the dogma of some authors is well exemplified in this case, viz: that when hemorrhage is so great as to require delivery, this operation may be safely performed.

Case XIII.—March 25, 1819, at the suggestion of Mr. Spence, I was called to Mrs. A., who was in the sixth month of her third pregnancy. She had been well up to this time; but she now had a profuse flooding, which had come on without any obvious cause. Cold vinegar and water had been externally applied, and cool air freely admitted into her apartment. She had taken a mixture with acidum sulphuricum dilutum and tinctura opii, and afterwards plumbi acetas and opium, in suitable doses, all without abating the discharge. She was pale; her skin felt coldish; her pulse was frequent and small; and she felt faintish. I found some coagula in the vagina, and fresh blood still flowed. The os uteri was high up in the pelvis, and was closed; the cervix was undeveloped. I could not prudently make further inquiries, and therefore I was ignorant as to the precise location of the placenta. I suspected it was fixed on the cervix. There was no pain. The circular abdominal bandage and the uterine compress, placed under it, was firmly applied. The vagina was well plugged with sponges, but I carefully avoided passing the first piece too high, so as to forcibly press against the os uteri. The retaining bandage was fixed. Stimulants and supports were cautiously administered. The external bleeding ceased; and we were convinced there was no internal loss. The plug was allowed to remain for about eight hours. At the expiration of this time, although there was no discharge, yet as she complained of irritation, it was removed. As nothing further occurred, I left the patient under the care of her medical attendant, who afterwards informed me that nothing unfavourable happened until she reached the eighth month, when she had a very slight discharge of blood, which was soon arrested by cold applications, etc.

She went on to the end of her pregnancy, and her labour was natural. The child was born alive. Mr. S. informed me that the membranes had ruptured before his arrival, and that he felt a small portion of the placenta hanging through the os uteri.

Remarks.—We have here a good example of the advantage of not meddling, beyond adopting suitable measures to stop the hemorrhage.

Case XIV.—May 25, 1824, Mrs. Such sent for me to see a hospital patient residing in Tib Street, who had been in labour for several hours, and was flooding. This was her tenth pregnancy. She was large in size, and the uterus seemed to project more forwards than usual. The pains were frequent, but they were very weak. When the midwife first visited her, the hemorrhage was very trifling, but afterwards it rather increased, but still not to any great degree; and therefore she did not send sooner for further assistance. Cold vinegar and water had been externally applied; the apartment had been kept cool; and the patient constantly kept in bed. Although the discharge had continued for some time, the woman did not appear to have suffered from the loss. I found the os uteri situated rather backwards; it was very soft, and dilated to more than the size of a crown-piece; along with the flaccid membranes I felt a small slip of placenta, and higher up I perceived the head of the child. On the accession of pain the membranes were only just made tense.

I had the patient placed on the back, and a regulating bandage applied and tightened. I now gave her half a drachm of secale cornutum, powdered and infused, and repeated the dose in half an hour; after which, the pains increased in power.

Having directed the midwife to tightly draw the bandage, I passed my hand, and, as far as necessary, I detached a portion of the placenta, and then ruptured the membranes. A very large quantity of liquor amnii soon escaped; and the head of the child rapidly descended (finding no obstacle from the os uteri) into the pelvis, and was born alive in about two hours. There was not the slightest bleeding after the completion of the operation. The placenta was immediately expelled. The uterus was well contracted. The bandage was now readjusted and pinned, with a large compress under it.

Remarks.—Why the hemorrhage was not very great, may be accounted for, partly from the comparatively small portion of the placenta which had been fixed to the os uteri, and partly from the very gradual separation of this organ from the uterus, in consequence of the weak pains, which necessarily effected the dilatation of the os very slowly. The atony of the uterus most likely arose from the large quantity of liquor amnii, and also from frequent pregnancy. It was thought prudent (there being no depression of the vital power) to administer the secale cornutum before the manual operation was performed, to guard against the risk of further bleeding. Obliquity of the uterus, to a considerable degree, existed, on which account I had the patient placed, to labour, on the back. The aid derived from the regulating bandage was very great; and when it was drawn tight, the fundus and body of the uterus were raised from the anterior dependent position, and retained in the line of the axis of the inlet of the pelvis.

Case XV.—March 11, 1824. Early in the morning, Mr. Dadley desired me to visit a hospital patient living in Miller's Lane, to whom he had been called by Mrs. Frost. She was in labour of her seventh child. Mr. Dadley found her very much reduced from hemorrhage, which had continued for some time previously to his being sent for, and which now recurred with greater violence during the pains, which were frequent and short. The os uteri was low down in the pelvis, soft, and dilated to about the size of a half-crown. He discovered a portion of the placenta with the membranes, and higher up, the head of the child. At this time a messenger was dispatched for me; but before I arrived, she was dead. Mr. Dadley stated the symptoms of exhaustion became so urgent, that he felt he should not be justified in waiting for me, and therefore he determined on immediate delivery. He passed his hand by the side of the placenta, and then ruptured the membranes: the patient immediately fainted and died.

Permission was obtained for a *post-mortem* examination. The aspect of the body was white and exsanguined. The abdominal viscera were pale. The uterus was flaccid and large in size; on cutting through its parietes, they were found thinner than usual. The placenta was also thin, and extensively connected to the right side of the cervix and body of the womb. The os uteri was nearly fully opened, and within it there was a narrow loosened portion of placenta.

Remarks.—Although I did not see the patient during her life, there can be no doubt the vital powers were very greatly exhausted from the hemorrhage, which had been incessant for a very considerable length of time.

The case is an example of an opposite character to some of those which are already cited. The atonic state of the uterus, evinced by the very feeble pains, and further proved by the *post-mortem* examination, no doubt mainly contributed to the fatal issue. If the fundus and body had acted energetically at an early period of the labour, the os uteri being so soft and unresistant, it is most probable the woman would have been saved under judicious obstetric management.

Case XVI.—April 25, 1825. Through the kindness of my colleague Mr. Fawdingtou, I was present at the *post-mortem* examination of a hospital patient. I was told she had lost a very large quantity of blood, which did not escape by large impetuous gushes, which sometimes immediately destroy a woman, but by an incessant dribbling discharge. As her dissolution seemed impending, it was deemed right to deliver her, although the os uteri was high, felt rigid, and was very little dilated. Mr. Fawdington stated that he performed the operation very slowly and carefully, but with great difficulty. The child was stillborn. She died on the second day after her delivery.

On inspecting the body, it was white and exsanguine. There was a little watery fluid in the peritoneal cavity. The uterus was soft and larger than usual. The os was ragged, there being several lacerations through its tissue, which appeared as if it was gangrenous.

Case XVII.—March 11, 1830. Early in the morning, Mrs. ——, midwife, sent for me to see a patient, whom the messenger stated to be in labour, and in great danger. She was in the eighth month of her sixth pregnancy. She had flooded, more or less constantly, for a fortnight. Her labour began the evening before, and she had strong pains during the whole of the night, which were accompanied by an increased discharge of blood. She was very much exhausted. Her countenance was extremely pale. The surface of the body felt very cold. Her pulse was scarcely perceptible. There was great restlessness, and she gasped for breath. The os uteri was soft, and dilated to about the size of a dollar. A portion of the placenta protruded through it into the vagina. As her death was inevitable, I deemed it right only to tighten the bandage, which was already about her, and to pass a piece of sponge *per vaginam*, more for the sake of satisfaction to her friends than to serve any other purpose. Brandy and water, etc., were ordered, but she had difficulty in swallowing. She died in about an hour.

Consent was obtained to examine the body the day following. It was white, as if altogether drained of blood. There was extreme paleness observable in the abdominal viscera. On cutting into the uterus, and opening the membranes, some liquor amnii escaped. The child lay in a natural position, and its body was very white, as if it had also lost its blood. The placenta was remarkably thin, and extensively connected; it covered the os, the cervix, and the body of the womb; it was more like a placental bag than like (as it is usually called) "a cake." That portion of this organ into which the funis was inserted was placed nearly over the centre of the os uteri. This opening was soft and considerably dilated, and was filled with the placenta, which was lacerated, and its tissue loaded with coagulated blood.

Remarks.—The midwife was most unpardonable in allowing this poor creature to bleed to death without earlier sending for further assistance. What individual efforts she might have ignorantly made to save the woman, I am unable to state; although I strongly suspect she (the midwife) had rudely meddled with the placenta. The extensive connection of this organ tended, no doubt, to increase the hazards which usually belong to a central positiou of it over the os uteri. An early and judicious delivery would have afforded her the best, and indeed the only, chance of being saved. The whiteness of the child's body showed that its blood had drained away; and there is no doubt that the source from whence it escaped was the lacerated placental tissue. (Vide *Lancet*, loc. cit.)

Case XVIII.—June 23, 1847. I received a note from Mr. Dunn, requesting me to see Mrs. L., who was flooding, in consultation with him, and to bring my galvanic apparatus along with me. He stated to me that she was now in labour of her fifth child, and had previously two attacks of slight hemorrhage, both of which had been arrested by quietude, cold applications, and an acid mixture. She was a delicate leucophlegmatic woman, about 40 years of age.

When Mr. Dunn first saw her, she had felt trifling pains; and the discharge, which at first was only moderate, gradually increased. There was no obvious cause to account either for this or the two former attacks. The os uteri was thin and partially dilated. The membranes and a portion of the placenta were felt, and a little above, the head of the child presented. An abdominal bandage had been applied, and cold water and vinegar externally used. As the pains continued to come on very frequently, and were very weak, and the hemorrhage was much greater, I was now sent for. I found this lady very feeble, evidently suffering the effects of loss of blood. Her countenance was pallid, especially the lips. The skin was pale; the pulse frequent and small; the os uteri was soft and thin, and dilated as nearly as possible to the size of a crown-piece. The pains seemed very weak and ineffective, and indeed the membranes were very slightly affected during their continuance; a considerable sized portion of placenta was felt in connection with them.

On applying my hand on the abdomen during the contraction of the uterus, I ascertained that this organ did not then become hard and resistant, but it continued softish. Under these circumstances, we continued first to pass the galvanic currents through the longitudinal and transverse axis of the uterus; and afterwards to adopt such measures as we thought best suitable for the case. After a very short time the uterus acted more energetically. The regulating bandage was now put on, and afterwards the hand was introduced, and a portion of the placenta was detached, and the membranes were ruptured. The waters being discharged, the head very soon came down, and pressed on the os uteri. The hemorrhage had now entirely ceased. Although the pains were much stronger, we considered it prudent to again pass the galvanic current through the uterus; and we continued to do so at intervals for about an hour. During this time the pains strengthened; and the head of the child descended and passed by the placenta, pressing this organ against the side of the pelvis. The child was born (alive) in about three hours after we first applied galvanism. The placenta was removed from the vagina in half an hour, and there was only an ordinary discharge of blood.

Remarks.—An atonic state of the uterus in cases of unavoidable hemorrhage is always to be deplored, for although the placenta is always more or less separated by each pain, yet active contraction of the fundus and body of the uterus, especially when there coexists a dilated and a dilatable os, is most advantageous, and tends, under proper obstetric management, to save the woman. The os was in this favourable condition, and by the application of galvanism, active and effective, uterine contraction was induced. The salutary effects of this powerful agent are not confined alone to giving energy to the uterus; but the depressed vital powers are raised by its use.

Case XIX.—April 13, 1848. I saw a poor woman residing in Canal Street, along with my respected friend and late pupil, Mr. Dorrington. She was in labour of her seventh child. He said he found her flooding excessively; the os uteri very little dilated and firm. The midwife informed him the patient had flooded very slightly twice before. Each of these attacks had come on without any assignable cause. The pains were regular, but very short and weak. Mr. Dorrington had a bandage, with a compress under it, tightly applied. He ordered her a drachm of laudanum. He remained with the patient for some time; and then, as there was no hemorrhage, he left, and in about three to four hours he called again to see her; and as there was no further discharge of blood, and as there was an improvement in her pulse, and the pains still were frequent and feeble, he determined to withdraw the plug. Some small coagula with the liquor amnii immediately came away, and soon afterwards fresh blood flowed. Mr. Dorrington found the os uteri considerably dilated, and very soft, and he now felt a portion of the placenta, and through the open membranes he touched the head of the child. At this time I was sent for, and requested to bring my galvanic apparatus. She appeared to have lost a large quantity of blood; she was very pale; her pulse was frequent and small; and she was faintish. I passed the hand and found the os uteri dilated to a considerable size and dilatable, and a portion of placenta loosely hanging through it. With Mr. Dorrington's concurrence, I further detached this organ before withdrawing my hand.

The galvanic apparatus having during this time been got in readiness, the conductors were successively applied on the abdomen, so that the current would pass transversely and longitudinally through the uterus. One conductor was also placed on the spine, and the other on the lower portion of the body of the womb, with the view of transmitting the galvanic current along the course of the nerves. We were well satisfied with the effects of each trial. Uterine action soon improved, and in half an hour was very effective. The head of the child was pushed through the os uteri, forcing the placenta aside. The hemorrhage had now ceased, and as the pains returned spontaneously, the labour was left to be finished by nature. The child was born alive in about three hours from our first essay with galvanism. The placenta was soon expelled. There was more discharge than usual. The patient recovered well.

Remarks.—The plug proved of great utility, as there is not much doubt the hemorrhage would have been much greater than it was, and not unlikely would have been fatal, if this mode of treatment had not in the first instance been adopted. The spontaneous rupture of the membranes did not arrest or even abate the discharge. The continuance of the bleeding was in some degree owing to the atonic state of the uterus, and in some degree to leaving the placenta to have its connections gradually broken. This organ was placed in a position favourable for the escape of blood, in consequence of the want of active uterine contraction, which would have quickly separated a necessary portion of the placenta by the head passing rapidly through the os uteri. These two important desiderata were obtained by artificially detaching a portion of the placenta, and the induction of brisk uterine contraction by the aid of galvanism.

Case XX.—Jan. 7, 1831. I was requested by Mr. —— to visit Mrs. L., from whom I received the following statement of the case up to the time I was called in. She was in the sixth month of her twelfth pregnancy, when she began to flood rather copiously whilst quietly sitting on a chair. She had several slight attacks at intervals of seven to ten days. Rest in the recumbent position, cool air, cold applications, and an acid mixture, with laudanum, were ordered. Notwithstanding she suffered from these repeated discharges of blood, she arrived at the end of the eighth month. On the evening of the above date, she had again a slight flow; but she had not been in bed above an hour before the bleeding became very profuse. She rose from bed, and stood leaning forwards over the edge of it, until she fainted, when she fortunately fell (forwards) on the bed.

Mr. —— was now sent for; he found her somewhat recovered, although she still remained rather faint. Her pulse was very weak; her countenance was very pallid; the surface of her body felt coldish. The os uteri, he said, was placed rather low, and dilated to about the size of a shilling, but it was very firm. The hemorrhage had been very great, for the body and bed linen were completely saturated, and there was a large pool of blood on the floor; and therefore, although the organic state was unfavourable, as he considered it hazardous to risk another attack, he proposed immediate delivery; but she determinately refused to allow it.

At this time I was sent for. The discharge continued to slightly dribble. The os uteri was not more dilated than before mentioned, and was firm and undilatable. The placenta I distinctly felt. Under these circumstances, I did not feel warranted to acquiesce in the necessity and propriety of delivery; but I preposed to plug the vagina, and to apply an abdominal bandage, and a compress under it, over the uterus. A drachm of tincture of opium was administered. The discharge was now completely arrested. Brandy and water and suitable support were given. She was well watched for eight hours, during which time she improved, and had regular pains. The plug was now withdrawn, and along with it some coagula came away, which was immediately followed by fresh blood. The os uteri was now considerably more dilated and dilatable; and as she consented to submit to delivery, I passed my hand (having had placed on a regulating bandage), and first separated a large portion of the placenta (which was centrally placed over the os), and then ruptured the membranes. I readily seized a foot, by which I brought the child's hips to bear on the os uteri, when I rested, and afterwards, as there was now no bleeding, I slowly extracted the body and head, co-operating in my efforts with the pains. The child was dead, and extremely white, as if it had also been drained of its blood. The placenta, being loose in the vagina, was immediately removed; its organization was a good deal broken up. There was only an ordinary discharge. A drachm of tincture of opium was administered. She continued to go on favourably for the first three days, at the end of which time she had a shivering, succeeded by a febrile heat. She felt pain in the hypogastric region, which was tender on pressure; and her right lower limb felt stiff, and began to swell; it was very pale; terminating in a slight attack of "phlegmasia dolens." Saline and suitable aperient medicines were prescribed. Leeches, poultices, and frictions, were applied. She gradually recovered.

Remarks.—The blood which had run on the floor was, as far as possible, taken up, and the quantity was very great. Her loss in the aggregate must have been very considerable. She bore a larger loss than most pregnant women could have endured without nearly completely exhausting their vital powers. It is, however, a fact, that every woman in this condition bears loss of blood much better than at other times. It was perhaps a fortunate, although not a very courteous determination, that she refused the proposition of her medical attendant, for then the os uteri was not in a fit state for delivery to be safely performed; and it is not unlikely if this operation had been forcibly undertaken, her life might have been sacrificed. The plug answered well to secure her until the os uteri became sufficiently soft and open. The child doubtless died from hemorrhage. It was very white, and had a very different aspect from that which is observed in children who die *in utero* from other causes, or during extraction after turning, in cases of preternatural presentations.

Case XXI.—Sept. 29, 1832. Mrs. O'Neil desired me to visit a hospital patient, residing in Pump Street, who was flooding. She was in labour of her sixth child, but not quite at the end of pregnancy. During the seventh and eighth months, she had a slight attack of the same accident, both of which were easily arrested by rest in bed, and the external application of cold vinegar and water. She had pains for about three hours before I saw her, but they were now more frequent and stronger. The discharge, at first trivial, had become very profuse. She was rather pale, and felt a little faintish. Her pulse was more frequent than natural, but was not very weak. The os uteri was dilated to about the size of a crown-piece; it was soft and yielding. I ascertained that the placenta was placed over it, but I could not find its connection with the membranes, and therefore I concluded that this organ was nearly (if not) centrally fixed over the os uteri. One drachm of tincture of opium was taken.

The local and general condition being favourable for delivery, and the child being alive, I concluded to perform this operation, having first had the regulating bandage put on, so as just to support the uterus, but afterwards to be cautiously tightened, as required, during the passage of the child. I now passed my hand slowly on, in a conical form, to the os uteri, and endeavoured to find the separated portion of the placenta, which (as I thought) I did. In carrying my hand onward, I moved it sideways, in opposite directions, so as to detach a considerable and an adequate portion of this organ; during which there was an increased discharge of blood. Having ruptured the membranes, I easily found a foot of the child, and readily brought it down. After I had drawn it so far as to bring the breech of the child, with one thigh bent upon its abdomen, to lightly bear on the cervix and os uteri, I rested, so that these portions of the uterus should not be too rapidly distended, before they were in some measure prepared for the passage of a bulk of such magnitude. The hemorrhage had now ceased, and as the child had not advanced so far as to expose the funis to dangerous pressure, I waited awhile longer, during which time the bandage was kept well tightened, and friction used over it, so as to induce uterine action. Shortly a strong pain occurred, when I cautiously drew down by the leg, and fortunately the child advanced; and as the pains continued, I co-operated in slowly extracting, and in the course of a very short time the child was born alive. The placenta followed immediately; on its maternal surface were to be seen the signs of the former and more recent separations. There was no more bleeding. A drachm of laudanum was given. She went on very well until the third day, when she had a slight attack of phlebitis, which readily yielded to treatment.

Remarks.—Both the local and constitutional condition were highly favourable for delivery; I therefore at once had recourse to it. Although the os and cervix uteri were tangibly in such a state of non-resistance to even a moderate force, yet I considered it both wiser and safer slowly and cautiously to draw down the child after having turned it. Its life, as well as that of the mother, would have been hazarded by too rapid extraction. The breech, with one thigh bent upwards and lying on the child's belly, is (as I have elsewhere stated) nearly equal in its measurement to the head; so that if this part is rapidly pulled through the cervix and os uteri before these portions of the uterus are prepared (which preparation must be gradually effected to permit its safe passage), this forcible distension then produces laceration and contusion of these parts, which in some cases has been found nearly in a state of sphacelus. Phlebitis and peritonitis not unfrequently occur after this mischievous practice.

Case XXII.—I am indebted to my respected friend and colleague, Mr. Masfen, for the following case, in whose words it is cited:—

"About 8 o'clock on the evening of Feb. 5, 1856, I was called in by Mr. Harris, to visit Mrs. N., of Silver Street, Hulme, who was stated to be eight months pregnant, but who had been in labour for two days, and was flooding considerably. On my arrival, I found her looking extremely pale, with feeble pulse of about 80, and was told she had lost a great deal of blood, but the hemorrhage had ceased; she had had two half drachms of laudanum, and described herself as tolerably comfortable. I ascertained a placental presentation, with the os uteri dilated to the size of a shilling, and there were moderate uterine pains. I gave her a drachm of laudanum, but as it did not appear to have any sedative action upon the uterus, I thought it desirable to hasten the delivery, and plug the vagina till such time as the os should be sufficiently dilated. I accordingly introduced a large oval sponge with some difficulty into the vagina, pressed it firmly against the os uteri, and secured it by a T bandage. I ordered four half drachms of powdered ergot to be given at intervals of half an hour; and having given directions to be sent for if the slightest hemorrhage should occur, or as soon as there had been sufficient action to produce dilatation of the os, I left the house. I was not summoned again till 10 o'clock the next morning, when Mrs. Harris informed me that the ergot had produced no apparent effect, that the pains had continued slightly through the night, that there had been no hemorrhage; but that on removing the bandage this morning, the sponge had come away, and she had immediately sent for me. I found the patient much in the same condition as I had left her, with feeble pulse, and deadly pallor of countenance. I gave a drachm of laudanum, and the os having been fully dilated, proceeded to deliver by turning. This was effected in a few minutes without any difficulty, and I ruptured the membranes after I had found the foot. The introduction of the hand appeared to give her considerable pain. The placenta came away in five minutes after the birth of the child, and the uterus contracted firmly. At the edge of the placenta, the portion which had been detached was easily distinguishable, about the size of the longitudinal section of a lemon, and on its centre was a darker coloured prominencnoc, about the size of a walnut, produced by the long continued pressure of the os. There was no hemorrhage. I applied a binder myself tightly over the abdomen; and the patient expressed herself as feeling very comfortable, and much delighted at having got over it so easily. The pulse at this time was scarcely perceptible, but it materially improved under the influence of a drachm of laudanum, which I ordered to be repeated. I remained in the house half an hour after the delivery, and she thought she should go to sleep, but complained of the tightness of the binder. It however was not slackened. On reaching home, about an hour afterwards, I found an urgent message had been left some time before, that I should visit the same patient immediately. I lost no time, but found that all was over. It appears that within five minutes of my leaving the house, she was suddenly seized with symptoms of dissolution. A neighbouring medical man was called in, but he said nothing was to be done, and she did not live many minutes. There had been no more hemorrhage, and the uterus, which I examined, was still firmly contracted.

"This case presents two points worthy of consideration. Would different treatment, or would additional treatment, have been attended with a satisfactory result? As regards the propriety of delivering under such circumstances, my friend, Dr. Radford, I believe, entertains doubts. It appeared to me, however, that to leave the patient with symptoms of labour, and an ascertained placenta prævia, would have been attended with imminent danger; and to have stayed an indefinite time, would have been out of the question, as actual labour might not have come on without interference for days or weeks. For loss of blood simply, I have almost invariably found opium a specific; and the quantities of this drug which exsanguined patients will tolerate, is only limited by the extent to which the hemorrhage has proceeded. The patient had half an ounce of laudanum in fifteen hours; she would doubtless have borne much more, but the symptoms did not appear to require it. The most direct and rational remedy—and, I think, the best—for extreme loss of blood, is transfusion. I performed this operation a few years ago in a somewhat similar case (vide *Lancet*, 1851, vol. i. p. 434) with perfect success. The gradual return of the pulse as the process was going on, at first wavering, then permanent, and afterwards the return of consciousness and the manifestation of interest in what was going on, establish this as a remedy of the highest utility. But what is the indication for its necessity? The patient on whom I performed the operation was apparently lifeless, utterly unconscious, and with no pulse at the wrist. In this case, the patient, when I left her, was lively and cheerful, and the pulse was improving under the use of opium. Dr. Radford speaks highly of the use of galvanism, and thinks it might have been advantageous in this case. Of this remedy, I have no experience; but one serious objection to either of these latter plans, in poor, not being hospital practice, is the difficulty of obtaining in time the proper instruments and efficient assistants."

Case XXIII.—Two cases were communicated to me by a medical friend, to be used as I thought proper; and as one (the following) illustrates an error of practice, I shall relate it in his own words:—

"About midnight, December 1, 1840, I was sent for to Mrs. M. N. L. I was informed on my arrival, that she had been flooding a considerable time, and had lost a large quantity of blood, which seemed to be true, from the state of exhaustion the poor creature was in; for her faintness was extreme, and she had every symptom of the most immediate danger. Upon examination, I found the os uteri a little dilated, and the placenta evidently presenting; but there had been little or no pain or uterine contraction. Having waited about an hour, during which time I tried to irritate the uterus with my finger so as to induce vigorous action, I obtained the desired effect of increasing the pains, and dilating the os uteri to its fullest extent, although I at the same time also increased the hemorrhage. I now resolved to give her the chance of an immediate delivery, which I effected by introducing my hand into the uterus, and turning and bringing away the fœtus; and this I did with greater facility than I could have imagined, as the resistance from the uterus was very trifling. I endeavoured to pass my hand through the placenta, but not being able to do it, I separated it on one side, until there was sufficient room for my hand to pass.

"Immediately after the birth of the child, which was dead, I detached the placenta, the uterus having but little power to expel it; and apprehensive, by its detention, of the risk of further hemorrhage from its extensive separation. The woman remained very faint and weak a long time after delivery; but being carefully nursed, she recovered by degrees, and was able to go out by the end of six weeks."

Remarks.—Great hazards were run by the injudicious interference with the os for the purpose of inducing uterine action. This practice was calculated to induce irregular contraction of the uterus, to produce a further separation of the placenta, and thereby an increase of flooding. The unsuccessful attempt to pass the hand through the placenta was, no doubt (and might have been still more), mischievous. We cannot positively say that the death of the child was caused by this procedure; but most assuredly its chances of being born alive were considerably lessened by it, as the tissue of the placenta must have been more or less injured by trying to perforate this organ.—*Assoc. Med. Journ.*, March 1 and 15; April 12, 1856.

31. *On the Depth at which the Placenta is implanted in the Uterus.*—Dr. Von Ritgen has given an elaborate and interesting illustration of the various seats of attachment of the placenta, other than to the neck of the womb. He refers to the method discovered in recent times, of determining after delivery the height at which the placenta was attached, by measuring the distance of the rent in the membranes made by the passage of the liquor amnii and fœtus from the margin of the placenta.

The bag burst at the edge of the placenta in 22 cases. It burst at one inch from the edge in 8 cases; between one and two inches in 12 cases; two inches in 7 cases; between two and three inches in 16 cases; three inches in 5 cases; between three and four inches in 4 cases; four inches in 6 cases; between four and five inches in 8 cases; five inches in 3 cases; six inches in 6 cases; and eight inches in 3 cases.

It follows, that since the distance of the edge of the placenta from the rent is absolutely decisive as to the distance of the edge of the placenta from the os uteri, that the edge of the placenta rested on the os uteri in 22 cases, and was within one inch in 32 cases, within two inches in 49 cases, and so on.

This proves that the placenta has commonly a much lower seat than has hitherto been believed.

It also appears that smallness of the ovum has a closer relation to lower seat of the placenta than is to be accounted for by the simple diminution of all the dimensions of the uterus.—*Brit. and For. Med.-Chirurg. Rev.*, April, 1856, from *Monatsschrf. für Geburtsk.*, Oct. 1855.

32. *Period of Exclusion of Placenta.*—Dr. Von Ritgen says, that instructions were given in the hospital for many years, not to remove a detached placenta without the express permission of the director. The reason was, to ascertain whether the leaving behind the detached placenta would cause mischief to the mother by absorption of the dead matter. This rule was followed for a time, so far as to allow the placenta to remain several days, and until the foul smell became insupportable; but at a later period it was not carried to this extreme, after it was ascertained that *no absorption of decomposing constituents of placenta ever took place, except in cases of fleshy growth of the placenta to the uterus.*

Summarily expressed, the detached placenta remained fifty-two times, or in about one-half the cases, less than four hours in the uterus; and in the other half, between four and fourteen and a half hours.

The spontaneously completely detached placenta was removed artificially in 3 cases on account of hemorrhage. In 1 case it was removed on account of spasmodic pains. In 2 cases after operations. In all the rest, the placenta was removed on account of severe after-pains, heavy pressure of the vagina, difficulty of micturition, disturbance of rest and sleep.

[We cannot but express the hope that the Professor is satisfied with these results, and that he will not consider it necessary to carry this experiment further.—Rep.]—*Ibid.*

MEDICAL JURISPRUDENCE AND TOXICOLOGY.

33. *Effects of the Humours of the Toad on the Animal Economy.* By M. Gavini.—It is a generally received opinion that the toad is venomous. Naturalists admit this; Buffon says that the toad and serpents are capable of killing one another by their bite and their poison. Experiments recently performed

on animals and detailed before the Society of Biology by M. Vulpian, have established the venomous power of the toad. The following case exhibits the action of the poison of the reptile on the human system:—

Towards the close of the month of June, which was hot and dry, a child, aged 6, in company with some other little boys, was throwing stones at a large toad, when he suddenly felt something spirted into his right eye. He was subsequently attacked with spasmodic pain in the same eye, which appeared only slightly injected with blood. About two hours after there was coma, continual yawning, incapability of keeping the eyelids open, subsultus tendinum; he carried such objects as were within his reach to his mouth to bite them; he frequently discharged an abundance of urine of the natural colour; his bowels were torpid; there was aversion to food and drink. When up the child's face was much altered; there was continual agitation of the head and arms. At one time he whimpered, at another he cried; subsequently, he fell into a state of coma. This condition lasted two days, after which alvine dejections, containing lumbrici, were obtained.

On the sixth day of his illness he was in a state of apathy, or sort of stupor; the pulse was regular.

After a period of calm he left his bed and ran like a mad person through the house. He was constantly howling, his eyes were injected with blood, the tongue was dry, the pulse regular, there was no febrile heat of body.

On the tenth day the only symptoms were stupor and inability to speak—a condition which has now lasted for two years.—*Dublin Med. Press*, April 9th, from *Gaz. Méd. de Paris*, March 22, 1856, and *Correspond. Scien. in Roma.*

---

34. *Method for the Detection of Phosphorus in Cases of Poisoning.*—E. Mitscherlich considers the following the most delicate method for the detection of phosphorus in toxicological cases: The substance to be examined is distilled with sulphuric acid and water from a flask, and the vapour conducted through a glass tube into a vertical glass receiver. This receiver passes through the bottom of a broad glass cylinder, filled with cold water, which is constantly renewed in the usual manner, so that the hot water escapes from the top, and the cold water enters at the bottom. Under the lower end of the receiver, which passes through the bottom of the cooler, a vessel is placed to collect the distillate.

If phosphorus is present, its vapour passes over with the steam into the receiver, and it may be seen where the vapour enters the cool portion of the receiver, as a distinct illumination in the dark, which long continues. Generally, an illuminated ring is observed. From substances, such as flour, which only contain one hundred-thousandth part of phosphorus, three ounces of fluid can be distilled off, and the distillation be continued for half an hour without the illumination ceasing. After such an experiment, the flask and its contents may be exposed to the air for fourteen days, and the distillation repeated with the development of the illumination.

When volatile bodies, as ether, alcohol, and oil of turpentine, are present, which destroy the illumination of the phosphorus, the ether and alcohol must be distilled off, and then the illumination will appear. Oil of turpentine prevents the illumination; but such an admixture is not likely to occur in forensic investigations. If ammonia be present, its detrimental influence may be prevented by the addition of sulphuric acid.—*Lancet*, April 26, 1856.

AMERICAN INTELLIGENCE.

ORIGINAL COMMUNICATIONS.

Indigo Detected in the Urine. By CHARLES FRICK, M. D., of Baltimore. (Extract from a letter to the Editor.)—*My Dear Sir:* I have lately had presented to me for analysis a specimen of urine, which contained a substance so rarely met with, that by some its occurrence in this secretion has been altogether denied—I mean indigo; and I believe that the present case is the first one reported in this country. Drs. Prout and Simon, and also Dr. Hassell, speak of having detected it in one or two instances where no indigo was taken into the stomach, as in the present case; and the latter observer proposes a hypothetical explanation of its formation in the human body. In the present instance it occurred in a patient fifty years of age, labouring under hemiplegia of some mouths' duration. The urine was slightly albuminous, specific gravity 1.011, full colour, and exhibited a few tube casts, and hypertrophied epithelium cells under the microscope. The reaction was faintly alkaline when I received it. On standing a few days, the colour changed to a dull leaden hue. On the surface, particularly around the circumference, and in some degree coating the sides of the vial, I observed a slight deposit of a deep blue colour. This hue also predominated in the deposit, which, under the microscope, was found to consist of urate of soda granules, and prisms of triple phosphate, mixed with an amorphous substance, in colour of a deep blue. I suspected this to be indigo, and was confirmed in my suspicions by an analysis made of it by my friend Dr. Steiner, of this city, as well as my own subsequent examination. The reactions it gave were as follows: The deposit was first digested in dilute acetic acid, and then washed in cold water. Muriatic acid neither dissolved it nor changed its colour. In sulphuric acid it dissolved, forming a solution of an indigo colour, but with nitric acid the colour changed from blue to yellow. On warming a portion of the sediment with dilute alcohol, to which grape sugar and potash had been added, the fluid lost its blue tint, and assumed a yellowish red colour, which, on shaking, was converted into a deep blood red, and then rapidly into a green. After resting some hours, the green tint disappeared, and the fluid became a yellowish red. Townes states that this change of colour is due to the sugar being oxidized, and the indigo reduced.

BALTIMORE, June 10, 1856.

Case of Monstrosity. By H. C. MARTHENS, M. D., of St. Louis.—I have lately met with an instance of the most remarkable deviation in the development of the human form, probably the most singular one on record.

The subject is a white male child, having a well-developed head and trunk, but with a total absence of the upper and lower extremities. The head is of good shape and size, perhaps a little too large. The eyes are bright and intelligent. The body is also well formed. The clavicles and scapulæ are in place, but there is not a rudiment of either arm visible. The skin is carried smoothly over each shoulder, except a small central dimple. The pelvis also is natural; here, likewise, there is no trace of a lower limb. The cuticle covers the acetabulæ smoothly, save a nipple-like projection in the centre.

The child was born in New Mexico, of American parents; is now sixteen months old; sprightly, active, and intelligent; has generally had good health. The mother is an educated and refined woman, as much attached to and interested in her offspring as if it were perfect in form.

SAINT LOUIS, Mo., *June* 10, 1856.

Experimental Physiology. BY DAVID R. WALTON, M. D.—Among the interesting lectures on Medical Science in Paris, none are pursued with more zeal and success than the several courses of Experimental Physiology.

M. Coste, at the College of France; M. Claude Bernard, at the same Institution, and at the Sorbonne; M. Flourens, at the Garden of Plants; MM. Wurtz and Verneuil, at l'Ecole College de Médecine; M. Brown-Séquard, M. Béclard, and M. Martin-Magron, at l'Ecole Pratique; M. Charles Robin, and others in private courses, each pursuing specialties, and all contributing to the discovery of elementary truths, are harmoniously developing the science of Physiology.

A circumstance which promises the most valuable results is the surrender of preconceived theories opposed by legitimate experimentation; the unanimous pursuit of facts as individualities, and a natural arrangement of analogical facts; thus establishing doctrines and practice as *spontaneous necessities*—*i. e.*, doctrines flowing from demonstrated facts. This characteristic may be easily illustrated by stating what passed this day before the pupils of M. Brown-Séquard, late Professor of the Institutes of Medicine and of Medical Jurisprudence in the Medical College of Virginia. Transfusion of blood formed the subject of experimentation in his regular course this day. The Professor first showed a dog, into the jugular vein of which had been, the day before, injected a mixture of blood drawn from two pigeons and a rabbit. The good state of this animal, in which circulated the blood of distant species, formed a contrast with the results obtained in the experiments reported, and the doctrines maintained by MM. Prevost and Dumas, who say the blood of a bird is poison if introduced into the vein of a mammal, and who maintain the incompatibility of the blood of different species. The following experiments show the grounds of error in said doctrine; and at the same time are suggestive of the true method of transfusion necessitated by dangerous hemorrhage.

It will be seen that it is the state or condition of the injected blood, rather than the species of animal from which it is derived, that determines its poisonous effects.

M. Brown-Séquard commenced by injecting into the veins of animals their own blood in different states. First experiment: blood was drawn from the right carotid of a dog, and as it flowed it was beaten by a feather brush to separate the fibrin and to oxygenate the liquid. A portion of this aerated blood was injected into the jugular vein of the same animal. At the expiration of an hour, more blood was taken from the dog, defibrinated and injected as before. This series was repeated eight times in six hours. The third abstraction was nearly devoid of fibrin, and the last five appeared to be destitute of any; but it was only when the blood had lost its power of being aerated, and when the black blood was injected, that fatal convulsions occurred.

In some animals blood was drawn from arteries, and in others from veins, and beaten from the commencement of the flowing till the same was injected into the veins of animals from which it had been drawn, or of animals of a different species. The injection of this aerated blood was not followed with fatal consequences, except in two instances, when it was found that air had entered the veins, and had been, as was supposed, the cause of death.

Finally, experiments were made by injecting into animals their own blood unoxygenated, which had been suffered to remain a few moments deprived of the contact of air, after it had been defibrinated; that is, the blood was first defibrinated, then placed in the syringe, and thus secluded from the air till its oxygen had combined with its carbon, and formed carbonic acid, rendering it black. This carbonated injection invariably produced convulsions and speedy death.

It is to be presumed that the doctrines of MM. Prevost and Dumas, concerning the transfusion of blood of different species, are formed from experiments made without due attention to aeration of the injected fluid. It is probable, also, that the general prejudice against transfusion of human blood as a remedy in case of dangerous hemorrhage, has arisen in part from the neglect of this oxydation, which all experiments prove absolutely necessary. It may be that in some cases too large a quantity has been transfused. It is found that the injection of blood equal to one-tenth the quantity lost is the standard proportion required.

Full details of these experiments will be given in a work composed of comparative and analogous cases by the several experimenters of Paris.

Paris, Feb. 15, 1856.

DOMESTIC SUMMARY.

Case of Erythema Tuberculatum et Œdematosum.—Dr. Silas Durkee records (*Boston Medical and Surgical Journal*, April 10, 1856) a case of this rare disease. The subject of it was a woman, 47 years of age, born of healthy parents, married at the age of 19, and the mother of six children. She was of medium size, dark complexion, black hair and eyes, of good moral character. She first consulted Dr. D. in July, 1855. There was then one tubercle situated on the inside of the left leg, midway between the knee and ankle. It was one inch in diameter at the base, and elevated one-third of an inch above the surrounding skin. It was of a deep-red colour, was perfectly round, and slightly elastic to the touch. It was not painful. It began to show itself in the month of March previous, making about four months before Dr. D. saw it. There were from eight to ten papulæ irregularly distributed in the immediate neighbourhood, and varying in size from mere dots to a pin's head; and two or three small tubercles, of the bigness of a split pea, near the inner malleolus. The appearance of the papules and the tubercle corresponded with the description and plate under the head of "Erythema Papulatum et Tuberculatum," in the *Illustrations of Cutaneous Diseases*, by Robert Willis, London, 1841.

"The leg and foot were somewhat swollen and œdematous. The general health was impaired. The woman had a poor appetite; looked thin and pale; and complained of severe constipation and debility. Pulse 65, and feeble.

"She stated that on the 4th of March, 1853, her right thigh was amputated in consequence of a disease on the right leg like that which occupied the left leg at the time I saw her in July. Both legs and feet had been more or less swollen, especially in warm weather, for six or seven years previously to the amputation. The tubercles on the right leg had existed eight months before the surgical operation was performed. They were fused together in one large mass, according to the patient's statement, and covered a portion of integument on the middle of the leg nearly as large as her hand. She had a favourable recovery from the operation, and for eighteen months afterwards enjoyed health. The malady never showed itself in the stump. The left leg was free from disease at the time the thigh was removed.

"Sept. 29, 1855. Foot and leg more swollen and œdematous than in July; and more than one hundred papules and tubercles were developed upon the leg. Some of them were entirely separated from others; some in close proximity at their bases, and some had coalesced into one common mass, especially in the neighbourhood of the first original tubercle. This aggregation of tubercles covered a surface nearly equal to the palm of my hand; and was elevated at some points one inch above the integument. Before any topical remedies had been applied, excepting the most simple, large sloughs had been cast off from this tuberculoid growth; and thus a cavity had been produced, one inch in length, one-third of an inch wide, and extending beneath the base of the tubercles into the subjacent integument. There was no purulent or serous discharge from this deep opening; and the patient stated that there never had been. I learned from the medical attendant that he had sprinkled bichloride of mercury upon portions of this large group of tubercles for the purpose of producing suppuration—an event which did not take place. He also stated that he had, with the same end in view, applied a solution of the nitrate of silver, ʒiii. to ℥i., but that no suppuration had been produced. The patient stated that from the time these local means were used, the limb became more painful, and that the disease advanced with greater rapidity than before.

"The largest isolated tubercle was imbedded in the skin just above the inner malleolus. It was more than an inch in diameter, and elevated half an inch. It had acquired this growth in about three months. The integument of the outer portion of the leg was, at this date, nearly free from tubercles and papulæ. The most minute specimens of the latter could be felt in the substance of the skin before they had scarcely risen above its surface. They were perfectly hard at this stage of their development, and of a bright red colour. On the summit of some of them the intensity of the red tint was a little obscured, as if the cuticle had been thickened, or partially detached from the derma. By pressing them with the point of the finger, the colour disappeared, and on the removal of the pressure it was quickly restored.

"The hairs had fallen out from the whole integument of the limb, excepting an irregular islet or patch, about five inches in length, and from two to two and a half inches in breadth, on the outer aspect of the lower part of the thigh and the upper part of the leg. Upon this district of skin most of the hairs were firmly retained in their sheaths until the patient died, although, in other respects, it was the seat of the same morbid changes that were displayed in its vicinity. All the follicles from which the hairs had escaped, were congested just sufficiently to attract attention; and by drawing the finger over the skin, many of them felt distinctly hard and solid; in others, the diseased action had been too feeble to produce such a condition, except to a very slight degree.

"Oct. 5, 1855. Three days before, the attending physician had applied a solution of nitrate of silver to many of the tubercles, and to the intervening integument. Vesication was thus produced, and, to-day, the serum is escaping from beneath the broken cuticle, and flowing in various directions over the limb. The swelling and œdema of the parts have increased since I last saw the patient, and she complains of more pain. The skin throughout nearly the whole range of the outside of the leg, where no nitrate of silver had been applied, and where no papules were developed, had a polished, shining appearance, with a bright scarlet colour; and the condition of the limb, apart from the tubercles, answered to the description given by Dr. Good, of Erythema œdematosum, or to what Professor Wilson calls Erythema læve. The redness vanished at once on pressure, and returned the moment pressure was removed. The intumescence of the foot, occasioned by the infiltrated fluid into the subcutaneous cellular tissue, was very great, extending even to the ends of the toes; but the colour of the skin, below the ankle, had not as yet undergone any change. To me it seems no misnomer to say, that two varieties of erythema existed in the present instance; that is, erythema œdematosum and erythema tuberculatum.

The latter variety, however, furnished by far the most interesting features of the case.

"The order of things in the progress of abnormal action, so far as relates to the tubercles, appeared to be this: First, there was defective nutrition of the hair pulp, or matrix; and hence the falling out of the hairs, or alopecia. The next phenomenon was a congestion of the plexus of capillaries of the proper hair sacs or follicles,[1] and this congestion constituted the minute red point or papule; and an aggregation of papules constituted a tubercle.[2] In many specimens, the individuality of the papulæ which were associated together in the formation of tubercles, was distinctly preserved until the latter reached their full maturity, and gave to them a slightly mammillated or dotted surface, which bore, in this particular, some resemblance to a red raspberry a little flattened. In other instances, the tubercles, especially before they had acquired their maximum size, presented a smooth, glossy surface; and in these the mammillated appearance was nearly wanting.

"Generally speaking, the tubercles were from one-fourth to one-third of an inch in diameter when at their full development. A few specimens, however, were three-fourths of an inch in diameter, and half an inch above the level of the skin. They were of a dark red or purplish colour, soft and elastic to the touch, and required for their maturity from eight to twelve weeks. Some of them, after they had ceased to increase in height, continued to augment by peripheral growth at the base.

"One papule appeared upon the very end of the great toe. In ten days it grew as large as twice a mustard seed, after which it began to diminish, and in five or six days more was gone.[3]

"Oct. 20, 1855. Patient reports that there is a constant dripping of watery fluid, occasionally tinged with blood, from the deep cavity already spoken of as having been prodneed by the sloughing of the large tuberculoid mass; and the mass itself is flattening down and diminishing in size. No abatement of swelling or pain in the limb.

"Small bullæ or vesicles formed upon the top of most of the nodules.[4] In four or five days the serum would burst through the cuticle; and it continued to ooze out for some ten or fifteen days. The daily amount of serum from any single tumour was comparatively trifling; but the aggregate quantity from the whole limb amounted some days, when most copious, to two or three ounces. No inconsiderable preportion of this, however, appeared to come from the excavation connected with the large aggregation of tubercles just alluded to. After the serous exudation had somewhat diminished in any individual tubercle, other changes soon took place. Its summit, which until now had been of a rounded form, began to flatten, and in a few days more became concave; and this condition proved to be the commencement of the putrefactive decomposition and wasting away of the tubercles. This process of decay, which pro-

[1] *Vide* Kolliker—Manual of Human Histology, vol. i. p. 183.

[2] *Vide* Wilson on the Skin. Also Willis.

[3] The anatomical distribution of the vessels of the part affords an explanation of this phenomenon. A single arterial twig is divided so as to supply quite a number (twenty or thirty) of the cutaneous papillary loops with blood, which is afterwards poured into one common venous ramuscule. When these vessels, as in cases of impeded circulation, are abnormally distended with blood, the entire group of congested papillæ will present the appearance of a single minute red point; and if the disturbance of the circulation extends to the contiguous papillary groups, the red spot will be greater or less, according to the number of papillæ involved in the congestion. Vide *Wedl's Pathological Histology*, p. 208.

[4] Dr. D. H. Bulkley reported a case of Erythema papulatum in the *New York Lancet* for 1842, page 363. He states that vesicles formed on the summit of some of the papulæ that appeared on the patient's face.

He also mentions the peculiar purplish discoloration of the skin in the same case, giving to the part the appearance of having been bruised.

Gibert also speaks of the formation of vesicles, or bullæ, on the summits of erythematous papulæ, &c. See Gibert, pages 72 and 74.

duced a peculiar mawkish odour, was very gradual, so that the larger lumps and masses required from eight to ten weeks for their obliteration. In some instances, as the cones began to diminish, their apex, now denuded of cuticle, began to assume a grayish or whitish appearance. This was usually due to the combined presence of pus and epithelium; and, occasionally, it was produced by epithelium alone. Sometimes the latter had a dirty gray colour, and was transformed into a soft, pultaceous substance. It would slip aside when touched with the probe, and, in order to obtain a bit for microscopic examination, it had to be cut with scissors. At other times, the epithelium thus lying in the cavity of the tumours was in a fluid state.

"The quantity of pus elaborated during the three months of my attendance upon the case was certainly microscopic; and ulceration, in the ordinary use of the word, did not take place. This fact, in connection with erythema tuberculatum, is mentioned by Prof. Wilson (p. 142). He states that the tubercles have no tendency to suppurate or ulcerate. But, in the case before us, we have the coexistence of erythema œdematosum also; and Dr. Good, speaking of this species of erythema, says: 'There is no difficulty in determining why œdematous inflammation should rarely, if ever, produce suppuration. Suppurative inflammation is, generally speaking, the process of a healthy part or habit taking place instinctively for the purpose of removing something that is dead, irritating, or otherwise mischievous, and of filling up the space hereby produced with sound living matter. In œdematous inflammation, the part or habit is unhealthy and debilitated; and hence, while there is necessarily less tendency to suppuration, there is less power of recovery.' Erythema œdematosum is the œdematous inflammation of John Hunter, who says that it seldom or never produces suppuration.—(*Hunter on the Blood*, Part II., ch. ii., sect. viii.)

"In the case under consideration, the whitish substance which reposed on the summit of the tubercles, and which, while *in situ*, bore a close resemblance to purulent deposit, consisted almost wholly of detrital matter; that is, of epithelial scales—solitary specimens of which were in a perfect state, and the rest in a broken down and decomposed condition. Pus globules were also found, although not in all cases, even with the aid of the microscope. But, admitting that pus had always been found, the fact would not impair the statements of Wilson, Good, and Hunter, and for the very reason that the quantity was microscopic. I think it is truth to say, that the amount of purulent matter, from July to January, was not equal to one ounce from the entire limb.

"It was by a slow process of sphacelation that some of the principal lumps, including the large mound of tuberculoid deposit, were finally obliterated; and a morbid action, similar to that which destroyed them, was excited in the subjacent tissues, and destroyed a portion of the derma just above the inner ankle as large as a penny, and a still larger amount of integument higher up on the inside of the leg. The texture of several other smaller portions of skin that was beset with tubercles, was also invaded in a like manner, and partial destruction brought about, as was seen at the autopsy.

"Another fact to be mentioned in this connection is the condition of the epidermis. On the 10th of November, the integument of the leg began to assume a dark colour, as if it had been stained with a solution of nitrate of silver, although none had been used for forty days. The colour continued to deepen from day to day until it became nearly black. The cuticle remained quite adherent after it had acquired its darkest hue; it could, however, be detached from the derma in small lamellæ or flakes, as the parts were washed from time to time in chlorinated water. When dry, it was as thick as very stout writing paper, and was very brittle. Under the microscope it appeared to be entirely disorganized, except where its under surface was attached to the cutis. Here a few epidermic scales were found in a normal state. On several occasions I examined the tissue now under consideration, and always found the above-named appearances. The cuticle cracked in all directions, and afterwards exfoliated—but was reproduced in a few days, and thus the leg looked as if covered with black scales.

"By the 20th of November, the anasarcous distension of the foot and leg began to subside, and the patient experienced great relief from pain. The limb continned to yield a serous discharge from numerous places with as much freedom as ever, until the 20th of December, by which time the quantity began to diminish, and by which time, also, the leg was reduced to nearly its natural size. During the ten days previous to death, the quantity of serum did not amount, by estimate, to more than four or five drachms for each twenty-four hours.

"Tubercles continued to be evolved, one after another, in pretty rapid succession, until not only the leg, but a large part of the integument of the thigh, was covered with them. Upon the latter, they were comparatively of recent origin; nor did they pass through the various metamorphoses which marked those of earlier growth upon the inferior portion of the limb. Those above the knee had, in most instances, an oval shape, with a base equal to the disc of a very small bean, and were raised but slightly above the skin. Other specimens were still smaller, and belonged to the papulate rather than to the tuberculate variety of erythema. A few papulæ appeared on the dorsum of the foot. These, like the ones that were seated upon the thigh, appeared at a late day, and, consequently, had not time to accomplish the entire cycle of development and decay which characterized the large tubercles on the legs.

"Three weeks immediately preceding death, all the tubercles then existing became very much flattened, and formed a striking contrast to the bold outlines which they presented at the time the artist was employed to take drawings of them (Oct. 11th). On and after the 22d of December, cerebral symptoms were present. Patient ceased to recognize her friends, except now and then; was rather stupid, although she could be roused so as to speak a few words; no paralysis of the vocal organs; no complaint of pain or suffering; said she could see scarcely any, and it seemed to her as if it was night all the time; pupils much dilated. I frequently asked her if she knew me; she would reply in the affirmative, but almost always gave the wrong name. The first thought I had that any cerebral affection had set in, was suggested by a singularly vacant stare which she exhibited—as if her vision were imperfect.

"At the *post-mortem* examination, five or six of the tubercles were about one-fourth of an inch above the skin, while nearly all the rest had so far disappeared as to be scarcely perceptible above the surface, and gave to it a mere knobby or rough aspect.

"During the height of the swelling and the pain consequent upon it, the patient required the free use of opiates, both internally and externally. For the last eight weeks of life, she lost all relish for food. Her pulse ranged from 100 to 108; tongue always remained clean. For four weeks before death she had great dyspnœa, severe gastric distress, and frequent vomitings, and she preferred the sitting posture to any other. On the second day of January she died, greatly emaciated.

"The diseased limb was the only part we were allowed to examine after the death of the patient. Some of the *post-mortem* appearances have already been spoken of. *Above the knee*, the skin was of a dirty, livid colour. Scarcely a trace of tubercles was to be seen. The only mark which indicated the spots where they had existed, consisted in the peculiar shrivelled or collapsed condition of the cuticle, from beneath which the tubercles had disappeared a few days before death. The integument of this portion of the limb was thickened to a moderate degree—say from a line to a line and a half.

"*Below the knee*, the skin had a very dark, reddish-brown colour; or a deep brown, with a purplish tint. So far as relates to the mere colour of this portion of the limb, a very tolerable representation of it may be seen in the London edition of Bateman's *Delineations of Cutaneous Diseases*, Plate XXXI.

"Dr. Ellis made several longitudinal sections through the integument, extending from the upper portion of the tendo-Achillis several inches along the external gastrocnemius muscle. Blood followed the track of the knife quite freely. The derma was much congested. It varied in thickness from four to six lines, by accurate measurement. It was thickest at the upper part of the leg. The line of demarcation between the derma and the subcutaneous cellular tissue was well defined. The substance of the muscular tissue was œdematous, and extremely tender, so that in handling it for examination it was easily torn.

The transverse striations were brought out in some specimens that were examined with the microscope; in others, none could be found. The cavity spoken of in connection with the large mass of tubercles, was found to have extended itself in different directions between the derma and the subjacent cellular membrane so as entirely to separate them. This space or cavity was filled with bloody serum."

The following report of the microscopic appearances of the morbid products, from time to time, was furnished by Dr. B. S. Shaw:—

[Fragments taken from the surface of the nodular masses, and the purulent fluid from the cavities in the centre of the larger elevations, were several times microscopically examined during the progress of the disease. The fragments proved to be composed of *epithelium*, nucleated, in large, flat scales, and in some the epithelium was very granular, and evidently in process of decomposition. The matter in the cavities was *pus*, presenting, in every instance, but one well-marked nuclei upon the application of acetic acid.

On microscopic examination of the parts removed at the autopsy, the following appearances were found.

The *epidermis* was composed, externally, of scaly epithelium, as in the normal condition; deeper, and in connection with the dermis, the epithelium was more or less globular, all the cells nucleated, many of them quite small, as in young epithelium, and accompanied by a large quantity of free nuclei. This deeper part of the epidermis was infiltrated with a serous fluid, which would account for the approximation to the globular form in the epithelium.

The thickened *dermis* was composed of the normal tissues, a great portion of it being more or less interspersed with fine granulations. In some of the reddened portions, blood globules were numerous, and, in other parts, the coloration seemed to be due to an infiltration of red colouring matter. The *cellular* and *adipose* tissues presented no well-marked microscopic deviation from their normal character, though their appearance to the naked eye was not natural; except, that in the *cellular tissue* as well as in the *dermis*, were large numbers of *free nuclei*, generally oval, pale, and free from granulations, and containing very large and pale nucleoli. These nuclei resembled very much some of those contained in the deeper part of the epidermis, and in some of the epithelium cells, though they were generally more oval, somewhat larger, and inclosed larger nucleoli. They varied so much in size, that no just estimate of their diameter could be obtained by measurement. Many of them were of the size of, and resembled cancer nuclei, but the indistinctness of their contour, and the paleness of their nucleoli (the highly-refracting properties of the cancer nucleoli being absent) seemed to distinguish them from cancer. Very few cells were found accompanying them, and these were very indistinct. To classify these nuclei under the name of cancer, epithelium, or other term, would seem at present impossible.

The *muscular* tissue immediately beneath the seat of disease was degenerated, consisting of granulated fibres, presenting only here and there traces of striæ.]

Necrosis of Inferior Maxilla from Vapour of Phosphorus.—Dr. JAMES R. WOOD has recorded (*New York Journal of Medicine*, May, 1856) an interesting case of this in a girl, 16 years of age, who had been engaged in a match factory. Dr. W. removed the entire lower jaw, and the patient made a rapid and favourable recovery. The contour of the face, he says, is preserved with remarkable accuracy.

Appended to the case are some interesting remarks on phosphorus disease.

OBITUARY RECORD.—It is with profound regret that we record the death of Dr. JOHN COLLINS WARREN, which took place in Boston on the 4th of May, at the mature age of 78 years. Dr. J. C. was the oldest son of Dr. John Warren, one of the most eminent physicians of his day, in Boston, and a nephew of Dr. Joseph, afterwards General Warren, who gallantly fell fighting at Bunker Hill in defence of our country.

Dr. J. C. Warren was born Aug. 1, 1778, graduated at Cambridge in 1797, and soon afterwards was appointed adjunct Professor of Anatomy at Harvard

College, and in 1815 succeeded, on the death of his father, to the Hersey Professorship of Anatomy and Physiology at Harvard College, the duties of which he discharged with eminent ability for thirty years. (1847.)

After his retirement from the active duties of his profession, Dr. Warren devoted himself to the study of the natural sciences with a zeal almost unparalleled at his advanced age.

The following account of Dr. Warren's last illness was given to the Suffolk Medical Society, by his old friend the venerable Dr. James Jackson.

"Dr. Warren's death could not be attributed, he said, to any disease which has a distinct name. For a long time his health had been bad, but there was no one marked affection. His friends had long observed a general falling off in his health. Some four years since he was induced to visit the South, and afterwards to go to Europe. From this last visit he derived some benefit. Two years ago he had an œdematous swelling of the feet. He had long before had some trouble about the heart, such as is common with old men, together with some other symptoms of disease, which were not regarded, however, as very alarming. In February last he sent for Dr. Jackson, on account of a slight ophthalmia, which he attributed to a sharp, cold wind. He had long been remarkably sensitive under such exposures. The ophthalmia continued to the time of his death, though it had then greatly diminished. This affection of the eyes seemed to be a slight affair, but it led him to keep his room darkened, and avoid out-of-door exercise as much as possible; and from the confinement, and accompanying depression, he became dyspeptic. He continued, nevertheless, to visit patients occasionally.

"On two occasions within a month of his death, he was seized suddenly with vertigo, followed by copious fecal discharges; but from these attacks he recovered, in each case within twenty-four hours. His last attack, a week before his death, was of the same nature, but with less of vertigo, and more abdominal pain. Dr. Jackson found him on the following morning low and weak, but with no extraordinary symptoms of disease. That day he remained in bed; but on the day following was so much better, that he rode out of town, and there he walked in the garden, on the damp grounds, an exposure unusual for him. In the evening he was attacked for the first time with chills and rigors, had pains in the head and limbs, but most in the abdomen. On Tuesday morning his symptoms were aggravated with alternate chills and heat, a high pulse, parched tongue, loss of appetite, but uncontrollable thirst, and great tenderness in every part of his body. From that time he grew worse daily. He complained of great soreness on the left side, in the trunk and limbs. The tenderness appeared to be confined entirely to the integuments. His nervous system was also affected in various ways.

"From this time his mind gradually failed, but he was at no time delirious. From 3 o'clock P. M. on Saturday, the day before his death, he ceased to pay attention to those around him, being, in the common phrase, "struck with death," and remained lying motionless on his couch, until 3 o'clock A. M. on Sunday, when he ceased to breathe.

"Dr. Jackson thought an examination would be very unlikely to show that death was caused by any local affection. He believed that distress of mind, added to the bad state of his heath previously, had exhausted his vital powers. Dr. Warren had sometimes been called cold, but his (Dr. J.'s) observation satisfied him that he possessed strong and deep feeling, though he seldom exhibited any outward emotion. The death of his first wife preyed on his feelings for a long time. When older and more feeble he was affected in like manner, more powerfully, by the loss of his second wife. At those times he did not show any outward marks of grief, but his vital powers were sinking under his mental suffering. Just so during the last few months he has been overcome by sad tidings respecting the health of his son, who is abroad. But Dr. J. refrained from the discussion of this subject."

The following remarks, made by Dr. Oliver Wendell Holmes, in offering to the Suffolk Medical Society some resolutions expressive of the feelings of the Society in regard to the loss they had sustained, present so eloquent and just a sketch of the character of Dr. Warren, that we cannot deny ourselves the gratification of giving them.

"*Mr. President:* Death has just removed from our midst one long known to us as a leading member of our various local associations; to this community as a most valued professional counsellor and honored citizen; to the profession itself as a master in one of its leading departments, and a laborious teacher of more than a whole generation of practitioners; to the country as one of its ornaments, and to men of learning everywhere as a liberal and enlightened student of Nature. The name of John Collins Warren is stricken from the roll of living men.

"There is no man here, whatever his age or standing, that can hear this brief announcement unmoved. To the old it is a sudden breaking up of associations that half a century of active life has been slowly knitting together. To the young it is one of those startling changes that shift the whole vista of the future; life slides forward a whole stage when those who stand in full relief upon its furthest confines drop beneath the horizon. We have all grown older in more than days since yesterday; we have lost a presence that filled no small space in our habitual outlook, and passed it over to the ever widening domain of memory.

"There have been few men in the time of the oldest among us who have stamped their character more distinctly on their associates than he whom we must now speak of as belonging to the past. He entered life with singular advantages. His father was the leading surgeon of the leading town of New England; had served his country faithfully in the camp and on the field; had founded a school, and was known as an eloquent and ardent teacher. His uncle had shed imperishable lustre upon the name he bore; his alliances gave him influence; his career was unimpeded by the embarrassments common to many who rise in spite of them to eminence.

"It is not much only to inherit advantages, as every day shows us but too clearly; we see the new men carrying off the prizes in every calling, in the face of the hereditary occcupants of power and position. But it is much to know how to bear the temptations of good fortune, or what is so called; to cast off indolence, to despise self-indulgence, to work from a high sense of duty, or even from a noble ambition, as others work from hard necessity.

"Whatever place Dr. Warren acquired or maintained in life, no man can say that he did not earn it and keep it by his own fair labour. In this great centre of life, where an overworking race sends its strongest muscles and its busiest brains to be worn out, it would be hard to name the man who toiled more unremittingly than he, during the busier years of his life. In his vast practice, at the hospital of which he was one of the founders, and where he passed so large a share of his time; in the Professor's chair, the offices of which he performed with signal fidelity and punctuality; everywhere, he was unsparing of his time and his labour. Those of us who met him at that busy period of his life remember him as grave, concentrated, often stern, a man of few words, and those apt to be peremptory, one who went his way bent on his own task, and not lightly to be turned aside from it.

"But neither all the advantages he inherited, nor all the toil he expended, could have given him the place he attained, without elements of personal superiority to lend vitality to both. Somewhere in the mind, or in the character, or in both, must be found the source of that remarkable influence which Dr. Warren exerted during a long series of years, amidst all the competition and the changes of city professional life. If we should look only at his purely intellectual qualities, we should not have reached the secret of his mastery. The varied intellectual power, the wide range of knowledge which belong to the scholar who lives in the world of thought, are not to be expected in the men whose lives are passed in the practical use of applied science. From them we can only demand accuracy instead of breadth of view, sagacity instead of erudition, readiness in the place of versatility. These are the qualities that must belong to the successful surgeon, and these, with a practised hand, and unshaken nerves, were generally granted by the profession and the public to belong to Dr. Warren. But to these qualities, which fitted him for superiority in his peculiar department, were added two other traits, which lay underneath all the rest, and gave them their consummate effectiveness: unswerving concentration of purpose, and unbending force of will. These gave him his unchallenged supremacy in the professional sphere he had chosen.

"To understand his character, we must compare that busy period of his life before referred to with its later years, after he had relinquished the most arduous portion of his daily duties. Then it was that the taste for natural science held sternly in abeyance during a long period of professional toil, was allowed to assert itself, and all might see how resolute must have been the purpose that could have kept it subjugated, and almost unsuspected. Then it was that the pleasant social qualities, overlaid for a time by the weight of severe occupation, found their spontaneous expression; and all could feel that the somewhat austere aspect of his overtasked middle age was only another proof that he had given his whole mind, and heart and strength to cares that might subdue his natural vivacity, and sadden his cordial smile.

"These last years of his life have softened all our recollections of his strenuous years of toil. He had got out of the brawling current, and as he neared the further shore, a quiet eddy carried him far back towards the fountains of his youth. A kindly old man, full of pleasant anecdote, busy with ingenious speculation, loving nature always, and studying her, not as once, in the fearful shapes in which she used to challenge his skill, but under the branches of the "Great Elm," or beneath the buttressed ribs of his huge Mastodon, or hanging over the sandstone tablets where the life of the eternity that is past has left its earlier autograph, he pursued his cheerful labors to the last, bent, but not broken, and so walked softly from among us into the land of shadows.

"I beg leave, Mr. President, to offer the following resolutions:—

"*Resolved*, That in the death of Dr. John Collins Warren, this Society acknowledges a Providential visitation, which has removed from their fellowship an honored and esteemed associate, to whom they have looked for counsel and assistance in all that tends to elevate the profession to which they belong.

"*Resolved*, That we gratefully recognize the hand of divine goodness, which has raised up in this community a succession of able and devoted men, who have identified the name they bore with the noblest acts of self-devotion, the advancement of the highest moral and religious interests, the diligent performance of duty, the promotion of humane and generous enterprises, the enlargement of the bounds of knowledge, and the cultivation of the graces of social intercourse, and that we trust this honored name may long be continued among us, in the children and the children's children of its departed representative.

"*Resolved*, That, as members of the medical profession, we express our sense of the great loss we have sustained in the death of one of its most distinguished members, who, by his natural gifts, his large acquirements, his indefatigable zeal, his untiring industry, his devotion to his calling, has raised the standard of professional excellence, and commanded the respect and confidence of his brethren throughout the country.

"*Resolved*, That, as members of this community, we recall with gratitude the many benefactions he has bestowed upon its public institutions, the labour he has devoted to its charities, the influence he has contributed to its various efforts for moral improvement, the Christian virtues he has exemplified in his life, and all that makes his example a guide to those who follow him in the same range of duties, or in any position of labour and responsibility.

"*Resolved*, That the heartfelt sympathies of this Society be respectfully tendered to the family of the deceased, and that while we assure them their sorrow is shared by all around them, we trust they may find consolation in the memory of the many good works which he did while with us, in the gratitude with which his name will be cherished, and in the trust that a useful and devout earthly existence has prepared him for a life of clearer knowledge and purer happiness."

These resolutions were unanimously adopted.

GRADUATES OF THE UNIVERSITY OF PENNSYLVANIA, 1856.

AT a Public Commencement held March 29th, 1856, at the Musical Fund Hall, the Degree of Doctor of Medicine was conferred by the Provost, HENRY VETHAKE, LL. D., upon the following gentlemen, after which the Valedictory Address was delivered by GEORGE B. WOOD, M. D., Professor of the Theory and Practice of Medicine.

NAME.	RESIDENCE.			ESSAY.
Allen, Joshua G.	Marple,	Delaware,	Pa.	Organic Life Force.
Arthur, Enoch	Frankford,	Philadelphia,	Pa.	Constitutional Peculiarities and their Pathological Tendencies.
Baird, Oscar H.	Petersburg,	Dinwiddie,	Va.	Enteric Fever.
Baldridge, John M.	Bigbyville,	Maury,	Tenn.	The Uterus.
Bannan, Douglass R.	Pottsville,	Schuylkill,	Pa.	Management of Labour.
Barrow, Samuel H.	Ringwood,	Halifax,	N. C.	Intermittent Fever.
Barret, Junius V.	Gainesville,	Sumter,	Ala.	Puerperal Fever.
Baxter, Joseph J.	Currituck C. H.		N. C.	Diseases of Eastern North Carolina.
Beattie, Wm. I.	Bennettsville,	Marlboro',	S. C.	Rheumatism.
Becker, Aaron D.	Bethlehem,	Northampton,	Pa.	Indigestion.
Bettis, Wm. J. F.	Camden,	Wilcox,	Ala.	Enteric Fever.
Birchett, Theophilus G.	Vicksburg,	Warren,	Miss.	Epidemic Cholera.
Blodgett, William J.	Savannah,	Chatham,	Ga.	Intermittent Fever.
Boyd, John M.	Knoxville,	Knox,	Tenn.	Anæsthesia in Labour.
Buck, Frederick J.	Bucksport,	Hancock,	Me.	Development of the Human Ovum.
Butt, H. Fairfield	Portsmouth,	Norfolk,	Va.	Muscular Tissue and Motion.
Byington, William C.	Newark,	Essex,	N. J.	Retroversion of the Uterus.
Capwell, Albert M.	Dunmore,	Luzerne,	Pa.	Pneumonia.
Christie, Robert J.	Stevensburg,	Frederick,	Va.	Fracture of the Patella.
Cohoon, John T. P. C.	Elizabeth City,	Pasquotank,	N. C.	The Tongue.
Coit, David G.	Cheraw,	Chesterfield,	S. C.	Pernicious Fever.
Coit, William N.	Plattsburg,	Clinton,	N. Y.	Anæsthesia.
Coleman, John F.	Uniontown,	Perry,	Ala.	Physiology of Respiration.
Cook, Joseph S.	Easton,	Northampton,	Pa.	Miasmatic Fever.
Cooper, John C.	Washington,	Washington,	Pa.	Epochs of Life.
Corson, Edward F.	Plymouth Meeting,	Montgomery,	Pa.	Vital Heat.
Crockett, Joseph	Wytheville,	Wythe,	Va.	Anatomy of the Ear.
Cross, Joseph F.	Chickahominy,	Hanover,	Va.	Cholera Infantum.
Cunningham, R. C.	Harrisburg,	Pontotoc,	Miss.	Southern Enteric Fever.
Dashiell, W. Bond	Shelbyville,	Bedford,	Tenn.	Auscultation and Percussion.
Dismukes, John L.	Nashville,	Davidson,	Tenn.	Abscesses.
Downes, Robert N.	Philadelphia,		Pa.	Diabetes.
Doyle, Oliver M.	Bounty Land,	Pickens,	S. C.	Congestion.
Drake, Nicholas T.	Hilliardstown,	Nash,	N. C.	Import and Dignity of the Medical Profession.
Dunn, Allen R.	Forrestville,	Wake,	N. C.	Enteric Fever.

NAME.	RESIDENCE.		
Flynn, John	Philadelphia,		Pa.
Fowler, Richard	Burnt Corn,	Monroe,	Ala.
Freeman, Edwin B.	Livingston,	Sumter,	Ala.
Freuch, Edward J.	Palestine,	Crawford,	Ill.
Frow, John G.	Mifflintown,	Juniata,	Pa.
Fuller, Francis T.	Kittrel,	Granville,	N. C.
Gillette, Fidelio B.	Shiloh,	Cumberland,	N. J.
Graham, John W.	Alexandria,		Va.
Grant, James F.	Bradshaw,	Giles,	Tenn.
Green, Richard M.	Princeton,	Dallas,	Ark.
Green, William J.	Rolesville,	Wake,	N. C.
Hall, William B.	Lowndesboro',	Lowndes,	Ala.
Hand, Daniel W.	Cape May C. H.		N. J.
Handy, William N.	Philada.,		Pa.
Harry, Samuel M.	Ercildown,	Chester,	Pa.
Haynie, R. Alpheus	Sperryville,	Rappahannock,	Va.
Hays, David S.	Hollidaysburg,	Blair,	Pa.
Helwig, Theodore A.	Philadelphia,		Pa.
Hildrith, Joseph S.	Somerville,	Middlesex,	Mass.
Holloway, Robert G.	Port Royal,	Caroline,	Va.
Hughes, James B.	Newberne,	Craven,	N. C.
Hutchison, James	Potter's Mills,	Centre,	Pa.
Jackson, Bailey	Elizabeth City,	Pasquotank,	N. C.
Jennings, Julius T.	Bennettsville,	Marlboro',	S. C.
Jones, Joseph	Riceboro',	Liberty,	Ga.
Jones, Joseph E.	West Chester,	Chester,	Pa.
Jones, Lewis H.	Milldale,	Warren,	Miss.
Jones, Thomas	Philadelphia,		Pa.
Jones, William K.	Petersburg,	Dinwiddie,	Va.
Kerlin, Isaac N.	Philadelphia,		Pa.
Kirby, William R.	Milldale,	Warren,	Miss.
Kitchen, Francis A.	Easton,	Northampton,	Va.
La Roche, C. Percy	Philadelphia,		Pa.
Lennard, Benjamin F.	Cuthbert,	Randolph,	Ga.
Leverett, Frederick P.	Pocotaligo,	Beaufort,	S. C.
Lewis, Richard H.	Chapel Hill,	Orange,	N. C.
Longstreth, M. Fisher	Philadelphia,		Pa.
Lowry, William M.	Lowry,	Bedford,	Va.
Lummis, George B.	Philadelphia,		Pa.
Lunday, William E.	Albany,	Dougherty,	Ga.
Mallory, Joseph B.	Memphis,	Shelby,	Tenn.
Mann, Theophilus H.	Henderson,	Granville,	N. C.
Marshall, Calvin P.	Newport,	Newcastle,	Del.
Marshall, Thomas	Markham,	Fauquier,	Va.

NAME.	RESIDENCE.			ESSAY.
Martin, Edwin G.	Allentown,	Lehigh,	Pa.	Moral and Physical Condition of Woman.
Maury, Thomas F.	Washington,		D. C.	Puerperal Convulsions.
Maynard, James G.	English Town,	Monmouth,	N. J.	Pneumonia.
Mazaredo, Ramon de	Cienfuegos,		Cuba.	Fractures.
Meaux, Thomas O.	New Orleans,		La.	Malignant Tumour.
M'Alpin, Sumner M.	Nixburg,	Coosa,	Ala.	Physical Diagnosis.
M'Cormick, Henry	Springfield,	Clark,	Ohio.	Homœopathic Remedies.
M'Elhiney, James P.	St. Charles,	St. Charles,	Mo.	Intermittent Fever.
M'Lemore, Sydney S.	Springhill,	Maury,	Tenn.	Crural Phlebitis.
M'Nairy, William J.	Pulaski,	Giles,	Tenn.	Dyspepsia.
Millen, George R.	Savannah,	Chatham,	Ga.	Morbid Sensibility of the Stomach.
Offutt, Thomas Z.	Rockville,	Montgomery,	Md.	Anatomy and Philosophy of the Brain.
Orendorff, Olcott	Columbia,	Herkimer,	N. Y.	Scarlatina.
Overton, Jesse	Columbia,	Maury,	Tenn.	Intermittent Fever.
Park, Robert W.	Aberdeen,	Monroe,	Miss.	Inflammation.
Parmer, Thomas J.	Pintlala,	Montgomery,	Ala.	Pulmonary Auscultation.
Peale, J. Burd	Pottsville,	Schuylkill,	Pa.	Influence of Emotion on Function of Secretion.
Percy, Robert	Trinity,	Concordia,	La.	Scarlatina.
Phillips, Albert L.	Raleigh,	Wake,	N. C.	Decarbonization of the Blood.
Pott, Samuel U.	Muncy,	Lycoming,	Pa.	Menstruation.
Riddick, William M.	Gatesville,	Gates,	N. C.	Scarlatina.
Ritz, Ambrose H.	Lewistown,	Mifflin,	Pa.	Asphyxia.
Rodgers, John H.	Springfield,	Clark,	Ohio.	Puerperal Convulsions.
Rowland, James S.	Hopkinsville,	Christian,	Ky.	The Human Mind.
Sandeford, G. Tyson	Bath,		Eng.	Yellow Fever in the British West Indies.
Sawyers, James H.	Knoxville,	Knox,	Tenn.	Vaccination.
Saunders, Dudley D.	Mobile,		Ala.	Action of Medicines.
Schultz, Solomon S.	Clayton,	Berks,	Pa.	The Study of Medicine.
Senderling, P. M.	Troy,	Rensselaer,	N. Y.	Insanity.
Shannon, Robert W.	Franklin,	Williamson,	Tenn.	Acute Muco-Enteritis.
Sheild, William H.	Yorktown,	York,	Va.	Bright's Disease.
Smith, Albert H.	Philadelphia,		Pa.	Influence of the Mind in Disease.
Snyder, Jno. J.	Bethlehem,	Northampton,	Pa.	Signs of Pregnancy.
Sterling, John	Morrisville,	Bucks,	Pa.	Intermittent Fever.
Taylor, De Witt C.	Philadelphia,		Pa.	Puerperal Fever.
Taylor, Thomas L.	Fredericksburg,	Spottsylvania,	Va.	Enteric Fever.
Thach, William T.	Mooresville,	Limestone,	Ala.	Enteric Fever.
Thomas, James Gray	Cedar Rock,	Franklin,	N. C.	Yellow Fever.
Thomas, Joseph	Milestown,	Philadelphia,	Pa.	Enteric Fever.
Tillum, B. Franklin,	West Chester,	Chester,	Pa.	Medicine.
Tutt, Charles Pendleton	Leesburg,	Loudon,	Va.	Endocarditis.
Tweedy, Robert E.	Courtland,	Lawrence,	Ala.	Enteric Fever.
Tyler, R. Bradley	Frederick,	Frederick,	Md.	Inguinal Hernia.
Vandyke, Edward B.	Princeton,	Mercer,	N. J.	Inflammation.
Vest, Nathaniel A.	Negrofoot,	Hanover,	Va.	Intermittent Fever.

NAME.	RESIDENCE.			ESSAY.
Walker, J. Newton	Marcus Hook,	Delaware,	Pa.	Pneumonia.
Walton, John Tompkins	Philadelphia,		Pa.	Experiments on Digestion.
Ware, John G.	Berryville,	Clark,	Va.	Typhoid Fever.
Warren, John L.	Newark,	Newcastle,	Del.	Origin of Vegetation.
Watts, Edward M.	Portsmouth,	Norfolk,	Va.	Anatomy of Mucous Membrane.
Wells, W. Lehman	Philadelphia,		Pa.	The Eye.
White, William W.	Aberdeen,	Monroe,	Miss.	Scarlatina.
Whitfield, George	Montgomery,	Montgomery,	Ala.	Acute Cystitis.
Whitley, Hillory M.	Forestville,	Wake,	N. C.	Cholera Infantum.
Wiggins, Alfred S.	Ringwood,	Halifax,	N. C.	Inguinal Hernia.
Williams, Charles J.	Pittsboro',	Chatham,	N. C.	Acute Dysentery.
Williams, Junius	Bolivar,	Hardeman,	Tenn.	Pneumonia.
Woodward, William E.	Cambridge,	Dorchester,	Md.	Enteric Fever.
Xaupi, Xenophon Xavier	St. Louis,		Mo.	Granular Conjunctivitis.
Young, Allen R.	Rolesville,	Wake,	N. C.	Miasma.
Zimmerman, Daniel A.	Darlington,	Darlington,	S. C.	Intermittent Fever.

At the Commencement, July 3, 1856.

Chas. B. Griffin,	Salem,	Roanoke,	Va.	Extra-Uterine Pregnancy.
Philip D. Grove,	Sharpsburg,	Washington,	Md.	Tubercular Melanosis.

TOTAL, 142.

PENNSYLVANIA COLLEGE—MEDICAL DEPARTMENT.

SESSION OF 1856–'57.

The regular Course of Lectures will commence on Monday, October 13th, and will be continued until the 1st of March.

FACULTY.

DAVID GILBERT, M. D., Professor of Obstetrics and Diseases of Women and Children.
ALFRED STILLÉ, M. D., Professor of Theory and Practice of Medicine.
JOHN NEILL, M. D., Professor of Surgery.
J. M. ALLEN, M. D., Professor of Special and Surgical Anatomy.
JOHN J. REESE, M. D., Professor of Medical Chemistry.
JOHN B. BIDDLE, M. D., Professor of Therapeutics and Materia Medica.
FRANCIS G. SMITH, M. D., Professor of Institutes of Medicine.

H. W. DE SAUSSURE FORD, M. D., Demonstrator of Anatomy.

Clinical Instruction will be given by Professors BIDDLE and NEILL, at the *Philadelphia Hospital, Blockley*, during the entire term of the session, in conjunction with other members of the Medical Board of the Hospital. The Students of Pennsylvania College—*both first course and second course*—will be furnished *gratuitously* with the ticket to the Philadelphia Hospital. Second-course students have the option of receiving gratuitously the ticket to the Pennsylvania Hospital. A Clinic will also be held at the College, every Wednesday and Saturday morning throughout the session.

FEES.

For the entire Course of Lectures	$105 00
Matriculation (paid once only)	5 00
Graduation	30 00

The Dissecting Rooms will be opened in September, under the direction of the Professor of Anatomy, and the Demonstrator.

Preliminary Lectures will be delivered during the fortnight preceding the opening of the session.

JOHN J. REESE, M. D., *Registrar*,
No. 342 Walnut Street, Philadelphia.

July, 1856.—4t.

PHILADELPHIA COLLEGE OF MEDICINE.

FIFTH STREET, BELOW WALNUT.

The WINTER SESSION of 1856–57 will commence early in October, 1856, and terminate in the following March.

The SPRING SESSION will commence early in March, 1857, and continue until the middle of July.

Degrees are conferred in March and July.

FACULTY.

JOSEPH PARRISH, M. D., Emeritus Professor of Midwifery and Diseases of Women and Children.

GEORGE HEWSTON, M. D., Professor of Anatomy.
B. HOWARD RAND, M. D., " Medical Chemistry.
HENRY HARTSHORNE, M. D., " Institutes of Medicine.
JAMES L. TYSON, M. D., " Materia Medica.
ALFRED T. KING, M. D., " Theory and Practice of Medicine.
GEORGE DOCK, M. D., " Surgery.
LEWIS D. HARLOW, M. D., " Midwifery and Diseases of Women and Children.

FEES: For one full Course, $84; Perpetual ticket, $150; Matriculation, $5; Practical Anatomy, $10; Graduation, $30.

Examinations are held daily by the Professors on each branch, and besides the usual Hospital advantages, advanced Students have the privilege of attending out-door patients, in connection with the Clinique, under charge of the Professors.

For further information, apply to B. HOWARD RAND, M. D., DEAN,
At the College, Fifth Street below Walnut.

JEFFERSON MEDICAL COLLEGE.

The Course of Lectures will commence on Monday, the 13th of October, and continue until the 1st of March.

Thos. D. Mütter, M. D., Emeritus Professor of Surgery.

Institutes of Medicine, etc.,	By Prof. Robley Dunglison, M. D.
Materia Medica and General Therapeutics,	" Prof. Robert M. Huston, M. D.
General, Descriptive and Surgical Anatomy,	" Prof. Joseph Pancoast, M. D.
Practice of Medicine,	" Prof. J. K. Mitchell, M. D.
Obstetrics and Diseases of Women and Children,	" Prof. Charles D. Meigs, M. D.
Chemistry,	" Prof. Franklin Bache, M. D.
Institutes and Practice of Surgery,	" Prof. Samuel D. Gross, M. D.
Demonstrator of Anatomy,	" Ellerslie Wallace, M. D.

Every Wednesday and Saturday in the month of October, and during the course, Medical and Surgical cases will be investigated, prescribed for, and lectured on before the Class. During the year ending March the first, 1856, *sixteen hundred and fifteen* cases were treated, and *two hundred and sixty-seven* operations were performed; amongst them many major operations—as amputation of the thigh, leg, and arm at the shoulder-joint, extirpation of the upper jaw, mammæ, &c., lithotomy, trephining and resection of the elbow-joint.

The lectures are so arranged as to permit the student to attend the medical and surgical practice and lectures at the Pennsylvania Hospital, and the Philadelphia Hospital.

On and after the 1st of October, the dissecting rooms will be open, under the direction of the Professor of Anatomy and the Demonstrator.

Fees:

Matriculation, which is paid only once,	$ 5
To each Member of the Faculty $15,	105
Graduation,	30

ROBLEY DUNGLISON, M. D.,
Dean of the Faculty.

Philadelphia: June, 1856.

UNIVERSITY OF LOUISIANA, MEDICAL DEPARTMENT.

The Annual Course of Lectures in this department will commence on Monday, November 19, 1855, and will terminate in the ensuing March.

James Jones, M. D.,	Professor of Practice of Medicine.
J. L. Riddell, M. D.,	Professor of Chemistry.
Warren Stone, M. D.,	Professor of Surgery.
A. H. Cenas, M. D.,	Professor of Obstetrics.
A. J. Wedderburn, M. D.,	Professor of Anatomy.
Gustavus A. Nott, M. D.,	Professor of Materia Medica.
Thomas Hunt, M. D.,	Professor of Physiology and Pathology.
Cornelius Beard, M. D., Samuel Choppin, M. D.,	Demonstrators of Anatomy.

The rooms for Dissecting will be open on the third Monday in October.

The Faculty are Visiting Physicians and Surgeons of the Charity Hospital, and attend this Institution from November to April.

The Students accompany the Professors in their visits, and, free of expense, enjoy extraordinary practical advantages.

There are, during the Session, about eight hundred persons prescribed for daily.

In 1854, the number of patients was thirteen thousand one hundred and ninety-two.

THOMAS HUNT, M. D., *Dean.*

The Administrators of the Charity Hospital elect annually, in April, fourteen resident students, who are maintained by the Institution.

UNIVERSITY OF NEW YORK.

MEDICAL DEPARTMENT—SESSION 1856-7.

The Session for 1856–7 will begin on Monday, October 13, and will be continued until the 1st of March.

Course of Instruction.—The Courses of Lectures given will be on Anatomy—general, descriptive, surgical, and pathological; Principles and Operations of Surgery; Materia Medica and Therapeutics; Institutes and Practice of Medicine; Obstetrics, the Diseases of Women and Children, with Clinical Midwifery; Chemistry and Physiology; Clinical Surgery; Clinical Medicine; Clinical Lectures on the Diseases of the Genito-Urinary Organs; Clinical Lectures on the Diseases of Women and Children; Clinical Lectures on Physical Diagnosis.

FACULTY OF MEDICINE.

Rev. Isaac Ferris, D. D., LL. D., *Chancellor of the University.*

Valentine Mott, M. D., LL. D., Emeritus Professor of Surgery and Surgical Anatomy, and Ex-President of the Faculty.
Martyn Paine, M. D., LL. D., Professor of Materia Medica and Therapeutics.
Gunning S. Bedford, M. D., Professor of Obstetrics, the Diseases of Women and Children, and Clinical Midwifery.
John W. Draper, M. D., LL. D., Professor of Chemistry and Physiology.
Alfred C. Post, M, D., Professor of the Principles and Operations of Surgery, with Surgical and Pathological Anatomy.
William H. Van Buren, M. D., Professor of General and Descriptive Anatomy.
John T. Metcalfe, M. D., Professor of the Institutes and Practice of Medicine.

Charles E. Isaacs, M. D., Demonstrator of Anatomy.
George A. Peters, M. D., Prosector to the Professor of Surgery.
Alexander B. Mott, M. D., Prosector to the Emeritus Professor of Surgery.

John W. Draper, M. D., LL. D., President of the Faculty.

Clinical Instruction.—Clinical instruction constitutes a prominent feature in the plan of education; and the unlimited resources of New York enable the Faculty to carry out the object which, to the practitioner, whether in surgery, medicine, or obstetrics, is the great end of medical study—namely, *familiarity with disease at the bedside.*

1. *Obstetric Clinique for the Diseases of Women and Children* every Monday P. M., by Prof. Bedford.
2. *Surgical Clinique* every Tuesday, by Prof. Mott.
3. *Medical Clinique* every Wednesday, by Prof. Metcalfe.
4. *Surgical Clinique, with the Diseases of the Genito-Urinary Organs,* every Wednesday P. M., by Prof. Van Buren.
5. *Surgical Clinique* every Saturday P. M., by Prof. Post.

Hospitals, Infirmaries, Dispensaries.—These well known Institutions afford ample opportunities to the Student. Professors Mott and Post are Consulting Surgeons, and Prof. Van Buren an Attending Surgeon at the *New York City Hospital;* and Prof. Metcalfe an Attending Physician at the *Bellevue Hospital.*

Practical Anatomy.—The study of Anatomy having been legalized by the Legislature, there will be an abundance of material. The Demonstrator's fee is five dollars, and the usual rates will be charged for the material, to defray the incidental expenses and to prevent waste.

Museum, Apparatus, &c.—The College is amply provided with all these facilities for instruction.

[Continued on next page.

MEDICAL COLLEGE OF THE STATE OF SOUTH CAROLINA.

The annual Course of Lectures in this Institution will commence on the first Monday in November, on the following branches:—

Anatomy by	J. E. Holbrook, M. D.
Surgery by	E. Geddings, M. D.
Institutes and Practice of Medicine by .	S. Henry Dickson, M. D., LL. D.
Physiology by	James Moultrie, M. D.
Materia Medica by	Henry R. Frost, M. D.
Obstetrics by	Thos. G. Pridleau, M. D.
Chemistry by	C. U. Shepard, M. D.
Demonstrator of Anatomy . . .	F. T. Miles, M. D.
Prosector to the Professor of Surgery .	T. F. M. Geddings, M. D.

CLINICAL INSTRUCTION.

D. T. Cain, M. D., Physician to the Marine Hospital and Clinical Instructor, lectures twice a week on the diseases of that Institution.

At the *Roper Hospital* Clinical Lectures are delivered twice a week by the Physician and Surgeon of the Institution, and operations performed before the class in the Amphitheatre of the Hospital.

The *Faculty Ward in the Roper Hospital.*—By the conveniences they have been able to furnish, a valuable addition has been made to the surgical practice of the city. Operations are performed before the class, and they have opportunities of being familiar with the subsequent treatment.

The anatomical rooms are opened the latter part of October, and the dissections conducted daily under the direction of the Demonstrator. Much attention is directed to this department; the material being abundant, and illustrations of various character being afforded for acquiring a competent knowledge of this all-important branch of study.

HENRY R. FROST, M. D., *Dean.*

Charleston, June, 1856.

PREMIUMS

OFFERED BY THE MEDICAL COLLEGE OF THE STATE OF SOUTH CAROLINA.

To promote scientific attainments, and to excite emulation in the youth of our College, two members of the Faculty offer to THE CANDIDATES FOR GRADUATION at the ensuing session of the College, premiums of $100 cash, or an equivalent, for any of the following productions:—

1. An original Treatise upon any subject in Pathology or Therapeutics. Or,
2. If no original Treatise is offered, for a production on the above subjects which will commend itself for its literary, scientific or practical applications to the wants of society, or the relief of suffering humanity. Or,
3. If without the opportunity of being practical in all its bearings, the production should commend itself by being suggestive, and thus likely to prove practically useful.

Communications will be classified as above, and a preference given to the order in which they stand—the decided merit in either will command a corresponding consideration.

The usual conditions to prevent undue partiality, will be observed, and the adjudication will be committed to three professional gentlemen of our community, who may be selected by Henry R. Frost, M. D., Professor of Materia Medica in the Medical College of the State of South Carolina.

The successful candidate will be declared upon the commencement day of the College, and the premiums then and there awarded.

UPON SURGERY.

By another Professor of the College, a Premium of $100 will, with similar motives and conditions, be awarded for the best Treatise upon a Surgical subject. All productions designed to compete for this prize, besides containing a fair summary of the existing information on the subject, should, as far as possible, be supported by original observations or experiments.

Communications to be addressed to E. GEDDINGS, M. D., Professor of Surgery in the Medical College of the State of South Carolina, and should bear a motto, with a sealed letter inclosing the author's name.

TO READERS AND CORRESPONDENTS.

The following works have been received:—

An Exposition of the Signs and Symptoms of Pregnancy: with some other papers on Subjects connected with Midwifery. By W. F. Montgomery, A. M., M. D., M. R. I. A., Ex-Scholar of Trinity College, Dublin; Professor of Midwifery in the King and Queen's College of Physicians in Ireland; lately President of that College and one of the Presidents of the Pathological Society; one of the Presidents of the Obstetrical Society, etc. Second edition. London: Longman, Brown, Green, Longmans, & Roberts, 1856. (From the Author.)

Report of the Recent Yellow Fever Epidemic of British Guiana. By Daniel Blair, M. D., Surgeon-General of British Guiana. London: John Churchill, 1856. (From the Author.)

Das Normalverhältniss der Chemischen und Morphologischen Proportionem. Von Adolph Zeiding. Leipzig: Rudolph Weigel, 1856. (From the Author.)

On the Diseases of Infants and Children. By Fleetwood Churchill, M. D., M. R. I. A.; Hon. Fellow of the College of Physicians of Ireland; Hon. Member of the Philadelphia Medical Society, etc. Second American edition. Enlarged and revised by the Author. Edited, with additions, by William F. Keating, M. D., A. M., Physician to St. Joseph's Hospital, etc. Philadelphia: Blanchard & Lea, 1856. (From the Publishers.)

A Review of the Present State of Uterine Pathology. By James Henry Bennett, M. D., Member of the Royal College of Physicians; Phys. Acc. to the Royal Free Hospital, etc. Philadelphia: Blanchard & Lea, 1856. (From the Publishers.)

A Treatise on Therapeutics and Pharmacology or Materia Medica. By George B. Wood, M. D., Late President of the American Medical Association; President of the College of Physicians of Philadelphia; Professor of the Theory and Practice of Medicine in the University of Pennsylvania; Senior Physician of the Pennsylvania Hospital, etc. etc. In two volumes. Philadelphia: J. B. Lippincott & Co. London: Trübner & Co., 1856. (From the Author.)

Lectures on Materia Medica and Therapeutics. Delivered in the College of Physicians and Surgeons of the University of the State of New York. By John B. Beck, M. D., Late Professor of Materia Medica and Medical Jurisprudence. Prepared for the press by his friend, C. R. Gilman, M. D., Professor of Obstetrics, etc. in the College of Physicians and Surgeons, New York. Second edition. New York: S. S. & W. Wood, 1856. (From the Publishers.)

The Physicians' Visiting List, Diary, and Book of Engagements for 1857. Philadelphia: Lindsay & Blakiston. (From the Publishers.)

Human Physiology, Statical and Dynamical; or the Conditions and Course of the Life of Man. By John William Draper, M. D., LL. D., Professor of Chemistry and Physics in the University of New York. New York: Harper & Brothers, 1856. (From the Publishers.)

New Elements of Operative Surgery. By Alfred A. L. M. Velpeau, Professor of Surgical Clinique of the Faculty of Medicine of Paris; Surgeon of the Hospital of La Charité; Member of the Royal Academy of Medicine and of the Institute, etc. Carefully revised. Entirely remodelled and augmented with a Treatise on Minor Surgery. Illustrated by over 200 engravings. Incorporated with the text; accompanied with an Atlas in quarto of twenty-two Plates representing the principal operative processes, surgical instruments, etc. Translated, with additions, by P. S. Townsend, M. D., Late Physician to the Seaman's Retreat, Staten Island, New York. Under the supervision of, and with notes and observations by Valentine Mott, M. D., Professor of the

Operations of Surgery, with Surgical and Pathological Anatomy in the University of New York; Foreign Associate of the Acad. Roy. de Med. of Paris, etc. Fourth edition, with additions by George C. Blackman, M. D., Professor of Surgery in the Medical College of Ohio, etc. In three volumes. New York: Samuel S. and W. Wood, No. 389 Broadway, 1856. Three volumes and one volume of plates. (From the Publishers.)

Hints on the Medical Examination of Recruits for the Army and on the Discharge of Soldiers from the Service on Surgeon's Certificate. Adapted to the Service of the United States. By Thomas Henderson, M. D., Assistant-Surgeon U. S. A., etc. A new edition. Revised by Richard H. Coolidge, M. D., Assistant-Surgeon U. S. A. Philadelphia: J. B. Lippincott & Co., 1856.

The Obstetric Memoirs and Contributions of James Y. Simpson, M. D., F. R. S. E., &c. Edited by W. O. Priestley, M. D., Edinburgh, and Horatio R. Storer, M. D., Boston, U. S. Vol. II. Philadelphia: J. B. Lippincott & Co., 1856. (From the Publishers.)

Obstetric Tables. By Dr. Pajot, Agrégé Professor in the Faculty of Medicine, Paris. Translated from the French, and arranged by O. A. Crenshaw, M. D., and J. B. McCaw, M. D. With three additional Tables on the Mechanism of Natural, Unnatural, and Complex Labour. By N. P. Rice, M. D., New York.

Transactions of the Seventh Annual Meeting of the Medical Society of the State of North Carolina. Held at Raleigh, N. C., May, 1856. Washington, N. C., 1856.

Memoir of Moreton Stillé, M. D. Read before the Philadelphia College of Physicians of Philadelphia, April 2, 1856. By Samuel L. Hollingsworth, M. D. Philadelphia, 1856.

Address to the Graduates of the Vermont Medical College of the Class of 1856. By Wm. Henry Thayer, M. D., Professor of Pathology and Practice of Medicine. Keene, N. H., 1856. (From the Author.)

History of the Ligature applied to the Brachio-Cephalic Artery; with Statistics of the Operation. (Paper read before the Tennessee State Medical Society, May, 1856.) By Paul F. Eve, M. D. Nashville, 1856.

Remarks on the Lunacy Laws, as also Asylums of Scotland and France. By John Webster, M. D., F. R. S., and F. R. C. P., Physician to the Scottish Hospital. (From the Author.)

Physicians' Tabulated Diary, designed to Facilitate the Study of Diseases at the Bedside. By a Physician of Virginia. J. W. Randolph. Richmond, Va., 1856.

Report of the Board of Managers of the Pennsylvania Hospital to the Contributors at their annual meeting, held fifth month 5th, 1856. Together with the Accounts of the Treasurer and Stewards. Philadelphia, 1856.

Annual Catalogue and Announcement of the St. Louis Medical College. Session 1856–57. St. Louis, 1856.

A Catalogue of all the Graduates of the Jefferson Medical College of Philadelphia; with Announcement for 1856–57. Philadelphia, 1856.

Annual Announcement of the Faculty of McGill College, Montreal, for the Session 1856–57. Montreal, 1856.

The following Journals have been received in exchange:—

Moniteur des Hôpitaux. June, July, August, 1856.

Revue de Thérapeutique Médico-Chirurgicale. Par A. Martin-Lauzer. June, July, August, 1856.

Gazette Médicale de Paris. June, July, August, 1856.

Annales Médico-Psychologiques. Edited by Drs. Baillarger, Cerise, and Moreau (de Tours). July, 1856.

Archiv. für Ophthalmologie. Herausgegeben von Professor F. Arlt, in Prague, Professor F. C. Donders in Utrecht, und Dr. A. Von Graefe in Berlin. Zweiter Band. Abtheilung, I., II.

Edinburgh Medical Journal. June, July, August, 1856.

The Dublin Hospital Gazette. June, July, August, 1856.

Association Medical Journal. Edited by Andrew Wynter, M.D. May, June, July, August, 1856.

The British and Foreign Medico-Chirurgical Review. July, 1856.

The Journal of Psychological Medicine and Mental Pathology. Edited by FORBES WINSLOW, M. D. July, 1856.

The Half-Yearly Abstract of the Medical Sciences. January to June, 1856.

The Glasgow Medical Journal. July, 1856.

The Retrospect of Medicine. Edited by W. BRAITHWAITE. January to June, 1856.

The Journal of Public Health and Sanitary Reform. Edited by BENJAMIN W. RICHARDSON, M. D. July, 1856.

The Indian Annals of Medical Science. April, 1856.

The Dublin Quarterly Journal of Medical Sciences. August, 1856.

The Medical Chronicle of Montreal Monthly Journal of Medicine and Surgery. Edited by WILLIAM WRIGHT, M. D. July, August, September, 1856.

The New York Medical Times. Edited by H. D. BULKLEY, M. D. July, August, and September, 1856.

Southern Medical and Surgical Journal. Edited by Drs. L. A. DUGAS and HENRY ROSSIGNOL. July, August, September, 1856.

Buffalo Medical Journal. June, July, August, September, 1856.

New Orleans Medical News and Hospital Gazette. Edited by Drs. CHOPPIN, BEARD, and BRICKELL, July, August, September, 1856.

Virginia Medical Journal. Edited by Drs. McCAW and OTIS. July, August, September, 1856.

The Louisville Review. Edited by Drs. GROSS and RICHARDSON. July and September, 1856.

The Medical and Surgical Reporter. Edited by S. W. BUTLER, M. D. July, August, September, 1856.

Nashville Journal of Medicine and Surgery. Edited by W. K. BOWLING and P. F. EVE. July, August, 1856.

The Ohio Medical and Surgical Journal. Edited by JOHN DAWSON, M. D. July, September, 1856.

The Peninsular Journal of Medicine and the Collateral Sciences. Edited by Drs. ZINA PITCHER, A. PALMER, WM. BRODIE, and E. P. CHRISTIAN. July, August, September, 1856.

The Western Lancet. Edited by T. WOOD. July, August, September, 1856.

Atlanta Medical and Surgical Journal. Edited by J. F. LOGAN, M. D., and W. F. WESTMORELAND, M. D. July, August, 1856.

The American Journal of Insanity. July, 1856.

The Northwestern Medical and Surgical Journal. Edited by N. S. DAVIS, M. D., and H. A. JOHNSON, M. D. July, 1856.

The American Journal of Dental Science. Edited by C. A. HARRIS, M. D., and A. S. PIGGOT, M. D. July, 1856.

The New York Journal of Medicine. Edited by S. S. PURPLE, M. D., STEPHEN SMITH, M. D., and H. D. BULKLEY, M. D. July, September, 1856.

The American Journal of Science and Arts. Conducted by Professor B. SILLIMAN, B. SILLIMAN, Jr., and J. D. DANA. July, September, 1856.

Charleston Medical Journal and Review. C. HAPPOLDT, M. D., Editor. July, and September, 1856.

American Journal of Pharmacy. Published by authority of the Philadelphia College of Pharmacy. Edited by WM. PROCTER, Jr., Professor of Pharmacy in Philadelphia College of Pharmacy. July, September, 1856.

The American Medical Gazette and Journal of Health. Edited by D. M. REESE, M. D. July, August, September, 1856.

Boston Medical and Surgical Journal. Edited by Dr. J. V. C. SMITH, WM. W. MORLAND, and FRANCIS MINOT. July, August, September, 1856.

New York Dental Recorder. Edited by CHARLES W. BALLARD, D. D. S. July, August, 1856.

The Cincinnati Medical Observer. Edited by Drs. MENDENHALL, MURPHEY, and STEVENS. July, August, September, 1856.

The New Hampshire Journal of Medicine. Edited by Drs. GEORGE H. HUBBARD and N. E. GAGE. July, August, September, 1856.

The Monthly Stethoscope. Edited by Drs. G. A. Wilson and R. A. Lewis. July, August, September, 1856.

St. Louis Medical and Surgical Journal. Edited by Drs. Linton and McPheeters. July and September, 1856.

The Medical Examiner. Edited by Samuel L. Hollingsworth, M. D. July, August, September, 1856.

Iowa Medical Journal. Edited by Drs. D. L. McGugin and J. R. Allen. May and June, 1866.

The Memphis Medical Recorder. Edited by A. P. Merrill, M. D. July, 1856.

The New Orleans Medical and Surgical Journal. Edited by Bennet Dowler, M. D. July and September, 1856.

The California State Medical Journal. Edited by J. F. Morse, M. D. July, 1856.

Communications intended for publication, and Books for Review, should be sent, *free of expense*, directed to Isaac Hays, M. D., Editor of the American Journal of the Medieal Sciences, care of Messrs. Blanchard & Lea, Philadelphia. Parcels directed as above, and (carriage paid) under cover, to John Miller, Henrietta Street, Covent Garden, *London;* or M. Hector Bossange, Lib. quai Voltaire, No. 11, *Paris*, will reach us safely and without delay. We particularly request the attention of our foreign correspondents to the above, as we are often subjected to unnecessary expense for postage and carriage.

All remittances of money, and letters on the *business* of the Journal, should be addressed *exclusively* to the publishers, Messrs. Blanchard & Lea.

☞ The advertisement-sheet belongs to the business department of the Journal, and all communications for it should be made to the publishers.

CONTENTS

OF THE

AMERICAN JOURNAL

OF THE

MEDICAL SCIENCES.

NO. LXIV. NEW SERIES.

OCTOBER, 1856.

ORIGINAL COMMUNICATIONS.

MEMOIRS AND CASES.

QUARTERLY SUMMARY

OF THE

IMPROVEMENTS AND DISCOVERIES IN THE MEDICAL SCIENCES.

FOREIGN INTELLIGENCE.

Anatomy and Physiology.

Materia Medica and Pharmacy.

Medical Pathology and Therapeutics, and Practical Medicine.

Surgical Pathology and Therapeutics, and Operative Surgery.

OPHTHALMOLOGY.

MIDWIFERY.

HYGIENE.

Medical Jurisprudence and Toxicology.

AMERICAN INTELLIGENCE.

Original Communications.

Domestic Summary.

THE

AMERICAN JOURNAL

OF THE MEDICAL SCIENCES

FOR OCTOBER 1856.

ART. I.—*The Physiological Effects of Alcohol and Tobacco upon the Human System.* By WILLIAM A. HAMMOND, M.D., Assistant Surgeon, U. S. Army.

THE present paper is intended to exhibit the action of alcohol and tobacco upon the system generally, and, more especially, upon the important functions concerned in the metamorphosis of tissue.

The experiments illustrative of the effects of these substances were performed upon myself, and were conducted with all the care and accuracy which my limited facilities permitted. Those only who are familiar with investigations of this character can appreciate the time and labour necessary to conduct them properly, and but for the improved and extended system of volumetric analysis now so much employed in physiological chemistry, I should probably have been compelled to refrain from inquiries necessarily tedious at the best, but incomparably more so when the older methods of quantitative analysis are observed. Yet, when we reflect, however tiresome and even disgusting physiological investigations often are, that it is only by actual experiments we can ever hope to lay the foundations of true physiological science, we can well afford, for the sake of accomplishing so noble an end, to labour cheerfully on, even though the way be not so nice as we might desire. The day of extravagant theories, unsupported by observation, has gone by, and he who has nothing better to offer than the unsustained creation of a dreamy mind, meets with but little attention, and merits still less than he receives.

The influence of *alcohol* upon the human system has recently been the subject of thorough investigation by Dr. Böcker, who, with a degree of zeal worthy the importance of the inquiry, performed a series of experiments upon himself which have rarely been excelled for completeness and accuracy; but as the conclusions derived from his observations have met with the opposition of several distinguished physiologists, additional investigation seemed not altogether uncalled for.

The experiments relating to the action of *tobacco* detailed in the present paper, are believed to be the first of the character which have been performed. Physicians have heretofore been content to decry its use as uniformly injurious, without seeking for a reason for its deleterious influence, or even attempting to show that it was so generally pernicious as they believed. That both it and alcohol, when used with discretion, are capable of exercising highly beneficial effects upon the organism, will be abundantly shown from the ensuing experiments. Their influence, however, is not constantly advantageous, and when employed under circumstances which do not justify their use (like many other articles of food of much less doubtful reputation), they may produce results which are far from conducive to health.

My own system was, I conceived, well calculated to exhibit the action of these agents satisfactorily. Not being in the habit of using either of them, I was peculiarly sensitive to their influence, and was able to perceive effects which, in a person more habituated to their use, might have escaped observation.

My manner of living during the succeeding investigations was as follows:—

I arose every morning at six o'clock, and retired to bed every night at eleven. I was thus awake seventeen hours, and asleep seven. The seventeen waking hours were thus appropriated: ten were assigned to study of as uniform a character as possible, five to daily duties, recreation, &c., and two to a uniform system of physical exercise. This course was rigorously insisted on throughout the whole of the experiments with both alcohol and tobacco.

ALCOHOL.—I had three objects in view in investigating the action of this agent.

1. To observe its effects upon a system in which the weight of the body was *maintained at a nearly uniform standard* by a sufficiency of food.

2. To ascertain its influence upon an organism where the body *lost weight* from a deficiency of food.

3. To determine its action upon a system where the body *gained weight* from an excess of food.

The experiments under these heads related to the weight of the body, the quantity of carbonic acid and aqueous vapour expired in respiration, the weight of the feces, the quantity of the urine, and the amount of its free acid, urea, uric acid, chlorine, and phosphoric and sulphuric acids. Besides these special determinations, I observed minutely every circumstance connected with my general health which could reasonably be ascribed to the action of the alcohol. I regret that I had no means at my command for accurately determining the amount of the cutaneous transpiration. Wherever this was sensibly affected it is noticed, but the liability to error when judging solely from sensation must not be forgotten.

The weight of the body was taken every day at 7 A. M., and at 2 and 10 P. M. The means of these observations are given in the tables. The carbonic acid and aqueous vapour exhaled from the lungs were determined by causing the expired air to pass through a tube containing chloride of calcium, and then through a saturated solution of baryta contained in two Woulfe's bottles. The excess of weight of the chloride of calcium tube indicated the amount of aqueous vapour, and from the quantity of carbonate of baryta formed, the carbonic acid was estimated. These determinations were made at 9 A. M., and at 2 and 10 P. M., and were continued one minute. From the mean of these observations the quantity for the day was calculated. As Vierordt has shown that the rate of respiration exercises a material effect upon the quantity of carbonic acid expired, I breathed during these observations uniformly fourteen times per minute, which is about the average natural frequency of my respiration. As comparative results were what I most desired, this method of estimation was sufficiently accurate.

The feces were weighed at 8½ A. M., immediately after their evacuation. The whole quantity of urine passed during the twenty-four hours was accurately measured. The acidity of this fluid was determined by a test solution of ammonia, and was estimated as oxalic acid, and the urea, uric acid, chlorine, and phosphoric and sulphuric acids were ascertained as in the experiments recorded in the April number of this journal.

In the following tables the weight of the body is given in pounds and decimals, the feces in ounces and decimals, and the quantity of urine in fluid-ounces and decimals. The weights of all the other substances are stated in grains and decimals. This system, though not so convenient as the French, has the advantage of being more commonly understood in this country, where the latter method is not yet generally adopted.

In the series of investigations previously detailed, ten days was the period fixed upon for obtaining average results. Further experience has, however, convinced me, that these can be obtained of sufficient accuracy in five days, and, where so many observations have to be made, the saving of time is an item not to be disregarded.

1. The action of *alcohol* where a uniform weight of the body was preserved.

After several trials, I found that food of the quality and quantity stated below, and taken as specified, kept up my weight to a nearly perfectly fixed standard.

I breakfasted at seven, lunched at one, and dined at five. At breakfast I ate five ounces of beefsteak, eight of bread, one half ounce of butter, and ten grains of salt, and drank six ounces of strong coffee, containing two drachms of cream, and two of white sugar. At luncheon, I ate three ounces of cold roast beef, six of bread, two drachms of butter, and twenty grains of salt.

At dinner, I took six ounces of strong beef soup, eight of roast beef, four of boiled beets, four of bread, two drachms of butter, half a drachm of salt, and drank four ounces of coffee. In addition to this food, I drank daily forty-eight ounces of water, twelve at each meal, and twelve immediately before going to bed.

I thus took daily into my system sixteen ounces of beef, eighteen of bread, six of soup, four of beets, one of butter, one drachm of salt, two of cream, and two of sugar, and drank ten ounces of coffee and forty-eight of water.

The following table contains the results of the experiments instituted under the foregoing conditions. The temperature of the atmosphere during their continuance was in the mean 73.06° Fahrenheit.

	Weight of body.	Carbonic acid expired.	Aqueous Vapour eXpired.	Feces.	URINE.						
					Quantity.	Free acid.	Urea.	Uric acid.	Chlorine.	Phosphoric acid.	Sulphuric acid.
1st day	226.41	11760.57	5115.07	8.10	43.42	31.43	664.20	15.37	139.62	55.36	41.56
2d "	226 40	11973 65	5286.25	8.05	43.05	32.86	658.31	15.41	142.86	55.16	42.53
3d "	226 35	11428.04	4963.41	8.11	44.10	30.19	666.00	14.29	148.54	56.92	40.60
4th "	226.44	11467.16	4895.50	8.08	45.03	33.15	673.29	14.03	142.75	54.79	43.26
5th "	226.43	11745.49	5004.26	8.09	43.69	30.52	682.58	13.81	146.52	53.65	40.35
Average	226.40	11674.98	5052.90	8.08	43.86	31.63	668.87	14.58	144.06	55.17	41.66

The above table, therefore, indicates the quantity of carbonic acid, aqueous vapour, feces, urine and its principal constituents excreted, when the weight of the body was nearly uniform, and when no alcohol was taken into the system. During the continuance of these experiments, my general health was excellent. My pulse averaged eighty-one per minute, and was of moderate strength and fulness. My appetite was good, and digestion was performed with regularity.

Having thus ascertained the state of the system as far as my inquiries advanced, when no alcohol was ingested, and when the food was sufficient to sustain the well-being of the organism, I next proceeded to investigate the action of the substance under consideration when all the circumstances which governed the preceding experiments were observed. On the day succeeding their termination, I commenced the second series by taking four drachms of alcohol at each meal, which course was continued for five days. The alcohol was diluted with an equal quantity of water. The other food, and the mental and physical exercise, sleep, &c., remained undisturbed. The mean temperature of the atmosphere was 72.44°.

The annexed table exhibits the results.

	Weight of body.	Carbonic acid eXpired.	Aqneous vapour eXpired.	Feces.	URINE.						
					Quantity	Free acid.	Urea.	Uric acid.	Chlorine.	Phosphoric acid.	Sulphuric acid.
1st day	226.64	10527.65	4729.52	7.11	41.90	30.17	591.10	13.21	112.15	33.29	30.87
2d "	226.95	10474.29	4853.27	6.91	39.71	29.29	585.17	13.18	119.10	35.40	25.84
3d "	226.80	10256.47	4825.33	6.79	40.24	29.78	562.20	13.96	94.70	28.47	30.19
4th "	227.06	10175.36	4893.68	6.76	39.88	31.65	586.52	13.24	105.38	30.17	26.24
5th "	226.81	10289.11	4975.19	6 75	40.45	34.26	583.41	13.12	101.04	26.18	28.18
Average	226.85	10344.57	4855.39	6.86	40.43	31.03	581.68	13.34	106.47	30.70	28.26

Thus, after the use of sixty drachms of alcohol in five days, my weight is seen to have increased from an average of 226.40 pounds to an average of 226.85 pounds, being .45 of a pound difference. The carbonic acid and vapour of water in the expired air had respectively decreased 1324.50 and 196.51 grains, the feces 1.22 ounces, the urine 3.43 ounces, the urea 87.19 grains, the chlorine 37.59 grains, the phosphoric acid 24.47 grains, and the sulphuric acid 13.40 grains. The free acid and uric acid (especially the former) were so slightly affected as to render it probable that the alcohol had exercised no influence upon them.

The cutaneous transpiration did not appear to be sensibly affected, except upon the third day, when I thought I perceived that it was augmented.

During these experiments, my general health was somewhat disturbed. My pulse was increased to an average of ninety per minute, and was fuller and stronger than previously; there was headache and increased heat of the skin, and my mental faculties were certainly not so clear as on the days when no alcohol was taken. There was also general lassitude, and indisposition to exertion of any kind. My appetite was variable. Digestion was effected as well as previously. The amount of flatus discharged from the intestines was sensibly diminished.

The metamorphosis of tissue and fat was evidently considerably retarded, as is shown in the decreased amount of urea, &c., excreted by the kidneys, and in the lessened quantity of carbonic acid and aqueous vapor given off in respiration. The diminution in the weight of the feces was doubtless mainly owing to the increased assimilation of food induced by the alcohol.

As this substance is incapable of being converted into tissue, the increase in the weight of the body was probably owing to the three following causes:—

1st. The retardation of the decay of the tissues.

2d. The diminution in the consumption of the fat.

3d. The increase in the assimilative powers of the system by which the food was more completely appropriated and applied to the formation of tissue.

From a due consideration of the foregoing experiments, I am disposed to think that, when the food is sufficient for the requirements of the system, alcohol is injurious by exciting the circulation and tending to produce a plethoric habit of body. In these respects, its influence is no worse than an excessive amount of food of any kind, or the omission of physical exercise when the system is habituated to its use.

It has been repeatedly shown that muscular exertion accelerates the destruction of the tissues, and Böcker has conclusively proven that the action of water is similar. When, therefore, the aliment ingested is sufficient to maintain the strength and weight of the body, alcohol, if indulged in, should be counteracted in its effects by one or other of the above compensating influences. The action of chloride of sodium is also antagonistic to that of alcohol, and might be similarly employed. By these means the balance of the organism would be preserved.

It is very evident, however, on a careful review of the preceding investigations, that under many circumstances in which man is frequently placed, alcohol might be productive of very beneficial results. The ensuing experiments tend to confirm this observation.

2d. The action of alcohol when the body lost weight from deficiency of food.

I ascertained, that, by reducing the amount of bread daily taken to twelve ounces, and the meat to ten ounces, the loss of weight in the body was sufficiently well marked. I, therefore, after allowing five days to elapse since the last experiments, instituted another series in which I took two ounces less of each of these substances at each meal. The remaining conditions of food, exercise, &c., continued as in the last series. On the evening previous to commencing these observations my weight was 226.73. The mean temperature of the atmosphere was 73.17°. The following table shows the results of the experiments in detail.

	Weight of body.	Carbonic acid expired.	Aqueous vapour expired.	Feces.	URINE.						
					Quantity.	Free acid.	Urea.	Uric acid.	Chlorine.	Phosphoric acid.	Sulphuric acid.
1st day	226.62	11125.54	4759.82	6.02	42.80	28.55	621.50	12.84	126.26	44.30	35.33
2d "	226.30	10862.29	4681.59	5.98	41.27	27.49	635.22	12.72	135.37	44.10	36.57
3d "	225.92	10555.70	4600.18	6.05	41.55	30.45	630.43	12.74	130.29	46.08	38.82
4th "	225.69	10641.65	4610.25	5.96	40.10	26.17	641.34	12.55	120.45	45.51	38.68
5th "	225.34	10686.90	4687.28	6.00	40.76	26.35	618.18	12.95	129.13	42.24	37.48
Average	225.97	10774.41	4667.82	6.00	41.29	27.80	629.33	12.76	128.00	44.44	37.37

During these experiments, my pulse averaged eighty-eight per minute. My general health appeared to be good, except that after exertion I was more exhausted than on the days when full food was taken. My desire for aliment was very much increased, and was never completely appeased by the quantity ingested. The sensible perspiration did not appear to vary from the quantity excreted during the first observations.

I proceeded in the next place to ascertain the effects of alcohol upon my system under circumstances similar to those which existed during the last experiments. With this view I took, on the ensuing day, twelve drachms of alcohol (four drachms at each meal), and continued it for five days. The mean temperature of the atmosphere was 73.34°. The accompanying table exhibits the results.

	Weight of body.	Carbonic acid eXpired.	Aqueous Vapour eXpired.	Feces.	URINE.						
					Quantity.	Free acid.	Urea.	Uric acid.	Chlorine.	Phosphoric acid.	Sulphuric acid.
1st day	225.45	10055.72	4426.18	5.85	40.22	30.10	584.75	14.01	119.17	38.50	33.17
2d "	225.56	9821.91	4252.75	5.81	39.52	28.56	561.52	13.82	115.24	36.42	34.29
3d "	225.50	10024.60	4385.90	5.82	39.10	26.14	575.19	14.05	116.91	32.19	31.42
4th "	225.52	9948.25	4449.68	5.80	40.00	27.19	570.28	14.00	118.14	37.10	29.86
5th "	225.48	9876.18	4364.36	5.76	40.77	31.24	582.35	14.06	120.43	34.48	27.57
Average	225.50	9945.33	4375.77	5.81	39.92	28.64	574.82	13.99	117.98	35.74	31.26

During the experiments immediately preceding these, my weight decreased an average of .28 of a pound daily, falling from 226.73 pounds to 225.34. In the present series, under the same conditions, except the use of the alcohol, this decrease has not only been overcome, but, there is an actual average daily increase of .03 of a pound, the weight rising from 225.34 to a mean of 225.50 pounds. The mean weight of the body is less than the mean of the last series, owing to the fact that the average daily gain is not so great as the previous average daily loss.

The carbonic acid expired is seen to have decreased an average of 729.08 grains, the aqueous vapour 312.06 grains, the feces .19 of an ounce, the quantity of urine 1.37 ounces, the urea 54.51 grains, the chlorine 10.08 grains, the phosphoric acid 8.70 grains, and the sulphuric acid 6.11 grains. The free acid of the urine, and the uric acid, were apparently slightly increased.

The sensible perspiration was not perceptibly affected through the day, but at night, it seemed to be somewhat increased. The general condition of my system was never better. My pulse had fallen to an average of 83 per minute, there was no headache, the intellectual faculties were clear, and of normal energy, the quantity of food ingested fully satisfied the appetite, sleep was sound and refreshing, and, in fact, all the functions of the organism were performed with regularity. The absence of any symptoms indicating derangement of the health cannot, I think, be ascribed to immunity by continued use of the alcohol, as ten days had elapsed between the two sets of experiments in which it was taken.

The good effects of this substance in limiting the waste of the body when the supply of food is not sufficient to maintain the vigour of the system, are here very evident, and stand in marked contrast to its influence when an abundance of food was ingested. The strength was not only sustained, but the body gradually, but noticeably gained weight. In short, the alcohol had taken the place of the bread and meat omitted, and at no apparent disadvantage to the general economy. As a compensating agent for a deficiency of food its power cannot, I think, be questioned.

3d. The effects of alcohol when the body gained weight from excess of food.

For the purpose of ascertaining the action of alcohol under the above condition of the system, I increased the quantity of meat daily eaten, from sixteen to twenty-two ounces, and the bread, from eighteen to twenty-four ounces. By this addition to the amount of aliment, I found my weight underwent a sensible and tolerably regular increase. The remaining food, and mental and physical exertion continued as in the first experiments. Five days were suffered to elapse between this and the last series of investigations. The mean temperature of the atmosphere was 72.06°. The annexed table contains the results of the observations made under the above circumstances.

	Weight of body.	Carbonic acid expired.	Aqueous vapour expired.	Feces.	URINE.						
					Quantity.	Free acid.	Urea.	Uric acid.	Chlorine.	Phosphoric acid.	Sulphuric acid.
1st day	225.61	11872.54	4895.32	12.10	43.30	35.63	698.70	17.25	152.18	58.29	50.67
2d "	225.85	12251.86	5824.48	12.98	45.61	34.71	721.62	16.82	155.21	64.06	50.18
3d "	226.15	12329.47	5250.79	12.74	45.23	38.23	710.43	17.86	150.59	62.10	51.50
4th "	226.36	12178.22	5387.20	12.76	46.18	35.45	735.84	18.05	158.25	66.75	48.15
5th "	226.59	12165.94	5419.68	12.65	45.56	39.28	728.37	18.10	161.03	62.38	49.05
Average	226.11	12159.60	5255.49	12.64	45.17	36.66	718.99	17.61	155.45	62.71	49.91

At 10 o'clock on the night before the commencement of the above experiments my weight was 225.50; a slight diarrhœa which occurred in the interval, had probably rendered it somewhat less than it would otherwise have been. On the last day of the series it was 226.59, showing an increase of 1.09 pounds, which, as all the excreted substances had increased in quantity over the amounts of the first series, could have arisen from no other cause than the excess of food. The sensible perspiration was, also, apparently augmented both by day and night.

Symptoms of derangement of the health were more or less present during the continuance of the observations. The pulse was increased in fulness and frequency, averaging 92 per minute. There was almost constant headache, indisposition to exertion, and increased desire for sleep, which was, however, frequently disturbed by unpleasant dreams. My appetite was not very good, and after eating there was occasional pain. There was an increased discharge of flatus from the intestines.

On the day succeeding the termination of these investigations, I commenced the following by taking, under the conditions of food, &c., of the last experiments, the fixed quantity of four drachms of alcohol at each meal, which, as previously, was continued for five days. The ensuing table exhibits the results. The mean temperature of the atmosphere was 73.60°.

	Weight of body.	Carbonic acid expired.	Aqueous Vapour expired.	Feces.	URINE.						
					Quantity.	Free acid.	Urea.	Uric acid.	Chlorine.	Phosphoric acid.	Sulphuric acid.
1st day	226.82	12015.87	5884.47	10.40	40.91	38.11	627.58	18.20	128.35	49 82	38.17
2d "	227.17	11523.19	5090.26	10.22	40.50	36.34	639.60	18.31	121.42	51.27	39.72
3d "	227.48	11452.71	4829.64	10.38	41.87	34.13	629.41	18.11	126.15	46.14	40.55
4th "	227.80	11514.28	4831.70	10.18	40.62	39.24	610.17	18.01	135.10	46.98	40.52
5th "	228.15	11382 50	4810.35	10.35	41.73	35.46	621.86	18.15	131.68	47.51	36.23
Average	227.48	11577.61	4989.28	10.30	41.02	36.65	625.72	18.15	128.54	48.34	39.04

During the series of experiments immediately preceding the present, the average daily increase of weight was .22 of a pound. By the above table, it is seen that, by the action of the amount of alcohol ingested, the average increase was raised to .31 of a pound per day. The average amount of carbonic acid excreted, compared with the mean of the last series, was reduced 581.99 grains, the aqueous vapour 266.21 grains, the feces 2.34 ounces, the urine 4.15 ounces, the urea 93.27 grains, the chlorine 26.92 grains, the phosphoric acid 8.29 grains, and the sulphuric acid 14.87 grains. The free acid and uric acid were but slightly affected. The perspiration was sensibly diminished.

Whilst these experiments were progressing, the healthy action of my system was very much disordered. Headache was constant, sleep was disturbed, the skin was hot, pulse full and bounding, averaging 98 per minute, and there was on two occasions after eating slight palpitation of the heart. My appetite was capricious. Sometimes disgust was created by the mere sight of food, at other times I ate with a good deal of relish. I think I should have been made seriously ill if I had continued the investigations longer. Upon a return, however, to my ordinary food, all unpleasant symptoms gradually disappeared. This fortunate termination was probably promoted by a diarrhœa of considerable violence, which commenced on the second day after the conclusion of the experiments, and continued forty-eight hours.

The inquiries into the actions of alcohol upon the human economy were now terminated. Upon consideration of the foregoing experiments collectively, I arrive at the conclusion *that alcohol increases the weight of the body by retarding the metamorphosis of the old tissues, promoting the formation of new, and limiting the consumption of the fat.* Viewed in detail, it is seen that, under the use of alcohol, the following effects constantly ensued :—

1st. The carbonic acid and aqueous vapour given off in respiration were lessened in quantity.

2d. The amount of feces was diminished.

3d. The quantity of urine was reduced.

4th. The urea, chlorine, and phosphoric and sulphuric acids were diminished in amount.

These effects, occurring when the amount of food was below the quantity required to maintain the weight of the body under the mental and physical exercise taken, were productive of no deleterious results to the system. On the contrary, when the food was sufficient to balance the waste from the excretions, and still more so when an excess of aliment over the demands of the organism was ingested, the healthy working of the system was disturbed, and actual disease almost induced.

The use of alcohol, even in moderation, cannot therefore be either exclusively approved or condemned. The labouring man, who can hardly procure bread and meat enough to preserve the balance between the formation and decay of his tissues, finds here an agent which, within the limits of health, enables him to dispense with a certain quantity of food, and yet keeps up the strength and weight of his body. On the other hand, he who uses alcohol when his food is more than sufficient to supply the waste of tissue, and, at the same time, does not increase the amount of his physical exercise, or drink an additional quantity of water (by which the decay of tissue would be accelerated), retards the metamorphosis whilst an increased amount of nutriment is being assimilated, and thus adds to the plethoric condition of the system, which excessive food so generally induces.

The foregoing experiments confirm those of Böcker so far as the diminution of the carbonic acid expired, and the reduction of the solids and water of the urine are concerned. This physiologist, however, found that under the use of alcohol the feces excreted and the water exhaled from the lungs were unaffected. The present investigations, on the contrary, indicate that both the fecal excretion and the water expired were materially diminished. These discrepancies are probably due to the difference in the quantities of alcohol imbibed, the preceding experiments being performed with a much larger amount of this substance than were Böcker's.

The perspiration not having been measured by direct experiment, I have not laid much stress upon the apparent results obtained. The temperature of the atmosphere was, however, unusually uniform during the continuance of the observations, and any alteration in the quantity of this excretion was doubtless owing to the influence of the alcohol. Yet the liability to form an erroneous opinion, when judging only from the sensations, leaves the action of alcohol upon the cutaneous transpiration still to be definitely determined.

It has been assumed by several late writers that the primary action of alcohol is the retention in the blood of the products of metamorphosis. I am inclined to think this opinion erroneous, and that alcohol, instead of preventing the elimination of the decayed tissues, acts by preventing, in a great measure, their primary destruction. No one will dispute the point that, if the first of these views is correct, alcohol must be uniformly deleterious, and that it must manifest such unmistakable symptoms as could not possibly lead to a misconstruction of its mode of action. If this had been its influence on my own system, what an immense accumulation of carbonized and nitrogenized substances would have been retained in the blood, and what a different set of symptoms would have been experienced! Besides, these symptoms would have been also present during the experiments conducted with alcohol when an insufficient quantity of food was taken; and yet on these days they were entirely absent, and my system was never in better order. Indeed, it may possibly be a question of doubt in the minds of some whether the unpleasant symptoms which were observed were not due as much to excessive food as to the alcohol.

The most strenuous supporter of the theory that alcohol causes the retention of the decomposed tissues in the blood is Dr. Carpenter, and it is with great diffidence that I find myself constrained to differ with so eminent a physiologist. Dr. Carpenter, also, whilst admitting (*Essay on Alcohol*) that there are occasions when it is of importance that an increased amount of mental or physical exertion should be made, and that under such circumstances alcohol may be temporarily beneficial, ascribes its influence in producing additional nervous force to the fact that it occasions more rapid metamorphosis of the nervous tissues. The experiments detailed in the present paper invariably show a diminished excretion of the products of nervous decay after the exhibition of alcohol, and consequently such cannot be its action.

I do not wish to be understood as at all contending for the propriety of habitual indulgence in alcohol. My experiments show that there are circumstances in which its use is injurious. I believe, however, that these circumstances can be so modified that alcohol may be moderately indulged in without the production of deleterious effects. Full food, insufficient exercise, and alcohol conjoined, will as certainly produce disease if the action of this latter agent is the retardation of tissue-metamorphosis, as though it prevented the elimination from the blood of substances injurious to the organism. On the one hand, however, the affection would be of a sthenic, and on the other of an asthenic character. Whilst, therefore, fully admitting that the use of alcohol requires prudence and discretion, I am not prepared to concede that it is essentially poisonous, or even that there are not conditions of the system in which its employment is not eminently to be commended.

Tobacco.—The experiments with this substance, though not so full as those with alcohol, were conducted upon the same general principles. They embraced the consideration of its effects under the following conditions:—

1st. When the food was sufficient to maintain the healthy balance of the system.

2d. When a deficiency of aliment was ingested.

I had previously instituted some experiments, which, though incomplete, were sufficient to indicate the general action of tobacco upon the organism. They were confirmatory of the present so far as they extended, which was principally to the relations of the substance under consideration to the urine and its constituents.

As in the experiments with alcohol, I fixed upon a definite and invariable amount of sleep and mental and physical exertion. This was precisely as has been previously stated in detail. The experiments related to the same determinations, and all the analyses were performed in exactly the same manner, and at the same periods of the day as formerly.

After the expiration of twelve days since the investigations into the action of alcohol, and when my system was again in a perfectly normal condition, I commenced the experiments with tobacco. I am not in the habit of using this substance in any form, but had, previous to my observations, smoked an occasional cigar without any perceptible effect resulting, other than slight nervous excitement. I have never in my life chewed tobacco or used snuff.

1st. The effects of tobacco when a sufficiency of food was taken to keep up the weight and vigor of the body.

I lived exactly as in the corresponding series of experiments with alcohol, except that I found it necessary, from, as I suppose, the greater heat of the atmosphere, and consequently the induction of a larger amount of cutaneous transpiration, to increase the quantity of water from forty-eight ounces daily to fifty-two ounces—thirteen at each meal, and thirteen immediately before going to bed. The observations under this mode of living were continued, as before, for five days. The mean temperature of the atmosphere for the period was 80.12°. The following table exhibits the results:—

	Weight of body.	Carbonic acid expired.	Aqueous vapour expired.	Feces.	Urine.						
					Quantity.	Free acid.	Urea.	Uric acid.	Chlorine.	Phosphoric acid.	Sulphuric acid.
1st day	225.84	11845.29	4827.50	8.12	40.54	29.43	643.18	13.10	151.62	57.42	39.52
2d "	225.78	11582.73	4855.91	8.10	41.66	27.82	662.27	12.78	155.16	54.38	36.18
3d "	225.76	11628.65	4986.70	8.11	42.13	30.51	650.30	12.64	144.25	52 29	35.27
4th "	225.80	11439.26	4758.37	8.07	42.76	26.17	665.14	12.82	142.51	56.77	35.40
5th "	225.76	11586.40	4994.85	8.09	41.35	25.39	667.58	12.80	150.52	60.06	38.22
Average	225.79	11616.46	4884.66	8.10	41.69	27.86	657.69	12.88	148.81	56.18	36.92

The heat of the atmosphere during the above experiments was 7.06 degrees greater than during the first set of experiments in the alcohol series. My pulse averaged 85 per minute. My health, notwithstanding the extreme heat of the weather, was excellent. My appetite was good, and my food was well digested.

Under the same conditions as the experiments just concluded, I proceeded in the next place to ascertain the direct effects of tobacco. With this object, I smoked one hundred and fifty grains of tobacco (nearly two cigars) after each meal, being four hundred and fifty grains per day. During these experiments, the mean temperature of the atmosphere was 78.11°. The annexed table exhibits the results.

	Weight of body.	Carbonic acid expired.	Aqueous vapour expired.	Feces.	URINE.						
					Quantity.	Free acid.	Urea.	Uric acid.	Chlorine.	Phosphoric acid.	Sulphuric acid.
1st day	225.81	11726.58	4658.22	8.10	40.21	30.84	628.41	18.29	135.43	88.60	40.59
2d "	225.87	11562.97	4473.18	8.11	39.63	32.26	610.93	18.80	118.15	84.10	43.17
3d "	225.86	11839.65	4485.41	8.09	39.80	35.18	614.11	19.03	127.84	75.33	38.65
4th "	225.90	11710.80	4627.64	8.06	39.45	31.59	604.50	19.01	117.25	81.52	40.10
5th "	225.85	11482.51	4681.57	8.10	40.02	34.57	618.68	18.45	130.21	70.49	44.15
Average	225.86	11664.50	4585.20	8.09	39.82	32.89	615.32	18.71	125.77	80.01	41.33

Under the use of tobacco, my weight had increased an average of .07 of a pound, the carbonic acid 88.04 grains, the free acid of the urine 4.93 grains, the uric acid 5.88 grains, the phosphoric acid 23.83 grains, and the sulphuric acid 4.41 grains. On the contrary, the quantity of aqueous vapour had decreased 299.46 grains, the feces .01 of an ounce, the urine 1.87 ounces, the urea 42.37 grains, and the chlorine 23.04 grains.

The general effects of the tobacco upon my system were exceedingly well marked. There was great nervous excitement, accompanied by irregular action of the muscles, more particularly of the eyelids, mouth, and upper extremities, which lasted for about two hours after each occasion of using this substance. The mind, however, was clear, and there was no headache. These sensations were succeeded by a pleasant feeling of ease and contentment, which also lasted about two hours. During the first part of the night, there was wakefulness, but this was always followed by a sound sleep, which continued till the hour for rising. The pulse was increased to an average of 92 per minute. My appetite was as good as usual. The perspiration was apparently slightly diminished.

After allowing five days to elapse, as in former experiments, in order that the system might have time to regain its natural condition, I commenced the observations under the second head, viz: the *effects of tobacco upon the organism, when an insufficiency of food was taken.* I reduced (as in the corresponding experiments with alcohol) the quantity of bread daily ingested to twelve ounces, and the meat to ten ounces. In all other respects, the conditions of the last experiments remained unaltered. During these investigations the mean temperature of the atmosphere was 80.92°. The results are contained in the following table:—

	Weight of body.	Carbonic acid expired.	Aqueous vapour expired.	Feces.	URINE.						
					Quantity.	Free acid.	Urea.	Uric acid.	Chlorine.	Phosphoric acid.	Sulphuric acid.
1st day	225.58	10672.86	4537.69	6.02	38.74	22.47	623.50	11.58	128.31	45.78	34.54
2d "	225.20	10384.61	4483.22	6.06	38.20	24.18	615.11	11.23	131.58	43.29	33.09
3d "	224.79	10350.92	4394.48	6.04	39.04	25.72	604.25	10.01	125.44	44.64	32.22
4th "	224.33	10526.45	4456.73	6.03	39.57	26.19	601.19	9.82	130.17	42.18	30.15
5th "	223.97	10347.81	4375.16	6.05	38.73	24.65	608.46	10.04	132.26	45.25	28.31
Average	224.77	10456.53	4449.45	6.04	38.85	24.64	610.50	10.53	129.55	44.23	31.66

The general effects observed, were of a similar character to those noticed during the experiments performed under like conditions in the alcohol series. The extreme heat of the weather, however, rendered the amount of sensible perspiration much larger. The pulse was 86 per minute. My appetite was always good; but as I always left the table with a feeling of hunger, I felt myself gradually becoming weaker day by day. On the night previous to the commencement of these experiments, my weight was 225.81. On the last day of the series it was 223.97. I had, therefore, lost 1.84 pounds, or an average daily of nearly .37 of a pound.

Under the condition of the system thus produced, I began, on the day following the conclusion of the experiments just detailed, and under circumstances every way identical, the concluding series relative to the effects of tobacco. I smoked, as previously, one hundred and fifty grains of cigars after each meal. The average temperature of the atmosphere was 74.09°.

The special results are exhibited in the annexed table.

	Weight of body.	Carbonic acid expired.	Aqueous vapour expired.	Feces.	URINE.						
					Quantity.	Free acid.	Urea.	Uric acid.	Chlorine.	Phosphoric acid.	Sulphuric acid.
1st day	223.80	10568.37	4382.28	4.50	37.85	26.81	569.70	14.91	118.36	72.86	40.21
2d "	223.65	10495.13	4417.30	4.48	37.29	25.14	541.28	15.11	111.53	75.71	38.02
3d "	223.55	10265.80	4293.74	4.49	37.15	28.16	536.12	15.29	115.83	78.60	39.00
4th "	223.56	10483.69	4150.83	4.53	37.48	28.73	552.10	14.80	112.40	74.22	42.23
5th "	223.54	10478.36	4203.41	4.62	36.92	29.54	540.61	15.17	114.66	70.91	40.58
Average	223.62	10458.27	4289.51	4.52	37.34	27.67	547.96	15.05	114.55	74.46	40.01

From the above table, it is seen that the loss of weight in the body, induced by the deficient supply of food, was lessened from the first, and entirely overcome on the fourth day—the average daily loss being less than .09 of a pound, against .37 of a pound, under the same conditions, except the use of tobacco. The excretion of carbonic acid from the lungs was not, in the average, perceptibly affected. The amount of aqueous vapour exhaled was reduced 159.94 grains, the feces 1.92 ounces, the quantity of urine 1.51

ounces, the urea 62.54 grains, and the chlorine 15 grains. The free acid of the urine was increased 3.03 grains, the uric acid 4.52 grains, the phosphoric acid 30.23 grains, and the sulphuric acid 8.35 grains.

The general effects upon the system were almost identical with those previously described as resulting from the former use of tobacco. There was the same nervous excitement, trembling, and wakefulness, but in a somewhat less degree. The pulse was an average of 90 per minute. The desire for food was not nearly so great as in the last experiments, neither was there so great a degree of debility. The cutaneous transpiration, whether from the diminished temperature of the atmosphere, or, as an effect of the tobacco used, was very sensibly lessened in quantity.

From these experiments the following conclusions are deducible:—

1st. That tobacco does not materially affect the excretion of carbonic acid through the lungs.

2d. That it lessens the amount of aqueous vapour given off in respiration.

3d. That it diminishes the amount of the feces.

4th. That it lessens the quantity of urine, and the amount of its urea and chlorine.

5th. That it increases the amount of free acid, uric acid, and phosphoric and sulphuric acids, eliminated through the kidneys.

These results differ in several essential points from those obtained with alcohol. The fact that the amount of carbonic acid given off in respiration was not diminished, would indicate that the consumption of the fat of the body is not lessened by the use of tobacco. The metamorphosis of the nitrogenous tissues, judging from the diminution in the quantity of urea and chlorine observed, would appear to be retarded, and yet the amount, both of the phosphoric and sulphuric acids excreted, especially the former, was very considerably augmented. As both phosphorus and sulphur enter into the composition of all the proteinaceous tissues, it is difficult to reconcile this apparent inconsistency in the results, unless by assuming (what there is great reason to believe) that the oxidation of the phosphorus, and sulphur of the brain, and nervous tissue, was so great in amount as to cause an increase in the elimination of phosphoric and sulphuric acids, even though the metamorphosis of the other nitrogenous tissues was lessened.

The effect produced by tobacco upon the excretion of the free acid, and uric acid of the urine, was also different from that caused by alcohol. Though both alcohol and tobacco diminish the quantity of urea, the latter only of these substances would appear to exercise any very material influence upon the amount of uric acid eliminated. If there are any definite and constant relations existing between these two constituents of the urine, they would appear to be farther from determination than ever.

Tobacco, when the food is sufficient to preserve the weight of the body, increases that weight, and when the food is not sufficient, and the body in consequence loses weight, tobacco restrains that loss. Unlike alcohol, this influence is unattended with any unpleasant effects upon the circulatory system, though its action on the brain and nerves is certainly not such as always to be desired. When used in greater moderation than in these experiments, this influence would, doubtless, be greatly lessened.

I refrain from entering into the discussion of the other physiological points connected with the foregoing experiments. A simple examination of the tables will show that these are many and of great interest, and that it is not only as exhibiting the actions of alcohol and tobacco upon the system that the investigations detailed in this paper are valuable; neither have I the time to discuss farther the immediate subjects of inquiry.

To that earnest band of physiologists who are constantly investigating the operations of nature, and who rely more upon actual observations than upon abstract theories, I submit these experiments. Though the deductions I have drawn from them may not stand before the progress of physiological research, the materials collected will, I am confident, never entirely lose their value.

FORT RILEY, *Kansas Territory*, August, 1856.

ART. II.—*Thoughts on Acclimation and Adaptation of Races to Climates.* By J. C. NOTT, M. D., Mobile, Ala.

THE following desultory remarks have been elicited by a perusal of the work of Dr. R. La Roche on *Yellow Fever.* It would be a work of supererogation in me at this late day to say anything in praise of this standard work, which has already taken its position in the classic literature of our profession; nor need I allude to the kind and gentlemanly tone which pervades it throughout. But there are a few points in these volumes on which I differ from the author; and, as they involve not only curious speculations but questions of deep practical importance, I will take the liberty of presenting certain facts and opinions of my own which are the result of thirty years' observation in southern climates. In so doing, my object is not controversy, but simply a desire to aid in developing the true history of southern diseases, which at this moment are so profoundly interesting to the people of the United States, north as well as south.

Although there are other opinions of Dr. La Roche with which I shall incidentally come into collision, the following paragraph is the only one to which I shall directly allude, as it expresses his opinions on the leading point which I desire to illustrate, viz: that of *acclimation*, or, to be more precise, the influence of southern climates on natives of the north. In vol. ii. p. 20, he says:—

> "In a word, habit seems to possess the power of modifying the system to so great an extent and so permanent a degree as to justify those who hold it in

the light of a second nature. In virtue of the influence it exercises, and the peculiar organic changes resulting from long exposure to the sensible and insensible qualities of the atmosphere, or to the extraneous materials by which that atmosphere may be contaminated, man enjoys the faculty to which I have alluded, of living under climatic influences of the most diversified characters. He resists the inclemencies of the elements, the insalubrity of the seasons, the extremes of temperature, as well as the action of malarial and other exhalations. With time, the native of the North acquires the privilege of supporting *with impunity* the scorching rays of a tropical sun, though the result is not obtained without inconvenience, suffering, and even danger, and without, in the greater number of instances, subjecting the individual to the ordeal of disease. Not so easy is it to become habituated to the baneful action of those modifiers—such as malarial exhalations—which exercise their agency on the principle of vitality. *But even here immunity is obtained*, either gradually and insensibly, without shock to the system, or more suddenly through the effect of an attack of fever. But whatever be the means by which the process is effected, that such protection is thus obtained, to a greater or less extent, in regard to *all malarial* and some other forms of fever, no one who has examined the subject with attention will feel disposed to deny. By long habituation to infectious localities and to the high temperature of hot regions, the system becomes acclimatized, and thereby acquires the power of *tolerating perfectly and permanently the poison*, or of eliminating it as soon as received, without succeeding reaction. The observation is of old standing. Pliny, nearly twenty centuries ago, called attention to the fact 'that they who are seasoned can live amid pestilential diseases;' and the statement has been confirmed by all subsequent observations. The immunity is more or less perfect according to the individual peculiarities of those exposed to the cause, and to the salubrity of the country whence they come; and is enjoyed at all future time, except when, from the concurrence of particular circumstances, the poison acquires unusual deleterious properties," &c. &c.

The doctor goes on to substantiate these opinions by references to Monfalcon, Lancisi, Pinkard, Sir Gilbert Blane, and other authorities of high repute.

I have given the above long quotation in order that Dr. La Roche might be fairly heard. The language to me is somewhat obscure, and, for fear of doing injustice, I shall simply give my own ideas, without attempting to define clearly the limits which he intends to set to the influence of *acclimation.*[1]

Dr. Rochoux has attempted a somewhat more precise definition of the term *acclimation*, and perhaps a better one cannot be given in the present state of knowledge. He says: "Acclimation is a profound change in the organism, produced by a prolonged sojourn in a place whose climate is widely different from that to which one is accustomed, and which has the effect of rendering the individual who has been subjected to it similar in many respects to the natives (*indigènes*) of the country which he has adopted."

This definition strikes at once a leading difficulty in this discussion, and one which should, as far as possible, be cleared away, before we attempt to estimate the influence of climate on mankind. Who are these "*indigènes*"

[1] Dr. La Roche prefers the word *acclimatization.* I prefer the common term, as it is adopted by Webster, by French writers, and it is shorter.

of whom Rochoux speaks? Are they, in all cases, really descendants of the same original stock as those who come to seek acclimation? Here, I repeat, are questions which have not been fully and fairly examined, even by Prichard, the great champion of the unity of the human race, and which embarrass our progress at every step.

My own opinions on the *original diversity of the races of men* have been long before the public, and need not be repeated here; nor, perhaps, does a practical view of the subject before us demand the reopening of that long mooted question, because recent discoveries have demonstrated that those well-marked races which are now scattered over the face of the earth have (unless where deteriorated by disease), with slight modification, preserved the same physical characteristics which marked them several thousand years ago. And if this *permanency of type* be, as it now universally is among naturalists, admitted, we have no reason to expect that climate will produce changes in races during the next thousand years which it has not been potent enough to effect in all recorded time of the past.

Moses, we are told, "was learned in all the wisdom of the Egyptians;" and, long before even his day, we know positively, through the researches of Lepsius, Champollion, Rosellini, and others, that the Egyptians had classed the races of men into the white, red, black, and yellow, each class representing a *group of races of kindred types.*

No one who has investigated the subject, will deny the antiquity of Egypt, China, and India, each of which existed as empires more than 2000 years before Christ, with populations presenting widely different physical characters, and speaking languages radically distinct from each other. Moreover, in Egypt, besides the millions of mummies which have been found in the catacombs of Thebes and Memphis, we see depicted on her time-worn monuments, authentic delineations of nearly all the races that the traveller now meets in his journey around the greater part of the Mediterranean. We there behold the portraits of Egyptians, Assyrians, Nubians, Abyssinians, Jews, Negroes, Tartars, Arabs, Berbers, &c.; and all, according to Lepsius, Bunsen, Birch, De Rougé, and other leading authorities, dating back at least 2300 years before the Christian era. Nor is evidence wanting to prove that Celts, Slaves, Teutons, Finns, Iberians, Pelasgians, and other types, inhabited Europe before the epoch of Moses. We might even go further, and produce evidence to show that America, Australia, and Oceanica had their *indigènes*, when Abraham and Sarah went to buy corn of the Pharaoh who then presided over the Egyptian empire.

We repeat, then, that the above races all existed, in their full developed types, 5000 years ago—that no known causes have ever transformed one race into another—and that nothing but amalgamation, or morbific causes, have ever greatly changed the physical characters of a race. So far we are sustained by facts; and *science* has nothing to do with the age of miracles beyond the starting point of my researches. The true origin of genera and species has proved a never-ending dispute among naturalists, and from the very nature of the case must ever remain so without a new revelation from the Creator.

The *antiquity* of the various types of man being conceded, let us next view them in connection with the other organized beings of our planet.

Naturalists teach, that while the surface of the earth presents an infinite variety of climates which influence animal and vegetable life, it may at the same time be divided into realms or regions, presenting totally distinct Faunæ and Floræ. These regions, which have been called *Zoological Provinces*, run so insensibly into each other as not to admit of precise boundaries, but each possesses an infinite variety of animals and plants that are peculiar to it, and which it is believed were there created. Prof. Agassiz, without pretending, in the present imperfect state of facts, to minute accuracy, has mapped off the earth into eight of these provinces, each of which contains not only peculiar animals and plants, but a *group* of human beings which seems to form an original element in the local creation, and to be *adapted by nature to surrounding climatic influences.* The following is the division of Prof. Agassiz: The *Arctic*, the *Asiatic*, the *European*, the *American*, the *African*, the *Malayan*, the *Australian*, and the *Polynesian Realms.* Now each of these realms has been shown to contain animals and plants that are found nowhere else, and also a group of human beings of peculiar type, which date back beyond human records, and which seem to be in perfect harmony with surrounding circumstances.

This is not the place to enlarge upon such a well-known law of natural history, and it may be sufficiently illustrated for the medical student, by a statement of the fact, that south of the arctic, at which the continents nearly touch, there is not an animal or plant that is common to the Old and New World. Every living thing (with *perhaps* a few rare exceptions) found in America at the time of the conquest, was here created.

Now, that the races of men, found in these respective realms, obey the same law of local creation as other organized beings, no doubt will be stoutly denied; but, leaving this point out of view, it will be admitted that these races have for ages been in harmony with the positions in which they are found, and cannot be removed to other zones without doing violence to their natures.

The animals and plants of different latitudes differ greatly in pliability of constitution, and are variously affected by changes. Those of the arctic and the tropic are each reared in extremes—are habituated either to very high or very low temperature, and cannot be transported far beyond their native climes, without injurious consequences. Hence, when the human beings or animals of the arctic or tropic are left to themselves, they rarely migrate much beyond the limits of their respective zones. Not so with the inhabitants of the middle temperate latitudes. Here the animals and plants are subject to cold winters and hot summers, and possess a pliability of nature which enables them to stand a wide geographical range. The races of men here are found to obey the same law, and have been the great conquerors, colonizers, and civilizers of the world; but even these have paid dearly for their migratory propensities. Though placed at the head of the animal kingdom, man is still an animal, and subject to the same physical influences as others. He is enabled to change his climate with more facility than most animals, simply because he is enabled to devise means by which he can protect himself against extremes of temperature and other unaccustomed influences.

Cabanis has justly remarked: "*Si l'histoire naturelle a besoin d'une bonne géographie physique, la science de l'homme, a besoin d'une géographie médicale.*" Much has been done since his day in the former department, but little progress has been yet made in the right direction in medical geography.

Every one admits that the negro cannot be carried to the arctic, or the Esquimaux to the tropic, without destruction of life. It is equally true that the natives of Europe and those of Africa brought to the United States are differently affected by the climate, which is equally new to each. We may go much further, and assert that various races of Europe, Asia, and Africa are influenced in different degrees by change to any given climate; and yet the element of race has played but an insignificant part in the question of acclimation. Much might be said on the relation of race to climate, but I can here do little more than call attention to its importance; and the few remarks I shall make, will be confined to the influence of our southern climate on exotic population.

All of our Southern States, as well as the tropical part of America, were covered by aboriginal tribes at the time of the conquest, which were everywhere a robust and healthy people. These races still inhabit the sickliest parts of Florida with impunity, and I meet others every day in the streets of Mobile, who present a vigorous and healthful appearance, though their bark tents are pitched around the town on the borders of pestiferous marshes. All testimony goes to show that these races suffer comparatively little from the indigenous diseases of the country, while they are terribly scourged by imported diseases, such as cholera, measles, smallpox, &c. In a word, it would seem that no foreign race can be placed, not even the negro, in such perfect harmony with our climate, as the Indian.

Writers on the physical history of man—Blumenbach, Prichard, Cuvier, and others, have made arbitrary classifications of races, which may be convenient, but which have no foundation whatever in nature; for example, the most commonly received division of races is the following: Caucasian, Mongol, Malay, Indian, and Negro. Let us take up the first division, and ask why has such a heterogeneous mass been grouped under the head of *Caucasian?* Slavoniaus, Teutons, Celts, Iberians, Finns, Pelasgians, Jews, Gypsies, Egyptians, Arabs, Hindoos, &c. &c., have all been thrown together under one name, though resembling each other no more than do dogs, wolves, foxes, jackals, and hyenas. Medical men have, in like manner, whilst discussing the subject of acclimation, thrown all these races together as amenable to the same physical laws, without stopping to inquire whether the principle be true or false.

All writers, in arguing this question, admit the broad division of *white* and *black races,* and although the study of climatic influences on the intermediate races may be attended with greater difficulties, it is none the less important.

The physicians of our southern seaports will not only tell you that negroes are much less susceptible to the influence of yellow fever poison than whites, but that the smallest infusion of negro blood into the white races diminishes their susceptibility. No facts can be better settled than these.

My own observation for twenty years in Mobile (where there is a very mixed population of Anglo-Saxons, French, Spaniards, Italians, Negroes, Mulattoes, Indians, &c.), has satisfied me thoroughly, that the susceptibility of Races to yellow fever is in direct ratio to the fairness of complexion. All the strictly white races are most susceptible; and in proportion as we descend through the dark-skinned descendants of the Iberian part of the population of France (Spaniards, Italians, Portuguese), the Mongols, Malays, &c., down to the negro, this susceptibility decreases. I know I shall be told, that these races are less susceptible because they are natives of warm climates; but my own conviction is that there is something in *Race* besides climate; and that the climate does not make the race, but that the race was originally made to suit the climate in which Nature placed it. The descendants of these dark-skinned races, born in Great Britain or in Germany, are less likely to suffer from yellow fever than the fair-skinned races; and we see the fact every year confirmed in Charleston, Mobile, and New Orleans, that negroes of the fourth, fifth, or even tenth generation in Virginia (where yellow fever does not prevail), enjoy almost perfect immunity against this disease. I have seen many hundred of these unacclimated negroes of Virginia exposed to yellow fever in Mobile; and until the memorable year of 1853, I never saw but two full-blooded negroes die of yellow fever. In the latter year more were attacked, but very few died. Negroes, too, possess a remarkable proneness to cholera, and to all forms of typhoid disease, typhoid fever, typhoid pneumonia, &c., as well as to the acute diseases of winter.

The statistics of Prussia show that Jews are much less liable to plica Polonica than the Slavonic, Teutonic, and other races of Europe; and we shall see further on that they are the only foreign population that can increase in Algeria.

But let us turn from this intricate problem of Races, and come down to the plain practical part of the discussion which lies within the reach of common observation. Let us inquire how far Dr. La Roche's ideas of acclimation are true, when applied "to *all forms* of malarial fever," and when he tells us that the native of the North, who comes to the South and inhabits "infectious localities," "*becomes acclimatized and thereby acquires the power of tolerating perfectly and permanently the poison.*"

Had the doctor lived at the South instead of the North he would have come to very different conclusions. He would have learned that the Anglo-Saxon easily becomes acclimated against yellow fever of the cities, but never against the marsh malaria of the rural districts: nay more, that susceptibility here increases with time, and that this race in "infectious localities" would, in time, if left alone, become exterminated by this "poison." A capital error has therefore been committed in grouping together yellow fever and the various forms of malarial disease.

I may be permitted to repeat that my conclusions are the result of many years' observation at the South, and that my attention has been closely called to the subject of acclimation by long connection with life insurance companics.

Yellow fever is, *par excellence*, a disease of towns and crowded population, while intermittents and remittents belong to the country; and wherever a large town is built in a malarial district, intermittent fever and its allies are driven to the suburbs, in proportion as grading, paving, and buildings extend. Charleston, South Carolina, may be selected from many others, as a striking illustration. This city was built in the midst of an "infectious locality," where marsh fevers exist to a terrible extent, in all grades, and yet it has become the most healthy town of the South. Its bills of mortality, for the last thirty-five years, will show statistics that compare favourably with those of any other city; and here among the causes of death bilious fever plays but a feeble part. The original disease of the spot has been expelled; and for it are substituted, at long intervals, epidemics of yellow fever; while the diseases of the suburbs and surrounding country are unchanged. The inhabitant of the town is fully acclimated to *its* atmosphere, but cannot spend a single night in the country without serious risk of life; nor can the squalid liver-stricken countryman come into the city during the prevalence of yellow fever, without danger of dying with black vomit. A stronger proof of the non-identity of yellow and marsh fevers cannot be demanded.

There are many difficulties in this subject which it is not my purpose to touch, for two reasons: 1st, because it would extend this paper too far; and 2d, because we are greatly wanting in accurate observations on many of the forms of disease, and the topography of their localities, in different parts of the world. I am inclined to think that not only has yellow fever been improperly considered as a mere grade of marsh fever, and attributable to the same cause which produces intermittents; but, that it is very questionable whether all the other endemic fevers of hot climates are attributable to the same poison. There is reason, for example, to believe that the fevers of the coast of Africa are different from those of the United States, and that although they are quite as violent, or even more so to the unacclimated, than ours, yet the native Africans withstand them better than they do our marsh fevers. So with the fevers of Spain and Portugal, which, during the Peninsular war, created such havoc among the English troops, while the *natives* seemed fully acclimated against them. We know that the Italians and the Anglo-Saxons never become accustomed to the endemics around them. I wish to illustrate more particularly the influence of the endemics of the Southern States on the Anglo-Saxon immigrants, and shall, therefore, not pursue this branch of the inquiry.

In treating the subject of *Acclimation*, two very distinct influences are to be considered: 1st, *Temperature;* 2d, *Malarial Exhalations.*

All writers on the diseases of hot climates inform us that, when the people of the North remove to hot climates, the system undergoes a great change from the heat alone. The robust, florid German or Anglo-Saxon in India, Jamaica, or in our Gulf States, perspires profusely, becomes attenuated, debilitated, tanned, and his whole external appearance and internal organism are greatly modified, independently of any malarial influence. This uncomplicated influence of heat may be well studied in our high healthy pine-lands of the South, at the Cape of Good Hope, and many places where intermittent or other malarial diseases do not prevail. Foreigners, in such localities, *do* undergo a positive acclimation. They, after a time, and particularly their descendants, become habituated to heat, and live in hot climates with a certain degree of comfort and health. There is ample reason to believe, however, that natives of the North never can become *perfectly* adapted even to high temperature, and that the duration of life is materially curtailed under such circumstances. The experience of the insurance companies of the United States seems of late to be confirming this view; and my own mind has long been made up to the belief that the Anglo-Saxon race positively deteriorates in hot climates under all circumstances. The population of the South nowhere presents the same vigour as that of Germany and Great Britain; and although they may not have attacks of fever, they are annoyed by many minor ills, which make them a physic-taking people, and curtail the average duration of life. Although Knox has pushed the idea to an extreme that I do not think warranted by facts, yet I do not believe that the climate even of our Northern States is so well adapted to the Anglo-Saxon stock as the temperate zone of Europe from which history derives them.

There is, then, a certain degree of acclimation to *temperature;* and it is equally true that persons so acclimated, and more especially their children, after having gone through this process, are less liable to *violent* attacks of our marsh fevers, when exposed to them, than the fresh immigrants from the North. The latter are more plethoric, their systems more inflammable, and although not more liable to be attacked by these endemics, they experience them, when attacked, in a more violent and more dangerous form. This fact holds good both with regard to remittent and yellow fever.[1]

[1] Dr. Boudin, in his "Lettres sur l'Algérie," after establishing the persistent influence of marsh malaria on French and English colonists, continues thus:—

"Reste à examiner l'influence exercée sur le chiffre des décès par le séjour dans les localités de l'Algérie, *non sujettes aux émanations paludéennes*, mais se distinguant

Leaving, then, the acclimation of temperature, let us come down to the main subject of our investigation, and inquire whether the white races can ever become acclimated against the influence of "malarial exhalations," or, in plain language, the morbific cause of intermittent fever. I recollect well the remark of my medical preceptor, thirty years ago, in South Carolina, that "Natives of the North, though subject to more inflammatory attacks, were *less liable* to intermittent and bilious fevers at the South, for the first year or two, than the natives who were born in malarial districts;" and my own observation leads me to the same conclusion.

The fact is so glaring and so universally admitted, that I am really at a loss how to select evidence to show that there is no acclimation against the endemic fevers of our rural districts. Is it not the constant theme of the population of the South how they can preserve health? and do not all prudent persons who can afford to do so remove in the summer to some salubrious locality in the pine lands or the mountains? Those of the tenth generation are just as solicitous on the subject as those of the first. Books written at the North talk much about acclimation at the South, but we here never hear it alluded to *out of the yellow fever cities.* On the contrary, we know that those who live from generation to generation in malarial districts become

de la France uniquement par une température élevée. A défaut de documents assez nombreux recueillis en Algérie même, nous invoquerons les faits relatifs à deux possessions anglaises ayant la plus grande analogie thermométrique avec notre possession africaine; nous voulons parler: 1°, du Cap de Bonne-Espérance; 2°, de Malte: l'un et l'autre proverbialement exemptés de l'élément paludéen.

"Au Cap de Bonne-Espérance, la mortalité de trois régiments anglais, de 1831 à 1836, a été représentée par les nombres suivants:—

En 1831	26 décès.
" 1832	26 "
" 1833	28 "
" 1834	28 "
" 1835	34 "
" 1836	33 "

"A Malte, où l'on peut considérer les hommes les plus jeunes comme les plus récemment arrivés d'Angleterre, la proportion des décès a suivi la marche ci-après.

Au-dessous de 18 ans	10 décès sur 1000 hommes.
De 18 à 25	18.7 " "
" 25 à 33	23.6 " "
" 33 à 40	29.5 " "
" 40 à 50	34.4 " "

"En résumé, les analogies puisées, non seulement dans les localités paludéennes, mais encore dans les contrées non marécageuses, ayant une plus grande analogie climatologique avec l'Algérie, se montrent peu favorables à l'hypothèse de l'acclimatment."

He then goes on to give statistics both of the civil and military population of Algeria, which show still more deadly effects of climate.

thoroughly poisoned, and exhibit the thousand protean forms of disease which spring from this insidious poison.

I have been the examining physician to several life insurance companies for many years, and one of the questions now asked in many of the policies is, "*Is the party acclimated?*" If the subject lives in one of our southern seaports where yellow fever prevails, and has been born and reared there, or has had an attack of yellow fever, I answer, "*Yes.*" If, on the other hand, he lives in the country, I answer, "*No;*" because there *is no acclimation against intermittent and bilious fever, and other marsh diseases.* Now, I ask if there is an experienced and observing physician at the South who will answer differently? An attack of yellow fever does not protect against marsh fevers, nor *vice versâ.*

The acclimation of negroes, even, according to my observation, has been put in too strong a light. Being originally natives of hot climates, they require no acclimation to *temperature,* and are less liable to the more inflammatory forms of malarial fevers, and suffer infinitely less than whites from yellow fever; they never, however, as far as my observation extends, become proof against intermittents and their sequelæ. The cotton planters throughout the South will bear witness, that, wherever the whites are attacked with intermittents, the blacks are also susceptible, though not in so great a degree. My observations apply to the region of country removed from the rice country. We shall see further on that the negroes of the rice-field region do undergo a higher degree of acclimation than those of the hilly lands of the interior. I know many plantations in the interior of Alabama, South Carolina, Georgia, Mississippi, and Louisiana, on which negroes of the second and third generation continue to suffer from these malarial diseases, and where gangs of negroes do not increase.

Dr. Samuel Forry, in his valuable work on the climate of the United States, has investigated fully the influence of our southern climates on our population, and uses the following decided language in relation to the whites:—

"In these localities, as is often observed in the tide-water region of our Southern States, the human frame is weakly constituted, or imperfectly developed; the mortality among children is very great, and the mean duration of life is comparatively short. Along the frontiers of Florida and the southern borders of Georgia, as witnessed by the author, as well as in the low lands of the southern States generally, may be seen deplorable examples of the physical and perhaps mental deterioration induced by endemic influences. In earliest infancy the complexion becomes sallow, and the eye assumes a bilious tint; advancing towards the years of maturity, the growth is arrested, the limbs become attenuated, the viscera engorged, &c." (P. 365.)

But leaving our own country, let us look abroad and see what the history of other nations teaches.

The best authenticated examples, perhaps, anywhere to be found on record, of the enduring influence of marsh malaria on a race, are in the Campagna,

Maremma, Pontines, and other insalubrious localities in classic Italy. The following account is given by Dr. James Johnson, in his work on *Change of Air*, and every traveller through Italy can vouch for its fidelity:—

"It is from the Mountain of Viterbo that we have the first glimpse of the wide spread *Campagna di Roma.* The beautiful little lake of Vico lies under our feet, its sloping banks cultivated like a garden, but destitute of habitations, on account of the deadly malaria, which no culture can annihilate. From this spot till we reach the desert, the features of poverty and wretchedness in the inhabitants themselves, as well as in everything around them, grow rapidly more marked. We descend from Monti Rose upon the Campagna, and, at Baccano, we are in the midst of it."

After describing the beauty of the scenery and its luxuriant vegetation, he continues—

"But no human form meets the eye, except the gaunt figure of the herdsman, muffled up to the chin in his dark mantle, with his gun and his spear—his broad hat slouched over the ferocious and scowling countenance of a brigand! the buffalo which he guards is less repugnant than he! As for the shepherd, Arcadia forbid that I should attempt his description! The savage of the wigwam has health to recommend him. As we approach within ten miles of Rome, some specks of cultivation appear, and with them the dire effects of malaria on the human frame. Bloated bellies, distorted features, dark yellow complexions, livid eyes and lips; in short, all the symptoms of dropsy, jaundice and ague, united in their persons." "That this deleterious miasma did exist in the Campagna from the very first foundation of Rome down to the present moment, there can be little doubt."

He then goes on to prove the fact from the writings of Cicero, Livy, and others; and makes it clear that the population of Italy are no nearer being *acclimated* against this poison than they were two thousand years ago.

Sir James Johnson makes the following just remark, which applies equally to the malarious districts of our country:—

"A glance at the inhabitants of malarious countries or districts, must convince even the most superficial observer, that the range of disorders produced by the poison of malaria, is very extensive. The jaundiced complexion, the tumid abdomen, the stunted growth, the stupid countenance, the shortened life, attest that habitual exposure to malaria saps the energy of every mental and bodily function and drags its victims to an early grave. A moment's reflection must show us, that *fever* and *ague*, two of the most prominent features of malarious influence, are as a drop of water in the ocean, when compared with the other less obtrusive, but more dangerous maladies that silently, but effectually, disorganize the vital structures of the human fabric, under the operation of the deleterious and invisible poison."

"What are the consequences? Malarious fevers; or, if these are escaped, the foundation of chronic malarious disorders is laid in ample provision for future misery and suffering! These are not speculations, but facts. Compare the range of human existence, as founded on the decrement of human life in Italy and England. In Rome, a twenty fifth part of the population pays the debt of Nature annually. In Naples, a twenty-eighth part dies. In London, only one in forty; and in England, generally, only one in sixty falls before the scythe of time, or the ravages of disease."

As is the case with all of our southern seaports, "the suburbs of Rome are more exposed to malaria than the city; and the open squares and streets, than the narrow lanes in the centre of the metropolis." "The low crowded and abominably filthy quarter of the Jews on the banks of the Tiber, near the foot of the capital, probably owes its acknowledged freedom from the fatal malaria to its sheltered site and inconceivably dense population." This immunity may arise, at least in part, from their position at the *foot* of the hill; for there is no exception to the rule at the South, that a residence on the bank of a river, or in low land, is less affected by malaria than the hill that overlooks it. At present the fact is inexplicable, although universally admitted.

We will here add some interesting facts from the writings of the distinguished military physician, M. le Docteur Boudin, derived from personal observation during long residence in Algeria, and from official government documents.

"On the 31st of December, 1851, the indigenous city population (of Algeria) amounted to 105,865 inhabitants, of whom there were—

Mussulmans	81,329
Negroes	3,488
Jews	21,048

"If we compare this census with that of the year 1849, the following facts appear:—

"1. By a comparison of births and deaths in the official tables, the Mussulman population is decreasing.

"2. The negroes have decreased, in two years, 689.

"3. The Jews, during the same time, have increased 2,020.

"The mortality among the European population in Algeria, from 1842 to 1851, has varied from 44 to 105 out of every 1,000; and, instead of diminishing from year to year under acclimation, *the mortality has steadily increased.*

Mortality according to Nationality.

"Heretofore we have given the mortality of the European population taken in mass. It is understood that this mortality must be greatly influenced by the *origin* of the different elements of the population. We have shown that the half of the European population is composed of strangers (other than French), and numbers over 41,000 Spaniards, and 15,000 Italians and Maltese. The official tables give the following mortality from 1847 to 1851, for the French and strangers (Spaniards, Italians, and Maltese):—

	Deaths for each 1000.	
	Strangers.	French.
1847	48.4	50.8
1848	41.8	41.7
1849	84.3	101.5
1850	43.4	70.5
1851	39.3	64.5"

Thus, on the one side we see that the mortality of the French greatly exceeds that of the other European population; while on the other, in 1850 and

1851, the mortality of the former rises to a figure three times greater than the normal mortality of France.

Jewish Population.

The official tables give the following *résumé* of the mortality of the Jewish population, during the years from 1844 to 1849:—

1844	21.6 deaths per 1,000.
1845	36.1 " "
1847	31.5 " "
1848	23.4 " "
1849	56.9 " "

This mortality is greatly below that of both the European and Mussulman population, and shows the difference of acclimation in Jews and Frenchmen: "Nulle part le Juif ne nait, ne vit, ne meurt comme les autres hommes au milieu desquels il habite. C'est là un point d'anthropologie comparée que nous avons mis hors de contestation dans plusieurs publications."

"According to the last tables of the French establishments in Algeria, the total number of births from 1830 to 1851, have been 44,900, and that of the deaths 62,768" ll! This fact applies to all the provinces, and shows that the climate tends to the extermination of Europeans.

The official statistics also show that the *Mussulman* (Moorish) population is steadily decreasing in the cities. Dr. Boudin asks: "Is this diminution the effect of want, or of demoralization? Is it to be explained by the cessation of unions between the native women and the Turkish soldiers? or finally, is it explained by that mysterious law in virtue of which inferior races seem destined to disappear through contact with superior races?"

Our space does not permit us to dilate on these interesting questions, but it would be an easy task to show that races are adapted to certain climates; and that the mingling of different stocks greatly influences the longevity of individuals, and the *longevity of races*.

As this subject of home acclimation is one of too much importance to be allowed to rest on the opinion of any one individual, I have taken the liberty of writing to several of my professional friends for the results of their observations in different localities and states. All the answers received confirm fully my assertion that the Anglo-Saxon race never can be acclimated against marsh malaria. I should remark that the following letters were written with the haste of private correspondence, and not with the idea of publication. The first letter is from Dr. Dickson, the distinguished Professor of Practice in the Charleston Medical College.

CHARLESTON, May 16, 1856.

MY DEAR DOCTOR: I hasten to reply to yours of the 9th inst., received by yesterday's mail.

1. "The Anglo-Saxon race can never become acclimated against the impression of intermittent and bilious fevers," "periodical," or "malarious fevers." On the contrary, the people living in our low country grow more liable to attack year after year and generation after generation.

We get rid of the poison in some places, and thus extend our limits of residence, but in no other way. Drainage, the formation of an artificial surface on the ground, and other incidents of density of population, such as culinary fires, railroad smokes, and the like, aid to prevent the formation of malaria, or correct it.

Boudin (*British and Foreign Rev.*, Oct. 1849) argues against the possibility of such acclimation, dwelling upon the little success and great mortality attending the colonization of Algeria, the European and English intrusion into Egypt and into Hindostan.

The French, he tells us, cannot keep up their number in Corsica. In the West Indies, the white soldier is twice as likely to die as the black; in Sierra Leone sixteen times more likely, and this continues permanently.

In *Bryson's Reports on the Climate and Principal Diseases of the African Station*, it is affirmed (p. 83) that on board the Atholl (a vessel kept some time on the station) the cases of fever have recovered much more slowly than formerly; so that, instead of its being an advantage to be acclimated, it is apprehended that it will be quite the reverse, as the system becomes relaxed and debilitated by the enervating influence of the climate.

2. "Do *negroes* in this country (rice-field) ever lose their susceptibility to those diseases?" Yes, in very great measure, if not absolutely. If they remain in the same locality, they are scarcely subjects of attack. I use cautious language—too cautious. It is my full belief that they become *insusceptible* of the impression of the cause of periodical or what we call malarious fevers. Who ever saw a negro with an ague cake? I certainly never did. Change of residence begets a certain but very moderate degree of susceptibility. If a house negro be sent to a rice-field he may be attacked. So in shifting along the African coast from place to place, the natives of one locality will be seized by fever sometimes at another. Bryson tells us that Fernando Po is so terribly insalubrious that negroes brought from any part of the African continent are always sickly there, "though the natives of the island itself appear to be a healthy and athletic race of people."

The same author tells us of the general insusceptibility of the particular race called Kroo-men, all along the coast. This class of people are therefore very useful and available, being hired in preference to others on board the cruisers.

3. Negroes increase in number on our rice plantations—nay, it is my impression that the rate of increase is greater than on the less malarial cotton plantations. The majority of deaths that do occur happen in winter and from winter diseases, few dying of fever, none or almost none from bilious, intermittent, or remittents, some from typhus or typhoid, or "typhous" fevers.

* * * * * * *

I remain, &c. &c. &c.,

SAMUEL HENRY DICKSON.

There is an interesting fact in the above letter to me, as I have no experience in the rice-field country. I allude to the acclimation of negroes in these flat swamp-lands, and their increase. As far as my observation goes, the *hilly* rich clay lands of the interior are with few exceptions more liable to malarial fevers than the swamp-lands on the watercourses. The hills in the neighborhood of our swamp-lands are always more sickly than the residences which are *on the river banks*. Professor Dickson says the rice-field negroes increase more than those on the cotton plantations. Certainly, negroes do suffer greatly on many cotton plantations in the middle belt of the southern States; and I have seen no evidence to prove that negroes can in this region become accustomed to the marsh poison, and my observation has been extensive in four States. A question here arises, is there any difference in types of those malarial fevers which originate in the flat tide-water rice-lands and those of the clay hills, or marsh fevers of the interior? I am inclined to think there is.

The following letter is from my friend Dr. Wm. M. Boling, of Montgomery, Alabama, who has had much experience in this region, and who is well known as one of our best medical writers.

MONTGOMERY, *Ala.*, May 17, 1856.

DEAR DOCTOR: Judging from my own observation, I am inclined to believe that there is no such thing as acclimation to miasmatic localities; in other words, that neither residence in a miasmatic locality nor an attack or even repeated attacks of any of the various shades or forms of miasmatic fevers confer any power of resistance to what we understand by the miasmatic poison—not regarding yellow fever, however, as belonging to this class of disease. On the contrary, one attack, it seems to me, instead of incurring an immunity from rather increases the tendency or predisposition to another. It would be no difficult matter, I think, to obtain histories of cases of persons born and continuing to live in miasmatic localities who have been subject to repeated attacks of miasmatic fevers occasionally during the entire course of their lives—say from a few days after birth to a moderate old age—"from the cradle to the grave." We do, to be sure, meet with persons who have resided for a considerable time in miasmatic localities without ever having had an attack of any of the forms of the fever in question. Such instances are more common, if I mistake not, among persons who have removed from a healthy into a miasmatic locality than among such as may have been born and reared in the latter. But it is a rare thing, indeed, according to my observation, to meet with a person residing in a place where miasmatic diseases are rife who has had *one attack and no more.*

Yours, &c. &c.,

WM. M. BOLING.

The identity or non-identity of yellow and marsh fevers has much to do with the subject of acclimation, but I must refer for my views on this subject to a paper of mine published some twelve months ago in the *New Orleans Medical News and Hospital Gazette.*

ART. III.—*Removal of the Entire Lower Jaw for Osteo-sarcoma.* By GEORGE C. BLACKMAN, M. D., Professor of Surgery in the Medical College of Ohio; Surgeon to the Commercial Hospital, Cincinnati, &c. &c. (With a wood-cut.)

MRS. V., æt. 60, corpulent, and of excellent general health, consulted me in May last in reference to an affection of the lower jaw, with which she had been troubled for about forty years. Its origin was attributed to an injury inflicted during the extraction of a decayed tooth on the right side. The swelling extended, at the time of my first visit, from near the external angle of the eye to the opposite ramus of the lower jaw. The mouth was enormously elongated and distorted, as represented in the wood-cut. The tumour extended downwards below the clavicle, and at its lowest point there was an opening some two inches in diameter, through which a bloody matter was discharged in large quantities. For many years the disease was very slow in its progress, but during the past two years the latter had been much more rapid. Of late, she had experienced much difficulty in taking nourishment, and, from the pressure of the enormous mass on the side of her throat, she was often threatened with suffocation. With the exception of the fungous opening already mentioned, the integuments covering the tumour presented a natural appearance. The glands of the neck were free from disease.

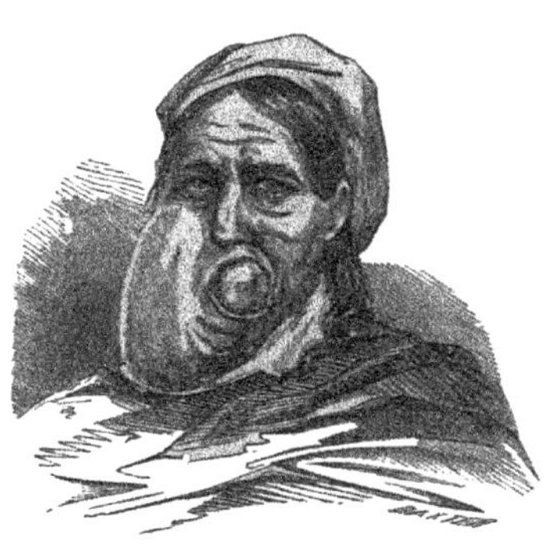

I advised an operation, and urged its performance before the commencement of the hot season. She failed, however, to arrange her affairs to come to the city until the latter part of June. At her request, chloroform was administered, or rather a mixture of one part of chloroform and two of sulphuric ether. She was very readily brought under its influence, when I made an incision which commenced just in front of the ear, on a level with the right eye, and extended to the angle on the left side. It passed about an inch and a half below the border of the lower lip, and the commissure was not divided on either side. Another incision was made which included the fungous opening, and the superabundant integument which required removal. The flaps were rapidly dissected, and the bony tumour exposed. The facial arteries bled freely, but were at once controlled by pressure until the ligatures were ready to be applied. With one of Luer's small saws I divided the bone at the left angle, detached the tongue, and disarticulated the right ramus. This was rendered less difficult, as the pressure produced on the condyles by the extension of the tumour beneath the zygoma, caused an absorption of their substance so that they readily separated, and the portions remaining at the articulation were easily extracted with the forceps. As the disease had already invaded the left ramus, this was also removed from the articulation. Retraction of the tongue, which had nearly proved fatal in several of my previous operations on the lower jaw, was guarded against at the very outset of the operation, by passing a strong cord through the organ, which was held by a trusty assistant. In this case, however, there seemed to be no tendency to any such retraction. The removal of the entire bone was accomplished in about fifteen minutes, and the patient lost not more than from six to eight ounces of blood. For an hour after the operation (at 3 P. M.), she seemed greatly prostrated, and until 8 o'clock that evening her pulse continued feeble. Beef-tea, wine, or brandy were regularly administered, at first through a tube, afterwards through the spout of a cup contrived for the purpose. There was no difficulty in swallowing, and her respiration was easy. She passed the night as comfortably as could have been expected, and at 8 o'clock next morning took her nourishment well, and even articulated some words distinctly. At 9 o'clock the heat was intense; no breeze was stirring, and as the sun approached the meridian, the thermometer rose in the patient's chamber to 98°. At 11 o'clock it became evident that her strength was failing, and at 1 o'clock P. M., when the heat had attained its greatest intensity (100° Fahr.) she died without a struggle.

I was assisted in the operation by several of the first physicians of Cincinnati, among whom I may name Drs. Carrol, Fries, Dandridge, Dodge, Foster, Armor, Muscroft, &c. &c., and I believe all agree in attributing her death to the exhaustion occasioned by the intense heat. Perhaps the anæsthetic likewise exercised a deleterious influence, but how much is due to that, it would be difficult to determine.

The tumour weighed 3½ lbs., and presented all the anatomical characteristics of osteo-sarcoma.

The removal of the entire lower jaw for necrosis has been performed by Perry, of England; Ganwesky, of Westphalia; Maisonneuve, of Paris; Pitha, of Prague, and Heyfelder, of Erlangen; also by McClellan, Carnochan, Marsh, and James R. Wood, of our own country. These cases are of interest, inasmuch as their results furnish us with illustrations of the wonderful reparative powers of nature, but they can hardly be classed with the operations for osteo-sarcoma executed by Professor Syme, Mr. Cusack, of Dublin; Mr. O'Shaughnessy, of India; by Dieffenbach, of Berlin; by Dr. Mott in the case of the negro "Prince;" by Dr. Ackley, of Cleveland, and I think I may add, by myself. In Professor Syme's case of removal of the entire lower jaw, the patient died suddenly the day after the operation, as was supposed, from suffocation produced by the retraction of the tongue. (*Contributions to the Pathology and Practice of Surgery*, p. 21.) Mr. Cusack informed me in June, 1853, that some fifteen years before, he had, for osteo-sarcoma, extirpated the entire bone, and that his patient died a week afterwards, during his absence from town, in a supposed epileptic fit. Dr. Signoroni, of Padua, is reported (*Phil. Med. Exam.*, vol. vii., 1844, p. 96), to have exhibited to the Medical Congress of that city, Sept. 27, 1842, a patient, from whom, by successive operations, he had removed the entire lower jaw affected with osteo-sarcoma. The patient was then in perfect health. Mr. William Hetling, Surgeon to the Bristol Infirmary, England, reported in the *Transactions of the Provincial Medical and Surgical Association*, 1833, p. 277, a case of very extensive osteo-sarcoma of the lower jaw, in which the greater part of that bone was removed, and in this report he makes the following statement: "Mr. Liston, of this city, lately removed the whole lower jaw in a case of this kind; and recovery would certainly have taken place had not an attack of the erysipelatous inflammation, then epidemic, supervened, and proved fatal."

For many years, Walther, of Bonn, has had the credit of having successfully removed the entire lower jaw, and as his claims have been questioned by some surgeons, we insert the following extract from a letter addressed by his nephew, Dr. J. E. Webber, to Dr. Perkins, of New York:—

"Suffice it to say, that I myself am acquainted with eye-witnesses, yet living, who saw the case before the operation, during the operation, and after the operation and subsequent recovery, and there is at this moment in the hands of the eldest son of Walther, a distinguished physician at the capital of Bavaria, a written account, minute in its details, affording a complete history of the case; which report, written by himself, at the request of his father a few days subsequent to the removal of the bone, will be published among the collected papers of Dr. Walther, which his family are about giving to the world."

I have been informed by Dr. Mott, that he has examined an individual who stated that his entire lower jaw had been removed by Mr. Hutton, of Dublin.

The most extraordinary operation on record is unquestionably that reported by Professor Syme, in the *Edinburgh Medical and Surgical Journal*, vol. xxx., 1828, p. 286. The illustrations there given present truly a frightful picture:—

"The mouth was placed diagonally across the face, and had suffered such monstrous distortion as to measure fifteen inches in circumference. The throat of the patient was almost obliterated, there being only about two inches of it above the sternum, so that the cricoid cartilage of the larynx was on a level with that bone. When the tumour was viewed in profile it extended eight inches from the front of the neck. It completely filled the mouth, and occupied all the space below it from jaw to jaw. The tongue was thrust out of its place, and lay between the teeth and cheek of the right side," &c. &c.

The jaw was removed from the right articulation to the left angle, and had a speedy recovery. The tumour weighed 4½ lbs.! In the 38th volume of the same journal (1832), Professor Syme states (p. 321) that the patient continued quite well, "masticating and articulating perfectly, and having nothing very disagreeable in his appearance." On the same page he refers to a preparation removed after death by Dr. Martin, of Chatham, in which the mass protruding from the patient's mouth measured at its neck twenty-one inches in circumference, and weighed 8 pounds!

I might notice in detail the successful operations of Cusack, O'Shaughnessy, Ackley, and others, in which nearly the whole bone was removed for osteo-sarcoma; but these are already familiar to the surgeon.

We will only add, that if in the terrible operation performed by Professor Syme, as well as by myself, but a few ounces of blood were lost, surely in operations of less magnitude in this region, the ligature of the primitive carotid must be unnecessary.

I have referred to the cases in which the entire lower jaw has been removed for necrosis, and, in connection with this subject, I would remark that I have in my possession the entire jaw affected with that form of the disease produced by the action of phosphorus among those engaged in the manufacture of lucifer matches. The operation was performed by Dr. Marsh, of Cincinnati, some three years since, at the Infirmary; but the patient survived it only a few months. This case was, therefore, prior to that in the practice of Dr. James R. Wood, which was reported in the May number of the *New York Journal of Medicine*. Dr. Marsh's patient came from Nuremberg, Germany, a place of considerable notoriety in consequence of the prevalence of the phosphorus disease.

ART. IV.—*On the Climate and Salubrity of Fort Moultrie and Sullivan's Island, Charleston Harbour, S. C., with Incidental Remarks on the Yellow Fever of the City of Charleston.* By JOHN B. PORTER, M. D., Surgeon U. S. Army. (*Concluded.*)

1853 was one of the most healthy years known on Sullivan's Island since the conclusion of the war with Mexico. Although diarrhœa was rather common, there was not a single case of cholera infantum at Fort Moultrie during the whole summer—an unusual event—though there were a good many cases of this disease on the island.

Fevers were more prevalent in April and May than in the usual fever months of August, September, and October. The great rains of 1852 had saturated the earth; there was considerable winter rain, and the last half of April, and almost the whole of May, were hot and dry. The action of the hot sun on the porous soil produced disease early in the season.

Variola, owing to the neglect of vaccination, prevailed in Charleston during the winter of 1853–54, but there were no cases on Sullivan's Island. Other eruptive fevers, as measles and scarlatina, were not uncommon in Charleston, but none of them made their appearance on the island. Here are a class of acknowledged contagious fevers—smallpox, measles, scarlatina—which are legitimate objects of quarantine. Smallpox was so prevalent in Charleston in 1853 and '54 as to affect the commercial interests. Country merchants and others were afraid to come to the city, yet no attempt was made at quarantine.

Abstract of the Meteorological Register at Fort Moultrie, S. C., for the year 1853.

MONTH.	BAROMETER.			THERMOMETER ATTACHED.				THERMOMETER DETACHED.					Highest degree.	Lowest degree.	Range.	Hottest day: mean.	Coldest day: mean.	Range.	Dew-point: mean.
	Max.	Min.	Range.	Sun-rise.	9 A.M.	3 P.M.	9 P.M.	Sun-rise.	9 A.M.	3 P.M.	9 P.M.	Av'ge mean temp.							
January	30.750	29.300	1.450	47.38	49.29	54.37	53.38	42.16	46.67	55.09	47.00	48.62	68	27	41	63.5	34.0	29.5	40.61
February	30.425	29.000	1.425	53.14	54.62	58 76	57.64	47.35	53.39	59.28	52.78	53.32	71	33	38	63.0	42.5	20.5	43.14
March	30.425	29.750	0.675	57.20	58.51	61.67	60.66	53.09	58.38	64.06	57.35	58.58	75	35	40	69.5	44.0	25.5	50.20
April	30.400	29.500	0.900	64.23	66.41	69.41	67.03	61.13	68.40	71.73	65.26	66.43	82	47	35	76.0	55.5	20.5	59.35
May	30.450	29.970	0.480	70.67	73.03	75.53	73.35	68.32	75.96	76.77	72.54	72.54	84	56	28	78.0	63.0	15.0	66.50
June	30.400	30.050	0.350	75.30	77.95	80.18	77.68	74.10	82.73	82.80	77.93	78.48	96	66	30	84.5	72.5	12.0	71.40
July	30.375	30.025	0.350	79.08	81.27	83.56	80.54	79.29	84.87	86.41	80.74	82.85	91	72	19	86.5	76.0	10.5	77.33
August	30.320	29.870	0.450	76.82	79.77	81.80	79.56	75.87	83.51	84.29	79.74	80.08	95	66	29	85.0	71.0	14.0	75.32
September	30.340	29.960	0.380	73.61	75.90	78.28	76.06	72.36	79.06	81.30	75.50	76.83	95	57	38	84.5	64.0	20.5	71.85
October	30.390	29.775	0.615	62.56	64.24	68.27	66.41	59.87	66.45	71.51	64.96	65.69	81	38	43	76.0	47.5	28.5	60.10
November	30.650	29.900	0.750	57.38	59.31	64.11	61.43	55.83	59.83	66.36	60.06	61.10	77	42	35	68.5	48.5	20.0	52.50
December	30.525	29.600	0.925	48.37	48.64	54.96	52.24	45.19	47.55	53.32	48.68	50.22	66	31	35	62.0	37.0	25.0	42.05

MONTH.	COURSE OF WIND AT SUNRISE.								Pre-vail-ing.	COURSE OF WIND AT 3 P. M.								Pre-vail-ing.	Rainy days.	Rain: quantity.
	N.	N. E.	N. W.	S.	S. E.	S. W.	E.	W.		N.	N. E.	N. W.	S.	S. E.	S. W.	E.	W.			
January	18	2	3	0	1	3	0	4	N.	6	9	2	2	2	2	4	4	N.	5	1.90
February	7	2	2	4	1	4	3	5	N.	1	2	3	7	5	3	4	3	S.	3	2.80
March	6	3	6	1	1	12	0	2	S. W.	2	4	2	4	4	5	3	7	W.	8	3.30
April	6	2	1	3	2	13	1	2	S. W.	0	5	1	9	7	3	3	2	S.	3	1.06
May	3	7	2	4	4	5	1	5	N. E.	0	5	1	3	14	4	4	0	S. E.	6	2.53
June	6	4	2	4	5	3	4	2	N.	0	3	1	6	10	1	9	0	S. E.	2	1.55
July	0	2	2	2	2	17	1	5	S. W.	0	1	0	11	13	5	0	1	S. E.	8	10.88
August	7	3	1	6	2	7	0	5	S. W.	0	7	0	5	8	5	6	0	S E.	8	2.20
September	11	1	0	2	3	4	5	4	N.	1	10	1	1	6	4	4	3	N. E.	8	8.10
October	18	2	1	1	1	4	1	3	N.	7	9	1	4	2	4	2	2	N. E.	8	4.05
November	14	8	4	1	0	2	0	1	N.	3	19	3	2	0	2	0	1	N. E.	6	4.89
December	2	3	7	0	1	6	1	3	N.	2	10	5	4	0	3	1	6	N. E.	8	2.39

Total quantity of rain, 45.65

Highest degree in the year, 96; June 24.
Lowest degree in the year, 27; January 28.
Range for the year, 69°.
Feb. 25. Peach-trees in blossom.
March 3. Plum in blossom.
Ther. from 90° to 96°, June 5, 6, 7, 17, and 21.

Ther. 90° and above, July 5, 6, 12; August 4, 5, 6, 14; September 7, 8, 9, 15.
Oct. 24. Ther. at sunrise, 71°.
Oct. 25. Ther. at sunrise, 38°.
Difference in 24 hours, 33°.
Oct. 25. Light frost.

No frost in the month of November.
Dec. 20. Ice ⅛ inch thick. First black frost.
Dec. 21. Thin ice.
Dec. 24. Thin ice.
Dec. 25. Rain, sleet, and snow.
Dec. 27. Thin ice.

Dr. Hume states:—

"The exemption of Charleston from yellow fever during the last summer [1853], is a subject of astonishment to all observers. That the season was unpropitious to health, the ravages of the fever on the southwestern waters, and other regions, fully exhibit. That we shared that general diffusion of unpropitious atmosphere, must be admitted, and our meteorological instruments testify to the same. Yet the devouring angel spared our city. * * * It is true that two attempts were made by the fever to invade our city, but it was rudely and unceremoniously repelled, and expelled on both occasions. As action was prompt, the history is short. Capt. P., of the Ellen Goldsborough, arrived from Baltimore on the 30th August, sickened on the 4th September, was sent to the Marine Hospital on the 6th, was declared to have yellow fever, and, on the 7th, was sent to the Lazaretto, where he died on the 10th. On the 23d September, Captain P., of the Barkelew, was reported under similar circumstances, and was immediately sent to the Lazaretto, where he also died. Thus ended both attempts of invasion, and we may here remark that it is the first instance of *Jacksonism*, in a matter of this kind, ever undertaken by a mayor to preserve the public health; and we have every reason to believe that to this prompt and decided action the health of the city is to be attributed. It is impossible now to say what might have been the result, if these vigorous measures had not been adopted, but we all know what has been the result when they have been neglected."

We will give some additional facts, a part of which Dr. H. might have included in his history.

The schooner Ellen Goldsborough arrived from Baltimore, August 30, 1853; lay at Accommodation Wharf. Two of the seamen were sent down to the Lazaretto from the same vessel, who recovered.

"Now the captain," says Dr. Simons, Port Physician, "was sick for some time in the Marine Hospital; had the black vomit, and, although staying in the same room with other mariners, yet the disease never extended, nor did any new cases occur in the vessel, or in any of the surrounding vessels."

It is desirable to learn if the Ellen G. carried the fever from Charleston to any other port; and the following, from Dr. Grafton, Port Physician of Baltimore, satisfies us on this point:—

"The Ellen Goldsborough, I find by reference to my books, passed quarantine on the 19th September last (1853), and, I presume, was free from disease of any kind, since she was not detained, and no cases taken from on board her. I cannot speak from personal knowledge, because of my absence from the hospital on sick leave. I never heard there were any cases on board, on or after her arrival at this port."

It is conclusive that the yellow fever was not carried from Baltimore to Charleston by the Ellen G.; and that the disease was not taken from Charleston by the same vessel, after the fever had occurred on board, to any other port. In connection with yellow fever, the Ellen G. is never heard of, after sailing from Charleston.

The schooner Barkelew (Berkelew), S. S. Kittridge, Master, arrived from Philadelphia on the 29th of August, 1853; lay at Accommodation Wharf. Dr. Hume might have easily given this information; and the date of arrival is a material circumstance, for without it we are left to infer that the Barkelew brought the fever from Philadelphia, particularly as the barque Mandarin, from Cienfuegos, Cuba, is brought into full view.

The Barkelew arrived at Charleston on the 29th August, and the first case of fever, the only case on board, occurred on the 23d September, twenty-five days after arrival, not in the person of Capt. P. (S. S. Kittridge), but in the person of his mate, or assistant. Why did not this patient communicate the fever to others? How could the mayor's "Jacksonism" protect the exposed persons?

Another important fact in relation to the sick of both vessels was obtained from the same medical gentleman, who has high character and standing. They had slept on deck without awnings. The same gentleman remarked that he could, in any summer, give a malignant fever to the most healthy northern man in a week, in the port of Charleston, provided his directions were strictly followed; to wit: heat himself during the day, drink a good deal of bad liquor, and sleep at night on the deck of a vessel, in the docks, without an awning. We have great confidence in the recipe. Dr. Simons alludes to this subject in his history of the epidemic of 1839.

Dr. Gilbert, Port Physician of Philadelphia, gives what follows:—

"The schooner Barkelew sailed from Philadelphia June 28, and arrived at Charleston August 29, having been out so long that she was considered, for a time, lost. She had arrived in our port from Charleston June 6, consequently she was here three weeks, and, during this time, lay at a pier between Market and Arch Streets. She did not again return to Philadelphia. Our yellow fever visitation embraced a period from about the 20th July to October 7, 1853; consequently she could not have received any infection whilst in this port, and her wharf was at least half a mile north of the locality in which the fever prevailed."

Abstract.

Barkelew arrived at Philadelphia, from Charleston, healthy,	June 6.
Barkelew left Philadelphia, on return to Charleston, healthy,	June 28.
Barkelew arrived at Charleston, healthy,	Aug. 29.
First case of fever on the Barkelew—only case,	Sept. 23.
First case of yellow fever in Philadelphia,	July 4.
Barque Mandarin arrived in Philadelphia,	July 13.
First fever case in vicinity of the Mandarin,	July 19.
Distance between the piers of the two vessels,	½ mile.

Dr. Gilbert's account settles the question in relation to the Barkelew.

We have thus, with some trouble to ourselves and others, collected the facts, many of which ought to have been presented by Dr. Hume. In investigations of this kind, nothing is more material than great attention to dates, which Dr. Hume seems to have almost entirely neglected in his history of the Barkelew.

We have two interesting cases, in 1853, from Dr. Robertson.

First case. "Arrived from New Orleans July 2. This patient, a lady, was taken at sea, and was brought up from outside the bar in the pilot boat. She had yellow skin, hiccough, constant nausea and retching, and bloody oozing from the gums. She was carried to a boarding house in King Street, where she remained until convalescence, when she left in the steamer for New York."

Here was a case of imported contagion, if there ever was one. The patient went through her illness without *surveillance*, unmolested by quarantines and lazarettoes, recovered, and "went on her way rejoicing." But why did not the contagion of this malignant case remain behind and spread? Simply because yellow fever is not contagious.

Second case. "On board the Isabel, July 25. Taken on the night of her arrival (24th) from Havana, where the disease prevailed. He was confined to the ship at Dry Dock Wharves, but free intercourse was allowed with him. It was a mild, but well-marked case."

If yellow fever is contagious, the disease should have spread in Charleston. No matter how or where the cases originated, the disease was introduced from the Ellen Goldsborough, the Barkelew, New Orleans, and by the Isabel from Havana; four points of origin, instead of "two attempts at invasion," as related by Dr. Hume, so that yellow fever ought to have spread over the city.

Regarding the barque Mandarin, in the port of Philadelphia, which vessel Dr. Hume attempts to give an account of, little will be said. In the first place, Dr. Jewell says that "in no instance can it be shown that the disease has spread from those labouring under the fever;" secondly, the disease was limited in extent; and, finally, Dr. La Roche has conclusively shown that it had a local origin, and that cases of it existed in the city anterior to the arrival of the Mandarin.

1854. Yellow fever prevailed in all parts of Charleston, but it did not spread on Sullivan's Island. Number of deaths: whites, 612—colored, 15, according to the report of the City Register. We do not propose to give the details of this epidemic, and only a few prominent points will be noticed.

Digging and excavating went on in the city during the warm season as usual. Church Street was being paved in April, and Anson Street in June. The work on the new custom-house was continued as heretofore; and the "filling in of the open space between the basin and street" with dock mud, at the new fish market (foot of Market Street), proceeded.[1] This "filling in" with dock mud was carried on during the hot season, and also paving the streets, and excavating at the new custom-house; and it was often remarked, as early as April, that if Charleston escaped yellow fever in 1854, the exemption must be attributed to the special interposition of a kind Providence. During the whole summer, the city was in bad police, and it would have been surprising if fever had not made its appearance, particularly in the vicinity of the docks and wharves. Fever did prevail, as by many was anticipated; and the disease was more severe after the gale of September 8th than previously, owing, probably, to the water and dock mud having been driven, by the heavy wind at high tide, into the streets and cellars nearly up to Meeting Street.

For the following facts in relation to the first cases of fever, I am indebted to the Report of Dr. J. L. Dawson, City Register, to the Board of Health, August 22, 1854.

[1] Proceedings of Council, February 14, 1854. Report of Market Board. (Vide *Am. Journ. Med. Sciences* for October, 1854.)

The first case occurred on the steamer Isabel, just from Havana. It is a singular fact that not one case of fever was traced from this, the first in the city, from the 11th of May to the 7th of August, a period of nearly three months.

Nor was a single case of fever traced from the second case, an Irish nurse on board the Isabel, from the 11th of July, although the patient went to a hotel, and mixed freely with all sorts of persons. Not a single case of fever was ever traced to these two first cases.

The ship Sullivan, from New York, arrived at Accommodation Wharf on the 21st July, one day before the Spanish polacres, and a case of fever (third case) occurred on board on the 7th August, 17 days after her arrival, a period of time amply sufficient, in the then state of the docks, for yellow fever to appear. If contracted from the sick of the polacres, the fever seems to have had a stage of incubation 16 days in duration, or four times as long as that of the old standard contagionists.

The Vesta arrived from Boston on the 16th July; lay at Union wharves, next to the Aquatic (which had fever on board), and no case of fever occurred until the 7th August, 22 days after arrival. Union wharves have been noticed as one of the worst localities in the city; and with or without the Aquatic, we are not surprised that the crew had yellow fever after laying 22 days at these wharves.

The brig Iris arrived from Maine on the 22d July, and lay at the new Custom House wharf until the 1st of August, 10 days, when she hauled round to Potter's wharf, on Ashley River. New Custom-House wharf is on or near Market Street dock, and on this dock (always filthy) the new fish-market was in process of construction, with the "filling in." Is it surprising that malarial fever, or even yellow fever, should affect the crew of this vessel?

The man who worked on board the Aquatic one month after her arrival at quarantine might or might not have contracted the fever on board. Pinckney Street, his place of residence, was in bad police. The man might have taken the fever on board the Aquatic, or on any other dirty and unhealthy vessel, and yet be unable to spread it in Meeting Street, or anywhere else.

But how came the Irish woman, residing in a respectable family on East Bay, near the Battery, to be seized with malignant yellow fever on the 13th of August? She had no communication with any person on the fever vessels; the wharves at which these vessels lay were at a distance from her place of residence, and no person on shore had been attacked with fever except the man in Pinckney Street (a great distance from East Bay and the Battery), he, having been taken on the 12th, died on the 14th, and the woman, attacked on the 13th, died on the 15th. We can account for the case only in this way; that the fever was already breaking out at different points in the city, as fully appeared on the 17th and 18th, only four and five days after this woman was attacked with the disease.

The barque Aura cleared from New Orleans on the 14th July, arrived at

Brown's wharf, where there had been no fever, on the 2d August, lay there until the 12th, and had a case on board on the 14th, just one month after clearing from a port where yellow fever prevailed.

We come to the cases at Central wharf. We find there were four cases of fever on as many different vessels from northern ports, these vessels having arrived on the 7th, 8th, and 9th of August, and all of these sick were attacked with the fever on the 17th of August. On the same day, a clerk on Central wharf was taken with yellow fever, making five cases on the 17th. No vessel with fever had been at this wharf during the season; these vessels brought no disease, yet five persons were seized with fever in one day, all of whom had been in this unhealthy part of the city at least eight days previous to the attack.

A seaman was sent to the Marine Hospital from brig Emily, Accommodation wharf, August 18th; taken on the 15th.

The wife of an Irishman was taken sick in Calhoun Street, near Anson; and died on the 18th, having been sick at least two days. This woman was in a part of the city not frequented by mariners, far from the wharves and shipping, and at a great distance from Pinckney Street. No case of yellow fever had yet appeared anywhere in the vicinity of this woman's residence.

A man residing at 33 Broad Street (one of the best streets in the city) was taken on the 18th August, two Germans at the foot of Hazel Street on the 19th, and one on the 21st, at the corner of State and Queen Streets.

Abstract of the Principal Cases.

Point of origin.	No. of cases.	Date of attack.
New Custom-House Wharf and Ashley River, brig Iris	2	Aug. 7th and 10th.
East Bay, near Battery	1	" 13th.
Brown's Wharf, Aura	1	" 14th.
Calhoun Street	1	" 15th or 16th.
Central Wharf	5	" 17th.
Broad Street	1	" 18th.
Hazel Street	2	" 19th.
State and Queen Streets . . .	1	" 21st.

It appears from Dr. Dawson's report that 23 cases of fever and nine deaths occurred in Charleston from May 11th to August 22d; 14 of these cases were on shore, or on board vessels at different wharves from the Aquatic and Spanish polacres, where there had previously been no fever. Nor is there a probability that the two women on East Bay and Calhoun Street had communication with any fever patient, nor those on Broad, Hazel, and State, and Queen Streets. We find several points of origin, and a majority of those attacked with fever were never exposed to the sick, nor to any malign influence on board the vessels reputed to be infected. From what source did many of these sick, particularly those near the Battery and on Calhoun Street, receive the contagion?

Our limits will not permit further remarks. Dr. Dawson's report is well worth a careful perusal.

In conclusion of remarks on the yellow fever of Charleston: There is no evidence that the fever was ever derived from imported contagion from the year 1699 to 1854; but, on the contrary, there is abundant proof that very many of the epidemics were of domestic origin. Similar views were entertained by Dr. Simons in 1851.

Yellow fever did not prevail on Sullivan's Island this year, but bilious fever was common, particularly after the gale of September 8th, when the island was nearly overflown, great damage was done, and large quantities of mud, sea-weed, &c., were driven on shore, where they soon took on the putrefactive process in the hot sun, and bilious fever was severe in consequence.

Two interesting cases of yellow fever occurred on the island this year. First case. Capt. W———, late of Augusta, Ga., an officer in one of the banks, removed from Charleston with his family to the island, on account of the fever in the last part of August, but his business required him to visit the city daily; he had yellow fever in September, black vomit, and died. It was a malignant case. His wife and several children, who did not go to the city, escaped fever, and not a single person on the island contracted the disease. Refer to Dr. F. M. Robertson, Charleston, for further particulars.

Second case. In the month of October, a discharged, dissipated soldier, went from Charleston to Fort Moultrie to enlist, and in two or three days he was attacked with fever, had black vomit, and died. Not a single man of the garrison had ever had yellow fever; not one of them had ever been exposed to it; not one of them took it from this case, not even the steward and nurses; nor was there another case in garrison during the year. Similar instances during this epidemic might be related.

Yellow fever prevailed on Sullivan's Island in the following years:—

1795. An aged gentleman, one of the most respectable and reliable men in Charleston District, informed me that he well recollects when yellow fever broke out in a certain locality on Sullivan's Island, east of Fort Moultrie, in Middle Street, and there were several deaths. The cause was this: A large lot was low, and quite wet, being little better than a marsh, and in the spring of this year the lot was raised by filling in with sedge and marsh mud instead of dry sand; in consequence, the fever broke out, and many deaths occurred.

1800. The fever occurred again this year. (*Med. Repos.*, vol. iv. p. 219.)

1802. "Charleston was afflicted with four epidemics; the smallpox, the measles, the influenza, and the yellow fever." This shows that there was "an epidemic constitution of the atmosphere," so much ridiculed by some; at any rate, four different diseases were epidemic. We would like to be informed what vessels imported these four diseases, and from what part of the world they were imported. "No instance can be recollected in which there was any ground to suppose that the yellow fever was either imported, or had been contagious." * * * "Five cases of the yellow fever (two of them fatal) occurred in one house on the island, while the other inhabitants were generally healthy." (*Med. Repos.*, vol. vi. p. 311.)

1807. "The disease in no instance proved contagious. It was carried from Charleston to Sullivan's Island, but whether they lived or died, the disease terminated with them." (*Med. Rep.*, vol. xi. p. 234.)

1817. Dr. Strobel's statement in relation to the yellow fever of this year has been sufficiently alluded to; and we will simply remark in this place that the large number of persons who went to Sullivan's Island to avoid the fever —" many of them in indigent circumstances," and crowded together in narrow, confined apartments"—may have engendered the fever as well here as in Lynch's Lane, in Charleston.

1824. "Independent of the distresses which occurred in the city, the disease broke out with dreadful malignancy among those who had sought refuge from its ravages on Sullivan's Island." (Dr. Simons, *Carolina Journ. Med.*, January, 1825.)

1827. Yellow fever occurred on the island and among the garrison of the fort. Assistant-surgeon C. F. Luce, U. S. A., died of this fever Sept. 27th, and there were several deaths among the officers and men. Major Lowd, U. S. A., informed me that it was very sickly at Fort Moultrie during this summer, and the cause was supposed to be that repairs were going on in hot weather; the lower floors were torn up, which exposed a large surface of wet or moist earth and rubbish. There was also much sickness, and several deaths, among the citizens on the island; and altogether, it was a year of much distress.

1834. Five cases of the fever (2 fatal) reported at Fort Moultrie; 2 of them originated in Charleston, 3 at Castle Pinckney.

1838. We refer to Dr. Lebby's letter for a case of yellow fever on Sullivan's Island, to which numbers were exposed, but "no other instance of it occurred in the family."

1839. We refer to Dr. Lebby's letter in full for an account of the fever on Sullivan's Island during this year. In this letter we find that "the Irishman who had not been in the city from May" and was taken last of August, did not come in contact with the other cases, and his fever originated on the island. Captain R.'s case and others originated on the island.

1852. This epidemic has been spoken of sufficiently; there can be no doubt that this fever was of domestic origin.

The diseases of Sullivan's Island are such as might be expected, considering the climate and other circumstances.

"Fevers are the proper endemics of Carolina, and occur oftener than any, probably than all other diseases. These are the effects of its warm, moist climate, of its low grounds, and stagnant waters. In their mildest season they assume the type of intermittents; in their next grade they are bilious remittents; and under particular circumstances, in their highest grade, constitute yellow fever."—Dr. Ramsay, *Hist. South Carolina*, vol. ii. p. 97.

All these fevers originate on Sullivan's Island—intermittent, remittent, congestive, and yellow fever—but the most common form of fever is the bilious remittent. Not a summer passes without more or less of it; sometimes it is mild, and at others severe. Fevers are so common on the east end of the island that this part of it is considered unhealthy.

Cholera infantum is indigenous, as might be expected from the proximity of the island to the city of Charleston, in the low country, in a hot climate, a humid atmosphere, and a high dew-point. Children who have had the complaint in the city have often been sent to the island to recover, and the benefit of the change is often surprising; and on the other hand, when the acute stage of the disease has been spent on the island, we have been solicitous that a change should be made—to Buncombe, N. C., to the North, or even to Charleston. We have known little patients to improve greatly by a removal to Charleston, the strong and damp winds of the island appearing to injure many of them. Change, of almost any kind, seems to work wonders in the chronic stage of this disease.

Chronic diarrhœa and dysentery are serious diseases in summer, and all persons affected by them should have a change of climate without delay.

The island is an improper residence for those who are affected with chronic bronchitis, or phthisis pulmonalis. In summer it is too hot, and the winds are too strong and damp, and in winter the cold and bleak winds render the island a very unadvisable resort.

Asthma is often greatly relieved by an island residence, even in winter. On the other hand, the disease is aggravated, and in some instances patients are obliged to remove when the winter winds come on.

Chronic rheumatism and neuralgic pains are not benefited by an island residence; the climate, both winter and summer, is too severe for such invalids.

Persons in a state of debility from almost any disease—fever, dysentery, cholera infantum, &c.—often come from Charleston to the island and recover their strength and appetite in a short time; and those who have suffered from the same complaints on the island are equally benefited by a change to the upper country, as already stated.

Vermes (the *ascaris lumbricoides*), during my residence at Sullivan's Island, were more common among children than in any part of the United States in which I have practised medicine.

From the physical character of the country around Charleston, it is evident that the summer climate is enervating, and most persons would improve by annually or biennially spending July and August in a more elevated region.

Apology for the length of these papers is necessary, but I could not permit the numerous errors of Dr. Hume (Report to Council, December 20, 1853) to pass unnoticed.

ART. V.—*Cases of Adhesion of the Placenta and Hour-glass Contraction of the Uterus.* By W. H. BYFORD, M. D., of Evansville, Ind.

CASE I.—I was called, November 1, 1842, to see Mrs. L., in the sixth month of her pregnancy with second child; she was 34 years old.

Mrs. L. had miscarried at early periods of pregnancy fourteen times, and for several years her health was much impaired on account of the flooding which usually attended them. She had been married eighteen years; had sometimes two miscarriages a year. Great difficulty was experienced in overcoming her almost constant tendency to abortion with the first child. She was attacked about one o'clock this morning with shivering, succeeded by febrile reactive pain in the right side a little below the umbilicus, of a dull character, which was persistent and aggravated by pressure. Soon after the chill had subsided she began to experience pains resembling "labour-pains." When I saw her the pulse was 105, full and hard; tongue with a white fur, some nausea, probably, resulting from the dose of laudanum taken during the night; costiveness; head, back, and bone-ache. The face was flushed, the skin dry and hot. Examined per vaginam; the os uteri was high up and tightly closed; the vaginal mucous membrane hot and devoid of secretion. The fœtal heart beat feebly between the left ilium and umbilicus, and the placental murmur was heard at the seat of the dull pain. She was bled sufficiently to affect the pulse in a sitting posture, took a saline cathartic, and had warm fomentations with tincture of camphor over abdomen, while absolute quietude was enjoined. Visited again at 10 o'clock P. M. The cathartic had acted pretty freely. Paroxysmal uterine pain relieved entirely; constant pain in side much better. Gave ten grains Dover's powders, ordered fomentations to be continued, and left for the night.

November 2, 10 o'clock A. M. The patient has perspired freely all night, rested well, and experiences no inconvenience but soreness in side when she moves. Pulse about 85, rather full. Spt. mindereri, quietude, and fomentations for the day. Called again at 10 P. M.; pain pretty nearly as severe as at first, with slight return of paroxysmal pains; pulse 100, full and tolerably hard; bowels not moved since day before yesterday; headache; back and boneache. Venesection again to about sixteen ounces; continue fomentations to abdomen; take two grains calomel and quarter grain sulph. morph.; repeat in four hours if not better.

Nov. 3, 10 A. M. Rested well, did not take the other powder, and says she feels better than since first attack. Gave a cathartic. After it operates take six grains Dover's powder every three hours.

It will be needless to pursue a regular account of the case further. With almost nothing else, in about a week she was quite well, except weakness. Mrs. L. required no further attention until she was, on Feb. 24, 1843, two o'clock A. M., taken in labour. I was called about six; found os uteri entirely open; the head engaged in the upper strait; pains active, frequent, and propulsive. All went on well, and in one hour and a half the child was expelled, the cord separated, and it removed. I should also state that the membranes did not give way until the head occupied the lower strait, and not more than thirty minutes before the head was expelled. The child being removed, I seated myself by my patient and waited for the uterus to expel the placenta. In a short time three pains succeeded each other, expelling more than ordinary coagula; but the placenta was not thrown down into the vagina, nor lower part of the uterus. I waited for several more pains; no placenta; much blood. The pains were described by the patient as cramps instead of throes, and being almost insupportable. Placing my left hand on the abdomen I found, to my surprise, that the fundus reached above the umbilicus, and instead of sinking, arose higher up during each pain. I introduced my hand into the uterus and found about the middle of the body a contraction, leaving scarcely room for the cord that resisted its farther progress; but as flooding was great I felt under the necessity of overcoming it and relieving the placenta. With my hand, made conical by the prescribed arrangements of the fingers, I was proceeding in a gradual and cautious manner when the patient fainted; relaxation immediately took place, and no further resistance offered. The placenta was implanted upon the side near the fundus, and adherent very firmly over an extent of about, as near as I could judge, one-fourth of its extent, so firmly as to require something more than mere *grasping* to remove it. After several minutes, cautiously "peeling up," it was separated and removed. The uterus followed, by more regular and normal contractions, until it contracted to its usual size after delivery. No farther hemorrhage occurred. The patient, however, was very much depressed by the loss she had sustained, and it was several hours before she recovered from it. About an inch of the edge of the placenta for nearly a third of its circumference was so condensed by the deposition of fibrin as to entirely obliterate the peculiar structure of the organ; no trace of the cavernous tissue being left. It was replaced by a firm, unyielding, almost cartilaginously bard substance. From appearances this must have been the point of adhesion between it and the uterus.

Case II.—I was called, December 6, 1845, to Mrs. J., pregnant with her sixth child. She was in the eighth month. Arriving at 2 two o'clock P. M., I received the following account of her case: She was attacked yesterday about six o'clock, while milking, with a dull pain in the left groin, reaching up towards the ribs, which she said distressed her very much. When she returned into the house it was necessary to take her to bed, in consequence of chilliness and paroxysmal uterine pains. After going to bed, placing a hot bag of ashes to her side, and taking thirty drops of laudanum in some warm tea, she soon became very much better. The paroxysmal pains ceased entirely. Towards morning the chilliness returned; it was succeeded by fever, pain in the head, back, and extremities. The febrile symptoms had constantly continued until my arrival. There was considerable pain in side, and soreness; pulse 104, tense, but not very full; nausea, constipation, dry skin, flushed face, coated tongue. I bled her until the pain was much relieved, the pulse reduced in force and frequency, and perspiration occurred. As she had taken castor oil in the earlier part of the day, and it had not operated, I gave another portion with ten grains of calomel, to be followed, if the bowels were not acted upon in six hours, by Epsom salts one ounce. Fomentations to the seat of pain, with hot spirits of camphor. After the medicine operated twice, she was to have eight grains of Dover's powders every three hours.

7th, 4 o'clock, P. M. Found her much relieved. The salts which was given her produced large green watery discharges; the Dover's powder produced perspiration; but yet there was some pain. Continue the fomentations and powders; give at bedtime two grains calomel and a quarter of a grain of sulph. morph., and repeat in four hours unless the first produces rest. Early in the morning sulph. mag. to produce purgation.

8th, M. Much better, some pain. As it was twelve miles in the country I did not see her again. But, by giving anodynes and mild mercurials until slight ptyalism occurred, she was so free from disease that she did not take anything more than laxatives to keep the bowels open.

I saw her husband five weeks after the attack, when he said Mrs. J. had some pain and soreness all the time since last visit, but that was all the inconvenience at present. Although she had always been attended by a midwife in her previous confinements, she was anxious to engage my services in this case, as she was apprehensive the *after-birth had grown fast to her side.*

Feb. 6, 1846, 8 o'clock A.M. A messenger arrived with a hurrying message from Mrs. J., who had been delivered at 6 o'clock, and was supposed to be dying from loss of blood. Nearly two hours elapsed before I saw her. She had been dead for half an hour. The placenta was undelivered, and the midwife said, "was not in the womb, nor did she know where it was." The husband desired me, if possible, to ascertain the cause of his wife's death. I passed my hand into the uterus and found the contraction of a portion of the circular fibres had divided the cavity into two chambers. In the uppermost was lodged the placenta. The contraction was dilated without much resistance. Arriving at the placenta I endeavoured to remove it, but the adhesion between it and the uterine walls was so extensive and firm that it required several minutes to "peel" it off. The whole uterus contracted so firmly and uniformly, after the withdrawal of the placenta and hand, that it awakened some hope of resuscitation. Accordingly, I caused her head to be removed off the bed and very much lowered, and her feet to be raised to an angle of forty-five degrees, so as to induce a flow of blood to the head, and, if possible, stimulate the brain to a discharge of its functions. I used the cold douche to head and chest, and, as well as I could, resorted to artificial respiration. But all produced no effect. It remained for me to examine the placenta. The same hard, compact appearance of its edge was present in this as in the first case. Not so dense, perhaps, nor so extensive, but contracted with the healthy structure, it was unmistakably fibrinous condensation. It occupied the edge, as in the former case, and extended about an inch towards the centre.

Case III.—Was called, July 6, 1846, four o'clock A. M., three miles, to see Mrs. M., who was moribund from hemorrhagic exhaustion. Extremities icy cold; gasping respiration; vomiting; frequent fainting; glassy eye; pulse imperceptible; husky voice; and delirium, jactitation, &c. The blood was still passing from the vagina, but to a very moderate extent. My first object was to cause the blood to flow to the brain. I turned her head and shoulders off the bed, and held them as much dependent as possible, and had the feet and legs raised. In this position, there seemed, for a few moments, some rallying. An attempt was made to administer stimulants, but she could not swallow in this position, and begged to be raised so that she could have a drink. Finding there was no other chance, I raised her head slightly above the horizontal position, when she fainted, and never revived.

The midwife told me that she was taken in labour at five o'clock the evening before. The labour progressed naturally, and the child was delivered about twelve o'clock at night. Everything promised well, for one so weak. The placenta being delayed, she examined but could not find it. Pains continued, of a crampy character, worked up, and the womb was so high that for a time she thought there was another child. Hemorrhage being very profuse, she became alarmed and perplexed, and desired to have me sent for. During the time the messenger was gone, flooding became still more copious; syncope occurred frequently, and ushered in the symptoms I have above described.

Upon placing my hand on the abdomen, I found it occupied with a long, irregular tumour, reaching above the umbilical region. I introduced my hand into the uterus, and found annular contraction near the middle, with the cord passing through it. Carrying the hand through it, the placenta was reached near the fundus, where it was pretty firmly attached. I removed it without much trouble, as the adhesion was not very extensive. As in the case of Mrs. J., the uterus contracted firmly upon my hand, and assumed its globular shape above the pubes. Upon examining the placenta, I found a portion of the edge, the circumferential length of about two inches, hard, thin, and shining when cut. A circumscribed spot of an inch, perhaps, near the hardened spot, was soft, and contained pus. The placenta, as a whole, was uncommonly large.

The history of Mrs. M.'s pregnancy was very interesting, although imperfect. In her sixth month, she fell down with a load of wood on her shoulder, and struck her abdomen against a plough handle. This caused her much pain in the place, and paroxysmal uterine pains for several days. These last gradually wore off, but she remained quite unwell during the remainder of her pregnancy. Had pain, some fever, night-sweats, diarrhœa, &c., the most of the time. She was very much debilitated at the time of her accouchement. So far as I could learn, she had had no medical attendance.

These three cases I regarded as placentitis, possibly complicated with local metritis. Sufficient proof, I think, of this was presented in the symptoms and appearance of the placentæ. Depositions of fibrin in all, and formation of pus in one, leave no doubt in the matter. How terrible the result in two! and, in the third, what imminent peril was incurred! Adhesion of the placenta was its effect. Does this adhesion ever occur only as a consequence of inflammatory deposition? I think not. Doubtless many cases of partial placentitis pass off in resolution, and are not recognized as such. Atony of the uterus may fail to throw off the placenta of ordinary attachment; but I think it next to certain, that all cases which resist pertinaciously powerful contractions, prevent the uniform subsidence of the uterine globe, and cause such horrible floodings as result in death in so short a time as two of the cases above detailed—and as must have been the case in the other, but for prompt and judicious management—are brought about by the plastic products of inflammation. Whether primary, or secondary to uterine inflammation, it is impossible to decide; that it may be primary is reasonable and probable.

Case IV.—I was called to Mrs. L., aged thirty, a stout, energetic woman, in labour with fifth child. The first intimation she had of the approach of labour, was an evacuation of liquor amnii, which occurred as she was getting in bed about 10 o'clock P. M.—now two hours since. It continued dribbling away, but she had no pain whatever. I quieted her apprehensions of danger from this, to her, unusual commencement, and went home, directing her to send for me when the pains should become urgent.

At eight o'clock next morning I was called again, and found the pains feeble but frequent, with constant draining of the water at each pain. The os uteri was open to the size of half a dollar, but high up. No propulsive tendency in the pains. I was absent again about two hours. When I returned, the os was entirely dilated, and the head was engaged in the pelvis. The pains had a slight propulsive effect at first, but, as they wore off, in the language of the patient, they "worked up" as each throe ceased. About high twelve, she was delivered of a large and healthy female child. This labour, for her, had been unusually tedious and painful. The placenta was found in the vagina, and was removed without any further aid from the uterus. Placing my hand upon the abdomen, I felt the uterus forming a long, narrow, irregular tumour, that reached above the umbilicus. While my hand was on the abdomen, a peculiar, sickening, and cramping pain, described as being very different from the ordinary after-pains, was experienced. It was of very long duration, and attended with a large discharge of fluid blood and coagula. I placed cold wet cloths over the abdomen, rubbed, washed, and *poured* a stream of cold water upon it, but to no purpose. The pain recurred often, the flooding continued, and an alarming state of exhaustion threatened. I now introduced my hand into the cavity. There was a contraction about the middle of the body, so tight that considerable perseverance was necessary to dilate it. This being done, a large body of coagula was set free that had been imprisoned in the upper division. The whole organ now contracted uniformly, until of its usual size and form in such cases. No further hemorrhage occurred. The patient, of course, was much prostrated, but recovered in a reasonable time and manner, and had a good "getting up."

Case V.—Was called June 4, 1848, to see Mrs. G. at 8 P. M., full term of pregnancy. About 5 o'clock, three hours before my arrival, while stooping, she experienced a gush of water from the vagina. For an hour it continued almost constantly to drain away. At the end of this time she began to feel, at intervals, a slight pain in the back. Things remaining so for some time I retired. About midnight I was called up; the pains had increased in frequency and severity, but, according to her own expression, "worked up" into her stomach. The os uteri was open only enough to admit the end of the index finger. Presentation good. At every pain a slight gush of water could be felt in the vagina. To be short, the pains continued slow, feeble, tearing, and "working up," until about 5 o'clock A. M., on the fifth, when the os uteri was fully dilated. The pains then became propulsive, but at the end of each pain the distressing sensation of "working up" was experienced, until the head was expelled. The child was delivered at 10 o'clock, seventeen hours after the rupture of the membranes. Apprehensive of irregular contraction, I placed my hand on the abdomen, and found the long hard tumour characteristic of these cases. Anxious to see whether nature would do anything for the relief of the case, I awaited the recurrence of pain, and I shall never forget the energetic epithets she employed to convey an idea of their excruciating severity. "They seemed like a cramping, that compassed all her capacity for pain; a rise, squeezing her bowels to a jelly." They were accompanied with profuse hemorrhage, coagula, and fluid. Although the placenta was felt, at the os uteri, it could not be removed by any justifiable means. When drawn down into the vagina it receded the moment the traction was relaxed. I introduced my hand. The placenta was grasped in the annular stricture, which existed about one-third up the body of the uterus, and so firmly held that it could not be removed without tearing. The stricture was slowly dilated and the upper chamber reached, which was very large, and filled with coagula. These, together with my hand, were expelled by the regular and uniform contraction of the uterus. It then contracted down to its usual size and shape. Much blood had been lost during this time, which, together with the protracted suffering and watching, reduced the patient to a great degree of prostration, and it was difficult to keep her out of syncope. The head was placed lower than the feet, brandy and laudanum were administered, and perfect quietude enjoined. In a few hours she was comfortable, and all the powers rallied so that it was safe to leave her. Her getting up was slow, and attended with the many nervous ailments so common to anæmia. No hemorrhage whatever succeeded the expulsion of the placenta, and normal contraction of the uterus took place. So soon as the stricture was dilated a uniform and simultaneous contraction of all the parts occurred, with remarkable energy, and put hemorrhage out of the question. The character of the pain which succeeded was declared to be "refreshingly changed," when contrasted with those which preceded, being simply after-pains, instead of the cramps experienced before, "so horrible to think upon."

In review of the above cases I desire to note—

1. The three first described cases all exhibited symptoms of abdominal inflammation, during some period of pregnancy, over a circumscribed locality.

2. The uterine pains determined the seat to be in the uterus.

3. In the first case the pain was ascertained to be in the same locality as the placental murmur.

4. All three of the placentæ contained the products of inflammation; the first two fibrinous, and the third pus.

5. In all three there was adhesion of the placenta and hour-glass contraction of the uterus below the place of adhesion.

6. The irregular contraction was supposed to be caused by the adhesion, and the adhesion by inflammation, causing plastitic effusion between the uterus and placenta.

7. The partial separation of the placenta was the cause of the hemorrhage, by opening the placento-uterine veins, and preventing contraction to an extent sufficient to close them.

8. In the last two cases the irregular contraction, no doubt, depended on the vamping of the uterine walls upon the uneven surface of the child's body for so long a time before delivery as to derange its contractile throes, and induce spasmodic action in the fibres most contracted.

9. The most effectual means of relief is the introduction of the hand to dilate the contracted part, and thus restore the uniformly arched shape of the organ, and remove the placenta and coagula from its cavity.

Is nature capable of relieving such cases?

10. Nature sometimes relieves such cases as the last two, by syncope. This relaxes the whole muscular organization, and with it, the spasmodically contracted fibres. The elasticity of the parietes of the uterus may, after the subsidence of the state of syncope, restore the regular rotund shape of the organ, and, upon the supervention of the next pain, it may contract uniformly.

ART. VI.—*Report of Three Cases of Ruptured Spleen; with Remarks on the different Organic Changes which give rise to this Lesion, and the different modes in which it may occur.* By JAS. J. WARING, M. D., Washington, D. C.

As the time again approaches for the prevalence of miasmatic influence and miasmatic disease, with their usual concomitants—anæmia, enlarged spleen, &c. &c.—it may not be amiss to communicate to the medical profession of this country the report of an accident which occurred in Washington City in the month of November, 1855.

CASE I.—Robert Johnson, aged 17, apprentice to R. M'C., a bricklayer, well formed, and always enjoying sound health till within the last three months of his life, was seized in August, 1855, with an attack of tertian intermittent, which continued with little interruption, for six weeks, that is, till September 26. At the latter date, he was seized with a bilious remittent, which continued nine days—that is, till October 5—accompanied with great enlargement of liver and spleen. Recovered from this severe attack, he continued well, with the exception of an occasional chill, till the evening of Tuesday, November 13, 1855, when he was picked up, in a dying state, on his employer's step.

A few extracts from the coroner's inquest will throw all the light necessary upon the further history of the case.

From the verdict of the jury we find "That the deceased, while engaged, about 7 o'clock in the evening of the 13th, in play with one R. T——r, and others, received a blow of the fist in the left side, from said T., and died about a quarter of eight o'clock of the same evening."

"Among a number of witnesses, sworn and examined on the evening of the 13th, was Dr. Du Hamel, who testified as follows: 'I was called from my office at a few minutes past 7 o'clock this evening, by the witness, M. W. I came round here, and found the deceased, just where he is now lying, nearly in a collapsed condition. I ordered brandy, which was given him. He seemed very desponding; said that he was going to die, that R. T. had struck him in the side. I then asked him where he was struck; he replied, under the ribs. *I examined, and found no cut nor bruise of any kind.* * * * I think, from his pulse at the time I saw him, his bloodless condition, and his present appearance, that there has been the rupture of some internal organ."

Then it was that the jury, in order that there might be no doubt of the cause of death, demanded a *post-mortem.* Invited to assist my friend, Dr. Du Hamel, it is in my power to give the results from my own observation.

Post-mortem, 13 hours after death.—Rigor mortis marked; abdomen tense and full. On opening the abdominal cavity, a slightly reddish-yellow fluid poured out rapidly, which darkened as it flowed. Eventually, large masses of coagulated blood were found in both iliac fossæ, and in the region of the spleen; none, however, in the region of the liver. These masses were in sufficient quantity to fill a large basin. The internal organs and tissues were found in a healthy state, except the spleen. This organ was very much enlarged, eleven inches in length by five in breadth, and weighed quite a pound

It was flaccid, and had, no doubt, diminished considerably in size from the loss of the blood distending it. The fibrous envelop was rather pale. The splenic artery and its branches were uninjured. No unnatural softening existed, nor other organic change of structure; nothing but the *ordinary weakening* from over-distention could be observed. The *hilum* was *ruptured* from the lower and outer border up one-third its length, and then at right angles across the *concave* surface of the spleen to the external and upper border, to one of those ridges marking the original lobular state of the organ. That portion of the hilum was ruptured which marks the attachment of the colico-splenic omentum. On regarding the rupture, it was plain that the strong fibrous envelop had ruptured where it was weakest, namely, at the hilum. The capsule so lacerated then seemed only to have gaped open, and put on the stretch the trabecular structure, tearing it very little, and that only superficially. This trabecular structure had the usual appearance and consistence of health.

Remarks.—It immediately occurred to me that the very delicate mesh-like tissue of the spleen is *yielding*, and adapted to receive within itself enormous quantities of blood, but that the fibrous capsule is unyielding, and, when put upon its utmost stretch, as it is at times, would be as liable to burst, on the application of an external force, as an ordinary bladder, and, like the latter, would burst at its weakest point. Thus, instead of being lacerated on its convex surface, which must have first received the impression of the blow, the rupture took place on the concave surface, which must have been impressed by *transmission* or *contre coup*, to use a French term. It is easily understood why the trabecular structure was only superficially torn; for, of course, the immediate and enormous outpouring of blood must have promptly relieved the tension: a hemorrhage, however, which would necessarily produce immediate death, even, as it did, in three-quarters of an hour.

I ought not to leave this case without one further comment; of interest, not merely to the medical advisers of communities, but to every member of those communities. There is a disease prevailing extensively in many, very many localities of our country, of so mild a type as to receive the sobriquet of *benignant*, and yet capable of producing such an enlargement or organic change of the spleen as to expose it to the constant danger of fatal rupture, even on the application of so slight a force as that given in sport.

CASE II. (Communicated by Dr. BOGAN, of Washington, D. C.)—"Was summoned, May 7, 1854, by the coroner to make a *post-mortem* on the body of Ty. Simms, æt. 40, found dead in his room at an early hour of the same morning. T. S. had been for some time intemperate in habit, he drank freely of ardent spirits, and kept irregular hours, retiring late, oftentimes after having drunk to excess. Parties residing in the same house, and beneath his room, state that he returned home late, and much intoxicated, on the night of the 6th inst. That some time after they were disturbed by hearing a noise as if some one had fallen, or had been knocked down, and that this was followed by the most distressing groans, which became more and more feeble, and at length ceased altogether. That the fall occurred about midnight, and the groaning ceased to be heard in about three hours. On the following morning, T. S. was found lying prostrate across the edge of his bed (a low wooden bedstead), in such a way that, the epigastrium resting on its edges, the head, superior extremities, and thorax lay on the bed, whilst the inferior extremities, rigidly contracted, rested on the floor.

"*Post-mortem.*—Upon opening the abdominal cavity, a large amount of partially-coagulated blood escaped; about *four pints.* The peritoneum was natural; the small and large intestines likewise. The stomach, however, was greatly contracted; so much so, indeed, that when dilated to its fullest extent, it could not have held over from four to six ounces. Its coats were hypertrophied and hardened, and the inner coat was of an almost uniform purple colour.

"The spleen was ruptured on its *convex surface*, in a vertical direction, at the junction of its middle with its external third. The laceration extended about two and a half to three inches in length, through the peritoneal and fibrous envelop, and through the parenchyma to the depth of three-fourths of an inch. The spleen was somewhat above the ordinary size, weighing from six to eight ounces, rather pale and mottled in appearance, *firm*, not *pliant*, yet *extremely brittle*, breaking down before the slightest pressure. Its vessels were enlarged in caliber, but quite empty."

Remarks.—The case, as just detailed, is in perfect contrast with the previous one. In the first case, the spleen was simply enlarged, and its fibrous coat put on the stretch, by an excessive engorgement of blood. No organic change, however, had taken place in its tissue, and, when exposed to a sudden violent blow, it did not give way and rupture at the point struck, but at a point diametrically opposite—the hilum, which is always the weakest point of the spleen unless modified by disease.

Not so in the latter case. The spleen was not much above the natural size, but its structure had been modified by *hypertrophy*, produced by an irritation or subacute inflammation long continued, so that, from its *brittleness*, the rupture naturally took place at the very point struck. This spleen, however, was abundantly supplied with blood, and, as in the previous case, death was sudden (though rather more prolonged to four hours instead of three-quarters of an hour), the immediate cause being an excessive hemorrhage.

CASE III. (Reported by ROBERT KING STONE, M. D., of Washington, D. C.)—"Numerous cases of fracture of the spleen, or rupture of its capsule, have been on record for at least a century and a half, and the able writings of Piorry, Kölliker, and others, render it unnecessary to do more than make statistical additions to medical science. The case which is here offered to the profession should have long since been presented for publication, but for a pseudarthrosis of the femur, under which the writer has suffered for nearly three years past. A recent case of injury and fatal hemorrhage from this organ, occurring in this city (Case I.), has induced me to turn to my note-book for this very interesting case.

"Wm. D——x, Esq., Chief Clerk of the Indian Bureau of the U. S. War Department, æt. 45, of genial habits, had supped with his friends on the evening of November 2, 1849, and, returning home in the dark night, slipped on the polished marble steps at his own door, striking his left side against one of their angles.

"He rose unaided, feeling at the moment no very great inconvenience from the fall, and entered his parlour. About an hour afterwards, he complained of feeling unwell and nauseated, and was, with a sense of weakness, assisted to his bed. Soon afterwards, he emitted the contents of his stomach, which were copious, from the recent meal. He continued much nauseated, with occasional retching, through the night. My friend, Prof. Thos. Miller, saw him at 3½ A. M., November 3d, aud found the patient in the following condition:—

"From the great tenderness in the left hypochondriac region, the patient imagined he had fractured a rib on that side; there was, however, no tumefaction of either thorax or abdomen. Great prostration ensued, the extremities became cold, and the surface was pallid and bathed with clammy perspiration. The pulse scarcely perceptible at times, and the respiration laboured. Occasionally there was great nausea, and the action of the heart very hurried and feeble. The patient became very restless, but was unable to move on account of the great soreness in the left side. The bowels were not moved, and the urine passed was of natural appearance. The occasional vomiting and retching continued from this time until death.

"Dr. Miller made the hopeless diagnosis of fracture of the spleen, or internal hemorrhage from injury of that organ. This distinguished physician remained with him until 7 A. M. of the morning succeeding the fall, and during this period, hot and stimulating applications were made to the general surface and extremities, whilst a cordial and anodyne treatment was directed internally. At 9 A. M., the learned and veteran Dr. B. S. Bohrer was called to the case, and found the condition still the same; saw that he had recently vomited more copiously, and still of undigested food. The symptoms varied little until death closed the scene.

"Having been requested to make the examination of the body, Prof. Miller called my attention at once to the region of the spleen, as he was satisfied I would there find the cause of death. As the patient had died in robust health, the external appearances were all normal. I found the abdomen filled with a large quantity of dark, coagulated blood. On reaching the spleen, it was found of *unusual size and thickness* and *extremely firm in texture*, with remarkable *brittleness*. The whole of its vertical diameter, on the *external convex surface*, was the seat of a *fracture* (*not a rupture of the capsule above*) as the fissure dipped into the stroma of the organ itself. The fracture was such as one would make in a firm coagulum of blood or in an Indian-corn cake. The organ was excessively brittle, fracturing under the slightest violence, and of a deep mulberry colour. The main trunk of the splenic artery was uninjured, and the hemorrhage came from the organic branches of that vessel.

"Mr. D. had often been in the southwest country and in the Indian territories, on official business, and had suffered severely with remittent and intermittent disease. The effects of this malarial cause on the spleen, and the bibliography of the accident, are too well known to need further dilatation. The effects of sudden and direct violence on a disturbed stomach, will also occur to every one."

Remarks.—The three cases here faithfully reported, point out two distinct conditions of the spleen in which that organ becomes unusually liable to rupture; they point out, also, two distinct modes in which that rupture may take place. In the first, the organ was simply distended to repletion with blood, and, on the application of an external force, its fibrous capsule alone gave way. In the second and third cases, there was a species of induration from hypertrophy, accompanied with a peculiar *brittleness*, which rendered both capsule and parenchyma equally liable to rupture.

As to the mode of rupture, it will be observed that the spleen, in the first case, was ruptured, not at the point struck, but at the directly opposite surface; whilst, in the other two cases, the spleens were ruptured at the points receiving the blow. It will be observed, too, that the rapidity of the hemorrhage varied in the three cases; for, as the hemorrhage was the immediate cause of death, the rapidity of its approach indicates the rapidity of the hemorrhage. In the first case, death took place in three-quarters of an hour. This is easily understood, as the spleen, as a diverticulum, was the seat of an unusual afflux of blood. In the second case, it took place in three or four hours, and in the third case in about ten hours. The difference between the last two may be due to the varying degree of hypertrophy; hypertrophy, according to Cruveilhier, having a tendency to pass onward to a degree of consolidation and compactness more and more incompatible with a free circulation.

The applicability of the following extract, translated from Cruveilhier's *Anatomie Pathologique du Genre Humain*, to the organic changes found in the spleens of cases 2 and 3, will, I hope, excuse its insertion. (Liv. 2, Pl. 5, p. 5.)

"Of all lesions of the spleen, the most remarkable, beyond contradiction, are its *induration* and *softening*. The first is always accompanied with augmentation of volume and weight, with a variable *brittleness;* which yet disappears, after a while, to give place to a *coherence* and a compactness such as I have never seen in any tissue or organ of the body. It becomes a dense flesh, in whose thickness is sometimes met an orange-yellow colour around the vessels—traces of sanguineous extravasation. This lesion is accompanied with filamentous, fibrous adhesions, sometimes cartilaginous, even ossified in little spots, or in the totality of the enveloping membrane. This state consists in an *hypertrophy* rather than an *inflammation.*"

To render complete any observations that may be made on the "organic changes" which give rise to "ruptured spleen," I continue the translation with a few comments:—

"In *softening*, the spleen never acquires a volume as considerable as in induration. It is rarely seen triple its natural volume, though softened spleens have been met with which weighed from seven to eight pounds. This softening is sometimes partial, more often general, presenting many degrees, so that at the height of this alteration, the spleen is converted into a muddy, disorganized pulp, contained in a sac formed by its membranes distended and weakened, to such a degree, indeed, that a very slight force suffices to tear it. M. le Dr. Balby, in his work on the pernicious fevers observed in the Hospital St. Esprit, at Rome, assures us that he has seen many *fissures* which occurred *spontaneously* during life. This *splenitic mud* (the French term) is sometimes little coloured, sometimes of a chestnut-brown. I have preserved, for several years, a piece of paper tinged with this liquid. It is not uncommon to meet with softening of the spleen in individuals who present other lesions capable of explaining the symptoms observed during life. I even think that it is this *so frequent* coincidence which has caused observers to overlook this alteration of the spleen as a thing of little importance, perhaps accidental, perhaps cadaveric. Hence it is that, in the range of observations, we read of examples of adynamic fevers, enteritis, and other maladies, acute and chronic, in which mention is made of softening of the spleen, without any effort being made to discover its relation to the principal disease."

In this connection, now, it may very properly be asked whether accidental rupture and sudden death have ever occurred in that organic change described above, under the head of softening or ramollissement? I am disposed to think it rare, and then occurring only in the very first stage of softening, occasionally to be found in spleens enlarged by slight attacks of miasmatic disease. In the more aggravated forms, however, it probably never occurs, for two reasons: 1st. Because this change usually accompanies disease which renders the patient incapable of attending to ordinary business or amusement, and hence prevents him from exposing himself to the ordinary casualties of life. 2d. Because, should a rupture take place, the hemorrhage would not be abundant, in the disorganized state of the spleen, and the cause of death would either be a *peritonitis*, should the rupture take place into the peritoneal cavity, or suppuration and abscess, should it take place into the direction of the abdominal parietes.

In conclusion, then, cases No. I, II, and III, stand as a fair type, in my judgment, of all cases of sudden death from ruptured spleen; and, as in these cases, the causes are in the great majority of instances: 1st. *Enlargement*, with *engorgement;* or, 2. *Hypertrophy* and *induration*, with *brittleness.*

ART. VII.—*Surgical Cases.* By F. HINKLE, M. D., Marietta, Lancaster County, Pa.

CASE I. *Extensive Compound Fracture of the Bones of the Face.*

On the 13th of December, 1853, between three and four o'clock A. M., I was sent for to see Thomas Russel, a labourer at an iron furnace. Upon inquiry, I learned that he had been injured in the following manner:—

A lump of coal had caught at the top of the shaft of a furnace at which he was working, so as to interrupt the progress of the elevators. These consist of a series of buckets revolving around a large piece of timber for the purpose of raising the coal. In attempting to remove the coal, he had placed his head between the timber and one of the buckets. As soon as the obstruction was cleared away, the machinery moved again, and, before he could withdraw his head, the edge of the bucket caught under the right malar bone, pressing the occiput against the timber. The force was so great as to draw him from the kneeling to the erect posture.

The men who supply the buckets, after waiting fifteen minutes, finding the impediment to their motion still continuing, and hearing groans, ran to the top of the shaft and found him in the above mentioned position. They procured a board, which was used as a lever to press down the bucket, and, after working twenty minutes, they succeeded in releasing him.

On examination, I found the malar and the superior maxillary bones of the right side pressed out *en masse* an inch beyond the inferior maxillary; the right palate, together with the nasal bones, crushed and displaced, lying obliquely across the sphenoid and frontal. The left palate bone was partially fractured. All the teeth of the right superior maxillary, except the molars, were pushed out, together with their fractured alveolar processes. The alveoli of the right side of the inferior maxillary were partially fractured; the cheek on this side was crushed to a jelly; the right ala nasi, upper lip and chin, were cut through to the bone, and the scalp was wounded severely in several places.

Treatment.—The eyebrow, which was laid open to the periosteum and thrown back, forming a triangular wound, through which the ball of the eye could be seen, was brought together by the twisted suture and strips of adhesive plaster. The wounds of ala nasi, lip, and chin, were then joined and retained by adhesive strips. I proceeded to adjust the dislocated and fractured bones, and commenced by replacing the malar and superior maxillary, which was easily effected. A probe was then passed into the nostrils, and the nasal bones elevated to their proper position. At the same time, I attempted to replace the right palate bone, but could not succeed, as it remained at least twenty lines from its normal situation. The right alveoli of the superior maxillary were then replaced, and held in their position by bringing the teeth of the lower jaw to press firmly against those which had been dislodged. A piece of linen, well greased, was laid on the bruised cheek, and over this was placed two pasteboard splints, softened in water and covered with muslin, to retain the superior maxillary and malar bones in their places; the lower jaw answered the purpose of a third splint. Cotton was inserted between the cheek and the splints to prevent their pressure. The face was covered with compresses dipped in cold water, and again over these a pasteboard splint. A bandage was then passed round the head and under the jaw in form of a figure of 8; this secured all firmly.

The hemorrhage was great, both before and during the dressing of the wounds; and I was frequently interrupted by his vomiting the blood which he had swallowed, the amount of which was almost incredible. He was now placed in bed on his right side, with the head thrown forward on the chest, to allow the blood to flow from his mouth.

While dressing the wound, and for some time after, his pulse was scarcely perceptible at the wrist. He was slightly delirious. Ordered him to be kept quiet, and the compresses to be wet with cold water every fifteen minutes; to have brandy and water in small quantities until reaction took place, after which he was to take a tablespoonful of the following mixture every two hours: ℞. Magnes. sulphat. ℥ijss.; tart. antim. et pot. grs. iss.; aqua fluvial. Oj.—M.

December 14*th.* Reaction took place six hours after dressing the wound. I found him as easy and comfortable as could be expected. There is great tumefaction of the face, which is almost jet black; blood still oozing from the nostrils; mind clear; bowels gently moved. The dressings retain their place. *Diet,* rice water. Treatment continued.

15*th,* ten o'clock, A. M. The patient is in much the same condition as at my last visit, except that his pulse is more frequent and quicker. Ordered the saline mixture to be given more freely. Dressings still untouched.

16*th.* Found the patient very restless, and complaining of an excessive pain in the left ear, and of the tightness of the dressings. I exposed the wound, and found the bones moved every time he breathed; the muscles were so relaxed that the lower jaw hung an inch below the lower. The parts were well cleansed, and new dressings applied in the same manner as those removed, with the addition of a pasteboard splint covered with muslin, which was placed inside the injured cheek. Over the eyes, nose, and left cheek, the only parts not covered with bandage, I applied wet compresses, and ordered all the dressings to be kept constantly moist. From this time the swelling gradually subsided. The wound was dressed every third or fourth day, at which time the lower jaw was moved to prevent anchylosis, and, with the exception of having twice an erysipelatous swelling over the scalp, he recovered without an unpleasant symptom.

By the fourth week he was able to sit up in a chair, and the bones and wound were well enough united to allow the removal of all dressings except the bandage, which was continued till the end of the fifth week. The wounds united by first intention, and, without a close examination, no visible deformity is perceptible.

CASE II. *Traumatic Tetanus successfully treated by local applications of Chloroform to the Spine.*—Mrs. D. E., æt. 38 years, of feeble constitution; the mother of six children, the last being but five months old when the following accident occurred: Having decapitated a large eel, preparatory to stripping off the skin, she attempted to hang the head upon a nail. While doing this, the jaws snapped and caught the index finger of the left hand upon its internal surface, between the second and third phalanges, directly over the joint. The contraction of the jaws was so firm, that she was obliged to open them by inserting a knife and forcing them apart.

The pain caused by the bite produced partial syncope. Upon examining the finger, she found that the skin was divided in several places along the line made by the jaws. The finger became purple and tumid on its internal surface, attended with an acute pain.

She engaged more or less in her household duties from this time until November 16, a period of three weeks, when she consulted me. She informed me that since the accident she had suffered pain of a dull, aching character, by times more or less acute, according as she had used the affected hand. She now presented the following symptoms: Pulse 58, very soft and slow; skin hot and dry; tongue slightly coated; bowels had not been moved for two days; acute pain, recurring every fifteen or twenty minutes, in the epigastric region, and extending into the hypochondriac region of each side. This affected her breathing, especially when the pain was severe, showing that spasm of the diaphragm was present. Eyebrows contracted; alæ nasi expanded, producing an anxious expression of countenance. It was impossible for her to open her eyes to more than half their extent.

Upon examining the finger, the punctures made by the teeth could be distinctly seen. Pressure over this surface caused acute pain, which darted along the arm, up to her neck, along the spinal column, head and face. There was not a nerve about the head or extremities but which was painful upon pressure. The stiffness, as she termed it, of her face and limbs, with difficult deglutition, had been coming on for four or five days before I was called; she thinking it was a bad cold. She could not sleep at night on account of spasms, which commenced at the diaphragm and extended to the head and extremities.

Treatment.—I directed her to take four compound cathartic pills, to be followed by a dose of castor-oil, if required; and to have her feet bathed in hot water, to which mustard had been added. A large pad of raw cotton covered with muslin to be laid along the whole length of her spine, and half an ounce of chloroform mixed with one drachm of ether, to be dashed suddenly along the skin; the pad then to be secured over the spine by tapes tied in front of her chest. The patient was now turned on her back and a drachm of the mixture was applied to the epigastrium, which was also covered with cotton. This afforded almost instant relief to the spasms, and mitigated the pain along the main nerves. The wounded finger was also bathed in chloroform, and well wrapped in cotton. I directed the chloroform to be repeated every two or three hours.

Nov. 17, 9 o'clock A. M. No improvement; symptoms the same, but yielded readily to the application of chloroform. When the applications were not made, her sufferings were very much increased. Breathing more laboured; bowels moved twice, but not freely. To use the chloroform more frequently and give the following powder: ℞.—Hyd. chlor. mitis grs. viii; Pulv. ipecac. gr. j.—M. To be followed by a dose of Epsom salts; also to take a teaspoonful of the following mixture every two or three hours. ℞.—Spts. æther. nit. f℥j; Ol. terebin. f℥j; Ext. cannab. ind. ℈j.—M.

18*th.* 8 o'clock A. M. Found the patient much better. She has had two or three dark-coloured dejections. Pulse 60; features less contracted. The pain in finger, cervical ganglia, stiffness of neck and jaw, are all much improved. Can bear more pressure on the spine and along the course of the nerves. To continue the applications of chloroform, particularly to the wounded finger and to the arm and neck of the affected side; and, in addition, to take the following pill every four hours: ℞.—Ext. cannab. ind. gr. j; Mass. hyd. gr. $\frac{1}{3}$; Pulv. rhei, grs. iss.—M.

19*th.* Symptoms continue favourable; pulse 60; tongue nearly clean; bowels moved; pain diminished, except in the arm and neck of right side. Countenance still indicative of the disease. Treat. cont.

20*th.* 9½ o'clock A. M. Symptoms improving; pain diminishing. Continue treatment.

21*st.* 11 o'clock A. M. Decidedly better; difficulty of deglutition nearly gone.

22*d.* Feels tolerably well, but says if she could only sleep at night she would be better; she finds her mind constantly wandering the moment she dozes. Pulse 65; skin moist; tongue clean. She can insert the end of her little finger between her jaws; pains have nearly left her. Treatment continued. Left the patient in good spirits, considering her nearly convalescent.

24*th.* Sent for in great haste at 3½ A. M. Found her sinking rapidly; pulse not perceptible at the wrist; features greatly contracted; eyebrows corrugated; jaws closed; eyelids closed, without power to open them; left pupil dilated; skin cool; finger painful; general muscular contraction, especially of the diaphragm; breathing laboured and painful; countenance anxious; deep livid hue of face; acute pain every ten minutes, commencing at diaphragm and extending to spinal column, ends of fingers and toes. Could not bear pressure on any part of the body without a jerk, like an electric shock. Gave brandy every fifteen minutes; applied chloroform freely to the epigastrium, spine, neck, arm and finger. Could not see her tongue; bowels moved yesterday. Gave three ounces of the best brandy with Hoffman's anodyne and tincture of valerian in an hour. Also two grains of Ext. cannab. ind. Pulse now gradually rose to 50. Chloroform controlled the pains.

7 A. M. Pulse 54, fuller; countenance more natural and less livid; pupils equal; better temperature of skin; breathing still difficult but not so painful. I now applied one or two ounces of chloroform every hour or two, just

as the pain returned, and thus again succeeded in checking the spasms, which were anticipated the whole day.

1 P. M. Applied caustic iodine to her finger every four hours, so as to blister it freely, but not expose it so much as a fly blister necessarily would do.

8 P. M. Pulse 55, rather feeble; skin moist and cool; bowels not yet moved; dyspnœa not so constant; otherwise the same as at last visit. Directed her to use brandy and beef-tea freely; gave pills composed of quinine, ext. cannab. ind., and mass. hydrar. every three hours, and to continue the local applications.

25th. 10 A. M. Tetanic symptoms milder; longer interval between the pains, and they are less violent; breathing improving; pulse 54, soft and feeble; voice faint; jaws still stiff, as are most of her muscles, yet the chloroform has removed all acute pain. Continued treatment, and, in addition, use twelve drops of the following mixture every two hours: ℞. Spts. æther. nit. f℥ss; ol. tiglii, gtt j; M. If dyspnœa returns to use Hoffman's anodyne and tinct. valerian.

A consultation having been agreed upon, Dr. J. Aug. Ehler, of Lancaster City, met me at 7 P. M. We found her slightly improved. Breathing not so painful; skin warmer; countenance more lively and less livid; features still contracted; the other symptoms remained as they were at my last visit. Pulse 54. She has taken half a pint of brandy, with beef tea. Continued treatment. Dr. E. ordered the cannab. ind. in larger doses.

She continued to improve and relapse for four days, supported with brandy, beef-tea, emulsion of carbonate of ammonia, and tr. musk.

The bowels were kept regular by castor oil. The ext. cannab. ind. was given to relieve pain and spasm, and the chloroform continued.

30th. The disease was now evidently checked, and from this period her recovery gradually took place. By December 10, she was perfectly well.

CASE III.—*Removal of a Tumour developed in the Posterior Wall of the Uterus.*—*March* 9, 1853. I was consulted by Mrs. Goodyear, æt. 64, who gave me the following history of her case: She commenced menstruating in her sixteenth year, and continued regularly and free from pain, except when interrupted by pregnancy, until she attained the age of fifty-two, when she became irregular, and the catamenia finally ceased.

She was married in her nineteenth year, and bore nine children, her labours being short and natural. Her general health was excellent from her youth up to 1848, when she had a severe attack of dysentery, which lasted two months. From this time until November, 1852, she enjoyed her usual health; was corpulent, but of active habits.

Her illness commenced in November, 1852, with a slight chill every day. This was followed by flushes of heat, violent frontal headache, tinnitus aurium, excessive pain starting from the sacral region and extending forward to the hypogastrium, and down the limbs to the toes. There were violent cramps of both legs. On the dorsum of the right foot there was a spot in which there was a constant burning pain.

Her tongue was always coated with a thick brown fur. Anorexia, irritable stomach with occasional vomiting, constant thirst, great irregularity in the action of the bowels and swollen abdomen, were other symptoms. In addition, there was a very irritable condition of the bladder, the voiding of its contents being accompanied with urinary tenesmus.

Her uterine bearing-down pains, she said, were far more severe than those of labour. These pains were, at the time of visiting her, nearly continuous, but had an exacerbation every twenty-four hours, coming on after the chill and lasting two or three hours, unless relieved by opiates; the passage of feces and urine also excited them.

She had been under the care of several physicians, but their treatment had been merely palliative, and chiefly directed to the removal of the intermittent pain, by quinia.

Present condition.—The symptoms mentioned in the above history still continue: pulse, 100. I made a careful examination of the abdomen, which was tympanitic, and contained a slight dropsical effusion. In the right iliac region, there existed a soft swelling, caused, apparently, by the cæcum being distended with gas.

Examination per vaginam.—The uterus occupied its normal position; no leucorrhœal discharge. In passing the index finger around the neck of the uterus, a tumour was discovered, pressing against the posterior wall of the vagina, and inclined to the right side. The lower border of the tumour reached to the point of insertion of the vagina into the uterus.

The uterine sound entered two and a half inches. By relaxing the abdominal walls, and using firm pressure, I could feel the upper portion of the tumour; and in moving the uterus with the sound, the tumour followed its motions. The tumour, which I supposed to be fibrous, rested on the right lateral half of the sacrum.

The *treatment* adopted was palliative and sustaining. After having recourse to most of the narcotic extracts, the following pill was found to give most relief, and was continued throughout the treatment: ℞.—Ext. cannab. ind. gr. ¾; quinia sulph. gr. j. M. ft. pilula. This was given three times per diem.

During the paroxysm, the following powders were used: ℞.—Morphiæ sulphat. grs. x; pulv. opii, grs. xxx; pulv. camph. grs. x.—M. Divide in chart. viij. One of these powders was given every three hours, until the pain was relieved, generally requiring three powders.

Chloroform was applied over the hypogastric region; injections of assafœtida per rectum, and a general alterative course of iodide of potassium and various preparations of iron, were all used without benefit. As her disease progressed her sufferings increased.

At my request, Dr. Washington L. Atlee, of Philadelphia, was sent for and met me in consultation, November 8, 1852. Wishing to give his opinion of the case in his own words, I recently addressed Dr. Atlee a note, requesting a description of what he found in examining Mrs. G., to which I received this reply:—

PHILADELPHIA, *Sept.* 28, 1855.

DEAR DOCTOR: I find, on referring to my notes of the case of Mrs. G., that I visited Marietta November 8, 1853, and saw the patient the same evening in consultation with you and Dr. Ehler. Immediately on my return, the next day, I made the following memorandum:—

The uterus is *in situ*. It is light and movable. The os admits the entrance of the mere point of the index finger. The sound enters two and a half inches, gives pain, and the uterus can be readily moved by it. The sound in the bladder causes great distress. By careful examination, a tumour can be felt through the posterior wall of the vagina, of an oblong shape, opposite the right sacro-iliac junction. This is partially movable. It is not hard and resisting in texture, as is fibrous tumour, but feels much like uterine tissue. It can be traced to the upper part of the cervix uteri, adjacent to the insertion of the vagina, and its pedicle is evidently attached to the uterus, as is proved by the sound, which, when moving the uterus, moves the tumour with it. The sound passes directly upwards in the uterus, at right angles with the long axis of the tumour, and its point can be felt above the pubis. Per rectum the tumour can be more readily felt, and the examination here also causes pain.

On surveying the bony surface of the interior of the pelvis through the vagina, an acutely sensitive spot was found on the inner face of the pubis, immediately to the right of the symphysis. Here the surface was elevated into a nodule or periosteal tumour which, when pressed upon, was intolerably painful. Indeed, the whole examination was accompanied with unusual suffering.

Agreeably to my instructions, you now introduced my "*bistourie caché*" into the uterus, and cut into its posterior wall, so as to incise the pedicle of the tumour, and you also nicked the os tineæ around its circumference. This had the effect of enlarging the os uteri, and also of bringing the tumour lower down in the pelvis. This proceeding was to be followed by ergot, and by subsequent operations.

I also advised you, should the periosteal tumour continue painful, to bisect it with a tenotome passed under the pelvic tissues.

Yours truly,
WASHINGTON L. ATLEE.

To F. Hinkle, M. D.

The operation was performed, as is stated in the above note, and the immediate effect produced was to bring the tumour down to the os internum, so as to be within reach of the finger. The patient suffered comparatively little during the operation, after which she was placed in bed, and three-quarters of a grain of morphia administered. This produced quiet sleep until 2 A. M., when she awoke, passed urine without pain, and was very comfortable.

3 A. M. Was suddenly seized with severe bearing-down pain, extending to the bladder; but the pain which she usually had in her limbs, was not so severe as before the operation. The nurse gave her morphia, but this failing to relieve her, I was sent for.

4 A. M. Found her suffering as usual; no febrile excitement, no tenderness of the os uteri, nor contiguous parts; repeated the morphia, and applied hot fomentations to the hypogastrium, which relieved her.

8 A. M. Accompanied by Dr. Atlee, I made an examination per vaginam. Found a slight mucous discharge, but no alteration in the state of the parts. No febrile excitement, but still complaining of constant pain in the hypogastrium and lower limbs. To relieve this, one fluidrachm of a mixture of ether and chloroform was directed to be inhaled, to take the place of the morphia; and the hypogastric and right inguinal region to be painted with strong tincture of iodine, once a day.

Nov. 10. Pains moderate; no febrile excitement; good appetite. Directed her to take five grains of ergot every three hours, until bearing-down pains should come on, and then to suspend the use of the medicine.

13*th.* 11 A. M. The patient has been occasionally using the ergot, but not continuously, on account of the intense pain it has produced. The anæsthetic and narcotics have been used, when required, to alleviate pain. A dose of ergot, taken this morning, brought on violent expulsive efforts, which still continuing, during my visit, I made an examination per vaginam.

The os uteri was found to be sufficiently dilated to permit the easy introduction of the index finger for half an inch, where it was arrested by the tumour, which was pressing against the internal os, and even slightly pushed into the cervical canal.

This being a favourable opportunity to proceed with the operation, I placed the patient in the proper position, and, using the index finger of the left hand as a guide, I introduced a blunt pointed bistoury with a long handle, and cut the uterine covering of the tumour, so as to enlarge the opening previously made.

The index finger could now be passed between the tumour and its uterine walls; but this proceeding gave so much pain that I had to desist. The patient was placed in bed, and directions left for her to continue the narcotic, and occasionally to use the ergot.

15th. She has been troubled with slight chills, headache, and furred tongue, for which was administered two grains of blue pill, followed by a dose of castor oil. These caused her bowels to be moved with less pain than she had experienced for a long time. I enlarged the incision in the uterus, and made a careful examination. The tumour was found to be adherent to its uterine walls, but the adhesions were slight and readily separated by means of the index finger. In this manner I had detached three-fourths of it, when I was compelled to cease from any further manipulation by the exhaustion of the patient. During the examination, &c., about two ounces of venous blood were lost. Ergot, narcotics, and anæsthetic continued.

16th. Ergot having previously been administered, I again attempted to dislodge the tumour by passing a tenaculum into it and then dividing its capsule, but the pain produced again compelled me to cease.

17th. Found the patient complaining of headache and nausea, tongue furred. Ordered her a mercurial alterative combined with quinia, to be followed by ol. ricini. *Evening.* The medicine has purged her, producing excessive pain, but has relieved the headache and nausea.

22d. The narcotics have been given very freely, and attention has been paid to supporting her strength by means of quinia and nourishing diet; but the narcotics have lost their effect, and the pain which she suffers causes her to lose sleep and strength, so that the symptoms call for speedy relief.

At 12 M., assisted by Dr. Ehler, I administered chloroform and examined per vaginam. The tumour was found dipping down into the cervix. In passing the finger between the tumour and the uterus adhesions could be felt, particularly at its posterior surface, but these readily yielded to the pressure of the finger. Having removed the adhesions, a tenaculum was inserted in the tumour and strong traction made which tore through it, and, to our surprise, gave exit to a quantity of serous fluid. The tenaculum was again inserted in order to drag it down, but without success, as the instrument tore through the cyst, which was partially disorganized. Forceps were then used, and we finally succeeded in removing the cyst in two. The patient was placed in bed and a little brandy given. She rested well for half an hour, when she was suddenly seized with pain so severe as to cause her to scream. This was followed by a slight rigor, which lasted but a few minutes; to this succeeded vomiting, and, when this ceased, the pain returned and continued until 9 P.M., when she fell asleep and slept well all night.

23d. Early this morning she was seized with severe pain in the right iliac region which readily yielded to morphia. She was free from pain during the day, and had a good appetite. Directed her to have the morphia if necessary.

24th. Has suffered all day with intense intermittent pains caused by uterine contraction, which could not be subdued by morphia. Examined and found the os uteri hot and swollen, and a free vaginal discharge. Ordered vaginal injections, and hot stupes to the abdomen.

25th. Was sent for in haste. Found her labouring under the most agonizing uterine pains; skin cool and covered with moisture. Having administered chloroform, I made an examination and found the cervix tumid and os closed; but by gentle pressure I inserted my finger up to the opening in the uterine wall, which was also closed. On pressing against this the adhesions gave way, and was followed by an audible puff of fetid gas. No sooner had this escaped than she fell asleep and rested well for three hours. When she awoke, the pain again commenced and soon became excruciating. I examined the cavity but it contained nothing to account for this. Morphia was given freely by mouth and rectum, but it afforded no relief. The anæsthetic was then used, and the patient kept sufficiently under its influence to control the pain. I directed her attendants to let her continue the inhalation when necessary, and as her tongue was dry and coated, and abdomen tympanitic, to administer one of the following powders every five hours: ℞. Magnesiæ grs. iij; hydrar. chlor. mitis gr. ss; pot. citrat. grs. vj; quin. sulphat. gr. ¼; carb. ligni grs. iss.—M. Also to inject into the vagina a dilute solution of chlorinated soda.

26*th*. The tongue is moist; pulse 120, and soft; the tympanitis still exists, and is accompanied by nausea. The excessive expulsive pains continue when not controlled by the anæsthetic; the discharge from the uterus is very free and fetid. Used the catheter and drew off a pint of clear urine; continued treatment, and use beef tea freely.

30*th*. Since the last report the patient has been gradually losing strength; her tongue has become clean; pulse 120. The pains have continued, but yield more readily to morphia. The anæsthetic has only been used when necessary. She has been taking quinia and beef-tea, both by mouth, and when the stomach has been irritable, injected into the rectum. The distention of the abdomen has disappeared, and there is no tenderness on pressure. She can now pass her water freely.

December 9. Notwithstanding the free use of tonics of various kinds and generous diet, the patient has been gradually sinking. Two days ago diarrhœa set it, and the abdomen again became tympanitic; but these symptoms disappeared under the use of acetate of lead and calomel. Without any other symptom worthy of note she continued to sink, and expired at seven this evening.

Post-mortem.—Assisted by Dr. Ehler, I examined the body at 10 P. M., three hours after death. The abdomen was swollen, but not uniformly so, as there was quite a prominence in the right iliac region. The peritoneum was healthy with the exception of an inflammatory patch of two or three square inches in extent in the right iliac region. A portion of the small intestines was inflamed, the inflammation extending to the colon and rectum. The prominence on the right side was found to be caused by the cæcum, which was enormously distended with gas.

The uterus was thrown back obliquely across the hollow of the sacrum. It was of the normal size, and, except the patulous cervical canal, of healthy appearance.

A section of the uterus was made, and the cavity which had contained the tumour exposed. We found it contracted so much as to form but a small prominence on the uterine surface, but by pressure we could distend it to its former size. The whole surface of the cavity was smooth and clean. To its upper surface was attached a small white pedicle about half an inch in length, and of about the same thickness.

There were no evidences of inflammation about the uterus or ovaries, death being apparently caused by enteric inflammation, attended by a fever of a typhoid type.

ART. VIII.—*On the Treatment of Delirium Tremens by Chloroform.* By W. R. RICHARDSON, M. D., late Assistant Physician in the Hospital, Blackwell Island, New York city.

A REPORT of the successful treatment of ten cases of delirium tremens with chloroform in the Penitentiary Hospital, on Blackwell's Island, New York, by W. M. Chamberlain, M. D., appeared in a recent number of the *New York Medical Monthly.*[1]

I was a member of the medical staff of the Penitentiary Hospital when nearly all these cases occurred, and for three months had charge of the delirium tremens wards under the Resident Physician, Dr. Kelly. During that time, I administered chloroform very frequently under his directions. Before the appointment of the present able and accomplished Resident, Dr. Wm. W. Sanger, scarcely a single case of delirium tremens occurred in its wards, in the treatment of which chloroform was not used. From several hundred cases thus occurring, Dr. Chamberlain has selected only *nine* in which it *seemed even* to have been successful, and in all of these, *except one,* I shall endeavour to show, that the recovery of the patients was due to the large doses of opium and diffusible stimulants administered internally, and not in a single instance to chloroform.

In two cases under my own charge, it produced fatal results almost immediately, and in many instances I have known similar results warded off only by the most assiduous exertions of the physicians in attendance.

I shall now proceed briefly to examine the ten cases which Dr. Chamberlain presents, "not," as he affirms, "as a challenge, &c., but in the hope that they may illustrate the power of that great narcotic, opium, and that *greater sedative, chloroform.*" Were I disposed to be hypercritical, I should question the correctness of Dr. C.'s nomenclature, when he classes chloroform among sedatives, as in that case, alcohol, ether, and ammonia would come under the same category together with the entire class of diffusible stimulants.

In the first case contained in Dr. C.'s report, I find that chloroform was not administered. The patient recovered under the ordinary treatment, opium and stimulants.

CASE II.—In this case the patient took five drachms of laudanum and "a small quantity of stimulus," how much is not stated, in five hours. On the following day "the same treatment" was continued until 1 o'clock P. M., when chloroform was administered "with happy effects."

[1] These remarks were written shortly after Dr. Chamberlain's report had appeared in the *New York Medical Monthly* for Jan. 1854; but from accidental circumstances were not published at the time. On perusing them afresh, the author, convinced of the importance of the subject they refer to, has thought it advisable to prepare them afresh for the press.

This was evidently a mild case, and the patient would undoubtedly have fallen asleep from the effects of the opium and brandy had the chloroform been omitted.

I wish to call attention particularly, in these cases, to the *vast* amount of opium given before chloroform produced its "happy effects."

Case III.—In this case, 900 *minims* of laudanum were given, and a large quantity of punch, the exact amount is not stated.

Chloroform was administered *seven times*, the sixth time producing almost fatal "*spasms* and laryngismus."

Case IV.—The patient took 395 minims of laudanum and 28 ounces of brandy. Chloroform was administered *four times.* Its second inhalation left him "greatly prostrated;" its third produced "great spasm and laryngismus;" during the fourth, "respiration was suddenly suspended," and "artificial respiration was resorted to." Fortunately, the patient was saved "to illustrate the power of that greater sedative chloroform."

Case V.—This, says Dr. C., "was in itself less severe, but tells a *similar story* for chloroform." 370 minims of laudanum were given in this case, 1 pint of ale, 2 pints of punch, and 10 ounces of brandy. Chloroform was administered *four times*, the third time producing "spasm and laryngismus." During the fourth inhalation, the patient "*ceased to breathe*," *the pulse at the wrist was imperceptible.* He was restored to life by means of "cold effusions," only *to die* in a few days with *pneumonia*, caused, undoubtedly, by the congestion of the lungs which this injudicious and repeated administration of chloroform had produced.

Case VI.—In this case, 1050 minims of laudanum were given, 1 gr. of morphia, brandy freely twice, the amount is not stated, and subsequently, half a pint of brandy. Chloroform was administered twice. After the first inhalation, the patient breathed stertorously, but did not sleep. The second time it was administered, "he was kept under its influence *one hour and forty-five minutes*" *without benefit, when it was determined* TO PUSH *its* EFFECTS. "After a few seconds of stertor, *respiration was suspended instantly, pulse* 0."

"Artificial respiration" was successfully resorted to, and the patient fortunately recovered.

Case VII.—In this case, 1240 minims of laudanum were given, punch and ale *freely* five or six times, and 12 ounces of brandy.

Chloroform was administered *three times.* After the first time, "violent spasms, opisthotonos and epileptiform convulsions occurred." The second time, "*laryngismus was so great that its administration was suspended.*" "*Respiration was slow and labored;*" "*became more and more difficult; finally ceased altogether;*" artificial respiration was resorted to *in vain;* he was at last restored by insufflation, and after this frightful exhibition of "that greater sedative," he slept—TWENTY MINUTES. After such a dreadful scene, one would suppose that no man would resume a treatment which had so nearly destroyed the life of a human being, but Dr. Chamberlain states, that in a few minutes after this, *chloroform was again administered.* After this third administration, "the patient slept—*a few minutes.*" For some time, his respirations were only *two, three,* and *four* in a minute. Fifteen or twenty hours afterwards, stimulants and opium having been freely and frequently given, the Doctor says, "I left him overcome with sleep." Since then I have carried the same man safely and successfully through an attack of delirium tremens as severe as that under which he labored when in Dr. Chamberlain's care, with the simple use of opium and brandy. And I have yet to see the case of *uncomplicated* delirium tremens, which will not yield to the *heroic* and *fearless* employment of these remedies.

Case VIII.—Patient took 1680 minims of laudanum, 10 ounces of whiskey, 1 pint of brandy, 2 pints of punch. Punch "freely" two or three times, and twice, "ad libitum;" and "egg-nog, as much as he could be made to take." Chloroform was administered four or five times. Once, inhalation was kept up "at frequent intervals" for two hours, and once, it was continued for an hour, each time producing "spasm, but no sleep."

Case IX.—In this case, comparatively little opium and brandy were given. Chloroform, however, was administered by inhalation three times. The first time, Dr. C. remarks, "we proceeded to administer chloroform to *deep anæsthesia,* resuming the administration whenever she (the patient) seemed about to pass from under its effects." "This was continued for half an hour." "During the progress of anæsthesia, subsultus came on, deepening in intensity, until it amounted to general spasm of the muscles." No sleep. After the second administration, she slept—*ten minutes.* In the third and last exhibition of this "*remedium magnum,*" Dr. Chamberlain states that "after a few inspirations the subsultus and respiration ceased simultaneously and instantly." "The head was thrown back on the pillow, the eyes were open and fixed, the face pale and cadaveric." "No pulse, no sound at the heart." Cold effusions and artificial respiration, successively tried, failed to restore her to vitality. Insufflation resorted to, as "the forlorn hope," after having been "maintained for ten minutes," fanned the feeble flame of life into a momentary flicker, and directly after this fatal inhalation of chloroform, says Dr. C., "she was watched in the hope that at the gate of death, the vicious cycle of her dreams might have been broken, but we were soon convinced that *delirium was as high as ever.*"

Soon after this the patient died. No post-mortem examination was made; had any been made, I am certain the lungs would have been found filled to engorgement with venous blood.

What was the cause of death in this case? I answer, Chloroform, decidedly. Any unprejudiced person will say the same; but what does Dr. Chamberlain say? "So far as we can trace the influence of the anæsthetic, it seems to have been favourable."

Case X.—In this case chloroform was "administered *three* times without permanent advantage." Stimulants and opium were then "given freely" for from twenty-four to forty-eight hours, and at the close of that interval the patient slept.

Among other diffusible stimulants chloroform was given internally. This case Dr. Chamberlain calls one "of SEDATION by the internal use of chloroform." It must appear evident to all *thinking* men that, to test any remedial agent in the treatment of disease, it must be given alone, otherwise the effects of other remedies used must necessarily complicate and obscure the results.

On carefully reviewing the cases in which chloroform has even the appearance of aiding in the cure of patients labouring under delirium tremens—and they form a very small proportion of those contained in Dr. C.'s report—it will be found that the anæsthetic *seemed* to produce sleep only after laudanum and alcoholic stimulants had been employed in large and frequently repeated doses previously to its administration.

In every case where it was given before the patient had been nearly narcotized with opium, it either produced fatal asphyxia, or its influence passed off in five or ten minutes, leaving the patient as delirious as, and often more so than, before its administration, and that, too, when cold aspersions, artificial respiration, and insufflations only proved equal to his *partial* resuscitation from asphyxia.

The pathology of delirium tremens is as well understood as that of any other disease of the nervous system. It is a waste of the brain and nerve substance, and a consequent exhaustion of nervous force, generally produced by excessive excitation of nervous phenomena by alcoholic stimulants, although it is not unfrequently caused by too long continued and too severe application to study, intense activity of the brain, or protracted watching without sleep. Whenever inflammation of the brain, serous effusion into its membranes or ventricles, or the formation and deposition of tubercles, occurs as an intercurrent disease, of course it complicates and obscures the symptoms and therapeutics of the primary malady.

In a pure and uncomplicated case of delirium tremens, we find that all the functions both of animal and organic life are inefficiently performed; the intellect is clouded, the appetite fails, digestion is impaired, all the secretions are scanty, the heart beats feebly, the pulse is small, and the tendency to local congestion is very great.

When chloroform is administered in such cases, it necessarily produces congestion of the lungs, since the blood, not being decarbonized, circulates more and more slowly through them until it ceases to circulate; hence the liability, in all cases where chloroform is inhaled, to death from what is sometimes called pulmonary apoplexy, or from subsequent inflammation of the lungs.

I have made autopsies in several cases of death following the administration of chloroform, in one of which it supervened immediately after the patient had ceased to inhale the anæsthetic, and I have invariably found the lungs completely gorged with dark venous blood.

Not only does chloroform produce congestion of the lungs, but also of the brain and nervous system generally. The stertorous breathing which is an index of complete anæsthesia, points out the deleterious effects of the poisonous vapours of the chloroform upon the medulla oblongata.

Without alluding more particularly to the danger attending the use of chloroform, increased as it must necessarily be when the patient is exhausted by sleeplessness and diminished vital force, it is almost entirely inefficient as a producer of sleep. Its soporific effects, even when complete asphyxia has been induced, are so evanescent that patients in whom stertorous breathing has been produced arouse from their semi-coma to a delirium as fierce as that from which they had been temporarily relieved by the subtle anæsthetic, in a few minutes after its removal.

These few remarks conclude what I have to say on the treatment of delirium tremens by chloroform.

My sole object in writing on this subject is to afford those of my brethren in the profession who have never witnessed the effects of chloroform in delirium tremens, the advantages of that knowledge of its deleterious results which an experience of several months in its almost daily use has afforded me. If I should, by this means, save a single unhappy wretch from a premature grave, and his medical adviser from the heart-rending consciousness of having caused, however innocently, the death of a human being, I shall have been sufficiently rewarded.

ART. IX.—*On the Yellow Fever in Baltimore in* 1819-22. By HORATIO G. JAMESON, M. D.[1]

IN the year 1819, we had a severe yellow fever epidemic in Baltimore. That year we had no regularly constituted Board of Health, but I was employed by the proprietors of the Maryland Hospital, I being then surgeon and one of the physicians to that institution, to attend the yellow fever patients. In the year 1820 a Board of Health was organized and a physician was appointed; the fever returned to a very distressing amount; the poor of whole neighbourhoods were removed to some rope-walks within one mile of the affected location, but the indigent sick were sent to the Maryland Hospital and placed under my care, so that I had special cognizance of the fever which prevailed in '19 and '20.

[1] [This paper was handed to us by its venerable author a short time previous to his death.—EDITOR.]

In 1821 I was appointed consulting physician; the epidemic again showed itself in great force, and also in 1822; after that year for two or three years there was a considerable number of sporadic cases occurring. I continued to discharge the duties of consulting physician till the year 1835—say from '21 to '35 inclusive, a period of fifteen years—during all which time I had ample opportunity of becoming acquainted with everything relating to the condition of the city, in respect to the state of health, and in respect to diseases.

In 1819 there was for several weeks a succession of yellow fever patients filling two or three large wards; these were mostly bad subjects for fever, and most of them advanced in the disease, so that a large proportion died. There was no apprehension in the institution of contagion, and there was the freest intercourse that the situation of the patients required. There was, of course, the steward and matron, their family of children, nurses, students, regular physicians, and physicians almost daily from the city, lunatics who were well enough to occupy the yard, and the washer-women. There was no unusual haste in the burial of the dead, bodies were suffered to lie in the dead-house as usual. Nevertheless, not a solitary case of disease occurred at the Hospital. We have said that the physician for 1820 caused the poor of the sickly districts to be removed to the rope-walks; here some sickened and some died. Citizens from other parts of the city had a free intercourse for several weeks. Not one case of disease occurred in any one who had not been an inhabitant of the sickly districts.

The present writer was consulting physician in 1821. The disease again assumed an epidemic form, and he being aware of the outrages, scenes of vice and debauchery carried on at the rope-walks, availed himself of an old ordinance, and caused several hundreds of the people to be removed from the fever districts to what is known as Old Town, on high ground, pure gravelly soil. Here the sick and the well were congregated together in such houses or parts of houses as could be procured, not more than from a half to one mile distance from the alluvial grounds where the malaria existed. This intermixture, with a fearless and unrestricted intercourse, was kept up for several weeks, there being almost no mortality after the removal. Now, again, we had the same state of things at the Maryland Hospital, and by the same physicians and assistants, the writer having again special charge of the yellow fever patients.

In the year 1822 the disease was more limited, and did not require a general removal, but there was the freest intercourse among the people. None suffered, except those who resided in the sickly parts of the city, which has never had an extent equal to one-tenth of the city. We have said sporadic cases continued to appear for some years after the epidemics above noticed, but, for the last quarter of a century or more, this scourge of mankind has disappeared, and Baltimore may justly be ranked among the most healthy cities.

We deem the following occurrence of much importance in one of our severe epidemics. The fever appeared in Commerce Street. This street runs north and south from the dock to what is termed *Exchange Place*, being about 100 feet wide. At the junction of these streets there was an old building called the Old Exchange. The building fronted on Exchange Place, but had also an entrance on Commerce Street from the rear of both ends of this building; a building extended back, perhaps fifty feet, and these were joined by a wall crossing on the rear of the lot. In this way was formed a sort of court, having no ventilation, except from above. This was a shed-like building, for it was only one-story high, and open on the inner side all around. All sorts of articles had been sold here, and not much regard paid to cleanliness. Things often lay exposed to the weather in this court; and the Board of Health, having been called to the premises, found a quantity of potatoes, onions, &c., in the cellars in a putrid condition.

Five gentlemen who did business in this building, and who occupied the Commerce Street front, were seized with the yellow fever before the Board of Health apprehended any danger in that quarter, and four of them fell victims to its deadly influence, whilst the fifth made a narrow escape. During that whole summer a family, consisting of a man and his wife and three or four children, lived in the Exchange, up stairs, in perfect health; but they had no connection with the Commerce Street doors, but used the Exchange front altogether. The roof of the shedding was flat, and the children were in the habit of playing on it. We do not recollect the exact height of the sheds, but we think from fifteen to twenty feet above the surface of the court, where much water was poured in times of heavy rain. It seems reasonable to suppose that the poisonous effluvia never rose as high as the roof of the shed, or the back door up stairs of the building; and we should think that to a contagionist it should seem stranger still, that, notwithstanding the mortality at the Old Exchange, on the south side of Exchange Place, not a solitary case of fever occurred on the north side of the "Place," one hundred feet distant only; and the whole square on that side was occupied by families.

We do not deem it necessary to enter upon any description of the disease in question at this time. We suppose it will not be doubted whether the medical faculty, and, indeed, the people of Baltimore, know the yellow fever when seen among them. Our object is to offer some information in relation to its non-contagiousness, and we have been led to believe that a stronger combination of circumstances cannot be found serving to prove the true character of the disease. Believe the facts, and there remains no room for doubt, were there no other corroborating accounts; and yet, up to the present time, the public mind is not disabused of the mischievous error: if facts are seen to disprove the contagiousness of the disease, it is alleged it must be so in some degree, or certain things must exist; and yet, whenever these are investigated, and the clearest proof obtained, the doubts, which are expressed from time to time, serve at almost every recurrence of the epidemic to beget mistrust, and almost conviction, that the hydra, contagion, is come at last. There is, perhaps, no other branch of human knowledge where conviction and abiding confidence have been so hard to prove and sustain.

ART. X.—*Resection of the Elbow-joint.* By CHARLES E. BELLAMY, A. M., M. D., of Columbus, Georgia.

WHILE house surgeon to King's County Hospital, Long Island, it was my good fortune to be instrumental in saving, by this operation, the arm of a woman, which would otherwise have been doomed to an immediate amputation. The fortunate result was exceedingly gratifying to the patient and her friends, as well as to the physicians who were present during the operation. It was the first case that had occurred in the observation of any of those present, and the case, as transcribed from my notes taken at the time, is as follows: Mrs. Cath. S———, aged twenty-eight, married, was admitted into King's County Hospital, ward 18, on May the 5th, 1855. She was sent here by her friends that she might undergo an amputation. When first examined, the elbow presented a very swollen and inflamed condition. From two sinuses, one on the side and one behind, there was a copious discharge of pus of a disagreeable odour. She states that, when quite a child, the arm was broken, and an abscess formed. She is unable to state when it was broken, but the inference is that the fracture implicated the joint, as the arm has ever since been anchylosed in a straight position. From that period up to the present time, there has been occasional pains in the region of the joint. About six weeks ago, it began to inflame and swell, and became painful in the extreme. After a while, she applied to Dr. Smith, of Williamsburg, who immediately made an opening, and a quantity of pus was discharged. The doctor informed me that at that time the bones were carious. She was then advised to be sent here. She suffers very much from hectic. Her lungs are pronounced healthy. Removal of the cause, a tonic treatment and generous diet are plainly indicated. She consents with reluctance to the attempt to save the arm. On the 12th of May, Drs. Turner, Ingrahan, Blanchard, and Holtzhauser, of the hospital, and Drs. Black and Smith, of Brooklyn, being present, I proceeded to the operation by first cutting down to the ulnar nerve, and isolating it from its attachments for the distance of two inches or more, and drawing it to the inner side of the elbow. The incision for this purpose extended along the inner posterior edge of the lower part of the humerus and the upper part of the ulnar. A similar incision was made along the outer side, and the two joined by a transverse cut, the whole forming an H-shaped incision. The flaps were turned back, and the olecranon separated with the saw from the body of the ulnar, the lateral ligaments divided, and the soft parts in front of the joint separated from the bones. A bandage being placed between to protect the soft parts during the action of the saw, the lower end of the humerus was cut off up to the point where the caries seemed to stop; afterwards, the head of the radius and the ulnar, as far as the coronoid process, where the disease seemed to have extended. The top in length to the bony skeleton was about two inches.

No arteries required ligation, torsion being sufficient. A gutta-percha splint was moulded to the front of the arm, the arm not straight, but forming a very obtuse angle at the elbow. The wound was brought together by the twisted suture, and cold-water dressing applied. The patient was narcotized with chloroform during the operation, and tolerated its use very well. She then took an opiate, and was put to bed. From the next day, she began to improve. She is three months advanced in pregnancy. On the 16th, most of the incisions had healed by adhesion. The patient continued to improve. Part of the wound remained open for several months, and from my not having taken away the entire amount of diseased bone, several small pieces separated and came away. In November, she was delivered of a fine boy, and soon after was discharged well, and with an arm capable of performing the motion of extension and flexion, volution and supination. The happy result of this case ought to induce others always to give this operation the preference when there is even a chance of saving the arm.

ART. XI.—*Hæmatemesis from a Tumour of Varicose Veins on the Stomach and Disgorgement of an Enlarged Spleen.* By G. B. HOTCHKIN, M. D., of Media, Pa.

THE patient in this case was a lad aged 10½ years, a son of my friend, Dr. J. Rowland, of this place.

He was an intelligent boy, of active and energetic habits, of a bilious temperament and sallow complexion, and had always been in delicate health, but had never suffered any severe illness since his infancy. When about six months of age he had an attack of intermittent fever, which, however, was not well marked; this left him with a very great enlargement of the spleen, which remained up to the time of his last illness, forming a tumour over the region of that organ.

At long intervals, from the age of six years upward, a small quantity of blood would be found on his pillow in the morning which could be traced to no cause, but during all this time his appetite, strength, and general health constantly improved. The hemorrhoidal veins were much enlarged from his infancy, and occasionally discharged blood. He suffered twice from a hoarseness amounting almost to total aphonia.

On Sunday, the 17th of February, ult., he was first attacked with hæmatemesis without any premonitory symptoms (his general health having been very good previously, except the hoarseness before mentioned), vomiting on that day a large amount of pure blood; and on that day and the next at least from two to three gallons of black tar-like fluid were discharged from the bowels, evidently decomposed blood mingled with mucus.

By the free use of astringents these discharges were checked, but the patient was left in a state of great prostration. Tonics and nourishing food were given, everything being cooled by ice before taken.

Under this treatment he seemed rapidly improving till the next Thursday, when the discharges reappeared, but with less violence and copiousness.

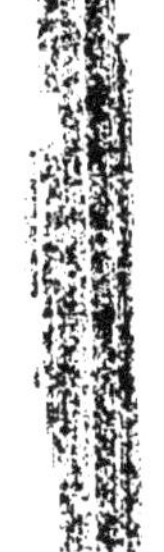

At this time we noticed that the tumour occupied by the spleen had disappeared, and that organ could not be felt at all. This fact, combined with the character of the discharges, satisfied us that there was serious organic lesion. Resort was had to eminent counsel in Philadelphia, by whose opinion our diagnosis was confirmed; and from that time but two principal indications were followed in the treatment pursued, *i. e.* supporting the patient's strength by tonics and nourishment, and holding the discharges in check by astringents.

On Sunday, March 2d, two weeks from the first attack, a third occurred; the discharge consisting from this time almost entirely of blood, fresh or in clots, discharged by the mouth.

These attacks were repeated occasionally till Sunday, March 16th, when, after a gush of blood from the mouth he sank rapidly, and died within an hour, just four weeks from the commencement of his illness.

The case was aggravated by ascites and suppression of urine during the last week, causing much suffering to the patient; these were, however, much relieved by appropriate treatment.

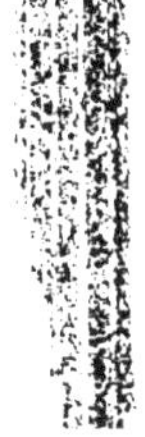

His mind was remarkably clear and calm through the whole time.

No exciting cause of this attack is known, except it be attributed to severe falls on the ice while skating a day or two previous.

We were indebted to the kindness of Drs. S. Weir Mitchell, and John Kane, of Philadelphia, for a very accurate and careful examination of the body.

Autopsy twenty-four hours after death. About eight pints of water in the peritoneal cavity; no abnormal collection in the thorax; the stomach filled with clotted blood. The tissues of the whole system white and bloodless, except a slight congestion near the cardiac orifice of the stomach.

A tumour on the stomach at the cardiac orifice about the size of a hen's egg, longitudinally divided, consisting of enlarged vessels filled with clots of blood; the largest spheroidal, and about three-quarters of an inch in diameter. These were traced through various convolutions into the gastric vein. These vessels seem to be perforated by minute orifices into the stomach.

The lymphatics about the pancreas and spleen were engorged and hypertrophied.

The investing membrane of the spleen was somewhat granular, and presented the appearance and feel called waxy, also shrunken. That organ was of natural size and its substance healthy.

There was no abnormal appearance of the vocal organs, except a slight thickening of the vocal chords.

Nothing more of interest was discovered.

ART. XII.—*Cases of Nymphomania.* By HORATIO R. STORER, M. D., one of the Physicians to the Boston Lying-in Hospital. (Read before the Boston Society for Medical Observation, July 21, 1856.)

CASE I.—For this case I am indebted to Dr. Sprague.

Margaret Murphy, aged 20, from Ireland; is of middle height, thick set, excessively plethoric. Countenance dull, unintelligent. Is shy and reserved, answering questions with great reluctance.

March 25, 1856. Complains of cough of three years' standing, leucorrhœa, dysmenorrhœa, and dysuria, with constant pricking in region of bladder. Thinks she has at times prolapsus uteri.

Is unmarried. Commenced menstruating at 14, since which time has always had more or less leucorrhœa. Recurrence of catamenia at first irregular, but of late less so. Always excessive pain at time of discharge, which usually lasts but a day, and is scanty. Character of discharge generally normal, sometimes clotty, never membranous. Has never had rheumatism. Has severe headache before catamenia, sometimes during intervals.

While a child was strong and healthy, and continued so till 1850, previous to her arrival in this country, when she had several fits, which were pronounced by her physician to be epileptic; these extended over a period of three months.

In 1853, she entered the Massachusetts General Hospital, coming under the care of Drs. Jacob Bigelow and Perry for uterine hemorrhage, consequent, as she then alleged, upon lifting a heavy tub of clothes. She subsequently re-entered the hospital in 1854 for cough and leucorrhœa, and was then treated by Drs. Shattuck, Bowditch, and Storer, Sen., getting cod-liver and fusel oils, her cervix touched with nitrate of silver, and with relief from neither.

Cough troublesome; but little expectoration. Has raised blood frequently, florid and frothy; still does so at times, not at menstrual periods. Upon auscultation and percussion, no evident signs of thoracic disease.

Appetite is capricious. Bowels free; relieved daily. Great difficulty in micturition; a small and interrupted stream, attended with urgent desire, and followed by excessive scalding. The pricking sensation already spoken of is constant. No tenderness about spine.

Upon digital examination by the vagina and rectum, an excess of heat in vagina, its calibre large. Uterus somewhat enlarged; no tenderness on pressure in its neighbourhood. Cervix rather broad and short, slightly abraded. Os largely fissured. In other respects genitals normal. Abdomen marked by parturition.

Upon asking patient to account for the puerperal signs, she acknowledged having got with child shortly after leaving the hospital in 1855. Was confined at Bridgewater seven months since; labour a very tedious one, lasting seventy-two hours, and delivery being effected by forceps. The child, a boy, died at four months of smallpox.

Menstruated for the first time since confinement on March 7th, a little over a fortnight ago; as much pain as ever.

April 3. Closely cross-questioned. States additionally that, while at the hospital, she was several times etherized by Dr. H. J. Bigelow; for what she pretends ignorance. Vaginal examination now repeated without further result. Her complaints of dysuria being still very great, the bladder was carefully sounded (without the use of ether), and nothing found. At one time an impression was given of the presence of a foreign body, but the sensation was only momentary. Sounding attended with great pain and shrinking. Patient was then shown to Dr. Hobbs, at my office, and sounded by him, with equal ill success.

The urine under the microscope gave no pus, no crystals, and but few epithelial scales.

Her statement concerning the etherizations sent me at once for further information to my father, from whom I learned that, while under his care at the hospital, suspecting stone or the like, he had requested one of the surgeons, Dr. Bigelow, to examine her, by whom several foreign bodies, pins and hair-pins, were removed from the bladder.

9*th*. At Lying-in Hospital, in consultation with my colleague, Dr. Dupee, ether was administered; the urethra was found free throughout its entire extent, but a foreign body was at length discovered in the cavity of the bladder. This, after some manipulation, was removed by Dr. Dupee. It proved to be a long piece of copper wire, broken and twisted upon itself several times, and seemed to have been imbedded in the anterior wall. It was without incrustation, and had the appearance of having been originally taken from the neck of a bottle, as, indeed, she afterwards acknowledged was the case. The operation was followed by considerable hæmaturia.

16*th*. Patient complained bitterly of being so soon again subjected to operation, asserting that at the other hospital she was allowed a much longer interval. This, however, did not now seem necessary; ether was given, and by a previous arrangement with Dr. Dupee, of alternation, I removed the greater portion of a hair-pin twisted upon itself.

23*d*. Again etherized, and another fragment of hair-pin removed; this time by Dr. Dupee.

29*th*. Again etherized, and bladder carefully sounded. After prolonged examination, both by Dr. Dupee and myself, nothing was detected, and her other symptoms, the cough, leucorrhœa, &c., having much improved, and menstruation having taken place more naturally than by her account ever before, she was, by arrangement with Dr. Walker, transferred the next day, on the 30th, to the City Lunatic Asylum, at South Boston, there being reason to fear that she might, unless restrained, do herself serious injury.

Her treatment while under my charge was sufficiently simple. I soon learned that her distress was, in part at least, overrated, some of it probably feigned. The cough, which, during her early visits to my office, was very constant, severe, and racking, and which then resisted a succession of expectorants, seemed immediately to yield after I had admitted her into the Lying-in Hospital, strangely enough showing a marked and sudden decrease with every removal from the bladder; the improvement was undoubtedly owing to her change to the warm moist atmosphere of the hospital. She certainly raised blood; this occurred more than once after her entrance, but I am inclined to think it was from the throat, and that, as was certainly the case with the hæmaturia, she overstated the quantity; in which opinion I am confirmed by an auscultation made of the patient by my friend, Dr. Borland, on April 27th, his results agreeing with my own.

The leucorrhœa, which seemed previously to have been treated in vain, at one time by merely constitutional measures, at another by local injections, was much benefited by vaginal suppositories, at first of oxide of zinc, and afterwards of alum and catechu, of each gr. xv to the ball. In so plethoric a patient, it did not seem advisable suddenly and entirely to check the discharge, and this was not attempted.

The dysmenorrhœa was lessened, perhaps partly by passage of the sound at the preliminary examination, although I have no doubt that the low diet on which she was placed contributed to the result. The diet, for nearly a month, was gruel. She several times eagerly desired to be bled; but I preferred keeping her on low diet, as equally likely to lessen her chance of peritonitis, and more so the chance of her persisting, if at all malingering.

Before my suspicions of the true state of the bladder were aroused, I endeavoured, as frequently with success, to allay the dysuria by throwing chloroform vapour into the vagina, and afterwards by a flexible catheter into the urethra and bladder itself; but the pain was not relieved.

The urinary tenesmus had been excessive, and I have no doubt that long continued expulsive efforts had at times produced a partial prolapse and protrusion of the anterior wall of the vagina, which she had supposed, as already remarked, to be prolapse of the uterus. It was noticed at every sounding of the bladder, the patient being thoroughly etherized, that in a short time most energetic contractions of the fundus vesicæ were invariably produced; as, indeed, had occurred at my early and unsatisfactory examination when ether was not used; which action, had the urethra been at all dilatable, as it was not, even under the stimulus of a powerful sponge tent, would have threatened partial inversion of the organ. These expulsive efforts, suggesting a transference of labour pains, were accompanied by a profuse flow of limpid urine, which was secreted with remarkable rapidity, or had else, though hardly probable, been collecting in the ureters, the patient generally passing but little in the twenty-four hours.

The hæmaturia subsequent to each operation was but slight, and lasted but a few hours; a fact rather remarkable when the sharp points of the foreign bodies are taken into consideration, they all having apparently imbedded, not merely entangled, themselves in the mucous membrane, and the difficulty of bringing such bodies through an urethra, whose diameter, though its coats had naturally become somewhat hypertrophied, was not above ordinary size.

For the twenty-four hours immediately succeeding each operation, she complained of considerable abdominal pain and tenderness. At first I had some fear of peritonitis, but soon found, upon experiment, that assafœtida, to which she had the usual repugnance, at once allayed her complaints and the pain. This proved invariably the case. My suspicions, hence, that these were rather the pains of hysteria, were strengthened by her general behaviour; and, subsequently, by learning of her convulsive seizures in 1850, and the details of the so-called peritonitic attacks at the Massachusetts General Hospital.

The pulse was generally somewhat quickened during the first day, but on the second used to sink to her usual standard, about 84.

The removal of the hair-pins and wire was in each case effected by ordinary dressing-forceps, and in each case only after much manipulation. They were not easily detected by the sound, or catheter, or forceps, particularly after the muscular contractions, which were very easily excited, had begun; getting lost between or covered by folds of the mucous membrane. When found, they were not easily dislodged from their position, and evinced a constant tendency to catch athwart the urethra before entering it, or having entered, to get entangled in some portion of its course.

From the outset she resolutely denied having introduced anything into the bladder subsequently to her discharge from the Massachusetts General Hospital, and asserted that what we removed had been introduced previously to that time and previously to her confinement, introduced merely to dilate the urethra for dysuria, and had slipped from her hand against her will. Neither of these statements can, however, be true. How she could have ever introduced such irregularly-shaped masses into the bladder, and how, once having had them removed, she could have dared to repeat the experiment, are mysteries which mental disease, a decided *furor uterinus*, can alone explain. It is impossible that so thorough a surgeon as Dr. Bigelow could have left anything in the bladder; it is impossible that she could have undergone so tedious a labour under these circumstances, instrumental as it was, without some one of the varieties of vesical fistula having been produced; and it is improbable that the alleged lapse of months, not to say years, would have left no incrustation.

The previous medical history of the patient, dating from her arrival in this country, is not uninteresting. The greater part of it she endeavoured to suppress; but, from chance words she let fall at various times, it became possible to ascertain her whole story from the several physicians who successively had charge of her; and, upon subsequently informing her of these discoveries, she acknowledged their truth.

On September 2, 1853, she called upon Dr. Salter, then complaining of severe expulsive pains, and stating that she had introduced a *cork* into the vagina some time previously, which, having forced it up by a bed-wrench, she was now unable to remove. This cork Dr. Salter could not discover either on that or on the following day. A third examination, however, on September 13, was more successful, and the cork was then removed. It was situated high up in the vagina, very near the os, a little back of and in contact with it, the smaller end being uppermost. "A strong effort was required to start it from its bed." The cork is now in my possession, and is of the size to fit a large jug.

Subsequent to this operation, the leucorrhœa, which had formerly been profuse, continuing and there being some symptoms of metritis, she was advised by Dr. Salter to enter the Massachusetts General Hospital, and did so October 14, 1853. She then stated, according to the hospital record as already quoted, entirely suppressing the fact as related to me by Dr. Salter, that having previously strained herself while lifting, she had felt something give way in lower abdomen, followed immediately by escape of blood from vagina. At her entrance, just a month after the operation by Dr. Salter, she was flowing, but not profusely, and had great pain in head, back, and limbs, with both dysuria and incontinence of urine. Abdomen full, tympanitic, exquisitely tender on pressure; but pulse only 92, and rather feeble. She left the hospital in November, 1853, not relieved, and sought a female friend, by whose advice "instruments" were introduced, which she found herself unable to extract; and shortly after, December 9, she entered Deer Island Hospital, where she was relieved.

Dr. Moriarty writes me, that at entrance she was suffering with pleurisy, and that when convalescent three pieces of German silver spoon, the "instruments" alluded to, were removed from the upper part of her vagina. She left Deer Island on April 8, 1854, the leucorrhœa and dysuria still continuing, and re-entered the Massachusetts General Hospital, June 13. At that time, according to her account, the urine had for several months regularly been withdrawn by catheter. While in the hospital, caustic was repeatedly applied to her cervix uteri for leucorrhœa.

On August 24th, a hair-pin and ordinary pin were removed from the bladder by Dr. Bigelow.

On September 3d, another hair-pin—this operation being followed by symptoms of peritonitis; and, on October 2d, a fragment of a third hair-pin. These specimens were at the time exhibited by Dr. Bigelow to the Society for Medical Improvement.[1] She was discharged November 5th, few of her symp-

[1] Extracts from Records, &c., vol. ii. p. 139, Am. Journ. of the Med. Sci., Jan. 1855, p. 57. Dr. Bigelow at the same time described a new method of operating; he had turned the points by vaginal manipulation. This, in 1856, I was unable to do.

toms having abated. For some time after leaving the hospital she continued under Dr. Bigelow's care as a private patient.

In June, 1855, she reapplied at the Massachusetts General Hospital as an out-patient, and was treated by Dr. Abbot, who did not sound her bladder, but auscultated abdomen, and from this diagnosed pregnancy, which at first she stoutly denied, but she afterwards admitted that her last catamenia had been in December, 1854. Dr. Abbot at one time discovered large vesications on the inner side of each thigh, which he supposed had been purposely caused for purposes of excitement, by blisters, though this was also denied.

She was confined in September, 1855, at Bridgewater, as already said. She next applied to Dr. Herrick, who, however, advised her again to enter the hospital; and finally, early this spring, she placed herself under the charge of Dr. Sprague, who prescribed expectorants for the cough, and introduced an India rubber pessary; the pressure of which, however, upon the bladder, she was not able to endure.

As previously stated, the patient was sent to the Lunatic Hospital at South Boston on May 30th; but, to my surprise, she again appeared at my office on June 21st, asserting that she had that day been discharged as "not insane." She again complained of pricking in the neighbourhood of the bladder, which was not the case when I last saw her. From this, my expectations that she would return to her old habit seem confirmed. I now refused to deal further with her, believing that merely palliative treatment without proper restraint would be useless. She then put herself under the care of Dr. Hobbs, who, it will be recollected, examined her with me at the outset, on April 3d, and I have since heard that she has lately been seen again among the out-patients at the Massachusetts General Hospital.

Each step in the above history but goes to confirm the very evident opinion that, if we forget her having imprudently got with child, "she is," to quote from a characteristic note by Dr. Bigelow, "a good girl, unfortunately biassed by genito-urinary proclivities."

I am inclined to think that she masturbates, though, as is usual, she denies it. Her manners are those of that habit. Her expression, when unconscious of being observed, is at times decidedly lecherous. She expressed great dislike of the various gentlemen who had previously had charge of her and of those who saw her with me; but yet, though she acknowledged that the catheter was not always necessary, and that she could pass it perfectly well herself, she was constantly asking that it should be done by others.

Her clitoris was not at all enlarged.[1]

[1] It would be difficult to decide upon the original exciting cause of irritation in this case. It has been ingeniously asked me by Dr. Buckingham, if she had been troubled by ascarides previously to her first experiment upon herself; a question that the patient would probably have been unable to answer, and which I carelessly neglected to put, although irritation of the vagina from the presence of ascarides in the rectum, both sympathetically and by actual transit of the parasites, is now recog-

Case II.—Mrs. B., American, aged 24, of under size, gross habit, pale and pasty complexion; is in easy circumstances; was married at 17, seven years since; no children, and has never miscarried; has enjoyed, she thinks, on the whole, tolerably good health. Bowels are now, and have been, freely moved daily. Appetite is, and has been, constantly good.

Menstruates regularly; has just done so; discharge continuing nearly a week, very scanty, attended on the first day or two after it commences with more or less aching pain in the back and head, and frequently throughout the period in the right iliac region. At times pain under the left breast, and frequently palpitation. Abdomen inclined to bloat; sudden tumefaction, and as sudden subsidence.

Has constantly trifling leucorrhœa, but hardly sufficient to require napkin.

Has during past three years been under the care of several physicians; one of whom thought necessary for a long time to apply nitrate of silver to cervix twice weekly. The probable effect, not an unfrequent one of this treatment, may easily be conceived from the further history.

Some little dysuria; scalding at and after flow.

For several months has been troubled by bad dreams, excessively lascivious in their character. Can hardly meet or converse with a gentleman but that next night fancies she has intercourse with him. Has frequently such thoughts by day, sometimes when in conversation; though thinks she would at once repel an improper advance on part of any man, and is not conscious of having over shown to such what was passing in her mind. Is much afraid that if further increase of malady, may not be able to restrain herself.

At such times is conscious of a "spasm" within genitals, and of the emission of a mucous jet, one or more drops, which stains linen. This emission did not occur at first, but now always takes place; whether awake or asleep, in the latter case, waking her; whether in bed or abroad; whether alone or with others.[1]

Husband has been a wine merchant; is still interested in the business; is a high liver, and has twice had attacks of apoplexy. Is much older than herself. Does not think he has missed having connection with her a single night since marriage, even at times of menstruation (this assertion repeated). Has frequently come to her three times in a night, and always with a seminal emission (this assertion also repeated). Has of late complained that he found physical obstruction to intercourse on her part, though she thinks it rather an increasing failure by him in erection.

Has herself always lived well, by his orders; meat three times each day,

nized as not uncommon; and a case illustrative of the latter class happened to be under my care at that very time.

[1] The questions upon this point were asked in consequence of a previous conversation with Dr. John P. Reynolds upon Duverney's glands, and similar occurrences in patients of his own. Dr. Herrick has since related to me another very interesting case.

brandy at dinner. Enjoys intercourse greatly; is conscious of excessive local excitement, so great that she not unfrequently faints during penetration; this, however, being no check to husband. Has, with him, always desired children; and thinks from that longing arose present excess.

Has not told these points of her history to former physicians; knew that she should, but such questions were not asked; though, as the answers prove, they were necessary to a correct understanding of the case.

Is sure that if husband should restrain himself, and keep from her, she could not keep from him. Has tried it.

Did not begin menstruating till just before marriage; was then ignorant of sexual matters, and innocent of impure thoughts. Had never masturbated, but was conscious of undefined but strong desire, which often led her to clasp in embrace her brothers more fervently than usual. Was on this account early married by advice of mother, who herself acknowledges similar warmth and precocity.

Has never had impure companions; has not been in habit of reading impure publications of any sort; has contributed tales, &c., to magazines, but has not overstated any of her symptoms in this history. Generally spends evenings at home; does not keep late hours, both having same desire to retire early.

Upon examination, heart and lungs apparently without disease; no tenderness along spine, nor in any part of abdomen.

Heat of vagina rather above standard; its size good; no obstruction. Uterus somewhat enlarged; this also evident by rectum; no displacement; cervix much elongated, and moderately thickened; signs to touch of slight abrasion. Os almost imperforate, not admitting sound; anterior lip much the larger. Speculum not used, because not needed.

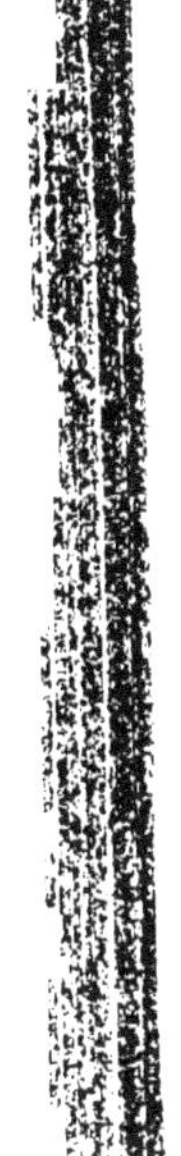

As in the other case, not the slightest enlargement of clitoris. Excessive irritability in its neighbourhood, gentle touch causing her to shriek out, not with pain, as she herself said, but with excitement. She now acknowledges constant itching in that region.

This first interview with the patient was had on May 16th, when the following treatment was prescribed, at the same time giving her fully to understand that if she continued her present habits of indulgence, it would probably become necessary to send her to an asylum —

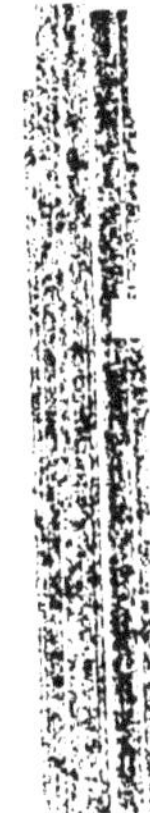

1. Total abstinence from husband; if not possible otherwise, by temporary entire separation.
2. Meat but once in the day.
3. Brandy and other stimulants not at all.
4. Novel writing to be given up.
5. Hair-pillows and mattress in place of feathers.
6. Cold sponge-bath morning and night.
7. Cold enemata at night.
8. Frequent lotion of anterior vaginal commissure with solution of borax.

9. Two-drachm doses nightly of equal parts of the tinctures of henbane, valerian, and lupulin; the last, as the others, given merely as a hypnotic, and not as an anaphrodisiac, its alleged effects in this respect being afterwards recalled to my mind by Dr. Read.

10. Iron; gr. iss of the sacch. carb. thrice daily in pill.

11. Exercise, fresh air, and occupation of mind by more and cheerful friends.

Mrs. B. saw me next on May 30th, two weeks later. Abstinence in accordance with my advice proving otherwise impossible, the husband had at once left the city. Patient found the change a hard one, but was endeavouring to follow out faithfully all my other directions. As yet no marked alteration, but thinks she is better.

June 17. Accompanied by sister, from whom I was able to verify her accounts of general health, &c. Now a little over a month since commencing treatment. Has had within a week a slight attack of dysentery; this now past.

Husband still absent. The lascivious dreams have not occurred for several days, nor the sudden vaginal emissions. The local irritation and heat have also much diminished, and as regards these most troublesome symptoms, she feels greatly relieved. Since last visit, her appetite for food, which was formerly voracious, has lessened; but the leucorrhœa has increased, the discharge being thinner and less tenacious. Is now compelled to wear napkins constantly. For this, ointment pessaries were directed, each to contain gr. xv of oxide of zinc.

Has again menstruated, more freely, and with less pain. To continue course formerly prescribed.

The patient is still under treatment. I now consider the case much more hopeful as regards the mental symptoms, which, however, will for some time require decided enforcement of very strict laws. Both the wife and the husband must be taught moderation, which done, there seems no very good reason why, after dilatation of the os, and perhaps, if it should be needed, application of potassa fusa, the patient should not realize her hopes, and get with child.

Most writers seem to consider that nymphomania must be attended, as cause or symptom, by ungovernable pruritus, though this I do not believe to be always the case. It was present as such in Case II., and in the immediate neighbourhood of the clitoris. It was also present in Case I., but in a different situation, and of rather different type, though to an equally great extent, "pricking," but here only far within the vagina, at its very end, and in the immediate neighbourhood of the bladder, the sensation, moreover, being that of all others which would have been expected from the peculiar bodies introduced. In both cases, the *effect* of unnatural or excessive stimulus became itself worse stimulus still, and so an active *cause*.

Apart from their furnishing different manifestations of but one and the same disease, these cases are of value as bearing upon two interesting questions.

They both go to prove Duchatelet's opinion, based upon frequent examination of prostitutes, to be correct, that excessive sexual appetite and excessive sexual indulgence are by no means necessarily attended in the female by a clitoris at all enlarged, while Case II. is a marked instance of that peculiar and forcible emission, still denied by many, of mucus from the female genital canals during heat, and under mental excitement alone, which, when occurring during intercourse, gave origin to the old and fanciful idea of a true "*semen muliebre.*"

7 Chester St., Boston, Aug. 1, 1856.

Art. XIII.—*Spina Bifida.* By Wm. H. Byford, M. D., of Evansville, Ind.

Within twelve months past three cases of spina bifida have been brought to my notice, in all of which a peculiarity has been observed which, so far as I know, has not been described by writers upon this subject. The peculiarity has reference to the genital organs mostly; and although in an affection of such general fatality it may not be a matter of much importance, so far as success in management is concerned, yet some interest may attach to it physiologically and pathologically. Two of the cases occurred in my own practice in this city, and the third in the practice of a respectable country practitioner (Dr. Thos. Runcie).

Case I.—Mrs. H. gave birth to her third child, female, June 6th, 1855. It was small, but to all appearances healthy and well formed, with the exception of a spina bifida tumour, occupying the place of the processes of the two lower lumbar vertebræ, about the size of an orange split in half. A circumstance worthy of note was a tendency in the lower extremities to draw up to the front of the abdomen and chest. They were, when not controlled by interference, extended somewhat rigidly and bent upon the abdomen, so that each foot touched the ear of the side opposite to which it belonged, and it required some force to restore them to their natural position. In about eighteen hours after its birth, the father came to my office and requested me to call, as the mother said something very uncommon was the matter with the child. Upon arriving, she directed my attention to a thick tenacious bloody mucus on the napkin, stating that it came from the vagina, that the child had cried a great deal through the night, and seemed to be affected with bearing down pains, as shown by its almost constant straining. Upon separating the labia, I found them and the thighs stained by the same discharge as was upon the napkin. The entrance to the vagina was large enough to admit the end of my thumb without obstruction. Protruding between the labia was the neck and body of the tiny uterus, with this mucous discharge issuing from the patulous os tincæ. After a moment's consideration, I oiled my thumb and pressed gently the latter organ upward and backward out of sight. A compress was bound over the closed labia with a T bandage. This afforded so much relief that the child rested better for several hours; but the descent was repeated, and the organs returned to their places several times before the death of the child. Bearing down pain invariably returned with the descent, and was relieved by the replacement of the uterus. The child lived about a week, when it died, worn out and exhausted by the suffering and pain, as I thought, from the prolapse. This case, although peculiar in this particular, did not cause any reflection other than a double malformation of any other kind. I supposed it a rare occurrence merely, and not worthy of special note.

Case II.—In less than two months I was called to see another child, delivered the day before, with a spina bifida in the same locality, though not quite so large as the one above described. I could not learn that the legs assumed the same position as in the first case, but the mother spoke to me of the sanguinolent discharge upon the napkin. The child was female, and upon examination I found the vaginal opening much larger than natural, and the uterus visible between the labia. It had been crying all night and straining fearfully. The uterus was made to ascend by very slight pressure upward. This handling did not give any uneasiness, as far as we could judge, and the replacement was followed by complete relief for several hours. This patient lived about ten days, and, as with the other, I thought was exhausted by the pain and watchfulness caused by the prolapse.

The case of Dr. Runcie (which was the third) was almost exactly like my first. The labia were separated by the prolapsed uterus, the vaginal opening much larger than natural, the same bloody mucus was discharged, and the child was distressed by the same sort of bearing down pain. In all these cases, the mucus discharged was of that thin tenacious kind furnished by the neck and cavity of the uterus, and in the first instance was seen issuing from the diminutive os tineæ. In a practice of nearly eighteen years, I had not before last June seen a case of spina bifida; in the last twelve months I have met with three—all females—all affected with congenital prolapsus uteri. Although unable to say, I apprehend, from the silence of all the authors I can at present consult, that the prolapse is rare. Certainly, however, when it is an accompaniment, it greatly embarrasses the management of the case, and renders the affection more surely fatal. Observing three cases of spina bifida with this peculiarity, occurring close together, induced me to think it might have possibly been hitherto overlooked, and determined me to send them to you for publication. These cases all proved fatal, the first in about one week, the second ten days, and the third three weeks. All of the little patients seemed to suffer a good deal of pain apparently from the uterine malposition.

Art. XIV.—*Laryngitis; Labour occurring during its Progress; Operation of Laryngo-Tracheotomy.* By G. B. Linderman, M. D., of Mauch Chunk, Pa.

Mrs. W. W. B., of Nesquehoning, Carbon County, Pa., mother of two children, at the end of her third gestation was attacked with acute laryngitis. She was first seen by Dr. Richardson, on the 19th of March, 1856, at which time she was suffering all the symptoms of laryngitis, and hourly expecting her confinement. He prescribed to meet the indications at the time. At 10 o'clock of the same day he saw her again, and found the disease increasing. He bled her freely, administered ten grs. hyd. sub. mur., nauseated her with tartar emetic, and applied tobacco cataplasms to the throat. This treatment was continued up to 3 o'clock of the 20th, at which time I first saw her. I found her with a flushed countenance; pulse 110, full and strong; skin hot and dry; inability to lie down; great difficulty of breathing, accompanied with a wheezing noise and a peculiar muffled cough. She could not speak above a whisper. Her bowels not having been moved, an enema was administered, which produced a copious fecal discharge. She was again largely bled, and took grs. ij hyd. sub. mur. every two hours, and kept nauseated with tartar emetic. The fauces were touched with arg. nitr. ℈ij to aqua ℥j. At 6 o'clock P. M. labour pains came on, and five hours afterwards she gave birth to a healthy male child, but with an increase of all her symptoms, and her attending physician thought that she would suffocate. After a desperate effort and violent coughing, some tough mucus was expelled and the paroxysm somewhat relieved. At 5 o'clock P. M. of the 21st of March, we found, to our regret, that all our efforts to arrest the progress of the disease had failed. In fact, she was in the last stage of asphyxia. Her face was purple, eyeballs projecting, veins distended, and lips blue. These alarming symptoms, together with the twitching of the muscles about the eyes, admonished us that death must soon close the scene. After a few minutes' deliberation, we determined to give her the chances of an operation, and accordingly, without loss of time (and with such instruments as are found in an ordinary pocket-case), I proceeded to operate. Placing the patient in the usual position, I commenced an incision along the median line of the thyroid cartilage and continued it to near the sternum, exposing the crico-thyroid membrane and upper part of the trachea. At this stage of the operation copious venous hemorrhage ensued. Three of the largest veins were ligatured, and the incision sponged with iced water, but the blood still continued to flow freely. Fearing that she would expire, I lost no further time in attempting to control the hemorrhage, but opened the cricoid membrane, cricoid cartilage, and first ring of the trachea, when a considerable quantity of coagula, tenacious mucus, and some false membrane were expelled. As soon as one full inspiration was taken, the hemorrhage ceased. One hour after the operation she was breathing quietly, pulse 90, small and feeble, and surface cold. The chest was covered with warm flannel cloths, and bottles filled with warm water were put to the extremities. At 8 o'clock P. M. she slept quietly.

The following notes will show the further progress of the case, and treatment of the same until recovery:—

March 22. Six o'clock A. M. Patient has slept some through the night and coughed considerably, expelling large quantities of tenacious mucus and false membrane. The incision was kept open by means of blunt hooks, and the expectoration removed with a small sponge mop. Six o'clock P. M., patient much the same except that the bowels are running off too freely; ordered opium to restrain bowels, and allowed beef-tea.

23*d*. Ten o'clock A. M. Slight ptyalism; complains of pain in the muscles about the chest and shoulders; system irritable; pulse 125; bowels tender to the touch, with some pain; secretion more profuse, but not so tenacious. There is also a limited secretion of milk. Allowed beaf-tea and gum-water to drink, and gave neutral mixture and morphia. Ten o'clock P. M. Swelling about the neck much diminished. Patient has slept most of the afternoon. Introduced a silver canula, dressed the wound with simple cerate, and covered dressing with oil silk. Continue beef-tea and gum-water.

26*th*. Wound is granulating; swelling nearly gone; respiration 30; pulse 110; tongue furred. Ordered bowels to be opened with citrate magnesia.

30*th*. Patient had continued to improve up to last evening, at which time she was seized with a protracted paroxysm of coughing and an abundant bronchial secretion. Her pulse is now 125; respiration 32; skin hot and dry; countenance anxious and dejected; tongue furred and moist. Ordered sulph. quinia grs. ij, pulv. opii gr. j, every three hours till she is composed, when the opium is to be omitted, and the quinia continued with neutral mixture.

31*st*. Pulse 95, respiration 25. Patient asked for, and allowed chicken-tea. She is now for the first time troubled with food lodging in the glottis when swallowing; but this is obviated by placing the finger over the tube when swallowing. Seems quiet and composed. Expectoration difficult on account of air passing through the glottis, which renders that through the tube less expulsive. Her tongue being furred, ordered grs. v mass. hyd., to be followed in the morning with cit. mag. and the following mixture: Syr. senega and spts. nitr. dulc. āā ℥j; tartar emetic gr. ½. Mix. A teaspoonful of which to be taken once in four hours.

Patient continued to improve up to 21st of April, when the tube was expelled during a paroxysm of coughing. The wound was allowed to heal.

May 20. The only vestige of the disease that now remains is the cicatrix. She speaks distinctly in a low tone, but cannot elevate her voice to any extent.

ART. XV.—*The Structure of the Eye examined in Connection with the Undulatory Theory of Light.* By EDWIN C. LEEDOM, M. D., of Plymouth, Montgomery County, Pa.

"As the eye is made for light, so light must have been made, at least among other ends, for the eye."—WHEWELL.

WHEN the structure of the human ear is exposed to view, we perceive a complex but exquisite contrivance. In the middle ear a system of machinery presents itself which is remarkable, on account of the obviousness of its adaptation to the purpose of receiving vibrations from the air, and transmitting them to the auditory nerve.

The organ of hearing, as every anatomist knows, consists of three principal parts: the external ear, formed by the pinna, lobus, and external meatus; the middle ear, or tympanum; and the labyrinth. The tympanum is separated from the external meatus by membrana tympani, which is connected with the labyrinth by four small bones, the malleus, incus, os orbiculare, and stapes, which last closes the fenestra ovalis by a membranous investment. These little bones are so connected with the membrana tympani, that the latter cannot vibrate in the smallest degree without its vibrations being transmitted by them to the fluid which fills the labyrinth, and thence to the ramifications of the auditory nerve, which are distributed through the vestibule, semicircular canals, and particularly the cochlea. The air within the tympanum is kept in equilibrium with the external air by means of the Eustachian tube, whereby the membrana tympani can vibrate more freely. Also, there are two small muscles which are connected with the ossicles, and serve to increase or diminish the tension of the membrana tympani; by which contrivance feeble sounds are rendered more readily perceptible, and violent sounds are prevented from acting injuriously on the auditory nerve.

The membrana tympani and the machinery within the tympanum are so completely adapted to receive vibrations, and to transmit them to the labyrinth, that, were we unacquainted with the important fact that a bell will not ring in the exhausted receiver of an air-pump or Torricellian vacuum, the structure of this part of the ear alone would be sufficient to convince the philosophical inquirer that sound is produced by vibrations of the air. Knowing that vibrations of the air excite corresponding vibrations of the membrana tympani—which vibrations are transmitted, by a most appropriate contrivance, to the ramifications of the auditory nerve in the labyrinth—we are naturally led to inquire whether—if light be the effect of vibrations in a subtle and elastic fluid or ether which fills all space and pervades all bodies, as eminent modern philosophers assert—the mechanism of the eye is as completely adapted to this ether as that of the ear is to the air? whether there is in the eye any organism capable of having imparted to it just as many distinct kinds of vibrations as there are primary colours in the spectrum, and no more? and, also, whether there is a system of machinery adapted to transmit such vibrations to the expansion of the optic nerve? If a person, ignorant of the formation of the eye, but acquainted with the mechanical properties of the air and the anatomy and physiology of the ear, should be told that light is produced by vibrations of an ethereal fluid, and that vision is caused by such vibrations acting on the eye, as hearing is by the vibrations of the air acting on the ear; he would no doubt, when he came to study the structure of the eye, expect to find a contrivance similar to what he had observed in the ear. He would, most probably, expect to find a membranous partition capable of delicate vibrations, and also having connected with it an organism adapted to transmit its vibrations to the optic nerve. But he would seek in vain for any part, or combination of parts, analogous to that observable in the ear. I dare assert that the keenest anatomist has never yet been able to detect a vibrating instrument in the eye; whereas in the ear, a mechanism for receiving and transmitting vibrations is so obvious that it cannot be mistaken. Indeed, there could not be any contrivance better calculated to arrest and stifle vibrations, should they occur, than that which is observable in the interior of the eye. Look at the consistence of the crystalline humour, which "has been compared to gum half dissolved." The vitreous humour, although its peculiar consistence, resembling melted glass, is owing to its membrane, the tunica hyaloidea, is also worthy of observation. How can any one possibly imagine that the use of these two bodies is to transmit vibrations to the expansion of the optic nerve?

On the other hand, is not the eye formed exactly as it should be formed, if light be, what Sir Isaac Newton supposed it to be, a substance composed of material particles which are emitted in straight lines from every visible point of a luminous or of an illuminated body, and which are reciprocally repellent in the course of the rays, but susceptible of being attracted by ponderable matter?

Light passes freely through the transparent cornea and humours of the eye to the retina, upon which an image of every visible object is painted. But it requires a nice contrivance to form the images of objects on the retina. The crystalline lens is mainly instrumental in effecting this. This lens acts upon the light which passes through the pupil in such a manner that the rays, which proceed from every visible point of an object, are converged to a point upon the retina. But this could not be accomplished if the crystalline humour were all of one uniform density; for the two faces of the lens are sections of the surfaces of spheres of different sizes, and it is well known to opticians that a double convex lens with spherical surfaces will not converge all the rays accurately to one focus, but that those rays which pass through the lens near its circumference are brought together sooner than those which pass through it near its axis. Now, this spherical aberration is obviated most simply by the central part of the crystalline humour being more dense than the part near its circumference. By this increase of density in the central part of the lens, the rays which pass near the axis of the lens are attracted more forcibly towards the axis, so as to be brought to the same point on the retina as those rays which pass through the lens near its circumference.

Could there be anything more simple, anything more beautiful, than this contrivance to prevent the spherical aberration? Does it not prove to demonstration that light is material?

There is a peculiarity of vision, which sometimes occurs in persons whose eyes are sound and perfectly formed, which appears to me to be inexplicable by the undulatory theory of light: I allude to cases of blindness to particular colours. Sir David Brewster, in his *Optics*, gives an account of eight or ten different persons who were blind to red light, but who were able readily to distinguish the other colours of the spectrum.

It is universally admitted, by the advocates of the undulatory theory, that the red colour is produced by the longest and strongest vibrations. Indeed, it has been long known that red light has more penetrating power than light of any other colour, and that, when there is any mere mechanical obstruction to the passage of light, the red rays will overcome a resistance capable of arresting all the other rays. Every one has observed that the sun presents a red appearance when the atmosphere is filled with smoke and vapours; and Cheselden asserts that all persons who have ripe cataracts can, for the most part, in a strong light, distinguish white, black, and scarlet. (*Anatomy.*) As scarlet is the only one of the primary colours mentioned, we may conclude that it is the only one perceptible.

If the undulatory theory be true, those vibrations of the ether which produce light must pass without impediment through the transparent cornea, aqueous humour, crystalline lens, and vitreous humour, till they reach the retina, at which membrane they must be arrested, so that each vibration may make an impression upon it proportioned to its strength; so that a vibration $\frac{1}{59750}$ of an inch in length may produce the sensation of violet, and a vibration $\frac{1}{37640}$ of an inch long the sensation of red.

Now, it is clear that, if vision were caused by any such mechanical operation as this, it would be impossible for such eyes as those mentioned above to exist, for the strongest vibrations would always be the most readily perceptible. Who ever heard of an ear that was very sensitive to a low and feeble sound, such as the murmuring of a rivulet or the humming of a bee, but totally insensible to the sound of a trumpet, or any other loud and powerful sound?

If we adopt the corpuscular theory of light, and suppose that bodies exercise an assimilating power over the light which enters their substance, that their particles attract and detain some rays, and allow others either to pass freely through the bodies, or to escape from their pores by radiation, as I have endeavoured to prove in another place (*Silliman's Journal*, vol. i., second series), the above-mentioned peculiarity of vision will admit of an easy explanation. If, owing to peculiarity of formation, or some other cause, the humours of the eye should possess the power of absorbing and rendering latent the red rays, those rays only which are complementary to the red would reach the retina, and no red colour would be perceptible. (*See*, also, Bache's ed. *Brewster's Optics*, note ix. of Amer. ed.)

If, in every case of blindness to particular colours, red were the only colour perceptible, that would be a strong argument in favour of the undulatory theory; for then it might be supposed that a degree of cloudiness of the humours might arrest all the vibrations except the longest and strongest, or those which produce the red colour; or that, owing to a less degree of sensibility than usual in the retina, none but the strongest vibrations would make an impression on that membrane, and therefore no colour but red be perceived. But as, in the cases recorded, the persons having the above-mentioned peculiarity of vision were blind to red light, some other theory than that of undulations must be resorted to for an explanation.

If the vibrations of an ether produce light, as those of the air produce sound, light and sound must both be reflected from objects, in the same manner, and with the same degree of regularity. Now, why does not the sound, which is reflected from an object, convey to the mind an idea of form, size, and position? I wish to call particular attention to the following passages from Dr. Whewell's *Bridgewater Treatise on Astronomy and General Physics.*

"The impressions of sight, like those of hearing, differ in intensity and in kind. Brightness and colour are the principal differences among visible things, as loudness and pitch are among sounds. But there is a singular distinction between these senses in one respect: every object and part of an object seen, is necessarily and inevitably referred to some position in the space before us; and hence visible things have place, magnitude, form, as well as light, shade, and colour. There is nothing analogous to this in the sense of hearing: for though we can, in some approximate degree, guess the situation of the point from which a sound proceeds, this is a secondary process, and distinguishable from the perception of the sound itself; whereas we cannot conceive visible things without form and place.

"The law, according to which the sense of vision is thus affected, appears to be this. By the properties of light, the external scene produces, through the transparent parts of the eye, an image or picture exactly resembling the reality, upon the back part of the retina: and each point which we see is seen in the direction of a line passing from its image on the retina, through the focal centre of the eye. In this manner we perceive by the eye the situation of every point, at the same time that we perceive its existence; and by combining the situation of many points, we have forms and outlines of every sort."

If we imagine light to be composed of material particles, which are emitted in straight lines from every visible point of an object, it will be very easy to conceive how "the external scene produces, through the transparent parts of the eye, an image or picture exactly resembling the reality, upon the back part of the retina," particularly, when we see that the cornea and humours of the eye are completely adapted to act upon the rays of light, so as to cause those rays, which proceed from any visible point of an object, to converge to a point upon the retina. But how an image of any object can be formed upon the retina, by the vibrations of an ethereal medium, is not so apparent, especially to my understanding.

Further on, Dr. Whewell, after speaking of the advantage of the faculty of perceiving the form and position of an object, makes the following remark: "Yet, in order to imagine ourselves destitute of this faculty, we have only to suppose that the eye should receive its impressions as the ear does, and should apprehend red and green, bright and dark, without placing them side by side." Indeed, if the eye received its impressions from the vibrations of an ether, as the ear receives its impressions from the vibrations of the air, would we not be destitute of the faculty of placing "red and green, bright and dark," side by side?

The narrow limits within which those vibrations of the ether which are said to affect the eye with the sense of light and colour are confined, present, it appears to me, another insuperable objection to the undulatory theory. A new colour has latterly been added to the spectrum, the lavender, which makes the number of primary colours eight. The undulatory theory requires each colour to be produced by vibrations of one invariable length and degree of quickness. But the ether must be susceptible of many more than eight kinds of vibrations. How is it that no others, but those within the above-mentioned limits, make any impression on the eye? If the eye were adapted to vibrations, as the ear is known to be, it would still be impossible to conceive that stronger vibrations, than those which produce the red colour, should make no impression on the retina. But it has been shown that the eye is not adapted to vibrations of any kind; therefore there is the best reason possible to believe that the ether has no existence, but that light is a substance, as maintained by Sir David Brewster. "It is," says he, "by the light of the sun that the coloured juices of plants are elaborated, that the colours of bodies are changed, and that many chemical combinations and decompositions are effected. It is not easy to allow that such effects can be produced by the mere vibrations of an ethereal medium; and we are forced, by this class of facts, to reason as if light was material."

Sir David Brewster, by his experiments, has rendered it highly probable that there are three primary colours only in the spectrum, red, yellow, and blue. Now, since it appears that light is material, and since these three primary colours have never been decomposed, may we not conclude that the white light of the sun consists of three different kinds of matter, and that each makes its own distinct impression on the retina, just as sugar, salt, or an acid does upon the nerves of the tongue; or musk, cinnamon, or bergamot upon the olfactory nerves?

Thus, I have endeavoured to restore to credit the corpuscular doctrine of the great Newton. The attempt has been a bold one; for, the undulatory theory "derives such powerful support from an extensive class of phenomena, that it has been received by many of our most distinguished philosophers." (Brewster.)

REVIEWS.

ART. XVI.—*The Microscope and its Revelations.* By WILLIAM B. CARPENTER, M. D., F. R. S., &c. &c. With an Appendix, by Francis Gurney Smith, M. D., Professor of the Institutes of Medicine in the Medical Department of Pennsylvania College, &c. Illustrated by 434 Engravings on Wood. Philadelphia: Blanchard & Lea, 1856.

THIS last book, from the fruitful pen of Dr. Carpenter, is not exactly a popular work, and yet can hardly be considered as of a strictly scientific character. It is intended to guide the amateur in the use of the microscope, not so much as a means of purely anatomical and physiological investigation, but rather as an instrument for the examination of all objects, interesting to the student of nature, which are too minute to be thoroughly appreciated by the unaided eye. The microscope is no longer a popular or even a scientific plaything; it excites our interest at the present day, not simply because it gratifies a trifling curiosity by magnifying the apparent size of minute objects, but because it brings into view what was before invisible, and, by giving us distinct and reliable information as to the minute structure of natural objects, enlarges the domain of scientific investigation. Nearly every department of natural science has been benefited at some time or other, as Dr. Carpenter remarks, by the invention or perfection of instruments; for nearly all natural objects, to whatever class they may belong, are so rich in details of structure, in the magnitude or the minuteness of their parts, or in the delicacy of their phenomena, that their study cannot be exhausted by means of our unaided and comparatively imperfect senses. In this way, the perfected *balance* has enabled the chemist to determine questions of the first importance as to the ultimate constitution of compound substances, but of such nicety that their solution would have remained altogether impossible without the assistance of the instrument. The *torsion balance* and *galvanometer* in physics, the *goniometer* in mineralogy, the *chronometer* and the *compensating pendulum* have all been of similar service. On the other hand, our information with regard to the size, form, and structure of natural objects is obtained mostly through the eye; but the eye is an optical instrument, adapted, as all optical instruments must be, to objects of a certain size seen at a certain distance. There is a somewhat extensive range of variation, both of size and distance, to which the anatomical structure of the eye enables it to adapt itself; but there are limits to this variation, in both directions, beyond which the unassisted organ fails to be serviceable, and requires the aid of artificial contrivances. Accordingly, our knowledge has been extended, in these two different directions, by two different instruments, the telescope for bodies which are too distant, and the microscope for those which are too minute to be appreciated by ordinary vision. As every powerful and delicate instrument requires, moreover, a corresponding care and precision in its management, it is an advantage to have some treatise like the present devoted to the general description of objects suitable for microscopic examination, and the mode of procuring, preparing, and preserving them, as well as the construction of the instrument itself, and the rules to be observed in its use and application.

The author's Introduction is mostly occupied with a rapid review of the principal branches of botany, zoology, and physiology, which have been more particularly benefited by the increased facilities of observation afforded by the microscope. One remarkable fact in the history of the instrument and the sciences to which it has been useful is that nearly the whole of the progress which we have made in microscopic inquiry has been accomplished during the second quarter of the present century. Previous to the year 1800 the instrument was so imperfect that it was capable of accomplishing but little. The compound microscope, indeed, was almost valueless, owing to the serious and apparently insurmountable difficulties of spherical and chromatic aberration. Nearly all the truly valuable discoveries of the older microscopists had accordingly been made with the simple microscope, and the limited capacity of this form of the instrument being more or less completely exhausted, microscopic investigation seemed to be arrested by a natural barrier that offered but little prospect of ever opening a way to further prosecution of the science.

During the first quarter of the present century, therefore, little or no advance was made, observations with the imperfect and deceptive compound microscopes then in use being so uncertain in their results as to give rise to fanciful and discordant opinions instead of conveying positive information. About the year 1825, however, the successful application of achromatic correction to the microscope, previously regarded as impossible, at once commenced the perfection of the instrument, and enabled it to be safely used in the examination of an entirely different and minuter class of objects.

Since that time, higher and higher magnifying powers have been constantly made available by modifications in the original principle of correction, and improvements in the number and application of the accessories, means of illumination, mode of preparing objects, &c. &c., until it now seems to be the general opinion of microscopists that we have nearly reached another natural barrier, similar to that which was broken through in 1825, and that any further increase of the available magnifying powers of the instrument must be preceded by the application of some new principle of which we are now altogether ignorant. The position, however, which we occupy at present is very different from that in which microscopic observers found themselves at the beginning of the present century; for, while they had already exhausted, in great measure, the limited field of investigation in which the simple microscope could be used, the compound instrument, on the other hand, has introduced us into so vast and fruitful a territory that twenty-five years of observation have only begun to make us acquainted with its varied and abundant contents. Even if the microscope, therefore, should not be essentially improved for many years to come, it would still remain a most valuable assistant to the student of nature, and continue to give him ample employment in the examination of new objects.

In fact, it has required nearly all the practice which the application of the compound microscope has heretofore given us to learn thoroughly the proper use of the instrument and the true limit of its capacities. During the first years of its employment the objects which, if presented for study, were of so novel a character that the observations of microscopists were naturally somewhat confused and rambling. The appearances which it presented were not unfrequently interpreted in a different manner by different observers—a discrepancy which for a time threw an undeserved discredit upon the instrument itself as a reliable means of investigation. This, however, as Dr. Carpenter justly remarks, is a danger to which every kind of study is more or less liable.

"It is a tendency," he says (page 39), "common to *all* observers, and not by any means peculiar to microscopists, to describe what they *believe* and *infer*, rather than what they actually *witness*. The older microscopic observers were especially liable to fall into this error, since the want of definiteness in the images presented to their eyes left a great deal to be completed by the imagination. And when, as frequently happened, physiologists began with theorizing on the elementary structure of the body, and allowed themselves to twist their imperfect observations into accordance with their theories, it was not surprising that their accounts of what they professed to have seen should be extremely discordant. But from the moment that the visual image presented by a well constructed microscope gave almost as perfect an idea of the object as we could have obtained from the sight of the object itself, if enlarged to the same size and viewed with the unassisted eye, microscopic observations admitted of nearly the same certainty as observations of any other class; it being only in a comparatively small number of cases that a doubt can fairly remain about any question of *fact* as to which the microscope can be expected to inform us."

This tendency in microscopic observers, however, though very much diminished since the perfection of the instrument, has not even yet entirely disappeared. The only safe and simple rule of investigation, viz: to describe exactly *what we see*, nothing less and nothing more, has only been recently adopted to its full extent, and is still sometimes inadvertently transgressed. A striking instance of this is to be seen in the existing remnants of Schwann's "cell-theory" of the minute anatomy of animal bodies. Schleiden had shown that every part of the vegetable fabric consisted of *cells*, or of some form derived from them by direct transformation; and that the vegetable cell consisted of a closed membranous sac, the "cell-wall," containing a fluid or semifluid mass in its cavity, and bearing a nucleolated nucleus on its internal surface. Schwann, seeing many points of resemblance between these vegetable cells, and their modifications, in the minute anatomy of man and the higher animals, inferred that the elementary forms were essentially the same in the two kingdoms; and when the structural details of the vegetable cell could not be fully made out in the animal cell or fibre, they were nevertheless inferred to exist, and described as though they had actually been seen. Subsequently, microscopic observers, following Schwann's lead, felt themselves, in a certain sense, under an obligation to believe from analogy what was not demonstrated by observation; and the vestiges of this mistaken idea are still to be found in some books on microscopic anatomy. The red globules of the blood, for example, and the epithelium cells of vertebrate animals, are still sometimes described as constituted, like vegetable cells, by a closed membranous cell-wall, the cavity of which is filled with a fluid differing, according to circumstances, in colour, consistency, and composition; and yet a single careful examination of either of these objects cannot fail to convince the unprejudiced observer that no such distinction between cell-wall and contents is visible, but that the animal cell, in the higher classes, consists, so far as can be ascertained, merely of a *mass* of animal matter of the same consistency throughout; the nucleus, when present, being simply imbedded in its substance, without occupying or projecting into any distinct cavity.

Another source of error for anatomical and pathological microscopists, which it has required some years to dissipate, was an under-estimate of the *number* and *variety* of the minute forms which naturally occur in the animal body, and which require to be studied patiently and in detail before making any inferences with regard to their origin or relations. The natural elementary forms were, at first, supposed to be few in number, and their study easily mastered; and any variation from the assumed type was hastily regarded as an indication either of developmental or of morbid changes. Thus, when Schwann saw, mingled in the same tissue, globular cells, fusiform cells, and slender fibres, he at once pronounced the fusiform cells to be an intermediate form, indicating that the globular cells were converted into fibres by gradual elongation. We have only learned since that time that fusiform bodies are, themselves, independent anatomical elements as much as the globules and the fibres; and that the simultaneous occurrence of the three forms is no satisfactory proof of their mutual conversion.

A similarly unfounded idea, as it appears to us, has been long obstinately adhered to, with regard to the physiological connection between the red and white globules of the blood. It was imagined that the red globules of the blood, in the adult, were produced from the white, by the direct transformation of the latter; and minute accounts of this transforming process have been given, from time to time, detailing the mode in which the white globule gradually alters its shape, becomes smooth instead of granular, acquires a red colour, and loses its opacity; terminating sometimes with the naïve remark, that "the conversion, however, must take place very rapidly, as its intermediate stages have never been satisfactorily seen." It required, in fact, several years of observation for microscopists to arrive at the apparently simple idea that the white and red globules, though mingled in the blood, might be as distinct and independent anatomical elements, as the capillaries and nerve-tubes which are mingled in areolar tissue.

Dr. Carpenter alludes to another source of error, which is, again, not peculiar to microscopists, but common to all observers and experimenters, viz: a neglect of the precise conditions under which the experiment or observation is made. Physiologists have often experienced the confusion which arises from two experimenters reporting different results of what was regarded as the same experiment. In reality, however, these discordant results belonged to two different experiments; the exact correspondence in the surrounding conditions, so essential to every delicate investigation, not being sufficiently provided for to insure a correspondence in the resulting phenomena. In using the higher powers of the microscope, a similar care is necessary that different observers, when examining the same object, should place it under absolutely the same conditions of magnifying power, illumination, mounting, focussing, &c. Many of the minute anatomical elements undergo, also, modifications in form, colour, and consistency, by very slight alterations in the media by which they are surrounded; and, if these alterations are not properly guarded against, a discrepancy of observation will naturally be the result. A marked illustration of this is noticed by Dr. Carpenter at page 40.

"Thus, one observer," he says, "described the human blood-corpuscles as flattened disks resembling pieces of money, another as slightly concave on each surface, another as slightly convex, a fourth as highly convex, and a fifth as globular; and the former prevalence of the last opinion is marked by the habit, which still lingers in popular phraseology, of designating these bodies as 'blood-globules.' Yet all microscopists are now agreed that their real form, when examined in freshly drawn blood, is that of circular disks, with slightly concave surfaces; and the diversity in previous statements was simply due to the alteration effected in the shape of these disks by the action of water or other liquids added for the sake of dilution; the effect of this being to render their surfaces first flat, then slightly convex, then more highly convex, at last changing their form to that of perfect spheres."

The distortion and varicosity produced in the smaller nerve-fibres by the pressure of the glass cover, the progressive coagulation of the white substance of Schwann in the larger by contact with air or water, and the unnatural accumulation of the white globules of the blood in the vessels of the frog's foot while the animal is under confinement, are all instances of the manner in which a neglect of the exact conditions, under which a microscopic observation is made, may vitiate its results or produce a discrepancy between the accounts of two different observers. It is but a short time since we have seen, in a somewhat elaborate treatise, a distorted and shrivelled condition of the blood-globules, in certain animals subjected to experiment, attributed to the effect of a poisonous substance which had been introduced into the circulation; while it was evident that these appearances were simply owing to the varying quantity of water with which the blood was mingled, and the greater or less rapidity with which evaporation took place under the microscope.

But such difficulties, as already remarked, are incident to every branch of scientific study, and are not at all peculiar to microscopy.

Dr. Carpenter begins, in his first chapter, with a history of the microscope, its optical principles and mechanical construction; its various accessories, with the mode of using them to the best advantage; and an account of the most approved patterns of the instrument now in use. He gives some directions, in the fifth chapter, for the collection, preparation, and mounting of objects, and then passes in review the objects of interest for microscopic examination which may be obtained from the animal and vegetable kingdoms. In describing these, he does not treat the subject as a professed botanist or anatomist; but his object is rather to illustrate the powers of the instrument for increasing our stock of information in every scientific department, and to guide the amateur to a knowledge of its general educational uses. He has omitted, therefore, as not falling within the scope of his work, all notice of the application of the microscope to pathological investigations, the detection of adulterations in food, and other similar topics, since an account of these, to be at all valuable, would require a more extended description of anatomical details than would be either interesting or useful to the class of readers for which the book is intended.

The fourth chapter, on the "Management of the Microscope," is full of valuable and judicious observations. It treats of the quality and arrangement of the light for microscopic observation, the care of the instrument, the management of direct and oblique condensers, precautions for avoiding errors of observation, rules for the selection and application of lenses of different powers, &c. &c. The author recommends very highly what is too often neglected, viz: the frequent use of object-glasses of *low magnifying power.*

The microscopist should, in fact, always commence the examination of a new object by a low power. Or rather, he should commence by ordinary dissection with the unaided eye, adopting, as he may find them useful, the same accessories, such as condensers, mirrors, transparent slides, &c., that he would employ with the microscope. It is remarkable, how much this preliminary examination is sometimes neglected by microscopists. The microscope is too apt to be regarded as altogether superseding ordinary vision for anatomical purposes; and, as enabling us to see, not only everything which is visible by the unaided eye, but a great deal more beside. This, however, is a great mistake. If we recollect that the eye and the microscope are both optical instruments, and that each is confined to its own limited range of objects, we shall understand at once that while, with the microscope, we can see much that is invisible by the unaided eye, so with the eye we can see many things, no less important, which are entirely invisible by the microscope. Whenever we magnify any object, just in proportion as we increase its apparent size, we lose in three important particulars, as follows:—

First. The field of view is diminished in size; so that a smaller part of the entire surface can be examined at once.

Second. The quantity of light is lessened; so that the object, if viewed as transparent, must be compressed or torn apart in a corresponding degree; and,

Thirdly. The plane of distinct vision is diminished in thickness; so that, while one surface of the object is in focus and distinctly visible, the parts immediately above or below will be out of the focus and indistinct.

While a magnifying instrument, therefore, enables us to see the minute elements of any object, it at the same time, and in the same degree, prevents our seeing the manner in which these minute elements are arranged with regard to each other, and to the outlines of the object as a whole. Now, the same difference which exists between the unaided eye and the microscope, exists also between the different powers of the microscope itself. The objectives of low magnifying power show us a comparatively large field, brilliantly illuminated, and include in their focus a tolerably thick stratum of the object. They show us the laminated or reticulated texture of the substance under examination, the meshes of capillary networks, the frequency and direction of the ramifications of nervous twigs, &c. &c. But in order to use the higher powers of the instrument, and to make out the form, size, and aspect of the smallest anatomical elements, we must first tear up the substance into such minute fragments, or reduce it to such thin sections, that the natural relation between these ultimate forms is lost; and if we have neglected the previous use of the lower powers, the knowledge we can gain from our examination will be exceedingly imperfect and unsatisfactory,

Take, for example, the anatomical examination of *bone.* With the naked eye we get not only the form and size of the entire bone, but the mutual relations of the compact and cancellated structures, the form and size of the medullary canal, and the situation of the medulla. With the help of the lower objectives, we then examine longitudinal and transverse sections of moderate thickness, and ascertain the size, direction, and inosculation of the Haversian canals, and the arrangement of the delicate spicules and lamellæ of the cancellated structure. With higher powers and thinner sections, we get the concentric laminæ of the bone-corpuscles or lacunæ, encircling the vessels of the Haversian canals, and the lines of separation between adjacent Haversian systems, and make out the fat-vesicles, bloodvessels, and nervous filaments of the medullary tissue. While, finally, with the highest powers, we can see only the forms and cavities of the lacunæ, with the hollow, branching, and inosculating canaliculi.

Suppose we are to examine a swollen and unhealthy-looking piece of human skin. If we at once tear it into shreds and subject it to examination with the highest powers of the instrument, we may see only a confused mixture of fibrous tissue, oily granules, and epithelium-like cells. But, if we have previously examined it with the lower powers, undisturbed by too much compression and laceration, we may have already recognized the anatomical characters of its hypertrophied sebaceous follicles; and can then interpret, in an intelligent manner, the appearances which are exhibited by the higher magnifying powers.

Dr. Carpenter makes a very convenient division of microscopic objectives three different sets, viz: those of *low*, *medium*, and *high* power. The *low* objectives are those whose focal length ranges from two inches to half an inch; the *medium* are those whose focal length ranges from one-half to one-fifth of an inch; while all those whose focal length is less than one-fifth of an inch are classed as *high* objectives. The author shows that these different sets of microscopic powers are not only applicable to different classes of objects, but require different kinds of illumination, different management of the accessories, and different preparation of the objects. All his remarks on this point, from page 192 to page 199 are exceedingly suggestive, and cannot fail to be of assistance to those who wish to use the microscope in an intelligent manner, and to obtain from it all the information which it is capable of affording.

The author speaks very fully of the importance and proper management of the *adjuster*, as part of the microscopic apparatus. Both the coarse and fine adjuster should be so arranged as to work freely, smoothly, and equably, without any "loss of time" or "backward spring," and particularly without any such disturbance of the centring of the microscope as will produce an apparent twisting or lateral sliding movement of the field of view. The necessity of a constant and proper management of the adjuster, and the amount of information to be derived from it, are fully insisted on. The adjuster, in fact, is the next most important part, in a microscope, to the objective. Its constant up and down movement enables the observer to bring into view, in succession, different *strata* of his object and to ascertain the natural connection between them. If the adjuster, therefore, be correctly employed, in connection with a proper attention to that change in the apparent outline of the object under different focuses, which may be called "microscopic perspective," it will give us much more information as to the structure of the object under examination than could possibly be derived from a single view or even from any number of separate single views. By this manipulation the microscopist examines, successively and in connection, every part of the exterior and interior of his object; and may, in fact, be said to *dissect* it by the microscope as thoroughly as though he had employed for that purpose the knife, scissors, and forceps.

It is with the higher microscopic powers that this use of the fine adjuster becomes more indispensable.

"A minute alteration of the focus," says Dr. Carpenter (page 164), "often causes so entirely different a set of appearances to be presented that, if this alteration be made abruptly, their relation to the preceding can scarcely be even guessed at; and the gradual transition from the one to the other, which the fine adjustment alone affords, is therefore, necessary to the correct interpretation of either. To take a very simple case: the transparent body of a certain animal being traversed by vessels lying in different planes, one set of these vessels is brought into view by one adjustment, another set by "focussing" to a different plane; and the connection of the two sets of vessels, which may be the point of most importance in the whole anatomy of the animal, may be entirely overlooked for want of a fine adjustment, the graduated action of which shall enable one to be traced continuously into the other. What is true even of low and medium powers, is of course true to a still greater degree of high powers; for, although the 'coarse movement' *may* enable the observer to bring any stratum of the object into accurate focus, it is impossible for him by its means to secure that *transitional* 'focussing,' which is often so much more instructive than an exact adjustment at any one point. A clearer idea of the nature of a doubtful structure is, in fact, often derived from what is caught sight of *in the act* of changing the focus, than by the most attentive study and comparison of the different views obtained by any number of separate 'focussings.' The experienced microscopist, therefore, when examining an object of almost any description, constantly keeps his finger upon the milled head of the 'fine movement,' and watches the effect produced by its revolution upon every feature which he distinguishes, never leaving off until he be satisfied that he has scrutinized not only the entire *surface*, but the entire *thickness* of the object."

In speaking of the rules which are to guide the amateur in the examination and selection of microscopes, the author enumerates pretty fully the different qualities which are essential to a good object-glass. The first of these is *definition* or *defining power*; that is, the power of presenting objects with a perfectly clear and well-defined outline. This is justly considered as the most essential quality of an object-glass, and of course as far more important than the mere extent of its magnifying power. For the only test of the true value of an instrument is not "how much does it magnify?" but "how much will it enable us to see?" and an objective of low power, but good definition, may be very serviceable in this respect; while another, though it very much increases the apparent size of an object, may yet give the outlines of its component parts so indistinctly, from imperfect defining power, that we may really not be able to learn so much from it as from the first. The excellence of the defining power of an object-glass depends upon the completeness of its correction for spherical and chromatic aberration; and it is to be judged of by the performance of the microscope with such objects as compound hairs, markings on the scales of Podura plumbea, Lepisma saccharina, &c. &c.

The next most essential quality is *penetrating power*; that is, the quality which enables us to see, with tolerable distinctness, those parts of an object which are a little out of focus; and to look, therefore, to some extent *into* and *through* its substance. This quality may be best judged of by the performance of the instrument with such objects as muscular fibre, injected preparations, &c.

The third quality in order is *resolving power*, the power by which closely approximated markings and ridges are separated from each other, or by which apparently continuous lines of demarcation are "resolved" into series of separate dots or depressions. The resolving power, in an object-glass, depends almost exclusively upon the extent of its angular aperture, since such markings and depressions as those which serve for its tests are to be seen, when minute and closely set, only by very oblique illumination; and the greater the angular aperture of an object-glass the greater, of course, is the degree of obliquity at which the light can be made to enter it through the object under examination.

Now, it happens that, of late years, it has been rather the fashion for microscopists to estimate the excellence of an instrument almost exclusively by the extent to which it possesses this "resolving power." Instruments of larger and larger angular aperture have been constantly manufactured, and a set of test-objects, covered with closely set eminences and depressions, chiefly the silicious coverings of minute *Diatomaceæ*, almost universally adopted as the means of estimating the comparative value of different microscopes. It is still no uncommon sight to see half a dozen microscopists sitting round a table, each with his favourite instrument before him, like a cock-fighter with his chicken, trying their respective powers on the lines and dots of some "Navicula" or "Pleurosigma," and awarding the palm of excellence to that which resolves the most difficult object.

This, however, as Dr. C. justly remarks, is a serious mistake. The "resolving power," to which this undue value is attached, is dependent, as already mentioned, almost entirely upon the extent of angular aperture, and has but little to do with a perfect chromatic and spherical correction. Moreover, it is really the least valuable of all the three qualities enumerated above. It is only adapted for showing superficial inequalities by oblique illumination, whereas the delicate intersecting lines in the substance of an object, which really do most towards showing its texture, particularly in the minute anatomy of animal bodies, are dependent much more for their exhibition on the powers of definition and penetration. The wide angular aperture, too, which is necessary for a strong resolving power, is unfavourable to definition and positively injurious to penetration. These points are presented by Dr. Carpenter in a very clear and forcible manner.

"The superiority in resolving power," he says (page 191), "possessed by object-glasses of large angular aperture, is obtained at the expense of other advantages. For, even granting that there is no sacrifice of that most important element, *defining power* (which can only be secured with a very wide angle, by the utmost perfection in all the corrections), yet the adequate performance of such a lens can only be secured by the greatest exactness in the adjustments. Only that portion of the object which is *precisely* in focus can be seen with an approach to distinctness, everything which is in the least degree out of it being imbedded (so to speak) in a thick fog; it is requisite, too, that the adjustment for the thickness of the glass that covers the object should exactly neutralize the effect of its refraction; and the arrangement of the mirror and condenser must be such as to give to the object the best possible illumination. If there be any failure in these conditions, the performance of a lens of very wide angular aperture is *very much inferior* to that of a lens of moderate aperture; and, except in very experienced hands, this is likely to be generally the case."

It should not be forgotten that, to the medical man at least, the microscope is an instrument for acquiring information, and not merely a scientific toy to play tricks with. The instrument he is to use, therefore, should be selected for those qualities which will aid him most in his anatomical, physiological, and pathological studies. Every other object is comparatively trifling and valueless. It is by forgetting these facts, and by allowing ourselves to think more of the instrument than of what we are to see with it, that we sometimes lose sight of our real objects of study as anatomists and physiologists, and come to resemble those *microscope fanciers* who are so justly hit off by Dr. Carpenter in the following passage:—

"It does not seem to me an unapt simile," he says (page 192), "to compare the devotees of large angular apertures to the gentlemen of the 'turf.' It is, I believe, generally admitted that the breeding of a class of horses distinguished by speed and 'blood,' which is kept up by the devotion of a certain class of our countrymen to the noble sport of racing, is an advantage to almost every breed of horses throughout the country; tending, as it does, to develop and maintain a high standard in those particulars. But no one would ever think of using a race-horse for a roadster or a carriage-horse; knowing well that the very qualities which most distinguish him as a racer are incompatible with his suitableness for ordinary work. And so I think that the 'breeders' of first class microscopes (if I may so designate them) are doing great service by showing to what a pitch of perfection certain kinds of excellence may be carried, and by thus improving the standard of ordinary instruments; notwithstanding that, for nearly all working purposes, the latter may be practically superior."

There is, also, a very useful section on the "errors of interpretation" to which microscopic observers are liable; such as the appearance of a faint colourless or slightly iridescent band about the edges of a transparent object, the "inflection" or "diffraction-band;" the appearances, caused by a highly refractive power in the object itself, combined with a globular or cylindrical shape, as in the case of oil-drops or the shaft of the human hair. In the case of the mixture of two fluids, of different refractive powers, the globules of the one which is in smaller quantity will always appear as minute lenses, the reason of which is easily understood, and the appearance itself partially interpreted with readiness by almost any observer. There is, however, a very simple rule suggested by Dr. Carpenter, for deciding whether the globules belong to the more or the less highly refractive fluid, which would not so readily occur to every one. If we have, for example, two mixtures, one composed of oil-globules in water, the other of drops of water in oil, the globules will present very nearly the same appearances in each case, viz: circles with a dark border and a bright centre. But the two can be distinguished by raising and lowering the objective. For if the drops are oil, they will become brighter as the objective is raised; since, being more highly refractive than the water, they act as convex lenses, and concentrate the light *above* the ordinary focus of the instrument; while if the globules be water they will become darker when the objective is raised, and brighter when it is lowered; since, having less refractive power than the oil, and acting, therefore, as double concave lenses, they cause the transmitted light to diverge from a focus *below* the plane of the fluid.

There is another common source of error of interpretation which is not distinctly alluded to by Dr. Carpenter, and which is not, in fact, of a strictly optical character, but which is more or less common to all anatomical investigations, viz: the alterations produced in the appearance of any object by the mode of its preparation, or the way in which it is mounted for preservation. This has been seen in the erroneous interpretation, and consequent erroneous nomenclature of some of the elements of bony tissue. When Purkinje first saw the black and opaque "bone-corpuscles," with their radiating filaments, he took them to be solid calcareous masses deposited in the soft animal substance of the intervening spaces. Subsequent examination, however, showed microscopists that these spider-shaped bodies and filaments were, in reality, cavities and hollow tubes, excavated in the solid, calcareous, and highly refracting bone-substance; their opacity resulting from their being filled with air, which was but slightly refractive in comparison with the calcareous substance, and from their acting, in consequence, like strong, double concave lenses. So the name given them by Purkinje was abandoned, and that of "lacunæ" and "canaliculi" adopted instead. But the anatomists still forgot that they were examining a dried section of bone, from which the soft animal substances had been removed by maceration and decay; and that, though the lacunæ and canaliculi were hollow and empty in such a dried section, they were, in the recent specimen, filled with an animal substance, forming bodies of the same shape and size; these bodies filling the cavities of the lacunæ and canaliculi during life, as the brain fills the cavity of the cranium. So we have again returned partially to the old name of "bone-corpuscles," or "osteo-plastes," according to the French anatomists.

A similar error is sometimes made in the use of vascular injections. For when the coloured fluid is forced into the vessels by long and steady pressure, the smaller arteries, veins, and capillaries, may be often so completely gorged with the injection as to crowd upon the intervening tissues, and to present an unnatural appearance of complete and uniform distention; whereas, during life, the different parts of the vascular system are almost always unequally filled—the tide of the circulation ebbing and flowing from one part to another, but hardly ever distending all the vessels of even the same part at the same time.

The "Brunonian" or "molecular" movement is also noticed by Dr. Carpenter under the above head. He describes its general characters and the conditions under which it is liable to appear. He does not attempt to explain its cause further than by hazarding the somewhat vague and unsatisfactory surmises that it may be owing either "directly to some calorical changes continually taking place in the fluid," or to "some obscure chemical action between the solid particles and the fluid, which is indirectly promoted by heat." We strongly suspect that the above phrases do not represent any idea. The molecular movement, however, is certainly not owing to evaporation, as has been suspected, since it will take place "with its usual activity," in a drop of watery fluid completely surrounded by oil; and has even been known to "continue for many years in a small quantity of fluid inclosed between two glasses in an air-tight case." The author recommends beginners to study the appearance of this movement in mixtures of different densities, and with different kinds of powdered substances, so that they may not be misled by it in the course of their ordinary investigations.

The body of the work is devoted to a description of the most interesting microscopic appearances to be found in the vegetable and animal kingdoms. The author commences with the "protophytes," or plants of the humblest rank, and treats in succession of the minute structure of algæ, lichens, fungi, and other cryptogamia, monocotyledonous and dicotyledonous phanerogamia, protozoa, animalcules, zoophytes, molluscs, annulosa, crustacea, insects, and arachnida, and, finally, of vertebrate animals. These portions of the work require no comment, except that they illustrate, in a remarkable manner, the extensive erudition of the author and his unusual industry, both as a student and a writer. He finishes with a very interesting chapter on the "applications of the microscope to geological investigation," followed by a short notice of the most interesting microscopic objects derived from the inorganic world. The Appendix, by the American editor, Dr. Smith, is chiefly occupied with the consideration of the microscope as a means of diagnosis, the natural and morbid appearances of the solids and fluids of the human body, urinary deposits, &c. &c., subjects which are sufficiently extensive to require a separate treatise by themselves. The work cannot fail to be a valuable one for the student of nature, both as a book of reference and as a guide to independent investigation.

J. C. D.

ART. XVII.—*Memoir on the Cholera at Oxford, in the year* 1854, *with considerations suggested by the Epidemic.* By HENRY WENTWORTH ACLAND, M. D., F. R S., F. R. G. S., etc., Fellow of the Royal College of Physicians, Physician to the Radcliffe Infirmary, Radcliffe Librarian, and Lee's Reader in Anatomy in the University of Oxford. 4to. pp. 172. London, 1856.

THE memoir of Dr. Acland presents a most able and interesting report on the cholera as it prevailed in Oxford, England, during the summer and autumn—from the beginning of August to the close of October—of 1854.

Everything calculated to throw light upon the etiology of the disease, is carefully recorded, and its history, from the appearance of the first cases to its decline and final disappearance, accurately detailed. Able and interesting, however, as the report before us unquestionably is, it tells us but the same story, with but little variation, we have learned from every preceding report of the epidemic wherever it has occurred. That it breaks out in the midst of a community, attains, more or less quickly, its acme, then rapidly declines, and ultimately disappears, without any one being able to identify the source from whence the disease originated, or the reason why that, for a certain season, the larger portion of a community should experience, to a greater or less extent, a special morbific influence, and then, without any appreciable cause, become entirely exempt from it. It is true, that every reliable history of the disease that reaches us records the fact that, under all those circumstances and conditions which, ordinarily, deteriorate the health of man, and while they give origin to various endemic maladies, invite the prevalence and augment the virulence of epidemics, the cholera prevails to the greatest extent and in its most malignant form. That these circumstances and conditions are incapable by themselves of generating the disease is, however, as satisfactorily proved as is their influence in increasing its prevalence and mortality.

The entire number of cases of cholera that occurred at Oxford, in 1854, was 194, of which 115 terminated fatally. The population of the town being 26,474, the cases per 1,000 were 7.33 and the deaths 4.34

Of the 194 cases, 108 were in females, and only 86 in males, of all ages. As the population of Oxford was composed of 13,197 males, and 13,277 females, consequently 6.52 in each 1,000 of the males, and 8.13 in each 1,000 of the females were attacked—and inasmuch as of the 115 deaths, 49 were males, and 66 females, it follows that the males died in the proportion of 56.9 to 43.1 recoveries, and the females in the proportion of 61.1 to 38.9 recoveries. There was, therefore, a greater tendency in females to be attacked by the cholera, and of those attacked, there was a greater chance of recovery than in the male sex.

We learn that in London, during the same epidemic, of 100 persons attacked between the ages of 15 and 25, 34.9 died. In Oxford, the mortality between the same ages, was at the rate of 42.85. In London, the mortality in those between 25 and 35, was 35.4 per cent.; in Oxford, 50 per cent. In London, the deaths in proportion to the cases, in those between 65 and 75 years, were 58.2 per cent.; in Oxford, in the proportion of 77.77 per cent.

Persons in easy circumstances suffered during the epidemic in Oxford the least; it was among the labouring, chiefly, that its ravages were experienced; of these fifty-six in each hundred attacked died. One medical man died—he had neglected serious diarrhœa, under which he had laboured for nearly a week. He was not engaged in attendance on cholera patients; another who had attended patients affected with cholera had severe and protracted choleraic diarrhœa, from which he recovered. Several other medical men suffered from diarrhœa. The nurses were tolerably exempt, only one died. The washerwomen did not suffer as a class. Dr. Acland remarks, that during the ninety days which may be said to have been the period of the epidemic, five men were engaged in emptying cesspools, during nearly forty nights. Not one of them had even diarrhœa. This last circumstance has been noted in other places, and suggests a very important question concerning the noxious or innoxious nature of collections of ordure, when freely exposed to the open air.

"However urgent the other symptoms, no case," it is stated, "was, as the author believes, returned as cholera in which the evacuations were bilious. Of the more serious forms of diarrhœa, wherein cramps, vomiting, and even more or less collapse would occur, there were many cases in the city. But the mortality was very small compared to that of the cholera. It appeared *generally* in the same localities, at the same times, and with nearly the same intensity at the different periods, as the genuine cholera."

"If we examine," says Dr. Acland, "what is certainly known of the amount of diarrhœa, we have some curious information. Dividing the epidemic into four periods of three weeks each, commencing with August 6, and ending October 22, it appears that we have no certain record concerning the first five weeks, or until the last week of the second quarter. In that week there were returned 1,313 cases of diarrhœa: in the third quarter 2,603 cases; in the last quarter 527. These cases, it will be remembered, do not include choleraic diarrhœa—nor do they include cases prescribed for at the infirmary. Now, in the sixth week there were, out of every 1,000 persons, nearly 50 persons prescribed for on account of diarrhœa alone, by the medical men, independently of the chemists: in the third quarter (the seventh, eighth, and ninth weeks), nearly 100 in every 1,000: in the last quarter, 19.90 in every 1,000. If then we assume that, in the second quarter, the attacked were the same as in the third—as they were nearly with respect to cholera, and there is reason to believe that there were actually a greater number of diarrhœa cases in that quarter—and that the first quarter had as many cases as the last, then it follows that, at the least, 6,260 cases were attended by the regular practitioners on account of diarrhœa alone. Some of the cases were perhaps relapses; but as I have stated, the applicants at the infirmary—more than 400—are not included. There cannot have been, therefore, less than a fourth of the population, at the lowest estimate, actually treated by the medical men for this form alone in the manifestation of the pestilence. That very many more were under its influence may with equal certainty be concluded."

"With respect to the severer forms of diarrhœa returned as choleraic diarrhœa, 123 cases are entered in the first table. The deaths among these 123 were 14—or the proportion of 11.5 deaths to 100 cases. But it is known that many more occurred whose names and addresses were not returned, and which therefore I could not tabulate in respect to their residences, etc. The numbers returned to the Board in the second quarter of the disease were 165: in the third quarter, 61 cases." "Taking the reported cases in the two middle quarters as 226, and the deaths 14, we find the deaths in choleraic diarrhœa to have been only 6.2 in every 100 cases."

Dr. Acland presents a general result of the choleraic visitations of Oxford during the years 1832, 1849, and 1854.

The first interval of freedom from the pestilence was seventeen years; the second interval was five.

The cases per 1000 of the inhabitants in 1832 were, in round numbers, 8; in 1849 only 5; in 1854, 7. If we exclude from each year the cases in St. Clements, whereon the disease fell so heavily in 1832, the years of pestilence claim, in the order of their precedence, 5.4, 5.8, 7.2 cases per thousand of the inhabitants. The recoveries in proportion to the deaths were in the proportion of 51.63 deaths to 48.37 recoveries in 1832; 52.08 to 47.92 in 1849; 59.27 to 40.73 in 1854. The disease, therefore, excluding the exceptional cases of St. Clements, was more severe, numerically, and more fatal in the last than in either of the previous epidemics, and returned, as has been noted, after a much shorter interval.

In reference to the spread of the cholera at Oxford, during the year 1854; in the first three weeks but 3 cases occurred; in the succeeding three weeks, 83; in the next three weeks, 91; in the following three weeks, 16; in the thirteenth and last week, *one* case. It may be said, therefore, that the first and the last quarters of the epidemic epoch were occupied by the onset and the decline of the disease respectively, while the two intervening quarters showed it at its maximum. Or, if we look at the ascent of the disease up to the end of the sixth week, or the middle of the epidemic, we shall find that there were 12 cases in the first week of the second quarter, 35 in the second, and 36 in the third.

"The epidemic did not decline from this central point at the same rate as it increased, for the seventh week had 35 cases, and there were 37 in the ninth; but then, in the tenth week, the new cases fell to 11, nearly the same number as occurred in the fourth week. There were only 5 new cases in the eleventh, none in the twelfth, and one in the last." "If we inquire into what was the mortality in proportion to the cases in each of the quarters, the following may be noted. In the first quarter, of the *three* cases *two* were fatal; of the 83 cases in the second quarter 48 died, or 57.8 per cent. In the third quarter, out of 91 cases, 52 died, or 57.1 per cent.; and in the last quarter, of the 16 cases, 12 died, or 75 per cent.; and the only case which occurred in the last week died—from which it would appear that, after the first three cases, of which two were fatal, in the first quarter, the *number of cases* increased greatly in the second quarter, slightly in the third, and greatly diminished in the last; the *mortality* in the third quarter was rather less than in the second, viz: 57.1 and 57.8 respectively; and the *proportional* fatality of the disease materially increased in the last quarter. Again, referring to the *weeks*, it seems proper to notice that in the seventh week the deaths were in the proportion of 65.7 per cent., but in the eighth and ninth 57.9 and 48.7 per cent. respectively of the persons attacked. In the small numbers with which we are dealing, much stress must not be laid on such statistics, and yet they are noticeable."

In regard to the local causes which may have influenced the progress of the cholera in Oxford, Dr. Acland remarks that the disease, as well as diarrhœa, was most rife among the poor and destitute of the city; in some alleys, when meat was distributed to the inhabitants, the diarrhœa was arrested.

The city of Oxford may be divided into an upper and lower level, one portion of it being 16.47 feet above the average water level, and another twenty feet below the summit. If the cases which occurred in the three epidemics collectively, including St. Clements, be reckoned, it is found that 141 cases occurred in the upper level, and 362 in the lower. Estimating the population in the upper level at 14,200, and that in the lower at 12,300, it will be found also that, on the average of the three epidemics, there occurred 33.09 cases in each 10,000 of the people in the upper level, and 98 per 10,000 in the lower. Estimating the deaths at 54.30 per cent., on the average of the three epidemics, the deaths were at the rate of 17.97 per each 10,000 in the upper level, and 53.26 per each 10,000 in the lower level.

The parishes of Oxford, which—if we except, perhaps, certain limited blocks of houses—are the densest, were also the most severely visited by the disease. This, however, Dr. A. remarks, cannot be attributed to the density alone, but to other causes also. In London, it was noticed that the densest parts of the population were not the most severely attacked; on the contrary, the mortality was far higher in some of the more open than in the denser districts.

In his description of the topography of Oxford, Dr. A. points out the fact that the lowest and poorest parts of the city are also those which are the least well drained; and Mr. Ormerod's sanitary map of Oxford points out most strikingly the way in which the epidemic and contagious diseases are collected round special centres, which, as is shown by a map accompanying the memoir before us, are in the neighbourhoods where the drainage is deficient. But it is not, as Dr. A. remarks, imperfect drainage alone which is the cause of ill health, though unquestionably a fundamental cause. "Where the drainage is bad the basements are damp and foul. In old towns, the ground is in some places saturated with liquid ordure to an amount scarcely to be estimated, and the wells are more or less impure;" "and in districts where the water is impure the diseases above referred to are the most rife." The notable instance of St. Clements may be instanced. In 1832 there were, out of 174 cases of cholera in all Oxford, in that parish alone 74 cases, and in 1849 only three. During the former epidemic the inhabitants had filthy water from a sewer-receiving stream, and in 1849 from the springs of Headington, conveyed thither soon after 1832. In 1854, out of 194 cases, but 18 occurred in St. Clements—a proportional increase which would tend to show, what indeed we have various other evidence of, that the water supply, though it may be one mode, is not the only one of conveying the cholera poison.

In 1854 the influence of the epidemic, as in former years, was not experienced by the inmates of the city prison, while among those of the county jail, in its immediate vicinity, choleraic diarrhoea and cholera made their appearance. Upon inquiry, it was found that the supply of water for the prison was derived from a pool filled with putrid and putrefying matter. The pipes through which the water was conveyed were immediately cut off. Previously there had occurred twenty cases of choleraic diarrhoea and *five* of cholera, *four* of which proved fatal. From the day after that on which the supply of impure water was cut off, only three cases of choleraic diarrhoea and *one* of cholera—none of which were fatal—were reported during the remaining three weeks of the epidemic.

In the city of Oxford the water of many of the wells was deficient in quantity and bad in quality, especially in some of the affected yards, while the water supplied by the waterworks was from the river, which was loaded with impurities.

From the meteorological tables given by Dr. A., it appears that in all the years of cholera the mean pressure of the atmosphere at Oxford was greater than the normal pressure. The year 1832 was distinguished by great regularity of temperature. Only one month, October, was abnormal, and that very slightly. In 1848 the months of February and April were abnormal, the former in excess, the latter in defect, as three to one and four to one respectively—that is to say, such differences are likely to occur every third and fourth year. The year 1854 presented greater irregularities. Six out of the twelve months were slightly abnormal; the low temperature of June and the high temperature of September are chiefly noticeable, the former in the proportion of five to one, the latter of six to one. The mean temperatures of all three years were normal.

In the year 1854 the deficiency of humidity, and the excess in the weight of the air are noticeable. There was great comparative steadiness of temperature in 1832, and the contrary in 1854. In 1832, in three months only was the range *greater* than the normal range—whereas in 1854 there were only three when it was *less*. The greatest excess was in September, 1854, which was abnormal in the proportion of 35 to 1. The same month in 1832 was also abnormal, but only in the proportion of $4\frac{1}{2}$ to 1. The range of the year was in both cases abnormal, in 1832 the proportion being as $3\frac{1}{4}$ to 1, in 1854 as 25 to 1.

In the neighbourhood of London there was, in 1832, a deficiency of 7 inches rain; in Oxford, there was an excess of $\frac{3}{4}$ of an inch. In 1849, the deficiency near London was $\frac{6}{10}$ths of an inch; in Oxford it was 2.14 inches. In 1854 the annual deficiency about London was 5.93 inches; in Oxford 9.57 inches.

In respect to the prevailing winds; during the severest period of the epidemic of 1832, the wind had a decided bias towards the N.W. The same was also perceptible in a still greater degree in 1854, but not so in 1849. The mean annual direction in 1832 and 1849 agrees nearly with the normal direction. In 1854, however, the annual deviation is as much as 39° towards the

N. In each of the three years there was a deficiency of S. wind, and in 1832 and 1849 a deficiency also of W., but in 1854 there was the large excess of 4.37 in favour of W. In December of that year there was no E. wind.

The subjoined table presents the principal results of the meteorological observations:—

	Atmosph. pressure.	Mean temperat.	Range of temperat.	Amount of rain.	Direction of wind.	Force of wind.	Days of hail.	Thund. and lightning.	Aurora borealis.
1832	Abn. +	Norm. +	Abn. —	Norm. +	Norm.	?	Abn. —	Abn. —	Abn. —
1849	Abn. +	Norm. +	?	Norm. —	Norm.	?	Abn. +	Norm.	Norm.
1854	Abn. +	Norm. +	Abn. +	Abnor.—	Abn.	Abn. —	Abn. +	Abn. +	Abn. +

"On comparing the details of this table," says Dr. A., "the reader will not fail to remark how few similar features the three years present. In fact, the abnormal excess of atmospheric pressure and the normal excess of mean temperature, are the only conditions common to them all. The years 1832 and 1854 are both very abnormal, but in every other respect except those just mentioned, in *opposite directions*. Hence, we might be led to infer, that meteorological excesses in either direction are equally favourable to the development of the disease. But then how are we to account for its appearance in 1849, which, viewed altogether, is by no means an abnormal year? There is, however, one point which the table brings out very strongly, that is, the extraordinary character of 1854. Except in the solitary condition of mean temperature, everything is abnormal. Excessive in atmospheric pressure, and daily variations of temperature, deficient in rain and wind, abnormal in the direction of wind, excessive in the display of electrical phenomena—as if to complete a meteorological paradox, this same year, remarkable for the abundance of harvest, was not less remarkable for pestilence and its consequent mortality."

Dr. A., in remarking on the relations between the atmosphere and the disease, observes:—

"The reader, on looking at the diagram placed at the end of the volume, will notice that in Oxford there were three distinct periods of increase in the number of cholera cases. The first from September 5, to September 13; the second from September 13, to September 28; and the third from September 28, to October 8. The diarrhœa recorded, followed nearly the same rule, as did also the choleraic diarrhœa. It would needlessly detain the reader to enumerate, in words, the numbers which he can see more graphically presented in the diagram; but, his attention should be directed to some coincident phenomena expressed by the sheet before him. 1st, It is truly interesting to see the way in which the general curves of the diarrhœa, choleraic diarrhœa, and cholera followed each other—suggesting, as far as one locality may suggest a theory, that there is some common agent concerned, more or less, in producing all three forms of disease. He should especially notice, for instance, how on September 18, when there was a great rise in the diarrhœa cases, viz: from 178 new cases to 226, this rise was coincident with the highest number of cholera cases in the second group, and with all but the highest of the choleraic diarrhœa—though this is not *always* the case. On the 22d, the diarrhœa cases fell when the cholera rose, but *the choleraic diarrhœa* was that day at its maximum. It seems as though the cause, whatever it be, which produced diarrhœa and choleraic diarrhœa, acted on that day rather with intensity on individuals, than extensively on the population. Again, the diarrhœa fell from 118 new cases, reported on the 27th, to 68 on the 28th; on this last day there was *no* new case of cholera. The diarrhœa rose again to 115 new cases on the 2d of October, and the cholera cases rose again to 9 new cases."

"Between the 27th of August and the 16th of October, which may be called the limits of the mass of the disease, excluding a few outlying cases at the beginning and the end, there were, as has just been said, three periods of increase, and of course two intervening periods of diminution. Exactly the same thing happened with the *ozone*, and at the same period—with this difference only, that whereas the greatest amount indicated by the ozonometer in the first period coincided with the worst cholera day; in the two subsequent periods the maximum of ozone followed the maximum of cholera. Of these facts, assuming a connection between them, there may be two explanations, either that the rise of the ozone caused the rise of the cholera—the first group—or that the rise of the ozone preceded or caused the subsequent period of cholera disease. This last view is scarcely applicable to the second and third group, for, as I have said, the maximum of ozone appeared while the cholera was on the decrease. It need hardly be said that one such coincidence is insufficient to establish a connection, still less to show its nature; whereas, on the other hand, it is quite impossible that the observer should not be struck with the fact of the coincidence of these four masses of diarrhœa, choleraic diarrhœa, cholera, and ozone. It may as well be added here, once for all, that in the collection of the statistics of these cases of disease, the medical practitioners were wholly unaware of the nature of each other's returns, and that, therefore, although the returns themselves may not represent with absolute accuracy the precise number of cases that occurred, it is most likely that any errors which may exist, mutually counterbalance each other, and that the curves really represent the actual course of the disease.

"On the 8th of September, the centre of the first period of increase of the disease, the temperature fell, and there was far less difference between the maximum and minimum of the thermometer than on any previous day for a week. From that day to the 13th, the maximum rose again, the cholera diminishing; but on the 18th, the centre of the next period of increase, it had again fallen. On that day, however, there was greater variation between the extremes of temperature than on the two preceding days. The maximum of the thermometer was on the increase on the day of the cessation of the second cholera period; but then, the minimum the day before had been lower than on any day for three months. At the maximum of the third period the thermometer was falling, and at the termination of this epoch it was again rising. So that we cannot predicate any one thermometric condition as common to these three periods.

"The weather was unusually fine, dry, and clear. In the first cholera period, and the third, the sky was comparatively free from cloud, on the day preceding and following the lull in the disease. After the second period there was no cloud, but at the next great lull, as in the centre of the second or middle period of increase, the sky was all but wholly overcast. Upon looking at the line formed by the degrees of moisture in the air, it will be seen that, on the days preceding the first two cholera periods, the air had been becoming more dry, and preceding the last period, more fully saturated. No rain fell on the maximum days of the two first cholera periods, or on the day of the material decline of the disease, September 27. But, a little fell on the maximum day of the third period, and on the minimum day which followed it.

"Contrary to the opinion which has been gaining ground on apparently sufficient data, we do not find that a general stagnation of the air is a necessary accompaniment of the epidemic. For although on the central day of the last period of increase there was scarcely any movement of the atmosphere around Oxford, it was blowing fresh during the central period—so fresh as to blow down the tents in the field of observation—as it did also during the decline of the disease. And the direction was by no means uniform. It was mainly northerly previous to the first period, southwest previous to the second, and northerly again previous to the third.

"During the first and third cholera periods the barometer was steadily falling, and continued to fall for some days afterwards. During the main central period it was steadily rising, and continued upon the whole to rise, excepting on one day of storm, Sept. 24, until the day before that of the great lull of the disease, Sept. 28, when it was falling, as it continued to fall chiefly during the height of the last period. It rose again, and fell an inch, in the fortnight during which the pestilence died out."

"The reading of the barometer here, as in London, is shown by Mr. Johnson to have been unusually high, as was the mean temperature, it being remarked by him that these two conditions were common to our three cholera epidemics, and the only conditions that *were* so. With us, as in London, the *range* of temperature was, this year, during a part, but not during the whole of the cholera period, less than usual. Of fog, mist, and haze, we here observed, I believe, less than is frequent with us. If, during the cholera period, we had two periods of calm, we had one period, and that the centre of the epidemic, of very considerable movement; in fact, the horizontal movement of the one or two periods before and after the centre of the epidemic exceeded that of any day in the previous ten weeks. And, lastly, especial attention must be called to the fact, that with us there was a greater amount of ozone shown on some days than on any previous day, for eight weeks, and that the total value of Mr. Johnson's ozone notation in the central week of the cholera—Sept. 17 to 24—amounted to nearly 37, and in no other week, for ten weeks, to 25."

We pass over the chapters on the treatment of the disease, on the theory of the cause or causes of the disease, and its mode of extension. From the first no important conclusions are to be deduced, and the second comprises views that can be considered in no other light than as mere hypotheses, neither borne out by the general facts on record having a bearing upon the etiology of cholera, nor by the special facts which the author has collected with great care, and recorded with much apparent candour, in reference to the occurrence, progress, and decline of the disease in Oxford.

No one doubts, according to Dr. A., that during a cholera period persons die of diarrhœa and of choleraic diarrhœa, without passing into cholera, and, also, that such cases do oftentimes pass into cholera. We have no disposition to dispute the general fact here stated. To us, however, it is very evident, that the diarrhœa and cholera are merely grades or stages of the same disease—the effects of the same morbific agent upon the system—acting with more or less intensity, or upon individuals more or less or differently predisposed to their action. The separating the initial diarrhœa from cholera has, we believe, been productive of not a little mischief—it has interfered with our investigations into the true pathology of the disease—retarded our acquaintance with its proper management, and led in numerous instances to a fatal security, and a careless and inefficient treatment, during the only period when the disease may with cetainty be controlled by the physician.

The hypothesis of Dr. Acland is, that the diarrhœa, simple and choleraic, prevailing during cholera seasons, is produced by atmospheric influence—meaning thereby the general cosmical conditions prevailing—without any specific poison, and genuine cholera by this same atmospheric influence, operating upon the discharges from the bowels, and producing from these a specific poison which is capable of generating cholera in the individual from whom the discharges came, susceptible of the change alluded to, or upon other persons: the discharges being innocuous, or incapable of communicating cholera until so changed; but when thus changed, either within or without the body, capable of distribution throughout the atmosphere—probably either in a dry or in a gaseous state, and absorbable through the lungs—or capable of solution in water and of absorption by the digestive organs. In other words, one cause—the atmosphere—produces the first group of disease, and along with the disease, an organic product—alvine discharge—which is innocuous until altered by the same cause which produced it, when it becomes the cause of the second group. "So that it might be theoretically, and perhaps truly, said," remarks Dr. A., "that if the cause which produced the diarrhœa ceased before the discharges could be acted upon, then they would remain forever innocuous."

From this hypothesis Dr. A. hazards the following general statements :—

"1st. Diarrhœa always coexists with cholera in any given locality, and is not communicated from person to person.

"2d. Cholera may arise without the suspicion of contagion.

"3d. Cholera may certainly be conveyed from place to place by human agency.

"4th. It can scarcely be any longer doubted that the evacuations of cholera patients are capable of communicating the cholera.

"5th. It is quite certain that in the majority of cases, the cholera evacuations do not communicate the cholera.

"6th. It is quite certain that in localities apparently exceedingly prone to development of cholerà, the cholera which is imported to them may not be propagated."

It is chiefly from the very excellent account presented in the memoir before us of the history of the rise, progress, and cessation of the epidemic of 1854, in the city of Oxford, and the careful collation of all those circumstances arising from the nature of the location, the character and condition of the population, and the prevailing atmospherical phenomena, by which the production and spread of the disease may have been more or less inflamed, or its character, as to mildness or malignancy, to a greater or less extent modified. In these respects, however, it constitutes a most valuable contribution to our materials for the formation of a correct theory of the etiology of cholera. It is true the data furnished by Dr. A. are insufficient of themselves to form the basis of any general conclusions, but are invaluable for comparison with observations of a similar character made at other places, during former, contemporaneous, or subsequent occurrences of the epidemic.

The following are presented by the author as a summary of the general conclusions deduced by him from the fact recorded in the present memoir.

"1. The history of both the city and the surrounding district unite in giving weight to the belief in the origin of cholera without communication with other cholera districts.

"2. Both the city and the district give evidence of the occasional communication of the disease from place to place, and from person to person.

"3. They both lead us to the conviction that places, and attendants on cholera patients, may enjoy a perfect immunity from contagion.

"4. From the survey of the city, we are inclined to believe that this immunity is less probable in proportion as less attention is paid to the destruction of the evacuations.

"5. Contact with the evacuations is therefore exceedingly dangerous.

"6. The hypothesis which refers diarrhœa to the state of the atmosphere, and cholera to the metamorphosis of diarrhœa evacuations by and in that atmosphere, derives support from these considerations.

"7. The poison of the evacuations may be conveyed through the air, or by the agency of water.

"8. Therefore, poisoned water, though one means of spreading the disease, is not the only means.

"9. For these reasons, and from the facts observed, we may conclude, and do assert, that crowded dwellings and imperfect ventilation are dangerous in the highest degree, during the presence of a cholera atmosphere, to those who are subjected to them, just as they are ruinous to health at other times.

"10. We must, therefore, conclude, that such dwellings, and such bad ventilation, are dangerous, not only to the persons exposed to them, but to the whole district or town which surrounds them.

"11. A low scale of diet favours diarrhœa, and a better diet tends to check it.

"12. Occupation exercised no marked influence in this district, and indeed persons in easy circumstances were more attacked, proportionally, than night soilmen, who work mostly in the open air.

"13. The lower half of this city was most attacked, but the lives of those who reside in the upper and drained portions are unquestionably endangered by the condition of the lower and undrained parts.

"14. Preparations for epidemic disease should not be left till the disease appears. There should, therefore, be wards, in every town, proper for receiving persons suffering from such diseases."

As an appendix to the memoir Dr. A. presents a brief sketch of the present sanitary condition of Oxford, and "the arrangements which a wise community would adopt beforehand to mitigate the terrible scourge of coming epidemics." Under the heads of ventilation, the construction and location of dwellings, drainage, provisions for the medical attendance of the poor, the connection between mental cultivation, physical improvement and health, recreation, etc., he treats, most pleasantly and wisely, questions of immense importance to the welfare, happiness, comfort and healthfulness of every community. It is true, he advances on these subjects but little that is new to those who have made themselves familiar with the well established principles of hygiene in all its several bearings—they cannot, however, be too often urged upon the attention of the municipal authorities of towns and cities, who, unfortunately, from their ignorance of them, either blindly perpetuate, by their acts, a state of things destructive of the health of their constituents, or blindly tolerate a condition of things prejudicial to the health and well-being of the community, and which invite the occurrence in its midst of the most severe forms of epidemic disease, or give to them, when they occur, increased extension and malignancy.

D. F. C.

ART. XVIII.—*The Medical Profession in Ancient Times. An Anniversary Discourse delivered before the New York Academy of Medicine*, November 7, 1855. By JOHN WATSON, M. D., Surgeon to the New York Hospital. Published by order of the Academy. New York, 1856. 8vo. pp. 222.

IT is of good augury that the attention of American physicians is beginning to be directed towards the history of medicine. The infant man, the infant state, the infant institution, takes no thought of its origin or genealogy, but, on reaching a maturer degree of development, recognizes the eternal laws which govern the world, and turns eagerly to the past for light to enlighten the present and the future. The medical profession in this country, if it may congratulate itself on a freedom from certain trammels which authority and custom impose upon the fraternity in Europe, has no reason to boast of its share in that precious legacy of knowledge which the past has bequeathed to it. In whatever else we may excel, we are certainly inferior to the rest of the civilized world in an acquaintance with medical history. Various indications have been given, however, that the defect is not unseen, and that there is a disposition to correct it. The recent translation of Renouard's history, and the present essay, are among these indications. The first named work professes to treat summarily of medicine from its origin to the nineteenth century, while the latter claims only to afford a sketch of its progress in the Greek, Alexandrian, and Roman schools.

In looking at the manner in which Dr. Watson has performed the difficult task of condensing his materials into a very narrow space, we cannot refrain from congratulating him on the interest with which he has invested the subject, and on the superior literary execution of his essay. The wide range and the marked accuracy of his research, the impartiality of his criticisms, the liveliness, perspicuity, correctness, and even elegance of his style, combine to suggest a regret that they should have been employed upon so scanty a performance. We will venture to express the hope and desire that this discourse may prove to be only the germ of a systematic and extended work which shall, by its native origin and intrinsic excellence, attract the general attention of the profession to the study of medical history. No department of literature demands a longer apprenticeship than this. Books, leisure, and the habitual occupation—or, as it were, saturation—of the mind with it, is an essential condition of excellence in the historian. Dr. W. has evidently surveyed the ground, and laid the necessary foundation of the edifice with caution, deliberation, and skill, and we feel persuaded that no one is, at the present time, more competent to complete it. In other departments of history, American authorship has achieved a classical position; why should not another name be added to those of Prescott and Bancroft, to illustrate the annals of science and benevolence, as theirs have done the records of political and social revolutions?

The first chapter of the essay treats of "the condition of medicine in the earliest organizations of society," points to its origin as an art in Egypt, and refers to its wider manifestations among other less cultivated nations. Herodotus, we are told, says that in Egypt "each physician applies himself to one disease only, and no more—all places abound in physicians; some for the eyes, others for the head, others for the teeth, others for the parts about the belly, and others for internal diseases." This fact, we may remark, indicates a high degree of civilization, for it is precisely what is observed in our own country and in Europe at the present day. Among the ruder provincial population one practitioner performs all the duties of the healing art, while in the populous and refined capitals we have physicians, surgeons, oculists, dentists, specialists devoted to diseases of the ear, lungs, heart, urinary organs, skin, &c. Thus do we see illustrated the essential sameness of human character and actions in all ages of the world. This chapter presents an instance of imperfect inference which we feel unwilling to pass unnoticed. We are told that Cambyses must have known something of the internal structure of the human frame, "for, having shot an arrow through the body of a child, to prove his skill in archery, he ordered them to open him and examine the wound; when the arrow was found to have pierced the heart." Now it will be remembered that, owing to its pulsations, the position of the heart is familiar to every one. Indeed, in Scripture language, "to stab one under the fifth rib," is equivalent to saying to stab him to the heart.

The second chapter treats of "the origin of medicine among the Greeks." Our author, following Littré, ascribes it to three sources: the Gymnasia, the Schools of Philosophy, and the Temples of Æsculapius. But in the first the only medical experience was derived from the occasional accidents produced by athletic exercises, and in the second, medicine was cultivated as a theory rather than as a profession. The temples of Æsculapius, or the Asclepions, were, however, the sources from which the stream of medical knowledge really flowed. They were numerous in Greece, and, indeed, were clinical institutions, where the priests acted as physicians, and gradually accumulated a fund of knowledge which they imparted to their pupils. But both, it would seem, practised among the general public. There must also have been two grades of lay practitioners, freemen and slaves; the former of whom were distinguished by their education, and, of course, by having a higher class of patients to attend. Plato thus contrasts them :—

"Do you not perceive that when there are both slaves and freemen sick in the cities, the slaves do for the most part go round and cure the slaves, or remain at home in the medical shops; and that not one of these slave-physicians either gives or receives any reason respecting the diseases of the slaves; but as if knowing accurately from experience, he orders as if he were a self-willed tyrant, what seems good to him, and then goes away, bounding off from one sick domestic to another; and by this means, he affords a facility to his master to attend to other patients? But the free-born physician for the most part attends to, and reflects upon the diseases of the free-born; and by exploring these from the beginning, and according to nature, * * * does at the same time learn something from, and, as far as he can, teach something to, the sick; and does not order anything until persuaded of its propriety; and then, after rendering the patient gentle by persuasion, he endeavours to finish the business by bringing him back to health." (P. 32.)

The course of education pursued by the Asclepiadæ extended through five years at least. They had not discovered that short path to knowledge which our countrymen follow, nor attempted that flying-leap to a diploma which some among our brethren are not ashamed to take, and which their teachers do not blush to recommend. The order of their study was systematic; theory, or "illumination," being followed by "inspection" or practical studies, including, "probably, the treatment of disease under the immediate supervision of the instructor." The whole course was conducted under religious sanctions; the commencement of the purely medical studies was hallowed by the well-known obligation called the Oath, and its conclusion was signalized by a public ceremony, in which the successful candidate for medical honours received a wreath in token of his conquest of the difficulties of science. The doctoral cap, or *bonnet* of modern times, is emblematical of the same idea. In spite of these safeguards against ignorance, the number of pretenders to medical knowledge was very great, and, as our author remarks—

"The regularly initiated were, then as now, disposed to look upon themselves as sufferers by the consideration occasionally bestowed upon impostors. 'Medicine,' says Hippocrates, 'is of all the arts, the most noble; but, owing to the ignorance of those who practise it, and of those who inconsiderately form a judgment of these, it is at present far behind all other arts. Their mistake,' he adds, 'appears to me to arise principally from this, that in the cities there is no punishment connected with the practice of medicine, and with it alone, except disgrace; and that does not hurt those who are familiar with it. Such persons are like the figures which are introduced in tragedies; for, as they have the shape, and dress, and personal appearance of actors, and are not actors, so also physicians are many in title, but very few in reality.'" (Pp. 44 and 45.)

How far this course of study was perfected, and what was its value before the time of Hippocrates, must ever remain doubtful; but the more probable opinion is that the greater part of the writings of the father of medicine represent the actual condition of the science and the art in his own day, rather than his original contributions to its advancement. As our author happily observes—

"The great among mankind are not merely those who set the first examples. Examples are often the result of accident; and the best of them, in a practical point of view, rarely the result of forethought. He who detects the rising spirit of the age, who first gives expression and embodiment, or the power of progress and endurance, to the wisdom, feelings, aspirations, customs, or hitherto undivulged opinions of his times, is even more worthy of regard than the innovator. Such a man was Hippocrates. He lived in an age of progress. The earliest historians, the earliest and ablest dramatists, the profoundest philosophers, the wisest legislators, the ablest generals, the greatest architects, painters, and sculptors of Greece, were all men of the same epoch. And while other arts and sciences were thus springing into life, and rising at once to maturity, it is not surprising that some man of genius should appear in the ranks of medicine, to give to its principles form and utterance. This man was Hippocrates.

"He was not, then, the inventor of the healing art, nor of the modes of teaching it. He was not the first to write upon it. But, familiar with its traditionary lore, with the science and philosophy of his day, and with the practical details of his profession in all its bearings, he was the first to combine such knowledge in systematic form, and to give to it a scientific value; yet not so clearly scientific, as to be sufficient of itself, in the form in which he left it, and independent of oral comment or practical illustration, to qualify the aspirant who would avail himself of it alone, for the proper exercise of his calling." (Pp. 47 and 48.)

Our author gives a summary account of the Hippocratic collection, which need not detain us; it is of more importance to inquire into the distinctive characters of the medical knowledge which was possessed by the sage of Cos. His great and imperishable renown is derived from the accurate descriptions which he furnishes of disease, and the importance of symptoms in diagnosis and prognosis. We think Dr. W.'s pen must have ill-expressed his thought when he tells us (p. 53) that Hippocrates "founds his system on *realities*," and then in the next sentence states that he adopted from the schools the doctrine of the primitive elements, and that of the primitive humours, and taught that disease is a process of coction in these latter, terminating in a critical discharge or in death. In close connection with this hypothesis, for it is nothing more, is the doctrine of critical days, a salient and capital element of the Hippocratic doctrine, but which, nevertheless, rests upon no better foundation than an assertion. It entered into nearly every system of medicine that has prevailed from time to time, and yet all strict observation fails to give it the slightest support. In accordance with his theoretical views Hippocrates perceives in diseases groups of aggregated but not necessarily affiliated symptoms, rather than phenomena naturally enchained and dependent upon a common organic cause. Hence it happens that the descriptions of Hippocrates are less remarkable for their completeness than for the fidelity with which certain symptoms are described, and the singularly accurate estimate which is given of their value in relation to one another, and to the ultimate issue of the diseases in which they occur. The school of Cnidos, which rivalled that of Cos, pursued the opposite, and, as we believe, the truer method. It seems to have regarded diseases as logical entities, always wearing the same essential features, and not as mere accidental groups of symptoms. "Thus," as our author states, "they enumerated seven different diseases of the biliary organs, twelve of the bladder, and four of the kidneys; they described four kinds of strangury, three kinds of tetanus, four of jaundice, and three of phthisis." Unfortunately, none of the Cnidian treatises have reached our time, so that we are unable to estimate the pathological knowledge which they may have displayed. It should be mentioned, incidentally, that the soundness of their doctrine may, to some extent, be inferred from the fact, that Aristotle favoured it much more than he did the principles of the Hippocratic school.

At a subsequent period, indeed more than four hundred years afterwards, the very same distinctions obtained among rival sects of physicians, in the Roman empire, and particularly between the Rationalists and the Empirics. The former, as Dr. Watson states (p. 106), held as essential to the proper management of diseases that the physician should inquire into their occult or constituent causes, as well as their evident and exciting causes. But, naturally enough, they differed as to what should be regarded as an occult cause, whether a redundance or deficiency of the four primitive elements, or of the four humours, or the quality of the inspired air, or some molecular derangement of the solids or fluids. They all, too, attached great importance to a correct knowledge of concoction, and yet no two of them probably had the same idea of this hypothetical process. On the other hand, the Empirics (or those who take experience for their guide) alleged that the inquiry after occult causes is fruitless. For, as Celsus pointedly remarks, even the philosophers must be allowed to be the greatest physicians, if reasoning could make them so; whereas it appears that they have abundance of words, but very little skill in the art of healing. Even in regard to a knowledge of the causes of diseases, they seldom help us to cure these latter. And as for its treatment, that is the result of observation and experiment merely, observation of the instinctive desires of the sick, and trial of those things which seem best adapted to allay their sufferings. When remedies are found, then men begin to discourse about the reasons of their use. For medicine was not invented in consequence of their reasoning, but theory was sought for after the discovery of medicine. On the appearance of any new disease the physician would not be obliged to have recourse to occult things; he would seek for its resemblance to diseases already known, and meet it by remedies analogous to such as had been successful in a similar malady until the true mode of treatment could be discovered. Not that judgment or reasoning is unnecessary to a physician, or that an irrational animal is capable of practising medicine, but conjectures which relate to occult things are of no use.

In our own age we cannot survey the medical profession without observing that it is still essentially divided into Coans and Cnidians, into rationalists and empirics. And although the immense and overpowering influence of experimental philosophy, illustrated by countless conquests in the field of observation, seldom allows the claims of the mere theorist to be heard, it now and then occurs that some dogma obtains a temporary and partial sway, to the disgrace of sound reasoning, and the grief of all who are devoted to the improvement of the medical art. The human mind tends no less in modern than in ancient times to form hasty generalizations, to discover causation where none exists in the relations of phenomena, and, among these latter, to apply reasonings to one class which properly belong to another. Hence the doctrines of disease have been allowed to shape and mould the forms of treatment, with which they had really nothing at all to do. Against this error the empirics contended, and it is even now far from being exploded, although oftentimes unconsciously entertained. We believe, as they did, that the *science* of medicine is expended chiefly on a knowledge of disease, that is, on pathology; and that the whole *art* of medicine is comprised in therapeutics. The improvement of the latter has no further dependence on the perfection of the former than this: pathology develops, defines, or limits more and more strictly the morbid conditions which we call diseases, and therefore presents to the therapeutist definite objects on which to test the powers of remedies. But although the science of medicine, in its department of special pathology, were perfect, it does not follow that therapeutics would partake of the same perfection. And the converse is equally true. Indeed, nothing is more certain than that the cases in which a cure is wrought with most certainty are those of whose pathological nature least is known. Witness syphilis and mercury, gout and colchicum, pain and opium, etc. etc.

Our author furnishes an apt illustration of the advantage resulting from keeping asunder fact and speculation, by quoting from Thucydides his famous account of the plague of Athens. This writer, with no pretensions to medical knowledge, and no guide but his own clear perception of facts and his freedom from the trammels of the schools, has furnished a description unsurpassed by that of any medical writer for its distinctness and completeness. It is remarkable that this account contains the first, and for a long time the only, statement of the communicability of disease from the sick to the healthy.

The reader of the essay before us will be interested by the sketch given of the mighty achievements of Aristotle in science, and with the description of Alexandria and its famous school, illustrated by Greek learning and genius. It was in that city that Herophilus first drew attention to the value of the pulse as a symptom, and that Erasistratus distinguished nerves of motion and nerves of sensation. Here Ammonius invented an instrument for crushing the stone in the bladder, when it was too large to be extracted by the incision made in lithotomy; and here, also, dissection of the human body was first performed. These physicians flourished about three hundred years before Christ. From that period until the Christian era no eminent medical writer appeared. Meanwhile the conquests of Rome had extended over the East, and she began to receive such civilization as she was capable of from the people of her subject provinces. To Asclepiades the Bithynian (B. C. 63), as our author informs us, belongs the credit of having first raised the medical profession in Rome to the confidence and respect of the people. He was the first to announce the doctrine of the self-limitation of diseases. Dioscorides, of Anazarba in Cilicia (A. D. 54), the great authority on the materia medica of the ancients; Aretæus, of Cappadocia (at the same epoch); and Galen, of Pergamus (A. D. 131), were all foreigners; while the only native Roman among physicians of eminence was Celsus, who lived in the earlier part of the first century. The work of this eminently clear and judicious writer, both as regards medical doctrine and practice, ought to be made familiar to every physician. It is readily accessible through the French and English translations. The following is from our author's account of the great Roman physician:—

> "Celsus, more than any other of the ancient Latin physicians, is celebrated for the purity and elegance of his style, and for a concise and judicious manner of handling his subject. The summary history of medical doctrines, of the materia medica, and of surgery, introduced at the commencement of his first, fifth, and seventh books, shows how carefully he had studied the great masters of the art, and how well he was prepared to furnish a thorough and reliable digest of their opinions; not indeed as a compiler of minute details, but as one able to grasp the philosophy of medicine, and at the same time not to overlook any facts essential to the guidance of the practitioner. While citing many authors, he holds Hippocrates, and next to him Asclepiades, in chief regard. In judgment he is too independent to acquiesce in all that had been advanced by either of these. He rejects the Hippocratic doctrine of critical days, and he differs from Asclepiades in many points; but whilst dissenting from those whose authority he usually respects, he gives sufficient reasons for his own opinions." (Pp. 112–113.)

The views of Celsus in regard to medical doctrines have been already referred to; of his practical knowledge and precepts it is sufficient to say that they are everywhere distinguished by precision and an air of candour which commends them to acceptance. Dioscorides was for many centuries the sole authority on the materia medica, and even now no writer on this subject can be regarded as well informed, who does not make a study of his treatise, particularly as it is presented by his commentator Matthiolus. In some respects, Aretæus occupies even a higher position than either of the preceding. As our author remarks:—

"Aretæus is one of the most original and elegant writers of antiquity. For truth and accuracy of description, some have even placed him above Hippocrates. There is perhaps no modern writer to whom he can be more aptly compared than Heberden. He appears to have written at that period of life when the mind, tempered and enriched by ample experience, is more disposed to rely upon personal observation than on the teaching of the schools, and to pay little regard to theories unsupported by the revelations of nature. Starting with a thorough acquaintance with the science of his day, taking Hippocrates as his model, and repudiating all futile speculations, he details the simple results of his own experience, in a systematic treatise of eight books on the history and treatment of acute and chronic diseases, and in a manner so striking and appropriate as rarely to have been excelled. His descriptions of marasmus, of phthisis, of angina, of asthma, and of mania, are frequently referred to as true to nature, and of poetic finish. Yet he himself acknowledges his inability to paint to his own satisfaction the ever-varying shades of disease, and advises every young physician to study for himself, and not to trust for all his knowledge to the commentaries of his instructors. In his practice he employs but few remedies, and never the monstrous compositions so much in vogue among the Romans. He makes frequent use of evacuants. Emetics, purgatives, and venesections are his main agents in the management of acute diseases; in these also relying much on regimen, and on cooling and refreshing drinks. But in the management of chronic diseases his practice is more diversified. His surgical is in keeping with his medical ability. He was the first, so far as I remember, to use the trephine for the cure of epilepsy. He employs catheterism in mechanical obstructions of the urethra, resulting from vesical calculus; for the removal of the stone, he recommends perineal section, by an incision immediately below the scrotum, and extending inward to the neck of the bladder until the urine and calculus escape. He employs the actual cautery for opening hepatic abscess, and cauterizes the scalp in certain diseases of the head." (Pp. 145–6.)

The reputation of all these writers has been eclipsed by that of Galen. Our author presents a succinct account of his life, showing how he travelled from Pergamus to Smyrna, and thence in succession to Corinth and Alexandria, in pursuit of knowledge, returning to his native place, which, however, in consequence of political disturbances, he quitted for Rome in the thirty-fourth year of his age. Here he ran a brilliant career, under the patronage of the imperial court, but ultimately retired to his own country, where he survived to an extreme old age. It is impossible even to enumerate in this place the improvements in medicine which are due to this great man; our author attempts to present only a summary of them, which is sufficient to show their variety and magnitude. They affected the fundamental as well as the applied branches; and, in fact, present an epitome of the entire circle of medical study. In all, he probably advanced as much of his own as he took from the existing sources of information, and by the vivid earnestness of his style persuaded men to adopt his theoretical conclusions. Indeed, for twelve centuries he reigned the autocrat of the medical world. Unfortunately, his prodigious acquirements appear to have overwhelmed his successors with awe, instead of inspiring them with emulation, and for a thousand years not more than two medical writers of original genius, or even of great critical acumen, appeared upon the stage. The estimate of Galen by our author appears to us unequal to his merit; it is in these words:—

"Galen wrote no work expressly on the practice of medicine; but he has left a complete code of medical science, the only complete code of which we read among the ancients. Possessing in its individual parts no great originality, made up of the doctrines of his predecessors of every sect, and disfigured by occasional incongruities, yet, as a whole, this code is remarkable for its general unity and consistency. But its fundamental doctrines are too often the creations of the imagination. In all his works, Galen delights to display his erudition; and, notwithstanding their vast number, they are mostly written in polished style. He professes to be the admirer and disciple of Hippocrates. Yet no two writers on medicine were ever in style and substance more dissimilar. Hippocrates wrote with the terseness of a philosopher; Galen with the flowing redundancy of the rhetorician, allowing nothing to remain unsaid, and adorning his discourse with criticism, biography, anecdote, sarcasm, vain-glorious boasting, personal narrative, and incidental allusions of every sort. But his brilliant errors, no less than his sterner truths, gave popularity and influence to his writings." (Pp. 172–3.)

The exceptions to a general torpor in the medical body, above alluded to, were Alexander of Tralles, who flourished in the sixth, and Paul of Ægina, who lived in the seventh century. Of the former it is said that, in point of originality, he ranks next after Hippocrates and Aretæus. The work of the latter (which is accessible to the American reader in the Sydenham Society's edition), although chiefly and avowedly a compilation, is a valuable because it is a logical one, and enriched by not a little of the author's original observations.

The decline and long stagnation of medicine may be ascribed, as it generally is, to the same causes which paralyzed the social and political world during the decay of the Roman empire, and the catastrophe which marked the irruption of the northern barbarians upon the civilized nations of the south. But there appears to be a special reason why medicine, more than any other department of knowledge, should have been subjected to decay. The Asclepions of Greece, which were at once temples, hospitals, and schools of learning and philosophy, had raised medicine to a height which it never attained elsewhere in the ancient world. The museum of Alexandria was of a more purely scientific character; and in it, as well as in the Grecian institutions, the ruling purpose was inquiry into the laws of matter and of mind. This research was clogged by no prejudices or superstitions, and its fruits were therefore, in their very nature, living, and growing towards perfection. But with the substitution of Christian for Pagan doctrine, human wisdom came to be undervalued, and everything else was sacrificed to the great object of working a moral reform. The Asclepions were temples of false divinities, and in the beginning of the fourth century they were closed by an edict of the Emperor Constantine. In their stead came hospitals and other charitable institutions, in which priests occupied the seats of philosophers, and devotional exercises took the place of philosophical discussion. The skill and wisdom of Hippocrates, and of his long line of illustrious successors, were discarded, and more reliance was placed on faith than on works in the cure of disease. The people were vastly the gainers by exchanging the contempt or indifference of philosophers for the tender solicitude of men and women who not only found a delight in charity, but, by its exercise, were striving to win immortal souls. But as charity abounded, skill declined; the new religion banished the old, and, with it, the philosophy which had thought it not impious to penetrate the darkest recesses of nature, and draw her secrets into the light of day. As our author states, the regularly educated lay physicians were gradually deprived of many of their prerogatives, and supplanted by the clergy, who, in their united capacity of priest and physician, were afterwards for many ages almost the only practitioners of medicine. Indeed, but for the preservation of Greek learning in the East, and the origin of the Arabian school of medicine in the eighth and ninth centuries, it is very doubtful whether medicine would have been prepared to take her place among the sister sciences, when at last the human mind began to shake off its fetters, and the dawn of knowledge broke upon the world in the fourteenth century.

In a concluding chapter, Dr. Watson gives some account of the laws and customs of the Roman empire in relation to the medical profession, and quotes from Galen a statement of the various elements of knowledge which in his time were regarded as essential to a medical education. These, the reader will perceive, included the whole circle of knowledge possessed by the ancient world; and when one considers it, he cannot help wondering how it came to be seriously supposed, in these modern days, that a young man can be qualified for practising the art of medicine by such scanty education as our present system affords.

"The importance of practical training," says Dr. W., "was, if possible, more highly estimated by the ancients than the moderns. Even the charlatans of Rome, who spurned all connection with the liberal arts, and professed to qualify their pupils within the short space of six months, were duly impressed with the necessity of clinical teaching, and were in the habit of ostentatiously parading through the streets, followed by a retinue of young men, with whom they made their daily visits to the sick." (P. 212.)

We shall quote but one passage more, and we offer it as a bit of consolation to those who mourn that the people have no appreciation of talent or knowledge, and that even the educated often lead the way in fostering quackery, and afflicting us with detraction or neglect. Our Roman brethren were not better off than ourselves.

"Of these illegitimate sons of Æsculapius, the numbers and pretensions were as great in ancient as in modern times; and they were quite as apt to receive the countenance and favour of the upper classes. Chosroes, of Persia, was the patron of Uranus; and Nero was the supporter of the audacious Thessalus, who, like Paracelsus, repudiated all learning as useless, and, like the still more recent mountebank, Hahnemann, modestly assumed to be above all, and opposed to all, who had ever gone before him. Pliny and Galen are justly severe on most of these ancient impostors. And, if we can credit their account of them, the host of industrialists, oculists, rhinoplasts, dentists, bone-setters, herniotomists, lithotomists, gelders, abortionists, and poison-venders, pervading Italy, France, and Spain throughout the middle ages—before whom the modern group of pretenders grow pale and insignificant—were at least equalled, if not exceeded, in ignorance, as well as arrogance, by the quacks of Rome." (P. 214.)

A. S.

BIBLIOGRAPHICAL NOTICES.

ART. XIX.—*Essay on Cholera Infantum, for which the Prize of the New York Academy of Medicine was awarded, March 5th,* 1856. By JAMES STEWART, M. D., Author of *A Practical Treatise on the Diseases of Children.* 8vo. pp. 66.

THERE is no disease incident to the period of childhood which, whether considered in reference to the extent to which it prevails every summer, in all the larger cities of the middle, southern, and many of the western States, or to the amount of mortality produced by it, claims so strongly the attention of the American physician as cholera infantum. Although a disease which has been, and we believe with propriety, ranked as an endemic peculiar to the United States;—although very full and interesting notices of it are to be found in the works of Rush, Currie, Mitchell, and other of our older physicians, and in our medical journals, especially those of the earlier period of the present century, in most of which the correct etiology of the disease is recognized—it was not until 1829, when Dr. Horner published his inquiry into the anatomical characters of infantile follicular inflammation of the gastro-intestinal mucous membrane, that its true pathological character was fully understood. It is in fact to the investigations of Dr. Horner and the series of carefully conducted dissections subsequently detailed by Dr. Edward Hallowell, in his paper on the endemic follicular gastro-enteritis, or summer complaint of children (*see* number of this Journal for July, 1847), that we are indebted for our present knowledge of the nature of the intestinal lesions in the disease under consideration. The paper of the last named gentleman, published in 1847, is the more valuable, inasmuch as in it he has traced, from a series of actual observations, carefully conducted, the relation of the morbid changes which take place in the intestines of those affected with cholera infantum, with the symptoms which mark the several stages of the disease from its inception until its close.

The inflammatory character of cholera infantum appears to have been admitted from an early period, and in some of the few dissections published previously to those of Dr. Horner, inflammation and congestion of the mucous membrane of the intestines is formally noticed as being met with—it was the latter, however, who first detected the seat of the inflammation and ulceration in the mucous follicles.

In the prize essay before us we have a very full and able account of the disease in question—presenting a faithful delineation of its symptoms, progress, etiology, pathology, and treatment. It does great credit to the author, and will, we are convinced, be favourably received by the profession. It presents clear and correct views of a malady which all who practise in the larger cities of most of the States will be called upon every summer to treat, and to whom, therefore, accurate conceptions of its causes, character, and proper management are essential to enable them to stay the truly frightful mortality of which it is every year productive.

After noticing the fact of the occurrence of cholera infantum at a particular period of early life and at a particular season of the year, and the foundation for the opinion that it is a disease peculiar to the United States, Dr. Stewart proceeds to investigate its etiology.

"That a clear idea of the causes of this disease may be obtained," he remarks, "with a view to investigate its pathology and the strictly practical application of remedial measures, it is proposed to subject all the circumstances which are observed to control its development to a careful examination. There is no disease which appears to demand so close an investigation of this nature, for there is none which has its pathology so intimately connected with the action of the agencies which are in constant exercise in its production, and in its maintenance throughout its course. The combination of these active agents —constituting what is known as climate, the more special local agents, and the physiological peculiarities of the period of life at which the disease occurs, it will be seen are all connected in the production and maintenance of the same pathological results, so formidable in their action, and so obstinate in their management. These circumstances are not to be regarded as mere isolated facts, but as an important group, which are essential, when connected with the phenomena of the disease and its morbid anatomy, to illustrate the morbid condition of the system: none of them can be separated without impairing the relation they bear to the nature of the disease."

The first cause necessary for the development of cholera infantum is a high atmospheric temperature. The invasion of the disease occurs immediately after a period of excessive heat sets in, and is one of its most marked effects. Hence it is during the summer months alone that cholera infantum prevails, and, all other things being favourable, the warmer the summer the more rife is the disease and the greater the extent of the mortality produced by it. As Dr. S. very correctly remarks, it appears scarcely to exist when the mean temperature is about 60°. Summers, the mean temperature of which is by no means considerable, may nevertheless be marked by a considerable amount of the disease, if there has been a prevalence of intensely hot weather during even a few weeks.

Dr. S. points out next the influence of excessive humidity of the air in the production of cholera infantum.

From a careful examination he has come to the conclusion "that ordinary climatic humidity has but limited influence on the development of cholera infantum.

"The same amount of moisture often exists in country places as is found in the city, and where the disease never is known to originate. We therefore directed our attention to the occasional state of the dew-point as it occurred where the disease was most prevalent, and discovered a great difference within doors, between it and the general dew-point of the external air, continuing often for a long time."

After noticing that his first observation was that the moisture was always greater nearer the surface of the earth and consequently in cellars and basements, he remarks, that his second observation was,

"That in very hot weather in excessively crowded houses, at night, when all are within, the dew-point is very nearly at the temperature of the air, consequently the air is saturated with moisture. With a temperature of 90° to 95° and a dew-point in a crowded room almost equal to the temperature, a feeling of suffocation is experienced, which is easily accounted for when it is known that the dew-point of the breath as it is expelled from the lungs is 94°, and that the mean dew-point of the atmosphere is 38°, and also, that in the hottest weather it rarely exceeds 70°. When the air is loaded with moisture and deposited easily at a temperature approaching to that of the living body, inspiration is difficult and unsatisfactory, while the system suffers great depression." "It is in such heated and moist places that we have found the greatest number of instances of cholera infantum."

In estimating the influence of such places in the production of the disease we must recollect that independently of the heat and moisture of the atmosphere, this is, also, rendered impure by the number who breathe it, by want of sufficient ventilation, from the exhalations of a number of living bodies crowded together, and most probably by personal and domestic filth. Now the malaria of crowded localities is very correctly ranked, by Dr. S., among the necessary conditions for the production of cholera infantum.

The disease is almost exclusively confined to cities. That it is not the product of that form of malaria, whatever may be supposed to be its nature and source, which gives rise to what have been termed miasmatic fevers, is proved by this, and by other views very clearly set forth by Dr. S. Not only is cholera infantum the especial disease of cities, but in these it prevails chiefly—always most extensively, and in its most unmanageable form—in the most crowded, badly ventilated and drained portions of the city, and where there exist the most abundant sources of atmospheric vitiation.

Another of those conditions the concurrence of which is necessary for the production of cholera, is a particular period of infantile existence—the period of teething. When children who have passed this age are exposed to the causes before referred to, the result, Dr. S. remarks, is dysentery. This he has repeatedly seen in the same house, during a hot season, where cholera infantum has prevailed.

"When the affection of the bowels that was excited in the older children continued for a few days, it always assumed the form of dysentery, and never that of the peculiar disease of infancy." This remark is a correct one, and is fully borne out by our own observations.

Pointing to the fact of the immediate dependence of cholera infantum upon disease of the mucous follicles of the intestines, which present an appearance of inordinate development, inflammation and ulceration, Dr. S. observes: "Their development is peculiar to the period of life at which cholera infantum appears —is the result of the natural movement of the system, and is simultaneous with the eruption of the teeth. The inflammation and ulceration of the follicles are, superadded morbid action, constituting the disease under consideration."

"When, in the order of the natural development of the infant's frame, these follicles for the first time show themselves, in connection with other parts concerned in nutrition, they are in a high state of activity, pouring forth an abundance of their natural secretion. Thus far the action is a natural one, and one of health. Should it become excessive, a serious diarrhœa takes its place, demanding the interference of the physician for its removal. This same condition of the development of the follicles, when complicated with other derangements of the system, and kept in a state of morbid activity by the continual operation of certain exciting causes, terminates in producing one of the most fatal diseases of our climate, the cholera of infants.

"Dissections of infants that have died of various diseases, have exhibited the development of the mucous follicles, commencing at the time of the appearance of the teeth, while before that time they are rarely to be seen. Numerous *post-mortem* examinations show that the follicles experience an increase of vital energy, which augments their secretion, and render their size larger, and their number greater, but which still does not produce any redness, tumefaction, or ulceration. Their activity in secretion during the time of dentition is the true cause of the ordinary diarrhœa in teething infants, usually ascribed to sympathy with the gums, and which, to a moderate degree, is not to be regarded as disease, but is the result of the physiological action of the period of life.

"The follicles, in the natural course of development, having just passed into a state of activity, are thereby prepared to have an additional or excessive development, on the application of a sufficient cause; and then the transition is both rapid and easy from a healthy to a diseased state."

Inappropriate food Dr. S. considers as an occasional exciting cause of cholera.

In regard to the modus operandi of heat, moisture, and malaria in the production of cholera infantum, Dr. S. supposes that their first effect is an interference with the freedom of respiration and the due change of the blood in its passage through the lungs; the depurative office of the liver is in consequence taxed to an extent far beyond the ordinary requirements when the respiratory function is fully and regularly performed—a diseased condition of the liver is quickly induced and its functions become disturbed—as is shown to be the case in cholera infantum, by the absence of the biliary secretions in the discharges from the stools after the disease is fully formed, and by the morbid condition of the liver almost invariably detected after death. The diseased state of the liver causing an obstruction to the passage of blood returned through it from the intestinal surface, congestion of the mucous membrane and its follicles ensues, to relieve which an inordinate secretion from these, already in a state of exalted action, is set up. When morbid action is thus once established, inflammation and ulceration is the course naturally to be expected.

The exposition of the pathology of cholera infantum, a brief outline of which we have here given, is reasoned out and illustrated by Dr. S. in a manner which would seem to give to it the semblance, at least, of truth. We have no especial objection to make to it; in its general outlines we believe it to be correct. We should be inclined, it is true, to account somewhat differently for the diseased condition of the liver, and to view this as less essential to the production of disease in the intestinal mucous follicles—which we believe may be more satisfactorily accounted for by the morbid impression made upon the capillaries of the surface, and the disturbances thence resulting to the exhalant and other depurative functions of the skin. The theory of Dr. S. is, however, ingenious and well supported—it demands a careful examination on the part of the profession.

A very good account is given of the general phenomena, distinctive of the disease, and a detailed and accurate description of its semeiology, in the incipiency, maturity and decline of the attack.

We come now to the important item of the treatment of cholera infantum. We may premise, that in no disease is prophylaxis of greater importance, more simple in its details, or productive of more decided results. The predisposition from age we have no means of removing, but the subjection of the teething infant to an intense atmospheric temperature, to crowded and ill-ventilated and foul apartments, to personal filth and the malarious neighbourhoods of a city may certainly be prevented, and improper kinds of food withheld from it. Could the children be removed during the excessive heat of summer into the cooler air of the country, or even into clean, capacious, well aired apartments, in the more open and less densely populated portions of the metropolis, and properly lodged, clothed, fed, and kept scrupulously clean, the annual mortality from the disease would be reduced to an insignificant number. Even after the disease has already commenced the same measures will in many instances be sufficient to arrest it, or generally to produce so favourable a change in its character, as to render it readily curable by a simple course of treatment. In fact, unless the infant be removed from the continued influence of the active agents in the production of the disease, as is properly remarked by Dr. S., " the use of therapeutic means is of little avail." Unfortunately, the condition and pecuniary means of the very class of the community among the children of which the disease prevails to the greatest extent, are such as to preclude the possibility of carrying out fully and effectually the measures referred to. Even the relief derived from their partial adoption during the day is productive, as Dr. S. points out, "of little benefit, by a return at night to the close and stifling air of the overcrowded dwelling." It is this, far less than the really unmanageable nature of cholera infantum, which renders it so destructive of life in our midst.

The hygienic treatment laid down by Dr. S. is particularly sound, and should be insisted upon in every case by the physician. In many of its details it may be carried out by every mother, be she rich or poor.

In respect to one point connected with the hygiene of young children as well as with the proper management of cholera infantum and other diseases of infancy, we would call especial attention to the remarks of Dr. S., and that is diet.

"Diet is a very important subject, both in the prevention and management of the disease. One of the greatest evils in its treatment is the use of vegetable food, either of a farinaceous or starchy nature. The last mentioned, so often given in the form of arrowroot on account of its soft, mucilaginous consistency, is especially objectionable. All vegetable substances are unsuited to young infants; but those of an amylaceous nature, being altogether insoluble, are with difficulty absorbed, and when the mucous membrane is diseased, scarcely ever are, but pass as foreign substances quite through the bowels, and may be detected in the discharges by iodine, the usual test for starch. Farinaceous articles are very likely to become acid, and excessively so in this disease. We regard all such articles for food in early infancy as highly pernicious, whether the child be sick or well. The food that nature supplies is best, and if there is no deterioration either in quantity or quality, should be the only food given. When, for any reason, it is necessary to make a substitute for it, milk, properly prepared for the child, should still be given.

"In cholera infantum, we have been in the habit of combining a solution of gelatine with the milk, as the most appropriate food for the child, and where the stomach is excessively irritable, to give nothing for a while but the jelly, prepared thick or thin, as the child will take it the most freely. The use of this substance has so frequently been followed by decided benefit, that we regard it as a valuable remedy. If gelatine comes under the class of respiratory food only, then it must be regarded as a therapeutic agent. It is so perfectly soluble that it is absorbed as easily as water, and no doubt has passed into the circulation before it could reach the diseased part, in which respect it contrasts very remarkably with arrowroot, so frequently given in this disease. As regards the indications of a want of proper nourishing or stimulating power in the nurse's milk, we have been much guided by the instincts of the child, which will cause it at times eagerly to seize some animal substance and suck it with avidity. Following this suggestion, we have directed cow's milk to be given, either diluted, pure, or combined with gelatine, changed occasionally for chicken water, and, when the child is especially eager for animal food, and has suffered much from debility, beef-tea, or a piece of fat pork, according to the instincts of the child. These last mentioned articles, and even salted meat, are especially beneficial in the more advanced forms of the disease and during convalescence. In some form, animal substances are necessary in every stage."

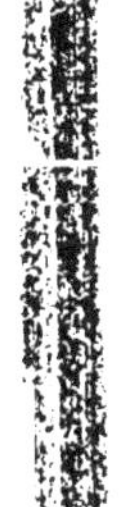

The views of Dr. S., in respect to the inappropriateness of vegetable substances as food for infants, were first made public in a communication which was inserted in the *New York Journal* for July, 1844. On its first appearance, the several po set forth in this communication strongly attracted our attention, and sitionsubsequent experience has convinced us that they are all well founded. We would very strongly urge them upon the attention of the profession. Their practical application will be found eminently useful in the prevention of many of those affections of the stomach and bowels of infants the foundation of which is often laid in the nursery, either before or at the period of weaning, as well as in the dietetic management of the more common of the diseases of the early periods of existence.

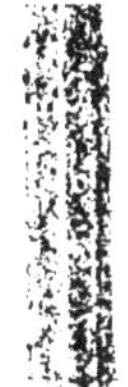

The plan of treatment of cholera infantum laid down by Dr. S., as well preventive as curative, is in its general outlines sound and judicious. In some of the details of his therapeutical directions we should perhaps differ from him; this difference would consist, however, rather in regard to a choice of individual remedies, than to the proper indications to be pursued, or the character of the general remedial measures by which these are to be fulfilled.

In every point of view we esteem the essay of Dr. Stewart to be a valuable contribution to the pathology and therapeutics of infancy, and as such recommend it to the notice of the profession. D. F. C.

ART. XX.—*Reports of American Institutions for the Insane.*

1. *Of the Ohio Lunatic Asylum, Columbus, for the years* 1854 and 1855.
2. *Of the Eastern Lunatic Asylum, Lexington, Kentucky, for the* years 1849, 1850, 1852, 1853, 1854, and 1855.
3. *Of the Insane Asylum of Louisiana, for the years* 1852 and 1853.
4. *Of the California Insane Asylum, for the year* 1854.
5. *Of the Bloomingdale Asylum, for the year* 1855.
6. *Of the Retreat, at Hartford, for the year* 1854.
7. *Of the Friends' Asylum, Frankford (Philadelphia), for the years* 1853 and 1854.

1. Dr. E. Kendrick, the Superintendent of the Ohio Lunatic Asylum, at the time of our last notice of a report from that institution, resigned his office in May, 1854, and on the 1st of July was succeeded by Dr. George E. Eels, the author of the documents now before us.

	Men.	Women.	Total.
Patients in the Asylum, Nov. 15th, 1853 .	115	138	253
Admitted in course of the year . .	113	133	246
Whole number in course of the year .	228	271	499
Discharged, including deaths . . .	106	132	238
Remaining, Nov. 15th, 1854 . . .	122	139	261
Of those discharged, there were cured .	59	71	130
Died	10	12	22
Applicants rejected in course of the year .	74	78	152

"In July," says Dr. Eels, "many of the inmates were affected with simple diarrhœa, which was readily controlled by the usual means. During the months of August and September, the intestinal disorder assumed more aggravated forms. Bilious diarrhœa and dysentery supervened. This in every instance subsided under the use of mild alteratives, such as blue mass, hydrarg. cum cret., and anodynes, conjoined with perfect rest, and a mild, fluid diet.

"We had also, during the same time, twenty-seven cases of fever. Seven of these were intermittent, nine remittent, and eleven continued. The two former varieties were very mild, and yielded readily to the use of anti-periodic remedies. The continued fever was of an asthenic character, and distinct from the other two varieties. It yielded neither to the tonic, alterative, nor antiphlogistic course of treatment, but continued uninterruptedly to run through a certain cycle of changes, and finally, at the expiration of from two to three weeks, slowly convalesced. This disease had not the well-defined symptomatology of typhoid fever. The surface was hot and dry, tongue moist and clean, pulse frequent, soft, and small. Diarrhœa was not generally a troublesome feature, although occasionally present. There were not present 'the lenticular rose-spots,' the tympanites, the dry mucous surface covered with sordes, nor the low muttering delirium, so peculiar to typhoid fever. This fever was treated by enjoining rest, acid drinks, rice-water for nourishment, frequent application of tepid water to the surface, with alkaline diuretics, diaphoretics, and occasional anodynes." Apparatus for lighting the building by gas was introduced in the course of the year.

From the report for 1855.

	Men.	Women.	Total.
Patients in the Asylum, Nov. 15, 1854 .	122	139	261
Admitted in course of the year . .	95	79	174
Whole number in course of the year .	217	218	435
Discharged, including deaths . . .	108	111	219
Remaining, Nov. 15, 1855 . . .	109	107	216
Of those discharged, there were cured .	50	48	98
Died	6	7	13

Causes of Death.—Maniacal exhaustion 3; phthisis pulmonalis 2; organic diseases of brain 2; apoplexy, suicide, intestinal hemorrhage, valvular disease of the heart, organic disease of stomach, and old age, 1 each.

"During the summer and autumn, the whole western country was afflicted with diseases having a malarious origin. The patients of this Asylum did not entirely escape this influence, although it is believed that they suffered less than any portion of the surrounding neighbourhood. A few cases of intermittent fever, not at all remarkable for their severity, constituted the sickness. These yielded readily to the usual anti-periodic remedies, and were in no instance rendered troublesome by complications. * * * A number of cases of cholera morbus, of extreme severity, occurred in the house." These were wholly among the employés, and soon yielded to treatment.

	Men.	Women.	Total.
Whole number admitted, from 1839 to 1855, both inclusive	1,428	1,348	2,776
Discharged, cured	714	697	1,411
Died	204	154	358

The insane of the United States cannot as yet congratulate themselves upon a complete redemption from association with malefactors. "Many cases," remarks Dr. Eels, "have been brought to the Asylum (in 1855) in chains, with their limbs lacerated and constitutions much impaired by protracted confinement in jails."

Dr. Eels makes the subjoined remarks upon the pathology and the treatment of insanity.

"In both male and female, whatever the original cause of their mental disease may have been, it is generally found that upon their admission they are debilitated, and that the strength which they exercise in their ravings is more apparent than real. The medical observer is in danger of being misled unless this general fact is constantly borne in mind. So far from the excitement exhibited by them being an evidence of a sthenic condition of the system, the reverse is the general rule. Antiphlogistic remedies, therefore, are seldom indicated, and only in exceptional cases; while nourishing food, tonics with anodynes, and the diffusible stimulants, properly administered, seem to allay nervous excitement, induce sleep, and restore the natural vigour of the worn-out frame. To these means we have generally resorted in cases of acute mania, due attention having been paid to the condition of the digestive functions, with decided benefit. A few such cases, reduced by depletory measures before admission, have required a long time to regain the vigour thus lost. The calmness by this (depletory) means obtained, has too often been as delusive as the original symptoms of excitement upon which such treatment was predicated, and instead of being a sign of returning reason, has been but the commencement of a prolonged and sometimes hopeless dementia."

If all that has been said be true, the heating of the wards of this institution, in years gone by, was far from being perfect. The method of warming by steam has been recently introduced, with much success. "During the last winter the mercury in the thermometer was never observed to fall below 64° in the most exposed wards, and ranged from that to 76°, with the capability of being elevated or depressed at will. So completely was the entire establishment warmed, in every part, that not only was no complaint made, but those catarrhal affections so common in this latitude, and to which the insane are peculiarly liable, were entirely unknown among us."

The comparatively youthful State of Ohio was the first in the Union to set the nobly philanthropic example of assuming the pecuniary expense of the support of such of her children as might be afflicted with mental alienation. The government caused an institution to be established, and after it was opened, was ready and willing to cancel from her treasury all the debts contracted in its current operations. The legislative appropriations for the support of the institution since 1847, have in no year been less than twenty-five thousand dollars. We perceive, with regret, that in the course of the year 1855, the pecuniary disability of the Asylum has been such as to compel the discharge of eighty-three patients, and to force its officers to singularly extraordinary financial manœuvres to enable them to provide for the subsistence of those who remained. We anticipated a dark day for this establishment, when, two or three years ago, we had occasion to record the fact that, with the other benevolent institutions of Ohio, it had been given over to the tender mercies of partisan politics. We fear that this financial trouble is among the fruits—if not the first fruits—of that unhallowed desecration.

12. We have the reports for six years, consecutive, with but one exception, of the Eastern Lunatic Asylum, of Kentucky, at Lexington. The annual changes in the patients, during the whole period embraced by them, are here presented in a condensed form:—

	1849.			1851.			1852.			1853.			1854.			1855.		
	M.	W.	T.	M.	W.	T.	M.	W.	T.	M.	W.	T.	M.	W.	T.	M.	W.	T.
Patients in the Asylum at beginning of the year . .	159	111	270	118	85	203	155	94	249	148	92	240	121	81	202	115	76	191
Admitted in course of the year	64	32	96	92	41	133	20	18	38	31	18	49	47	27	74	70	33	103
Whole number in the year .	223	143	366	210	126	336	175	112	287	179	110	289	168	108	276	185	109	294
Discharged, including deaths	87	56	143	55	32	87	27	20	47	58	29	87	54	32	86	81	27	108
Remaining at end of year .	135	88	223	155	94	249	148	92	240	121	81	202	114	76	190	104	82	186
Of those discharged, were cured	27	6	33	28	13	41	14	13	27	29	15	44	21	5	26	29	7	36
Died	52	46	98	20	14	34	7	6	13	13	8	21	14	12	24	43	13	56

The causes of death will be mentioned as we examine the several reports in succession. It should be remarked that this is an old institution, and that while on the one hand, comparatively few patients are received while their disease is yet in its acute stage, so, on the other, they generally make it a permanent residence, unless they are restored to their normal mental condition. Very few are discharged otherwise than by death or recovery.

Since the above was written, a letter has been received from Dr. Chipley, in which the following statement is given, as explanatory of the large mortality at the Asylum:—

"The law makes this institution the receptacle for the insane, idiots, and epileptics; nor have we any right to discharge them because they are found to be incurable. Much the larger number of cases of insanity committed to our charge are of some years' standing, and not a few of the patients arrive so far exhausted as to perish within the first week.

"The law provides that idiots may be taken care of at home, for which the State pays a sum not exceeding fifty dollars—or they may be sent to the Asylum. The effect of this law is to impose upon us only those idiots who have reached the last stage of life; who have become so far exhausted by disease, or so debased and filthy that no one will consent to take care of them for fifty dollars. These necessarily add to our mortality. The same may be said of epileptics. They are sent here, generally, to be taken care of in their last illness. Many of this class die in this institution annually. Nearly 250 of the aggregate number of deaths were caused by cholera, in the years 1833, 1849, 1850, and 1855."

The most important part of the report for 1849, is that which embodies a history of the appearance, progress, and effects of Asiatic cholera, within the precincts of the Asylum. As this epidemic was one of the most remarkable in the annals of institutions for the insane, we quote the record with but little abatement:—

"Anticipating the approach of cholera, we had spent weeks in precautionary measures to avoid its invasion. The whole establishment had undergone thorough cleansing, ventilation, and whitewashing. Disinfectants and antiseptics were everywhere applied. No spot whence it was thought possible the cause of disease could emanate, was left untouched; and if its cause is to be regarded as local in its origin, we are yet unable to account for its generation here. Indeed, those wards in which it was most prevalent and most fatal, were those which, if the disease is of miasmatic origin, should have been most exempt. They are high, dry, and airy, and occupied by a class of inmates least exposed to that cause of disease. The epidemic appeared on the 21st of May, and continued until the 25th of June. There were 280 patients in the Asylum, of whom not more than fifty entirely escaped its effects.

"When cholera invaded us, measles had been prevailing to some extent, but with the exception of two cases, which seemed to run into the epidemic, none died. During the few weeks that the epidemic raged, there was a large number of deaths from epilepsy, or, rather, among our epileptic patients. This class of patients usually composes (furnishes?) about one-third of the deaths annually reported by us, but they generally drop off gradually, in the course of the year. This season, however, no less than twelve died while the cholera was in our midst. How far the pestilential poison may have influenced these attacks, I know not; but I am persuaded that it had something to do in augmenting their violence and fatality, as it apparently modified every other disease which co-existed with it. The diseases proving fatal during the year may be classed as follows: Cholera 60; fever, sequel to cholera, 12; dysentery, sequel to cholera, 4; measles 2; epilepsy 14; chronic diarrhœa 6.

"There were many obstacles to the successful treatment of the disease (cholera) in our inmates. * * * Few (of the insane) regard its attacks. Still fewer submit willingly to treatment, and the kind attentions of friends are received as officious interference. In a number of patients, though vigilance was enjoined upon all, the malady had progressed to a fatal extent before it was made known. Several would be found of a morning, who had lain still, suffering diarrhœa to go on to exhaustion, without moving from bed, or uttering a complaint, thus eluding the night-watch. Some resisted all remedies, and many would not be persuaded to the use of sufficient medication. Besides their mental condition, their physical state lessens their power of resisting exhausting maladies. The crowded condition of our wards at the time, and the great difficulty of obtaining adequate nurses, also, no doubt, diminished the number of recoveries. * * * * The influence of the ravages of the cholera has been felt, and is apparent in every department of our domestic concerns. The labour of the institution is mainly done by lunatics. With the exception of cooking, in which they lend some help, everything may be said to be done by them. The washing, ironing, farming, and gardening, entirely so. The epidemic made sad havoc among our working class of patients, leaving the burthen upon others less accustomed, and less able to bear it."

The report for 1851, gives the following bill of mortality: Epilepsy 19; chronic diarrhœa 5; old age 3; pulmonary consumption 2; apoplexy 2; gastro-enteritis 1; gastritis 1; typhoid fever 1.

The large proportion of fatality from epilepsy will be perceived. "It is almost universally the case," Dr. Allen remarks, "that this class of patients are brought to us labouring under the disease in its most hideous and unmanageable form." They are generally retained at their homes until it becomes complicated with mania, phthisis, or some other malady, aggravating the epilepsy, or abbreviating the life of its victim.

"Early in the spring smallpox was introduced into our midst, by a patient from a neighbouring city." He was in the febrile stage when admitted, and hence the disease was unrecognized until "contact with a large number of inmates had occurred." But seven were seized with the disease, and in no case was it fatal.*

The original buildings of this asylum were very defective in architectural arrangement. At the suggestion of Dr. Allen, and in accordance with plans designed by him, additions and alterations were made. Their near approach to completion is mentioned in this report.

The medical history of the institution for 1852 and 1853 is embraced in one report. The deaths, in the course of the two years, were from "pulmonary disease" 12, epilepsy 5, old age 4, chronic diarrhœa 5, inflammation of the brain 2, pneumonia 1, traumatic gangrene 1, marasmus 2; and two were caused by a conflagration of which we shall give an abbreviated description.

Between 12 and 1 o'clock on the night of the 14th of February, 1852, a fire was discovered upon the roof of the building occupied by men, at a point nearly "the most remote from chimneys or hot-air flues, and the most hidden from observation. * * * The day had been inclement, and some pains must have been taken to ignite the materials; and a watchman, who was under an engagement to be (at the asylum) failed to come that night, the only one of the winter in which regular rounds had not been kept up." The conflagration is, therefore, attributed to design, but the incendiary has not been discovered. "At one time," remarks Dr. Allen, "I believe every patient was removed from danger, and the one who was afterwards known to perish, seems to have re-entered the house, and to resist efforts for his rescue. A second inmate, of whom we never heard afterwards, we fear was also lost, though it is not certain." The adjoining building was saved by the exertions of the attendants and the patients. The fire destroyed "about seventy lodges (dormitories?), three long halls, as many day-rooms, and three latticed verandas." It consequently became necessary to overcrowd other apartments, and to place patients in rooms the windows of which were unprotected. Yet, at the date of the report, there had been "but two or three elopements, and but a single, and not a serious injury received in attempts of the kind. * * * We have much yet to learn of the capacity of the insane for self-government, and the restraint which hopelessly impaired reason may be taught to exercise over the impulses of the lunatic."

In the report for 1854, we are informed that Dr. John R. Allen, who had been connected with the institution, as superintendent, upwards of ten years, dissolved that connection, by resignation, on the 1st of October. From that time, until the 1st of April, 1855, the vacancy was filled by the former assistant physician, Dr. Perrin, the author of the report for the year. "The health of our family," he writes, "has been generally good. Of the deaths, five were caused by exhaustion, six by consumption, seven by epilepsy, five by chronic diarrhœa, two by old age, and one by suicide." Dr. Perrin's report is brief. He complains that some persons send their relatives to the asylum not only "when, from extreme old age, or from some chronic affection, they have become filthy and unwilling to take food, or when their attendance has become hopeless and disagreeable, but even when they are actually in a dying condition." In this connection he contributes to the domain of psychologic science, a sweet ebullition of filial affection which may be worthy of preservation. We make the extract *verbatim* and *punctuatim*. "I will take the liberty to quote a few lines from a letter received by me, a few weeks ago, from a gentleman (?) who wished to send us his aged father: 'If I pay only three months of his board would it not satisfy the managers? I do not think that father will live long, and this is my reason for not wishing to pay six months in advance.'"

Of the 190 patients remaining in the asylum at the end of the year, it was believed that 165 were incurable.

The report for 1855, was written by Dr. W. S. Chipley, who entered upon the duties of superintendent on the 1st of April of that year. It contains an account of another, the fourth, invasion of the asylum by the epidemic cholera. It commenced "about the first of July." Several of the patients who were attacked "became pulseless and icy cold; the skin was shrivelled, the surface of the body blue, the tongue and breath cold; and yet, of some twenty-five cases that occurred between the 1st and the 20th of July, not one proved fatal." From the 20th to the 24th, there was no new case. On the latter day, however, "five patients fell victims" to the disease. "Every effort was made to prepare for the worst." Several of the patients, who, it was believed, might with safety be at large, were discharged. One of them died of cholera at his home. "Few of our inmates," says Dr. Chipley, "escaped an attack, and thirty-four perished. It is, however, worthy of remark, that of all those who were the subjects of the malady before it assumed a malignant aspect, not one suffered a second time. * * * Of twenty employés, we lost seven: two female attendants, one male attendant, the assistant matron, the baker, and the watchman. Besides these, several deaths occurred among those who came to our help in the hour of trial. * * * Few persons remained in the house twenty-four hours without an attack." Dr. Steele was acting-assistant physician; Drs. York, Clark, and Proctor, recent graduates, and the Rev. Mr. Adams and Mr. Fox, medical students, volunteered their services and rendered valuable aid. "Of all these gentlemen, Dr. Clark alone escaped an attack; and one of them, Dr. York, died. Dr. York did not remain in the institution more than twenty-four hours, when he returned to the city with symptoms of the disease upon him, and died the next day a martyr to the cause of humanity." One temporary nurse died at the asylum, and two ladies of Lexington who took charge of a ward, one of them but one day, the other but three days, contracted the disease and died after they left. In answer to the entreaties of friends to fly from the infection, one of the employés said, "No consideration would induce me to assume the post I now occupy during the prevalence of this terrible disease. I now believe I shall contract the malady, and that I shall perish of it; but I will not desert the poor creatures committed to my charge. If I must die, I will perish in the faithful discharge of my duty." His fate was in accordance with his alleged belief.

The causes of mortality and their several effects, in the course of the year, were: cholera 34; epilepsy 9; exhaustion 8; consumption 3; apoplexy 1; injury by leaping from a window, before admission, 1.

In giving the supposed causes of the malignant form which the cholera has assumed at each of its several visits to the asylum, Dr. Chipley states, that "the condition of the water-closets is such that the air of all the wards is more or less tainted;" and that the water, with which the establishment is abundantly supplied, "is very strongly impregnated with limestone, and rarely fails to produce severe purging with new patients from other counties."

This institution presents the anomaly of legal obligation to defray the expense of removing pauper patients from their places of residence to itself. When convenient to do so, an attendant is sent for the patient. But if this cannot be done the patient is "usually brought under the order of court, in charge of two or three persons, whose compensation becomes a charge upon the institution. * * Several have been compelled, by those appointed to convey them to the asylum, to toil their wearisome way from distant counties on foot, and unprovided with shoes. An old lady, over fifty years of age, was thus brought by three stout men. Up to the period of her death, which occurred a few weeks after her arrival, she never gave the least evidence of a disposition to do violence to any one. A child might have governed her."

Horses and a carriage are devoted to the use of patients, and dancing parties, concerts, and festivals upon holidays are given; but it appears that the asylum is very deficient in newspapers, periodicals, books, and most of the other manifold adjuvants in the moral treatment which are now to be found in the best conducted institutions of the kind.

Whole number of patients since the Asylum was opened	2113
Discharged recovered	777
Died	852

Of the remainder, who are not now in the institution, no less than 129 eloped. Twenty-three elopements occurred in the course of the six years embraced by these reports. These numbers are large, very large. No institution of the kind is free from this method of subtraction from its inmates, yet in no other within our knowledge does it exist to the same extent. The report states, that the fences upon the grounds are imperfect, and both Dr. Allen and Dr. Chipley advance the idea that it is better to incur the risk of elopements than the hazards of detriment to the patients by too close confinement.

A building has been erected in the place of that which was destroyed by fire. It is heated by steam.

Dr. Chipley devotes several pages of his report to an argument in favour of the establishment, in Kentucky, of an institution for idiots.

Thus closes our glance at the six annual cycles in the history of the Eastern Lunatic Asylum of Kentucky. Rarely, if ever, was a public institution visited by so rapid a succession of misfortune. Cholera, conflagration, measles, variola, cholera! such are the scourges which we have witnessed at their work among the alienate of reason. We have never looked upon the like before; may we never look upon the like again.

3. The reports from the Insane Asylum of Louisiana are biennial. The one now before us is for the years 1852 and 1853. Since the last preceding report "the eastern detached building" has been completed, and is now occupied by the violent female patients, and the eastern wing of the main edifice has been erected. The latter is occupied by the better classes of females. The asylum now has apartments for 140 patients.

	Men.	Women.	Total.
Patients in the Asylum, Dec. 31, 1851 . .	33	45	78
Admitted in 1852	25	15	40
Admitted in 1853	50	33	83
Whole number in the two years	108	93	201
Discharged in the two years, including deaths	40	29	69
Remaining, Dec. 31, 1853	68	64	132
Discharged cured, in 1852	2	7	9
Discharged cured, in 1853	2	2	4
Died in 1852	6	7	13
Died in 1853	17	10	27

Deaths, in 1852, from chronic diarrhœa, 5; marasmus 2; old age 1; chlorosis 1; "disease of lungs" 1; "fits" 1; chronic dysentery 1; not stated 1. In 1853, from diarrhœa 8; cholera 4; cholera morbus 3; yellow fever 2; phthisis pulmonalis 3; "fits" 2; dropsy, general palsy, marasmus, lead colic, and "flux," 1 each.

"The two patients who died of yellow fever came through an infected district on their way here, and arrived with the disease in them. It did not spread in the Asylum.

"We received patients from the city (New Orleans), on the 21st of November, among whom there were two decided cases of cholera; and, on the 24th of the same month, we received more patients from the city, with two more cases of cholera, all of which proved fatal. Others had premonitory symptoms, which were checked. The disease did not spread."

Jackson, the township within which the Asylum is situated, was visited, in the autumn of 1853, by an epidemic called, by some, yellow fever; by others, dengue. No case occurred at the Asylum.

"Diarrhœa is the most troublesome disease we have to contend with. * * * Some cases have recovered, some have been improved, and life prolonged. But, generally, when a disposition to chronic diarrhœa is manifested, the disease, although checked, recurs again and again, until it finally terminates in death."

Whole number of patients since the Asylum was opened . .	325
Discharged, cured	53
Died	95

Nearly all the patients are from the pauper and indigent classes.

4. It is with peculiar interest that we take up the report from the Asylum of California, and trace the progress of the development of mental disease under the unique and unprecedented influences operating upon the inhabitants of that newly settled State. As with the preceding report from this institution, noticed in a former issue, so with the one before us, we shall deviate from our usual course of review, constrained thereto by the special circumstances of the case:—

	Men.	Women.	Total.
Patients in the Asylum, Dec. 31, 1853 .	93	10	103
Admitted in course of the year	179	23	202
Whole number in course of the year . .	272	33	305
Discharged, recovered	132	18	150
Died	20	1	21
Remaining, Dec. 31, 1854	120	14	134

It will be perceived that all who were discharged, living, from the institution, are reported as cured; and that this number (150 of 305) is within a very small fraction of fifty per cent. of the whole number who received the benefits of the Asylum in the course of the year. The only explanation of this remarkable result is found in the supposition that a very large proportion of the cases were of but recent origin—a supposition which might almost be assumed, *a priori*, as a fact, based upon a knowledge of the manner in which California received the mass of her population, and the proximate period within which her settlement has been effected. The following classification of all the cases treated within the year throws some light upon the subject:—

Acute mania 104; chronic mania 52; periodic mania 25; epileptic mania 14; puerperal mania 12; nymphomania 4; monomania 32; dementia 34; melancholia 28.

Of the 52 cases of chronic mania, it is probable that nearly all were among the patients received in former years. The proportion of cases of acute mania is very large, and as they doubtless originated from other acute diseases, or from causes the origin and influence of which were but slightly remote, they were necessarily eminently curable. The same remarks are equally applicable to the cases of puerperal mania, and, though with diminished force and generality, to those of melancholia. It may be remarked that, according to our ideas of the classification of mental disorders, there is a discrepancy or inconsistency in the report, which we do not understand. The foregoing classification includes the whole 305 cases under treatment in the twelve-months. Nothing is mentioned therein of *mania-à-potu*. In a subsequent part of the report, however, Dr. Reid remarks that the "table of mortality is somewhat greater than last year, owing to a variety of causes, but principally from the admission of persons not proper subjects for an asylum for the insane, such as mania from typhoid fever, *mania-à-potu*, and epileptics." The table of mortality is as follows:—

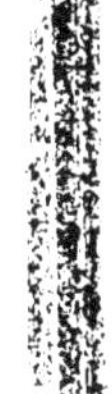

Acute mania 2; mania-à-potu 2; typhoid fever 3; puerperal fever 1; marasmus 2; erysipelas 1; epilepsy 4; dropsy 1; dysentery 4; ramollissement 1.

"The general health of the establishment has been good. No epidemic, no acute disease of any kind, unconnected with the brain, has prevailed to any extent. No suicide has occurred within the past year, nor, indeed, at any time since the organization of the institution. *These cases of self-destruction have become so numerous lately—have swept over the State almost like an epidemic—that the Asylum is considered exceedingly fortunate that nothing of the kind has happened within its walls.*" A remarkable comment upon the psychological condition of a people!

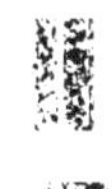

"Several homicidal cases have also been under treatment, yet no accident of a serious or dangerous character has taken place. Of the 305 cases, 25 were suicidal and 12 homicidal."

It must be well known to those who have read our *notices*, that we place but little confidence in the tables of alleged causes of mental aberration. The reasons for our distrust have heretofore been given. We believe, however, that the subjoined, which is extracted from the report under review, is worthy of its space. The reader may himself judge of the probabilities of its accuracy, from its similarity or dissimilarity to that which, with a knowledge of the manner in which the State was peopled, and the difficulties, the dangers, the sufferings, and the various other mind-disturbing influences to which that people have necessarily been subjected, he might be led to expect.

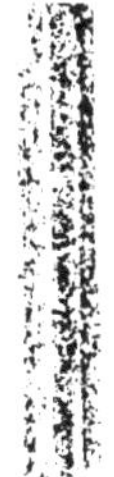

Moral Causes.		Physical Causes.	
Mental excitement	7	Intemperance in the use of spirits	42
Domestic affliction	21	Intemperance in the use of opium	2
Pecuniary disappointment	28	Intemperance in the use of tobacco	1
Political disappointment	2	Masturbation	28
Disappointed affection	5	Amativeness	3
Desertion of wife	3	Consequences of parturition	10
Desertion of husband	3	Suppressed menstruation	2
Desertion of mistress	2	Congestive fever	2
Seduction and desertion	2	Typhoid fever	6
Jealousy, &c.	2	Injury of head	6
Grief and fear	5	Epilepsy	10
Sudden wealth	2	Syphilis	4
Religion, &c.	3	Coup de soleil	2
Fanaticism	3	Ill health	23
Spiritualism	4	Hereditary	10
Mormonism	1	Unknown	12

Some of the most prominent peculiarities of this table are the very large proportion of cases from pecuniary disappointment, domestic affliction, masturbation, and parturition; and the very small proportion of those from anxiety in respect to religion, as compared with similar tables in the reports of institutions in the older States.

"The temperature of our climate," says Dr. Reid, "is so equable, the atmospheric changes so regular and gradual, that they exert but little influence in the production and development of the disease. During the six hottest months of the dry season, 272 patients were admitted, and 214 during the other months." The last observation applies to the whole period of three years since patients were first received.

"The attention of the public, of medical men, and of legislators, should be constantly directed to the fearful and alarming increase of insanity in this State. The productive causes of this disease should be sought for and investigated with minute care and attention; the method of prevention and cure should be pointed out, and, especially, of its curability in the early stages."

Age, at time of Admission, of 305 Patients.

	Men.	Women.	Total.
Between 10 and 20 years	21	2	23
" 20 " 30 "	142	12	154
" 30 " 40 "	68	10	78
" 40 " 50 "	26	6	32
" 50 " 60 "	9	2	11
" 60 " 70 "	4	1	5
" 70 " 80 "	2	0	2

The predominance of numbers in the decade 20 to 30, is much greater than in most other similar institutions. "The average age was only 32 years."

Relation to Marriage.	Men.	Women.	Total.
Single	213	4	217
Married	38	18	56
Widowed	21	11	32

The ratio of the number of the single to that of both married and widowed, is as 2.11 is to 1.

Occupation.—Miners 102; *no occupation* 43; sailors 14; carpenters 12; traders 12; clerks 11; farmers 10; blacksmiths 10; merchants 8; soldiers 8; labourers 7; cooks 6; peddlers 5; tailors 4; gardeners 4. The remainder of the 305 were divided, in small numbers, among twenty-four different occupations.

Nativity.—United States—Maine 6; N. Hampshire 2; Vermont 5; Massachusetts 24; R. Island 4; Connecticut 3; N. York 34; New Jersey 5; Pennsylvania 8; Delaware 2; Maryland 4; Virginia 4; N. Carolina 3; S. Carolina 2; Georgia 2; Alabama 1; Mississippi 3; Missouri 10; Louisiana 4; Arkansas 2; Texas 3; Kentucky 6; Tennessee 7; Ohio 14; Indiana 5; Illinois 8; Michigan 3; Wisconsin 2; Iowa 2; Oregon 1; Utah 1; *California* 4.

Thus, every State, excepting Florida, is represented, and only thirteen of them by a smaller number than California herself.

Europe.—Ireland 24; France 22; Germany 18; England 16; Scotland 7; Italy 5; Spain, Portugal, Russia, Prussia, and Poland, 2 each; Switzerland, Denmark, Norway, and Sweden, 1 each.

Other Foreign Nations and Dependencies.—Mexico 10; Canada 2; Australia 2; Chili, Peru, China, and Hindostan, 1 each. "We have also admitted 9 Africans—six males and three females."

It is remarkable that, with so many Chinese as there are in the State, only one has become a patient in this Asylum.

In view of the large accession of females to the population of the State within the past two years, and the increased number who have become insane and sent to the Asylum, Dr. Reid recommends the erection of an additional wing to the buildings, for their special accommodation.

The subjoined extract is from the meteorological register for 1854, kept at the Asylum, which is in the city of Stockton, latitude 37°, 57′ north; longitude 121°, 14′, 26″ west of Greenwich.

"The coldest month was January, the mean temperature being, at 8 A. M., 34°, at 2 P. M. 58°, and at 8 P. M. 40°. The warmest month was July, the mean temperature at 8 A. M. 69°, at 2 P. M. 90°, and at 8 P. M. 73°.

"The coldest morning was January 20th, the mercury standing at 18°; the coldest noon was January 20th, 36°; the coldest evening was January 20th, 24°.

"The warmest morning was July 23d, 78°; warmest noon, July 8th, 98°; warmest evening, July 15th, 80°.

"On January 14th, at 8 A. M., the barometer was 29.12, and on December 10th it stood at 29.90 all day. These were the extremes during the year.

"There were only 67 cloudy and rainy days in the year; the remaining 298 days were clear and cloudless.

"The whole amount of rain during the year was 19.2 inches."

5. The report by Dr. Brown, of the Bloomingdale Asylum, for 1855, is circumscribed by very narrow limits, furnishing to the medical reader but little of interest, other than the numerical results for the year:—

	Men.	Women.	Total.
Patients in the Asylum, Jan. 1, 1855	50	77	127
Admitted in the course of the year	59	48	107
Whole number " " "	109	125	234
Discharged, including deaths	53	54	107
Remaining, Jan. 1, 1856	56	71	127
Of those discharged, there were cured	27	25	52
Died	14	5	19

"Five patients died within a week after arrival, and two others within twenty days. The various deaths may be referred to pulmonary consumption in *two* cases; to epileptic apoplexy in *one;* to serous apoplexy in *one;* to gradual decay incident to some forms of insanity, in *three* cases; to disease of the kidneys in *one;* to suicide in *two;* to general paralysis in *four*, and to exhaustive mania in *five*.

"Two persons who had long been supported here by the Trustees of the Sailors' Snug Harbor, being unobjectionable as inmates of their institution on Staten Island, were removed thither. One of them had been domiciliated here more than thirty years. Besides several of his contemporaries, there still remain four who antedates his admission from eight to fifteen years. All of these, after passing from forty-one to forty-eight years in the institution, continue in good physical health, witnesses to the salubrity of this region."

When passing under review the report of the Bloomingdale Asylum, for 1854, we remarked, in effect, that since the enlargement of the "lodges," and the introduction of the new system of heating and ventilation, this institution has few equals in the United States, in regard to the physical comforts surrounding the patients. We were at that time under the impression that the method of heating by steam had been introduced into the principal edifices, as well as the lodges. This, however, has not been done. On a recent visit to the Asylum, we found the old system of heating that edifice by furnaces still retained. In this respect, then, the assertion above-mentioned is incorrect; and therein the institution is far behind many others, especially as there are no flues leading the warm air into the dormitories. This defect supplied, the assertion holds good.

It will be observed that our remark applied—and intentionally so—to physical comforts alone. Let us follow this suggestion. The Bloomingdale Asylum was one of the first institutions established upon this side of the Atlantic for the special custody and curative treatment of the insane. Its founders, the Governors of the New York Hospital, were actuated by an enlarged and enlightened philanthropy, which will ever command the admiration of all to whom it shall be known. They prosecuted their work with a zeal worthy of all commendation and imitation. Their idea of the proper Lunatic Asylum was in advance of their times. They were gifted with a prescience of which the building erected by their direction remains a monumental witness. No other structure for similar purposes, erected at so early a period in this country, approaches by far so nearly, in most respects, to the idea of the present day.

The establishment went into successful operation. Years passed by, and governors who controlled it rested too long upon their original work. They did not keep progress with that scheme for meliorating the condition of the insane, which, in its career of improvement, acknowledges no parallel in the history of philanthropic science and art. For a long time, comparatively few improvements were introduced into the Asylum, and those generally more tardily than at other institutions of the kind. It is now but twelve years since, from the floors of the patients' rooms in that establishment, between two and three dozens of staples, which had been inserted and used for the purpose of strapping down the patients, were removed.

Since that time, numerous and important improvements have been rapidly adopted and carried into effect; but yet, in many instances, at a later period than elsewhere. At this moment, however, aside from the mentioned defect in heating, the Bloomingdale Asylum stands, in most that Nature can contribute to constitute a beautiful site, and most that Art can perform to embellish it and make it a delightful residence for the insane, with but few equals, scarcely a single rival, in the world. This is much. But it is not everything. Executive authority, in public institutions for the insane, whatever may obtain in other human associations, loses much of its vigor and force by diffusion. Its true vitality consists in concentration. "No man can serve two masters." In order that power may exert its proper influence, the source of that power must be integral. Allegiance and obedience are truly faithful, only when they are yielded to a unit. To produce a harmonious result from the combination of diverse elements, it is necessary that those elements be arranged and adapted, each to the other, with a single eye, and a single hand, or by eyes and hands acting in subordination to a single mind. In recognition of these important truths, the founders of all the recently established American institutions for the insane, each for their particular hospital, have delegated the sole administrative power, both within doors and without, to the Superintendent. The long array of our State institutions, the extremes of which are in Maine and California, are organized, without an exception, upon this principle. Convinced of the superiority of this organization, the Trustees or Directors of some of the older Asylums which were originally conducted upon a different plan, have not long hesitated in the adoption of it. Several years have elapsed since its introduction into the Friends' Asylum, at Frankford (now Philadelphia) and a similar change has recently been made at the Asylum in Columbia, South Carolina. In short, of all the existing institutions devoted exclusively to the insane, throughout our whole country, the Bloomingdale Asylum is the only one which still clings to that relic of the past, a collocation of executive officers, acting nearly independently each of the other. Of these officers, there are three, Physician, Warden, and Matron. None but they who have learned from experience, can comprehend the amount and the variety of the evils which, in its practical operation, flow from this system. We cannot believe that the governors of that institution will long adhere to it. Observation, reason, a knowledge of human nature, the experience and the action of others, all are against them in their persistence in retaining it. Their institution will never attain the position which it ought to hold; it will never rank with several others in the United States; it will never be conducted so well as it might be, until it shall be guided by that integral power which is the essence of that organization which they see fit still to reject.

Intimately allied to the foregoing question, and perhaps second to it in importance of all the principles upon which, alone, an institution for the insane can be conducted in a manner as nearly approaching perfection as human capabilities will permit, there is another, in regard to which we believe that general usage, and the almost unanimous opinion of persons versed in the subject, are in advance of this Asylum. We allude to the propriety of including, among the officers of every public institution of this description, an Assistant Physician.

In the course of the last twelve years, the number of patients in the Bloomingdale Asylum has fluctuated between one hundred and one hundred and fifty. The average for the whole period will not vary materially from one hundred and twenty-five. Other than this institution, there is none in this country, among those which are usually ranked as independent and unmixed establishments, and where there is so large a number of patients, in which the medical staff does not consist of more than one person. The same is true of the continental European institutions. Indeed, throughout the German States, it is believed there is no one that is regularly organized, and that accommodates more than one hundred patients, in which the Superintendent is not aided by *two* Assistant-Physicians. So much for usage; and usage is the practical expression of opinion.

Of all descriptions of public institutions for the invalidate, it may be safely asserted that there are none, in which there is a more urgent necessity for the constant presence of a physician, than there is in a curative hospital for the insane. The visits of the relatives of the patients; the decision in regard to the propriety of interviews between those relatives and patients; the admission of new patients, and the importance of obtaining an accurate history of their cases; the sudden paroxysms of violence which may occur at any moment among the inmates; and, most especially, the attempts at suicide to which every establishment of the kind is continually liable; these, each and all, and more which might be added, testify to the great importance of having official medical assistance to which there may be an immediate resort.

It is not in the nature of things that one man, holding an office like that of superintendent, or physician, to a large public institution, can, at all times, hold himself prepared for immediate obedience to a call upon his time and his services, within the precincts of that institution. Should any man attempt it, it must be through a sacrifice of his own health. This is not to be asked, not to be expected, from any one. It is not the duty of any one, how benevolent or how philanthropic soever he may be. The institution, therefore, which is under the care of but one physician, must, at times, be devoid of medical assistance.

But at the Bloomingdale Asylum, the contract with the physician has always contained, if we mistake not, the stipulation of absence, after the morning visit to the patients, one day in every week. Now, if the only medical officer of an institution may have leave of absence from the premises, after his morning visit, on *one* day in the week, why not, in pursuance of the same principle, on *two* days? And if the privilege be granted for *two* days, wherefore not for *three*, or *four*, or *five*, or, in short, for the whole hebdomad? Just how far does the principle hold good? Where is the line at which it fails?

It is believed that every one who fully understands the nature of a hospital for the insane, will not fail to perceive that, in its default of an assistant-physician, the institution in question exhibits a second defect, which must be remedied before it can take its stand in the foremost rank of its American compeers.

Where shall we find an irrefutable argument in favour of the principles and practice which we have thus briefly, and but too feebly, advocated? Look over our various establishments for the insane. Which are the most flourishing, the most generally known for their superiority, the most nearly perfect in all the details of medical and moral treatment? We answer, and answer proudly as truthfully, it is those in which the executive power is vested solely in the Superintendent; those in which that officer is the least untrammeled by superior authority; in which his time is not regulated by antecedent negotiation, but in which he is left at liberty to use it, as a conscientious man should use it in his position, agreeably to the exigencies of the moment; those in which his absence is compensated by an efficient assistant, in which it is practically acknowledged that he more fully understands the wants and the necessities of the patients than it is possible for any other person officially connected with the institution to understand them; and in which his suggestions, derived from experience, observation, reading, or his own inventive talent, have been the most generally adopted, and the most cheerfully and immediately carried into effect. We cannot justly close these remarks without acknowledging our belief that Dr. Brown, of the Bloomingdale Asylum, is eminently worthy of precisely such a position. We hope to see him, ere long, in the enjoyment of it.

6. The report by Dr. Butler, of the Retreat for the Insane, at Hartford, Conn., makes the following exhibition of the movement of the patients of that institution:—

	Men.	Women.	Total.
Number of patients, March 31, 1854	89	97	186
Admitted in the course of the year	69	100	169
Whole number " " "	158	197	355
Discharged, including deaths	73	89	162
Remaining, March 31, 1855	85	108	193
Of those discharged, there were cured	26	47	73
Died	9	8	17

Causes of Death.—Exhaustion and general debility, 7; diarrhœa, 2; consumption, 2; paralysis, 2; old age, 1; apoplexy, 1; general paralysis, 1; "disease of the stomach," 1.

Whole number of patients, from April 1, 1824	2804
Discharged recovered	1404
Died	282

"The large number of female patients admitted into the Retreat for the past few years," remarks Dr. Butler, "is worthy of notice. This is too marked to be considered a mere casualty. During the past year, 31 more females than males were admitted, and nearly as many (though mostly from other States) were rejected for want of room. The character of the cases admitted may be seen from the fact that, of the recoveries, nearly two to one were females. The daily average of excess of females over males, for the year, has been 27. For the twenty years from 1824 to 1844, there were admitted 692 males and 635 females, or an excess of 57 males. During the past ten years, there have been admitted 587 males and 785 females, or an excess of 198 of the latter."

There is probably no institution for the insane which has been in operation for any considerable time, that has not suffered, to some extent, from unjust and injurious reports of the treatment of its patients. After remarking that he knows not that the conductors of the Retreat have been more annoyed in this manner than those of other institutions having no legal authority to retain their patients, Dr. Butler arrives at the following conclusion: "I see no other remedy for this trouble but to continue our unwearied vigilance in the enforcement of the wise and humane rules you (the Directors) have adopted for the care and treatment of the insane, and to wait patiently for the time when the love of the marvellous shall cease to invest everything connected with a lunatic asylum with an unreal mystery, and (people) shall put more confidence in the full and frequent inspection of candid, sane and intelligent persons, than in the honest delusion of half-cured patients, or in the revengeful misrepresentations of discharged attendants."

The Retreat was, if we mistake not, the fifth public institution for the insane established in the United States. In its early history it attained a widely-extended, and, undoubtedly, well-merited celebrity. During the administration of Dr. Butler, the buildings have been much enlarged, and all the means for successful treatment greatly improved. But none of its earlier improvements contributed more towards making it a complete establishment than the "Lodge" for the violent female patients, which was finished in the autumn of 1854. This building combines all the modern conveniences of heating, ventilation, and baths, together with such advantages of arrangement as may have been suggested to the mind of Dr. Butler, in the course of a tour of observation to the recently-erected edifices for the insane in England. The rooms for patients—a class formerly, and, but too frequently, still placed in "cells"—are 11 feet high, 11 in length, and 8 in width, and they have a hall of reunion, or parlor, 28 feet by 16.

"The system for heating and ventilation," remarks Dr. B., "has more than equalled my most sanguine expectations. We are enabled by it to maintain, at all conditions of the atmosphere, a free and abundant ventilation of each and every room, while any one or all of the rooms can be kept at the temperature of any degree of heat, rising from that of the external air to seventy or eighty degrees. All offensive effluvia from the close-stools is by the same system of ventilation prevented from rising into the room, by being carried downward into the foul-air flue, in the cellar. The rooms are spacious and cheerful, so constructed as to admit of easy supervision, and yet also of entire seclusion from the unnecessary observation of other patients or of any one else." The construction of the building is explained by several engravings of ground-plan and sectional views, at the beginning of the report.

7. The "Asylum for the Relief of Persons deprived of the Use of their Reason," is now, through the recent action of the municipal authorities, within the limits of the city of Philadelphia. Its thirty-seventh annual report exhibits the following movement of its population during the fiscal year ending on the 1st of March, 1854:—

	Men.	Women.	Total.
Patients at the beginning of the year .	30	26	56
Admitted in course of the year . .	20	20	40
Whole number " " " . .	50	46	96
Discharged, including deaths . .			39
Remaining, at the close of the year .			57
Of those discharged, there were cured .			15
Died			8

Causes of Death.—Suffocation, 1; marasmus, 1; dysentery, 1; disease of brain, 2; pneumonia, 1; general paralysis, 1; epilepsy, 1.

Dr. Worthington relates several cases of recovery, from which we select one of the most interesting.

"A middle-aged man, a carpenter by trade, for about twelve years had been a constant source of anxiety and distress to his friends. He was under treatment for nearly a year before any signs of improvement were manifested, at the end of which time he was induced to take a part in the labour of the patients in the garden. He soon began to improve, and to show a desire for regular employment. He was then taken to the carpenter's shop, and work put into his hands which he took pride in doing in the best manner. After a period of probation, he was regularly discharged, and has now been employed, for nearly a year, as carpenter to the Institution; is active, industrious, and rational, earning for himself a respectable living, and is altogether a very valuable member of our Asylum community."

Treating of the causes of mental alienation, the Dr. says that "a fruitful source of insanity is the neglect of that kind of training which, at the period when the mind is most capable of receiving them, aims at the inculcation of those principles of religion and morality, and the formation of those habits of self-control, which are the surest safeguards against the evils of life. How often do we see children indulged by their parents in every whim and caprice, or permitted to follow their own inclinations, until their self-will gains such an ascendency that finally the restraints, not less of moral principle than of parental authority, are entirely set aside. * * * * These evils are greatly augmented by the reading of works of fiction—often of a positively immoral tendency—by which the imagination is fostered at the expense of the reason and judgment, and the sentiments and passions stimulated to undue activity. False ideas of men and things are thus engendered, in consequence of which individuals thus placed in a kind of opposition to the realities about them, become suspicious and misanthropic, and often fall victims to insanity.

"Of a somewhat similar character is the neglect of training the young to habits of industry in the pursuit of some occupation by which they may be able, without undue care and anxiety, to provide for themselves a maintenance, and secure a respectable position in society. How many young men are there whose parents, desiring for them some easier way than what they have themselves walked in, send them from the workshop or the farm, to throng the various professions, in the delusive hope that they will thus be able to earn their bread without the sweat of their face. How large a number of these are sure to meet with disappointment; and, becoming disheartened and dispirited, lose the mental and physical energy they once possessed, and fall into a state of hypochondriasis or melancholy; or, if successful, how many are induced by the desire of wealth or pre-eminence, and in the excitement resulting from the fluctuations of trade, to overtask their brains, until, worn out by excessive and long-continued application, this organ becomes incurably or fatally diseased. * * * * The history of cases which have been sent to the Asylum within the last few years, shows an increasing number of patients who are rendered insane by the causes which have been thus briefly depicted."

The thirty-eighth annual report is embellished with two new and beautifully executed engravings, apparently upon steel. One represents a front view of the Asylum; the other a bird's-eye view of the garden and library. A third plate shows the ground-plan of the Asylum.

The largest number of patients in the course of the fiscal year was 73; smallest number, 57; monthly average, 64⅝, which we believe is the largest in the annals of this Institution.

	Men.	Women.	Total.
Patients, March 1, 1854	26	31	57
Admitted in course of the year . .	15	27	42
Whole number " " " . .	41	58	99
Discharged, including deaths . .			40
Remaining, March 1, 1855 . . .			59
Of those discharged, there were cured .			17
Died			8

One who was discharged much improved, recovered soon after.

Causes of Death.—Marasmus, 1; diarrhœa, 3; paralysis, 1; phthisis, 1; old age, 1; inanition, 1.

Two of the persons who died had been in the Asylum about five years, one nine years, and two about twenty years. Two were between 40 and 50 years of age, one between 50 and 60, two between 60 and 70, two between 70 and 80, and one between 80 and 90. These few statistics furnish no argument in favour of the idea—probably a correct one—that insanity abbreviates human life.

The largely predominating number of women over that of men, among the patients, will be noticed. It is remarked that the highest number of the former, in the course of the year, was 43; that of the latter, 30.

Dr. Worthington remarks that "at one time insanity was commonly regarded as the effect of an inflammatory condition of the brain and its membranes, and consequently the disease was much more actively treated than would now be considered necessary or proper; yet we still occasionally meet with cases in which it has been aggravated, and rendered much more difficult of cure, by the injudicious use of exhausting remedies."

In his remarks upon treatment, he says "the female patients, of all classes, enjoy the benefit of healthful daily recreation, in pleasant weather, on the extensive grounds containing thirty acres of lawn and woodlands, laid out with walks which, being sheltered from the rays of the sun, afford a delightful place of resort in warm weather. Within doors they are engaged in sewing, knitting, and other suitable occupations; and during the past few weeks have made up more than a hundred garments for the destitute poor, the materials having been kindly furnished by benevolent individuals in the city. The library continues to be resorted to, daily, by the convalescent and quiet. * * * * It is situated at the end of the garden, in the midst of a pleasant lawn which is planted with shrubbery and ornamental trees. It is fitted up with cases containing a neat collection of stuffed birds and animals, minerals, shells, corals,

&c., and a library of about five hundred volumes. The books are used, by all the patients who desire the privilege, in their own rooms. * * * * I may mention, as an evidence of the interest that has been manifested by the patients in mental occupation, a weekly periodical called *The Pearl*, which was issued by one of them, with such assistance as he could procure in the family, during a part of the past year. It was well filled with original and selected matter—the contributions of the patients and their friends—and illustrated with neatly executed drawings, by one of the former. A few have taken considerable interest in the subject of phonography; and one has made such progress in the study, as to be able to read it with facility. * * * * The amusements with which they have heretofore been furnished, such as exhibitions with the magic lantern, games and puzzles of different kinds, have been continued during the past year."

P. E.

ART. XXI.—*Hints on the Medical Examination of Recruits for the Army, and on the Discharge of Soldiers from the Service on Surgeon's Certificate. Adapted to the Service of the United States.* By THOMAS HENDERSON, M. D., Assistant Surgeon, U. S. Army, late Professor of the Theory and Practice of Medicine in Columbian College, D. C., etc. A new edition, revised, by RICHARD H. COOLIDGE, M. D., Assistant Surgeon U. S. Army. 12mo. pp. 211. Philadelphia, 1856. Lippincott & Co.

THE first edition of these hints was received with marked favour. They were acknowledged, by those for whose instruction they were mainly intended, as an excellent compendium of the important and responsible duties of the Army surgeon, in the passing of recruits, and the discharge of soldiers from the service on account of ill health or physical disability.

Dr. Henderson was qualified in an eminent degree for the preparation of a work of the character of the one before us, as well from the extent of his general medical acquirements, as from the experience he had acquired as a medical officer of the army, during upwards of twenty years of faithful service. Previously to his death, which happened two years ago, he was engaged in the preparation of the present improved and enlarged edition, which has received a further revision at the hands of Dr. Coolidge, and is published in accordance with the known wish of the author.

The work, though primarily intended for the use of the army surgeon, cannot fail, however, to interest and instruct the medical practitioner whose sphere of duties is circumscribed within the limits of civic life. He may be called upon to certify to the freedom from disease or from any marked predisposition to disease, in applicants for life insurance or annuity, or in candidates for admission into beneficial societies, and from the volume of Dr. Henderson he may find a few useful hints to direct him in his examination. Nor is the physician, in his course of civic practice, entirely exempt from occasions when his judgment may be demanded to detect feigned from real disease or infirmity. Cases occasionally happen in which disease or infirmity is assumed to obtain exemption from service on juries, or the cancelling of indentures by apprentices; to impose on beneficial associations, or to enjoy the benefits conferred by charitable institutions. In such cases the work before us will assist him in his examination.

There is a curious circumstance connected with the subject of feigned disease which is not noticed by Dr. Henderson, it having no immediate connection with either of the questions discussed by him. We allude to a disposition that is occasionally met with in individuals to represent themselves as the subjects of some strange and anomalous malady. We do not allude to those instances of monomania in which the patients actually imagine themselves to be labouring under certain diseases of which they present no symptoms, but where much trouble and occasionally some ingenuity is practised to invent circumstances confirmatory of the malady under which they pretend to labour. We have met with instances in which persons pretended that they passed daily an amount of sabulous matter by the skin, or large masses of lime per urethram, or that they vomited insects, or voided small animals from the bowels, and carefully invented the circumstances which they supposed necessary to confirm their statements. In none of these cases have we been able to detect any other motive for the deception than a desire, perhaps, in the individuals to render themselves objects of wonder and attention. They neither solicited alms, nor ceased to follow their ordinary occupations, by which one or more of them supported their family quite comfortably. They were all very ignorant persons, of weak intellects, and extremely credulous. D. F. C.

Art. XXII.—*Des Phénomènes de Contraction Musculaire observés chez des Individus qui sont Succombé à la suite du Cholera ou de la Fièvre Jaune.* Par George Henry Brandt, M. D. Thèse pour le Doctorat en Médecine, presentée et soutenue à la Faculté de Médecine de Paris, le 21 Août, 1855. 4to. pp. 46. Paris, 1855.

On the Cause of the Muscular Contraction observed in the Bodies of those who die of Cholera and Yellow Fever. By G. H. Brandt, M. D. A thesis presented to the Faculty of Medicine of Paris for the Degree of Doctor in Medicine.

The muscular movements which are often observed to occur after death in the bodies of those who have fallen victims to the cholera or yellow fever, would appear to be of a special character; they are unquestionably of a different character from those we observe at the moment of death, as well as from those which occasionally take place upon the occurrence of the cadaveric rigidity.

Although the occurrence of very marked muscular contractions of the limbs and even of the trunk, after death from cholera, is noticed by many of those who have described the disease during its wide epidemic spread since the year 1818, and the same phenomenon is stated to have been frequently observed after death from yellow fever, by writers of unquestionable authority, no one appears to have attempted to explain the cause of its occurrence, or even to examine into the particular circumstances under which it usually, or invariably takes place. It was not until the year 1849, that this phenomenon attracted any further attention, than the simple record of its not unfrequent occurrence, when Dr. Brown-Séquard first pointed out some of the leading circumstances which favour its manifestation, and subsequently attempted to explain its nature and cause. The observations made by this gentleman in 1854, in the large cholera hospital of the Island Maurice, of which he had the sole charge, have, he assures us, furnished him with additional proofs of the correctness of the views originally advanced by him five years previously.

According to Dr. B.-Séquard, the muscular movements referred to are always restricted to cases in which the individuals, of great physical vigour, have died within twenty-four hours from the commencement of the attack of cholera, and without having experienced paroxysms of cramp sufficiently violent or numerous to exhaust muscular irritability. The three circumstances, therefore, which, according to his observations, favour the production of muscular movements in the dead from cholera, are—

1. Strongly developed muscular force.
2. Short duration of the disease.
3. Absence of cramps, or, when present, slight or of short duration.

All these circumstances being united, the muscular movements after death are the most marked. Most frequently two only of them occur, namely, the first and second. It is seldom, indeed, that robust individuals are attacked with severe choleric symptoms, without the occurrence of violent cramp, but as in these cases death occurs early, the cramp, though severe, does not last sufficiently long to exhaust the muscular irritability. Occasionally the movements after death are observed in bodies with but moderately developed muscles, but only in cases in which the duration of the disease has been very short. The rapid occurrence of death is considered by Dr. B. S. as the circumstance most favourable to the occurrence of muscular contractions in the corpse. It is, he considers, essential that the muscles should retain after death, a considerable amount of irritability. This irritability, when not exhausted by long continued disease or poisoning, attended by violent and lingering convulsions, continues in the dead body much longer than is generally supposed. In two criminals, observed carefully by Dr. B. S., he observed it to be apparent in the one, thirteen, and in the other fourteen hours after decapitation. Under the same circumstances, we know that Nysten had in one instance known it to continue for twenty-six hours after death.

The duration of muscular irritability in the dead body being in inverse proportion to the extent to which it has been exhausted during life, it is to be concluded, therefore, that the muscular movements so often observed after death from cholera, will take place only in cases where the disease has been of short duration and has not had time to wear out the irritability of the muscular system.

"It may be objected," Dr. B. remarks, "to the position that there exists a direct relation between the muscular energy of the patient, and the duration of the movements which occur after death, that it is precisely in individuals of great bodily vigour, the disease is attended by cramps of extreme violence, which always exhaust muscular irritability. If it be objected, that as it is necessary for the existence of the movements after death, the muscles should still retain a large amount of their irritability, it would be impossible for these movements to be observed in the bodies of such as have had cramps, the answer is very easily given; in individuals of great bodily vigour, when the cramps have lasted for twenty-four hours, no movements occur after death; even when the cramps have existed for a few hours only, the movements observed after death are but slight in the muscles that had been the seat of cramp, while in the other muscles they may be very considerable."

The persistence of a large amount of irritability in the muscles being assumed as the condition necessary for the occurrence of the movements that take place in the bodies of those who have fallen victims to cholera; Dr. B. S. supposes that the exciting cause of these movements is the accumulation of carbonic acid in the blood and muscular tissue. He believes that, besides this, it is probable that there exists another agent which, during the epidemic prevalence of cholera, is generated in the blood and by its action on the spinal chord, or upon the muscles, produces the cramps characteristic of that disease, as well, perhaps, those also of which individuals, within the sphere of the epidemic influence, but not labouring under cholera, are often the subjects.

That carbonic acid is an excitant of the nerves and muscles, is shown by the sourish and pungent taste imparted to the tongue, when fluids strongly charged with carbonic acid gas are swallowed. Its action upon the nasal mucous membrane is evidenced by the well-known pungent sensation it excites in the nerves of this part when eructation occurs after drinking mineral water, beer, or champagne.

Wharton Jones has shown that in causing a current of carbonic gas to pass into the lungs of a frog, the bloodvessels contract, the blood globules become united to each other and adhere to the parietes of the vessels; upon arresting the current of gas the circulation resumes its normal condition; now these are precisely the phenomena that occur when the bloodvessels are subjected to galvanism, as the brothers Weber have shown.

Dr. B.-Séquard adapted to the trachea of an animal recently dead, of which the lungs had collapsed upon opening the thorax, a tube, the other extremity of which was connected with the body of a syringe. By retracting the piston of the latter the air contained in the lungs of the animal was removed, and then a quantity of carbonic acid, equal in amount to the air extracted, was slowly injected into the trachea. The flame of a candle being now brought opposite to the outer orifice of the tube was blown aside by the jet of gas coming from the lungs. The jet is produced by a contraction of the bronchi resulting from the contraction excited in them by the carbonic acid, as may be proved by substituting hydrogen or nitrogen gas for the carbonic acid, neither of which will excite the bronchi to contract, and consequently no jet from the lungs can be detected after they have been injected.

The heart of a frog removed for some minutes from the body, and contracting, in the atmospheric air, some 25 to 30 times in the minute, was placed in an atmosphere of carbonic acid. Almost immediately its pulsations increased to 40, 50, or even 60 in the minute.

From these facts it is evident that carbonic acid is an excitant of the nervous system and muscular tissue.

M. Herpin, of Metz, in a recent communication to the Academy of Sciences, thus describes his own experience of the effects of the carbonic acid: "The first impression that is experienced in plunging into a stratum of the gas, is a sensation of mild, agreeable warmth, similar to that produced by a thick clothing of fine wool or wadding; to this there succeeds a peculiar sense of pricking or formication, and, later, a sort of burning that may be compared to that produced by a sinapism when it commences to draw. Pains formerly experienced, especially those from old wounds, are revived; the skin becomes red; an abundant perspiration occurs, which exhibits an acid character on those portions of the surface that are exposed to the action of the gas. The sensation of heat and the perspiration continue during many hours after retiring from the bath. At first, the movements of the heart are but feebly accelerated, but after the immersion in the gas has continued some time, the action of the heart is increased; the pulse becomes full, quick and accelerated; the sensation of heat is more intense, and is attended with turgescence and redness of the skin, headache, oppression of the chest, etc."

Dr. Struve, on exposing his leg to the action of a stratum of carbonic acid gas, experienced, at first, a sense of formication and an agreeable warmth, which augmented until an abundant perspiration broke out over the limb.

M. Boussingault informs us that he experienced, in his own person, similar phenomena to those described by M. Herpin, on exposure to the carbonic acid which is largely disengaged from certain excavations in New Grenada.

"In all cases in which there is an increased quantity of carbonic acid in the blood, there takes place an excitation of the nervous system and of the muscles.

"*a.* In cases of asphyxia, general convulsions develop themselves, and it is evident that in these cases there is a coincidence between the augmentation in the blood of carbonic acid and the excitation of the nervous system and perhaps of the muscles. The convulsions in such cases have been vaguely attributed to a pretended desire for respiration. To show, however, that there is actually a direct excitation of the spinal chord, Dr. Brown-Séquard performed before the Biological Society the following experiment. He divided transversely the chord at the lumbar region, and then asphyxiated the animal. Convulsions ensued as well in the posterior as in the anterior limbs.

"*b.* Dr. Brown-Séquard has ascertained that the irritability augments in the muscles after the section of their nerves, and this augmentation continues to last for several weeks. If a mammiferous animal, in which the sciatic and crural nerves of one of the limbs had been divided ten days previously, be asphyxiated, we find that movements continue to occur in the paralyzed limb for some time after the cessation of general convulsions. This is an important fact, because it shows that in a part where the irritability is augmented, movements are produced, although there is the same condition of the exciting agent as in those parts of the body where the muscular irritability is in its normal state, but in which no movements take place.

"*c.* If we divide the phrenic nerves, the diaphragm ceases to contract rhythmically; upon asphyxiating the animal and destroying the spinal chord in the cervical and dorsal regions, the rhythmical movements of the diaphragm reappear, and only under the direct excitation of that muscle by the blood charged with carbonic acid.

"*d.* The movements which take place in the intestines when we open the abdomen after death, have been attributed to a pretended exciting action of the cold air. Dr. B.-Séquard has shown that the contraction referred to is the result of the excitation of the blood charged with carbonic acid. If, without opening the abdomen, we asphyxiate an animal, very violent movements take place throughout the intestines. If, on the other hand, we lay open freely the abdomen, the intestines will not be found to contract so long as the respiration is unrestrained; on asphyxiating it, however, almost immediately the intestines will commence to contract, and very soon their entire mass will become agitated. Similar experiments show that the same is true in respect to the bladder.

"*e.* If we asphyxiate a female guinea pig about to bring forth, it very often occurs that the uterus contracts and expels its contents. If we open the abdomen of a pregnant rabbit, on the 25th or 28th day of gestation, and expose fully the uterus to the action of the air, there will be found not to occur any contraction of the organ. If now the respiration of the animal be suspended, contractions will be seen to take place in the cornua of the uterus. The impediment to respiration being removed, these contractions will diminish or even cease. Asphyxia being again produced, very violent uterine contractions will again occur and sometimes expel one or more of the fœtuses.

"*f.* Relatively to the heart, the facts observed by Dr. B.-Séquard, and other physiologists, are more numerous, and perhaps still more decisive. When we divide the par vagum on both sides, the respiration diminishes and the quickness of the heart's pulsations increases. When we cut the great sympathetic on both sides, we find, also, that the pulsations of the heart augment in number, but, as R. A. Wagner has shown, to a less extent, and Dr. B.-Séquard has ascertained that in this case, as in the former, respiration is diminished.

"If any one will have the courage to arrest during one minute his respiration, he will find that during the last twenty seconds, the number of the heart's pulsations are more frequent than they were during the twenty seconds preceding the experiment.

"*g.* By injecting into different parts of the body blood charged with carbonic acid the contractile tissue of these parts are thrown into action. If, on the contrary, we inject red blood, or that charged with oxygen and containing little carbonic acid, contractions do not immediately take place, but, at the end of a certain time, when the blood injected has become changed into venous, the movements occur."

Thus having seen from the foregoing facts that the carbonic acid is an excitor agent of the nervous system and the muscles, it follows that, if we find very powerful excitation of these parts in all cases in which there is asphyxia, we have the right to attribute this to the augmentation of carbonic acid in the blood which then occurs.

The explanation proposed by Dr. B.-Séquard of the occurrence of muscular movements in the bodies of those who have died of cholera, is founded upon the two series of facts that we have just passed in review: 1st. The persistence of muscular irritability, in a very high degree, after death, in the cases in which these movements take place; and 2d. In such cases there is a considerable accumulation of carbonic acid in the blood, in other words, the blood has become excessively black, a condition, as has been shown, coexistent with exciting properties of a high grade. Hence, it is only in subjects of strongly developed muscular frames, that have been rapidly destroyed, in a state of asphyxia, that movements are observed after death.

It may be asked, why is it that in the cases referred to, movements occur in certain of the muscles and not in others? To this it is replied, that it is especially in those muscles which have not been, or only partially exhausted by the cramps by which the disease had been attended that the convulsions are observed. Besides, the bloodvessels of certain of the muscles which, during the lifetime of the patient, like those of the skin, were in a state of contraction, at the moment of death, dilate and allow the blood to flow into them, the excitation of which causes them to act.

In explanation of the fact that the muscles which are the seat of the post-mortem movements, cease their actions and resume them at a latter period, it is remarked that the excitor agents of the muscles of animal life are capable of acting, also, upon the muscular fibres of the bloodvessels. Hence, when the muscles of animal life are thrown into action by the carbonic acid, or other exciting agent existing in the blood of those attacked with cholera, their bloodvessels are excited to contraction at the same time, and the blood is, in consequence, expelled from them. Now as this contraction cannot continue for any time, when the cause of excitation is in this manner removed from them, they relax and the blood returns into them again, when, of course, the excitation is renewed.

Why is it that muscular contractions do not occur after death in individuals that have fallen victims to other diseases than cholera and yellow fever?

"We must exclude from the cases in which these contractions are liable to take place all those in which the muscular irritability, either from the long duration of disease, or any other cause, has been greatly diminished before death. It is only in cases in which muscular irritability still persists to a considerable extent at the moment of dissolution that muscular movements present themselves in the dead body. These cases are those in which life has been extinguished by decapitation, submersion, strangulation, certain poisons, etc. But, in all these the second of the two conditions essential for the production of post-mortem muscular movements is wanting, namely, a sufficient quantity of the excitant agent in the blood for the production of those movements. Besides, as has been already remarked, Dr. B.-Séquard considers it probable that there exists in the blood of those affected with cholera or yellow fever a special excitant agent, which is, perhaps, the very poison by which these diseases are produced, or, at least, which is generated by the action of the poison upon the system. It may, however, be replied, that if there exists a special exciting agent in the diseases indicated, it is useless to invoke the action of carbonic acid in the blood, especially as this acid exists in the blood of individuals destroyed by asphyxia, who, also, possess, often, very great muscular irritability, and in whom, nevertheless, no muscular movements occur after death. This objection is easily refuted. In the first place, there is a larger amount of carbonic acid accumulated in the blood of such as fall victims to cholera or yellow fever, than in those destroyed by asphyxia, and the muscular irritability may be equal in both cases; consequently the movements are the result in the one case of an adequate amount of the excitant agent, their absence, in the other, is the result of a deficient amount of this agent. Again, even admitting that no such difference in the amount of carbonic acid exists in the two classes of cases, it merely requires the addition of another exciting cause in the instances in which the post-mortem movements occur, one, namely, special to the diseases after which they are ordinarily observed. Finally, even though it should be shown that this special exciting agent is alone sufficient to give rise to the muscular contractions that occur after death from cholera and yellow fever, it may not be the less true that the carbonic acid accumulated in the blood plays a part in the production of these contractions, inasmuch as it has been shown to be an excitor of the muscles."

We have presented a tolerably full exposition of the views of Dr. B.-Séquard in relation to the cause of the movements observed in the bodies of those who have fallen victims to cholera and yellow fever, as detailed in the thesis of Dr. Brandt. They are ingenious and plausible, while the facts and arguments by which they are supported and illustrated are replete with interest. The position assumed by Dr. B.-Séquard, that, in the cases in which the post-mortem movements are observed, there is an increased irritability of the muscles, Dr. Brandt pronounces to be certainly not sustainable, and we think that in this he is correct, for it is extremely improbable that an increased irritability of the muscles can occur after diseases in which the normal condition of the blood is so greatly changed, and where especially its amount of oxygen is so notably diminished.

D. F. C.

Art. XXIII. *Varicose Veins; their Nature, Consequences, and Treatment, Palliative and Curative.* By Henry T. Chapman, F. R. C. S., formerly Surgeon to the St. George's and St. James's Dispensary, and sometime Lecturer on Surgery at the School of Medicine adjoining St. George's Hospital. London: John Churchill. 1856.

In the monograph before us, a reprint of several articles which have already appeared in the *Medical Times and Gazette*, the author publishes his experience and views relative to the curability of varicose veins. The chapters on his treatment are prefixed by a general survey of the pathology of varix, and by a review of the methods of cure hitherto adopted.

Varix, Mr. Chapman defines to be "every—the smallest—dilatation of the vessel, whereby its caliber is increased to a degree which may augment unduly the influence of gravitation in retarding the blood's current, or which may render the valves inefficient." The sources of obstruction to the saphenic current are considered in detail, and the views of Sir Benjamin Brodie, relative to the superficial veins being alone the seat of the disease, are substantiated. We would remind our readers, however, that this fact has recently been denied by M. Verneuil, of Paris, who affirms that the deep muscular veins are always affected synchronously with the superficial ones; and that they even may be diseased without the latter being at all involved.

The general and local predisposing causes of varix form a most interesting section in Mr. Chapman's book. As the most powerful and constant of the latter, he enumerates the presence of subacute or chronic inflammation. This fact he considers as not having been enunciated with sufficient distinctness heretofore. In the summing up of the causes of varix, we find the following passage: "In estimating the comparative influence of mechanical and constitutional causes in the production of the disease, the foregoing details will, I think, indicate sufficiently the share borne by each, namely, that whereas the former are often powerful enough alone to generate it, in the majority of cases they would not be competent to originate dilatation unless certain conditions of the venous tissues preparatory thereto already existed. The first may be immediate and active in their operation, the others are remote and predisposing; but it is to the combination of the two causes that varicosity is ordinarily due."

In part second of the work, Mr. Chapman considers the palliative and curative treatment of the disease. The curative treatment of varix, he pertinently remarks, has hitherto been conducted more with a view to the obliteration of the vessel, than with regard to the re-establishment of its circulatory function. Such an object our writer deprecates, assuming, it seems to us with justice, that even were such an object accomplished, it could not properly be called a cure, inasmuch as a compensating increase in the caliber of collateral vessels must ensue, and the result be simply a change as to the locality of the disease. All operative interference in the treatment of varix, Mr. Chapman positively discards, whether it be by subcutaneous section, by ligature, or by the application of caustic to the veins. His reasons for so doing are twofold. In the first place, he alleges the danger of extensive phlebitis; and secondly, he affirms that even should no danger from phlebitis ensue, every operation hitherto devised fails in the great majority of cases in accomplishing the object in view; for he remarks, "The authors of such proposals too often overlook the circumstance that *permanent* obliteration can only be effected by a high degree of phlebitis; and consequently that the ultimate success of these attempts must always be directly proportionate to the risk incurred; and that, in the same degree in which they contrive to diminish it, the chances of cure will also be lessened."

In the pages devoted to the palliative treatment of varix, the author considers the application of the ordinary laced stocking, and whilst admitting its efficacy in the earlier stages of the disease, or during pregnancy, he still thinks that little in the way of a permanent cure is to be hoped for through its agency.

The main object, however, of the publication seems to us to be to bring before the profession the treatment of varix adopted by the author, and which he denominates curative. This treatment by wet strapping and bandaging, Mr. Chapman considers as applicable to the disease in three stages. First, to simple uniform varix—the ordinary plaster strapping he asserts is, under certain circumstances, inconvenient, heating to the skin, apt to produce excoriation, and preventive of the application of lotions. These unfavourable results Mr. Chapman obviates by using instead of plaster, a bandage of linen resembling the ordinary bandage of Scultetus. This being soaked in cold water, is applied so as to envelop the limb from the sole of the foot to the knee. Over this bandage of strips a roller bandage is applied, and the whole directed to be kept continually moist. The advantages possessed by the application of wet straps are asserted to be, the exertion of an even, equable compression, the absence of all danger of excoriation, and the great permeability of the apparatus to the passage of fluids.

In cases of long standing, vesicular, or sacculated varix, the same general method is recommended, with the addition of firm compresses of lint upon each venous cluster. Should the varix be complicated by the occurrence of inflammation, the employment of the usual antiphlogistic local and constitutional remedies is advised, combined with the wet strapping and bandaging.

At the termination of the work a series of selected cases are introduced, in support of the views and treatment previously enunciated.

In conclusion, we cannot lay aside this modest little monograph, without testifying to the pleasure we have derived from its perusal. We regard it as a useful and practical contribution to the study of the pathology and treatment of an affection, troublesome and vexatious both to surgeon and patient.

J. H. B.

Art. XXIV.—*A Review of the Present State of Uterine Pathology.* By James Henry Bennet, M. D., &c. &c., 8vo. pp. 76. Philadelphia, 1856: Blanchard & Lea.

The leading object of this review is to sustain the correctness of the views in reference to uterine pathology, advanced by the author, originally in the *London Lancet*, and subsequently, more fully developed and enforced in his work on inflammation of the uterus, its cervix and appendages, by the results of his own subsequent experience, the facts adduced by others, and the admissions of those by whom the validity of his views are denied. He examines at the same time, the objections that have been brought against these views, and the opinions respecting uterine pathology generally that clash with them.

The doctrine, that to inflammation of the mucous membrane, or of the proper tissue of the neck or body of the uterus, with its varied sequelæ, are to be referred the great majority of instances of confirmed uterine suffering that come under the observation of the medical practitioner, although when first announced by Dr. B., favourably received by a few, was by the more authoritative of the profession, opposed and rejected. The number by whom it has been since adopted, and acted upon in the treatment of permanent functional derangements of the uterine organs, and the general conditions of dyspepsia, debility, and morbid cerebro-spinal innervation by which these are usually attended, has greatly increased—including some of the most distinguished members of the profession in America as well as in Europe—still, however, there are not a few of equal eminence, from whom the doctrine receives but little or no support.

It is a curious circumstance, that upon a question which would appear to be one easily solved by a series of cautious observations, there should continue to exist so wide a discrepancy of opinion among the members of the medical profession. That while, with Dr. Bennet, many refer to inflammation and inflammatory lesions of the uterus as the primary cause of most of those forms of confirmed vital and functional uterine derangement described under the names of leucorrhœa, amenorrhœa, dysmenorrhœa, menorrhagia. &c. &c., others deny entirely the existence of inflammatory and ulcerative lesions of the neck of the uterus as the cause of uterine functional diseases and the usual train of general symptoms by which these are attended; while others, again, who admit that the lesions of the cervix and body of the uterus, ascribed by Dr. Bennet to inflammation, are of frequent or occasional occurrence, differ from him as to their causes, symptoms, and pathological importance, and deny that they exercise the influence over the general health that he has ascribed to them.

These several views of uterine pathology in opposition to, or in discordance with, the doctrines he advocates, Dr. Bennet has submitted to a very concise but satisfactory review, in which he has shown either their want of correspondence with well established facts, or their origin in partial or erroneous deductions from correct premises.

In his review of the very able Croonian Lectures of Dr. West, "on the pathological importance of ulceration of the uteri," Dr. B. remarks:—

"The key to Dr. West's lectures, the explanation of the frame of mind under the influence of which his researches were carried out, and the *résumé* of the results to which they have led him, are to be found in a paragraph at the foot of page 27, which runs as follows: 'The really important question is, whether ulceration of the os uteri is to be regarded as the first in a train of processes which are the direct or indirect occasion of by far the greater number of the ailments of the generative system, or whether, on the other hand, it is to be considered as a condition of slight pathological importance, and of small semeiological value—a casual concomitant, perhaps, of many disorders of the womb, but of itself giving rise to few symptoms, and rarely calling for special treatment?' The first part of this paragraph may be considered a concise statement of the views Dr. West attributes to his antagonists, of the scientific error he thinks he has to encounter. The second part may be considered a concise enunciation of the opinions with which he rises from the investigation.

"Dr. West wrestles with an imaginary enemy—combats a foe of his own creation. No pathologist, to my knowledge, at home or abroad, has described ulceration of the os uteri as a morbid entity—as a disease existing *per se*. On the contrary, all who have written on the subject have spoken of ulceration, and described it as a result of the inflammation which invariably, necessarily, precedes and accompanies it, and which may exist without it for years, in the uterus as elsewhere. Dr. West has been apparently misled by the discussion to which Dr. Lee's extraordinary assertions gave rise. Dr. Lee, in his anxiety to crush the modern views of uterine pathology, boldly denied the existence of ulceration. He thereby thought to destroy doctrines which announced inflammation and inflammatory lesions as of constant occurrence, and ulceration as the most frequent secondary lesion of all, and the one that more especially necessitates instrumental interference. Thence it was that the discussion took place on this one point: Is there, or is there not such a condition as ulceration? Thence, also, I presume, the origin of Dr. West's error in thinking that his antagonists impute to ulceration alone all the pathological influences which they ascribe in reality to inflammation and to inflammatory lesions generally. At least, I can say, most assuredly, that I have never in my writings for a moment attempted such a separation. If Dr. West will substitute in the paragraph I have quoted, the words 'inflammation of the neck and body of the uterus and their sequelæ,' for the words 'ulceration of the os uteri,' I will accept his proposition as a true exposition of my opinions; but as long as it remains as it is, I cannot possibly thus accept it.

"This fundamental error, made at the very threshold of Dr. West's inquiry, appears to me to thoroughly negative its value. It has induced him to establish a comparison, which runs throughout his essay, and on which his statistical tables are based, between two groups of patients who, in reality, do not admit of being compared. This is at once apparent, when we reflect that one group contains 125 females, presenting inflammatory ulceration of the cervix, and the other group 110, who present morbid uterine conditions, by far the greater part of which are also the result of inflammation."

"I cannot myself see what scientific advantage can possibly accrue from the minute comparison of the symptoms, local and general, presented by 125 women having ulcerated uteri, and by 110 women in whom the cervix uteri is not ulcerated, it is true, but who are mostly suffering from other modes of manifestation of the same inflammatory disease. It can only make confusion worse confounded, and so far from clearing up the subject, involve it in impenetrable darkness. Indeed, to me it appears incomprehensible that a pathologist of Dr. West's powers of observation and analysis, should, in studying a disease, have thus isolated one of its morbid conditions; should have laboriously compared the cases in which it is present, with those of the same generic nature in which it is absent, and because he could find no real substantial difference between them, have denied its pathological importance."

Notwithstanding the pathological character, relations, and value of ulceration of the cervix uteri may, by Dr. Bennet and many others, be correctly estimated, it is very certain that there are not a few practitioners who view this condition of the uterine orifice as the primary and sole cause of all the local and uterine symptoms, as well as of the disordered states of the chylopoietic viscera, of the nutritive and assimilative functions, and of the cerebro-spinal system, indicated by dyspepsia, debility, anæmia, hysteria, &c., they may detect in the female patients who apply to them for advice. Whenever such symptoms are present ulceration of the os uteri is diagnosed, the speculum is introduced to obtain a confirmation of that diagnosis, and the local application of caustic promptly employed to cure the ulceration, and in this manner, to relieve all the symptoms of diseased action under which the patient may happen to labour. How often the diagnosis is erroneous in these cases we need not inquire. We have reason to believe that ulceration of the os uteri is more often inferred than actually detected, and caustic applied often when its effects are rather injurious than beneficial; certainly without any very decided relief of the proper uterine symptoms, and the general indications of impaired health by which these are attended.

The views of uterine pathology entertained by Dr. Bennet appear to us to be, in the main, correct, and to be sustained by the observations of those who under the most favourable circumstances, have carefully studied the phenomena and progress of the several morbid conditions of the uterus and its appendages. The treatment based upon these views, so far as our own experience extends, is unquestionably the one best adapted for the removal of uterine diseases, when judiciously applied and carried out.

It is to be recollected that Dr. Bennet ranks ulceration of the os uteri as one of the results of inflammation, and the one which more especially calls for instrumental interference; whether he has overrated the frequency of ulceration of this part is a question that can only be settled by an extended series of observations. To dispute the propriety of his applying the term ulceration to certain denuded pus secreting patches often met with upon the os and cervix uteri as the result of inflammation, would be a discussion as to words and not as to facts. Dr. Tyler Smith, who at first denied the proper ulcerative character of the patches referred to, has, in a more recent work, recognized them as true superficial ulcerations.

The most interesting portion of Dr. Bennet's review is the fifth chapter, in which he discusses the opinion entertained by those who refer to displacements of the uterus as the principal and often sole cause of uterine disturbance and the suffering attendant upon it. This opinion Dr. B. repudiates entirely. To show its untenableness he directs attention to the smallness of size and lightness of weight of the uterus; to the great laxity of its means of support and fixity; to the extreme mobility which it consequently evinces, to the ease with which it obeys many physiological causes of displacement to which it is subjected, and to the complete immunity from pain, or even inconvenience, with which these displacements are borne. Like all the other viscera, the uterus is capable of bearing, without inconvenience, any amount of displacement compatible with its means of fixity, and any amount of pressure to which it can be subjected by the proximity and functional activity of surrounding organs. This capability of our organs to bear considerable pressure without inconvenience is not only observed in the temporary physiological conditions described, but is also found to exist under the permanent pathological pressure of non-inflammatory morbid growths, such as tumours, aneurisms, &c.

Having thus shown that mere displacement of the uterus and the pressure to which it is, in consequence, subjected, is not, as a general rule, productive of pain and inconvenience, Dr. Bennet points to the important fact that when once inflammation supervenes, this immunity from pain and inconvenience on pressure, as is the case in all the other organs of the body, ceases, and the slightest amount of pressure or even the normal movements of the part is tolerated with difficulty.

Flexion and displacement of the uterus, simple or combined, including prolapsus, more or less complete, of the entire organ, are generally found to coexist with uterine suffering and the ailments thence resulting, and to the presence of these dislocations of the organ the extreme partisans of "*the displacement theory*" attribute primary importance—as in the majority of cases the real cause of the existing mischief—as the morbid condition which principally requires treatment. In their eyes, the coexisting inflammatory lesions—the ulcerations, hypertrophies, and indurations, are, in many, if not in the majority of cases, epiphenomena, either occasioned by the displacement, or merely complicating it.

"The reasons," remarks Dr. B., "which have led me to the conclusion that these views are erroneous; that the displacement is, on the contrary, in most instances, really the epiphenomenon, and that it does not require, generally speaking, actual treatment of any kind, may be divided into physiological, pathological, and therapeutical.

"*Physiologically*, we have seen that the uterus bears pressure and displacement, when perfectly healthy, without pain or inconvenience. We have seen also in the married state the neck of the uterus is very frequently mechanically retroverted; thrust on the rectum, into the sacral cavity—the body of the uterus being at the same time, anteverted—and yet that all goes on normally, without either distress or discomfort being experienced. We have seen that slight anteflexion, or anteversion, is probably a natural condition during life, and that very decided flexions of the uterus may exist congenitally, or be produced by accidental causes, such as violent efforts, habitual rectal constipation, or even menstruation, and remain for a time, or for life, without producing any morbid symptoms. Such being the case, on what reasonable grounds can we be called upon to attribute to a slight flexion or to a slight displacement of the uterus the symptoms of uterine suffering presented by a female in whom one or the other coexists with inflammatory lesions. Is it sound logic—is it rational to do so? Is it not much more consistent with physiological observation and common sense to attribute the uterine and general disturbance to the inflammation, and to consider the displacement as the epiphenomenon—as the secondary, comparatively unimportant, element? And if this reasoning applies to slight displacements, does it not also apply by extension, although in a minor degree, to the more decided uterine displacements when connected with inflammatory lesions?

"*Pathologically*, there are many valid reasons for considering moderate displacement of the uterus a phenomenon of secondary and not of primary importance, in the cases of uterine suffering in which it is observed. The inflamed uterus, instead of bearing, without inconvenience, as the healthy uterus does, pressure and displacement, often becomes extremely tender, and like the inflamed finger, suffers not only from pressure, but from mere contact. Thus, even when there is no deviation or displacement of any kind, we frequently find that females who are labouring under slight uterine inflammation, complain greatly of weight, heaviness, and bearing down, and are unable to stand or walk with ease. The mere physiological weight of the inflamed uterus or cervix uteri, its mere contact with, and pressure against, the surrounding organs when in the erect position, becomes all but unbearable, and the recumbent position is sought with eagerness. Why, therefore, should we attribute uterine suffering to displacement only, or even principally, if on the one hand, we constantly find all the symptoms, local, functional, and general, that characterize such suffering, existing in cases where there are inflammatory lesions only, without either deviation or displacement, whilst, on the other hand, mere displacement, unattended with inflammatory disease, fails to produce these symptoms?

"This train of reasoning becomes the more cogent when we consider that, setting aside the physiological and accidental displacements to which I have alluded—uterine displacements are generally the immediate result of enlargement of the uterus or of its cervix, and that enlargement of the uterus is generally the result, direct or indirect, of inflammation."

"*Therapeutically*, the secondary nature and importance of uterine displacements, when not carried to an extreme degree, may be undeniably proved by the results of practical experience. For very many years I have completely ignored, as far as direct treatment is concerned, the existence of displacement in the numerous cases of uterine ailment which I have been called upon to treat. Looking upon the displacement as a mere congenital, physiological, or pathological concomitant of the inflammatory disease which I, all but invariably, find to exist when uterine suffering is present, or considering it to be the direct result of enlargement of the body or neck of the uterus, inflammatory or other, I have generally looked upon it as a mere symptom, and acted on this view. Thus as a rule, I have thrown aside pessaries, bandages, and all artificial or mechanical agencies for the sustentation or straightening of the prolapsed or deviated uterus, accepting these conditions, and the distress they may occasion, as symptoms not in themselves requiring any particular treatment beyond partial rest. My great aim has been to remove what I consider the cause of the pathological prolapsus, retroversion, or anteversion, be that cause relaxation or disease of the vagina, congestion, induration, and hypertrophy, or passive enlargement, either of the body or neck of the uterus. I find that when these morbid conditions can be thoroughly and completely removed by treatment, and when time has been allowed to nature to restore the integrity and functional activity of the recently diseased organs, one of two things occurs—either the displacement ceases—the uterus ascending to its natural position if prolapsed, and returning to its normal intra-pelvic situation if retroverted or anteverted, or it does not. In either case, however, in the immense majority of instances, the patient is freed from pain, or even discomfort, and ceases to complain of the symptoms of uterine suffering. When the uterus returns to its physiological position as a result of the removal of the morbid condition which produced the displacement, the subsidence of pain and discomfort is a fact which may be explained either by appealing to the displacement or to the inflammatory lesions which accompanied it. This alternative, however, is no longer admissible when the displacement—prolapsus, anteversion, or retroversion—remains after the removal of the inflammatory lesions, all pain and discomfort at the same time disappearing, and this I am constantly witnessing. I speak within reasonable limits when I say that scores and scores of my former patients, who had for years suffered from uterine ailments before they were treated by me, are now living like other people, perfectly free from inconvenience of any kind—walking, standing, running, and going through all the ordinary ordeals of life, *although the uterus has remained displaced.* It has either remained lower than normal, or has kept in anteversion or retroversion, and in some to a considerable extent. These women are, however, otherwise sound, free from any inflammatory lesion, and the displacement consequently gives no more trouble than do the congenital and physiological displacements described above."

The views briefly set forth in the foregoing sentences have a most important practical bearing—that they will be borne out to their fullest extent by the results of experience we feel confident. We have for years practised upon them with the most happy results. Our own observations, which have been by no means of very limited extent, nor we hope carelessly made, enable us to indorse the general conclusions of Dr. Bennet, "that uterine displacements, in the immense majority of cases, require no special treatment; that in those extreme cases of anteversion and retroversion in which it would be desirable to straighten the uterus by mechanical means, the intra-uterine pessary, when borne, is of but little, if any use, as the displacement usually returns as soon as it is extracted, and that in complete prolapsus, vulvar bandages afford the support the easiest borne, and the most efficacious, combined occasionally with an abdominal bandage, with a view to take off intestinal pressure."

Dr. Bennet is far from asserting that displacements of the uterus are never productive of inconvenience or distressing symptoms when unaccompanied by inflammation or its immediate sequelæ. Both prolapsus and retroversion may, when extreme, very materially impair the comfort of the patient, without giving rise, however, to the same train of local or general symptoms which are attendant upon the proper inflammatory affections of the uterus and their results.

"There are," remarks Dr. B., "cases of prolapsus or procidentia uteri, in which all the means of sustentation which the uterus naturally presents have become so strained or weakened, and in which the vaginal outlet is so loose and open, that the uterus will fall when the patient is in the erect position, and no treatment can restore the healthy tone of the parts involved so as to admit of the uterus being retained *in situ*. When this is the case, like other practitioners, I resort to mechanical agencies, but principally to extra-vulvar pressure and support. All intra-vaginal pessaries, in my experience, give rise to irritation, and are consequently objectionable, and to be dispensed with if possible. Complete procidentia uteri is principally observed in the lower classes, and is evidently the result, generally speaking, of their being up and about too soon after their confinements, when the uterus is much too heavy.

"Retroversion, when extreme, and attended with considerable non-reducible enlargement of the uterus, is also a most unmanageable form of ailment, and must likewise be excepted from the above remarks. It may remain as a serious morbid condition when all inflammatory disease has been removed, blocking up the rectum, and occasioning considerable distress by pressure, as does retroversion in pregnancy when the displaced uterus has attained a certain size." D. F. C.

ART. XXV.—*The Obstetric Memoirs and Contributions of* JAMES Y. SIMPSON, M.D., F. R. S. E., Professor of Midwifery, in the University of Edinburgh, etc. etc. Edited by W. O. PRIESTLY, M. D., Edinburgh, etc., and HORATIO R. STORER, M. D., Boston, U. S., one of the Physicians to the Boston Lying-in Hospital, etc. Vol. II. 8vo., pp. 773. Philadelphia: J. B. Lippincott & Co.

THE contents of the present volume are both valuable and interesting. It comprises the essays and contributions of Dr. Simpson on various subjects connected with the pathology of the puerperal state; the physiology and pathology of the products of conception; the pathology of infancy and childhood, and the use of anæsthetics in midwifery, surgery, etc. These, it is true, have already appeared in the professional journals of the day; several of them have, however, been added to, or in a great measure remodelled and re-written by the author expressly for the present work. Besides the essays and contributions on the subjects above enumerated that had been already published, the volume before us contains some that now appear for the first time—namely, "Pathological researches on puerperal arterial obstruction and inflammation," "On the rudimentary reproduction of extremities after their spontaneous amputation"—"On the practical application of chloroform as a topical anæsthetic to mucous and cutaneous surfaces," and "On carbonic acid gas as a local anæsthetic in uterine diseases, etc."

The entire collection presents a series of essays rich in facts, suggestions, and practical observations on some of the most important and interesting topics in the domain of physiology, pathology and therapeutics, and the profession cannot but be thankful to the editors for their agency in the collection and arrangement of these memoirs and contributions of the industrious, talented and experienced Edinburgh professor and practitioner, in a form that renders them easy of access to all, whether for the purpose of careful study or of occasional reference.

We should be tempted to enter into a somewhat extended analysis of some of the leading papers contained in the volume before us, were we not convinced that the work itself will be in the hands of every practitioner. The reputation of Dr. Simpson as a teacher and practitioner, and the frequent reference made to his views on questions connected with obstetrics and the pathology and management of uterine diseases, cannot fail to render American physicians desirous of a more intimate acquaintance with the professional memoirs and contributions he has, from time to time, presented to the medical public.

The present notice will, therefore, be confined to a very brief survey of a portion of the contents of the present volume.

In the essays on the analogy between puerperal and surgical fever, and on the communicability and propagation of the first named disease, Dr. Simpson discusses questions of deep interest to every practitioner of our country.

In a note to the first of these essays the author, after remarking that puerperal fever has often been denominated, in accordance with the special notions which the writer happened to entertain of its pathological nature, puerperal peritonitis, or metritis, or phlebitis, peritoneal fever, etc., observes, that any name thus drawn from pathology must ever change with the changes and advances of pathology itself, while a nosological name—such as puerperal fever—never requires to be varied, but is always fixed and intelligible. The danger to be apprehended from the denomination, puerperal fever, is its being apt to lead to the supposition that the pathological conditions upon which the phenomena of the disease depend are so intimately connected with the puerperal state as to differ essentially in their origin, character, progress, and general results from any occurring out of that state, or in the male subject, a supposition, the falsity of which, we believe, can be readily established—which in fact is shown by the observations adduced by Dr. S. in the very essay under consideration.

"Medical literature," he remarks, "does not possess a sufficient series of data to enable us to institute a full comparison between all the elements of puerperal and of surgical fever. But the consideration of a few points may prove enough to indicate at least a strong analogy, *if not an identity*, between these two forms of disease."

Dr. S. then goes on to show in what respects puerperal and surgical fevers are assimilated to each other: 1. In the anatomical conditions, and constitutional peculiarities of those who are the subjects of them; 2. In the pathological nature of the attendant fever; 3. In the morbid lesions respectively left by either disease; and, 4. In the symptoms which accompany each affection.

Under the second of these heads, Dr. S. remarks—

"Two opinions were formerly held with respect to the pathological nature of puerperal fever. One class of pathologists—as Puzos, Levret, Hamilton, White, etc.—regarded it as an idiopathic or putrid fever, *sui generis;* another class—Hey, Armstrong, Mackintosh, Campbell, etc.—still more earnestly maintained that the disease was essentially a local inflammation—that the fever was merely a consequence of, and attendant upon, this local inflammatory inflammation—and that the malady was to be treated and cured by venesection and other active antiphlogistics. The first of these doctrines became generally abandoned with the advances of pathological anatomy, because local inflammatory lesions in the uterus, peritoneum, chest, etc., were, after death, found far too frequently, and of far too marked and intense a character to be explained upon the doctrine of a previously existing fever alone. But, again, on the other hand, the idea that the disease was essentially a local inflammation, and that the fever was merely an effect symptomatic or sympathetic of that local inflammation, has been in turn gradually disproved also, as the pathological anatomy of the disease has been, of late years, more completely investigated. For it has been found that—1st. There is no general uniformity of relation and sequence between the degree and intensity of their supposed cause—the local inflammatory lesions—and the degree and intensity of their supposed effect—the attendant fever; 2d. Sometimes the supposed cause—in the form of simple peritonitis, or metritis, etc.—may exist, without these inflammations exciting the usual phenomena of their supposed effect, namely, the symptoms of puerperal fever; and 3d. We see occasionally cases of true and fatal puerperal fever, without discovering on the dead body any traces or evidence of the local inflammation which had been considered the origin of the disease. In other words, under this last class of cases we have the existence of the supposed effect without the existence of the supposed cause. And this observation holds good with regard not only to the individual local inflammations, which have been illogically dogmatized into the alleged invariable origin of puerperal fever, but it holds good with regard to the whole class of local inflammatory causes."

"Some authors, while they maintain the disease to be a fever entirely symptomatic of some local inflammation, at the same time hold that this local inflammation may be seated in different parts, in different cases, and different epidemics; and that the disease originates, in one case, in metritis; in another, in ovaritis; in a third in peritonitis, and so on. Without remarking on the illogical nature of imagining that the same disease may have such varied origins, we may once more pointedly observe, that—as sometimes happens in continued fever—occasionally though very rarely, no inflammatory lesions whatever can be traced upon the bodies of patients who have died of puerperal fever. Dr. Locock has observed several cases of this kind, and, in the practice of the late Dr. Beilby, I saw one very marked and rapidly fatal case of puerperal fever, in which my colleague, Professor Bennett, was unable to detect anywhere in the abdomen, or in the uterus, its appendages or vessels, any traces of inflammatory action or effusion. The great rarity of such instances is no sufficient argument against their important bearing upon the question of the nature of puerperal fever.

"The evidence which I have thus briefly sketched has induced, of late, most of our best pathologists to reject the idea, either that puerperal fever is an idiopathic fever *sui generis*, or a disease originating in and identical with peritonitis, or with any other local inflammation. And, on the other hand, many investigations and experiments made during the last ten or twenty years upon the effects of an acquired, or artificially excited, state of vitiation or poisoning of the blood, have inclined them more and more to adopt the doctrine, that the real source and cause of puerperal fever is to be found in a toxæmia or morbid state of the circulating fluid. The direct injection of pus, and other morbid secretions and matters, into the blood of the lower animals by Gaspard, Cruveilhier, Castelnau, and others, have produced a series of symptoms during life, and a series of lesions on the dead body, showing a very strong analogy to those of puerperal fever. The commixture of pus with the blood in the human subject, in cases of phlebitis, etc., in which pure pus enters directly into the circulation, gives rise to a similarity both of febrile functional lesions as seen during life, and of inflammatory organic lesions as seen after death. And in the puerperal female, there exist such conditions as facilitate the infection of the general circulation, by pus and other morbid matters contained in the uterine cavity. For they may obtain easy access to the general circulation—1. Through the orifices of the utero-placental veins, that open upon the internal surface of the uterus, which are, perhaps, not always completely closed, and which have their mouths constantly in contact with the contents and secretions of the uterine cavity. 2. Through the innoculation of morbid and contagious matters upon the abraded surface of the vagina; and, 3. By any accidental inflammation commencing in the lining membrane of the maternal passages—which are distended and contused during delivery—readily passing, by the law of continuity alone, through the venous orifices opening on the interior of the uterus, and thence along the lining membrane of these vessels. Under the now generally adopted view, that puerperal fever originates in a vitiated condition of the blood, we can solve more easily the problem with respect to the relation of the two elements, constituting puerperal fever—namely, first, the febrile action, and, secondly, the internal inflammation, which are present during it. For under this pathological view we see that the fever is not itself the cause of the attendant inflammations, nor these inflammations themselves the cause of the attendant fever; but that both of them—that is both the fever and the inflammations—are the simultaneous sequences or effects of one common cause—namely, the original vitiated or diseased condition of the general circulating fluid. And further, the same doctrine enables us to perceive how, in one set of cases, or one epidemic of puerperal fever, the febrile effect or element may be more marked than the inflammatory; and how, in others, and these generally the most amenable to treatment, the inflammatory element or effect may be more marked and more prominent than the febrile."

We may be excused the presentation of the foregoing long extracts from an essay published nearly six years ago, but in a form not readily accessible to the mass of the medical profession in this country, when the vast importance of the subject to which they relate is taken into consideration. The views advanced by Dr. S., in reference to the pathology of puerperal fever, are, we are convinced, in their general outlines, correct. They are certainly borne out by a careful analysis of all the facts connected with the etiology, history, phenomena, and morbid anatomy of the disease, as we have attempted, on more than one occasion, for many years past, to prove. They lead to a prophylactic and a curative treatment, which press themselves forcibly upon the attention of the medical profession.

In the essay just noticed, and the one which succeeds it, Dr. S. fully recognizes the communicability or propagation of puerperal fever, by—1st. A materies morbi, inoculated into the dilated and abraded lining membrane of the maternal passages, during delivery, by the fingers of the attendant; which materies morbi may be derived from contact with the inflammatory effusions in the abdomen and elsewhere, of patients who have died of puerperal fever, or with the morbid secretions coming from the bodies of such patients whilst alive, or with the inflammatory effusions produced in erysipelas and gangrenous inflammation of the limbs, scrotum, vulva, or other parts of the body, or in cases of the more subacute forms of disseminated or phlebitic inflammation which sometimes occur after delivery; 2d. He refers to one or two recorded instances which seem to prove that some varieties of febrile exhalations, received, by inhalation, into the blood of a newly delivered woman, are capable of producing in her a disease analogous to, if not identical with puerperal fever, these febrile exhalations being conveyed in the clothes of the medical attendant, or by the bedclothes, etc., used by puerperal patients, not properly washed and aired; 3d. By the morbific air generated in a small ill ventilated ward or hospital, crowded with puerperal patients; 4th. By certain epidemic influences; 5th. By the same causes which give rise to erysipelas. Dr. S. had long believed and taught that there was a pathological connection between erysipelas and puerperal fever, as to their pathological nature, their pathological anatomy, their symptomatology, and their causation. The two diseases had, in Britain, been repeatedly observed to prevail at the same time, in the same town, in the same hospital, or even in the same wards. There were various accurately recorded instances in the British journals showing that when the fingers of medical men were impregnated with the morbid secretions thrown out in erysipelatous inflammation, the inoculation of these matters into the genital canals of parturient females produced puerperal fever in them, in the same way as the inoculation of the secretions from patients who had died of puerperal fever itself. The effused morbid matters in the one disease, as in the other, being capable of producing the same effect when introduced into the vagina of a puerperal patient. In an instance recorded by Mr. Hutchinson, two surgeons, living at ten miles distance from each other, met half way, to make incisions in a limb affected with erysipelas and sloughing. Both touched and handled the inflamed and sloughing parts; and the first parturient patients that both practitioners attended within thirty or forty hours afterwards, in their own distinct, but respective localities, were attacked with, and died of puerperal fever. The late Mr. Ingleby mentions an instance of a practitioner making incisions into structures affected with erysipelas, and going directly from this patient to a woman in labour. The patient took puerperal fever and died. And within the course of the next ten days, seven cases of puerperal fever occurred in the practice of the same practitioner, almost all of them proving fatal. Various other cases, similar to the preceding, are well known to the profession.

Dr. S. alludes to the converse fact, namely: that there would appear to be sufficient evidence to warrant the belief that the secretions and exhalations from puerperal fever patients, are sometimes capable of producing erysipelas.

The evidence adduced in support of the several positions, above referred to, in respect to the communicability and propagation of puerperal fever; as well as that adduced by Dr. S., and the immense mass, in addition, which might be collected from medical works and the professional journals, demands a candid and serious examination on the part of every practitioner. It comes to us from too many independent sources, from authorities of too respectable and reliable character to permit it to be lightly set aside on the plea of its being the result of inaccurate or imperfect observations, or that it has been manufactured to support a favourite theory, or suggested from the love of opposition to received doctrines. The entire subject is one of paramount importance, in reference to the prophylaxis of puerperal fever. As Dr. S. very correctly observed: "In a disease like puerperal fever, it is the means of prevention that we are to look to, and to expect success in, more than the means of cure. It is here, as elsewhere, evident that human life would probably be saved to a far greater extent, by studying the means of preventing the causation of disease, than by any study of the means of treatment, after disease has once actually commenced."

The memoir on Peritonitis in the Foetus in Utero is one replete with interest, though the facts detailed in it are of less practical importance than those of many of the other papers which compose the present volume.

The causes productive of peritonitis in the fœtus are not well understood. In some of the cases observed by Dr. S., the mother had been exposed to severe labour, or fatigue, and exposure to cold and moisture, or bodily injury during gestation; in two cases, there existed general ill health during the whole of that period, in one of which the mother was herself twice attacked with peritonitis during the course of pregnancy. In two cases the mothers had an attack of gonorrhœa during the period of utero-gestation, along with a syphilitic eruption in one instance, and ulcers in the other. It appears to him highly probable, from investigations he has made, that a great proportion of the children of syphilitic mothers that die in the latter months of pregnancy, will be found to have perished under attacks of peritoneal inflammation. In other instances, however, adduced by Dr. S., the mother was not aware of being, in any way, exposed to any known morbific influence, and had not been the subject of any particular indisposition either before or during pregnancy. That the disease may originate in the fœtus, from causes strictly originating in, and confined to the fœtal economy itself, would seem to be shown by a case related by Dr. S., where, in a case of twins, *one child only* was affected, whilst the other was healthy and lively, although they were connected to the mother by one placenta, and consequently were both exposed equally to any morbific influence, which the state of her economy might have been capable of exerting on them.

In some instances, peritonitis in the fœtus would appear to be directly induced by morbid physical conditions of the abdominal viscera, and by irritant fluids accidentally applied to the peritoneal surface itself; as by internal strangulation of the intestines, by a rupture of the bladder, from accumulation of urine, in consequence of an impervious state of the urethra, etc. Cases are referred to by Dr. S., in which peritoneal inflammation in the fœtus was, in all probability, similarly induced; he having repeatedly observed an effusion of patches on the peritoneal surface of the intestines and other abdominal viscera, in instances of monstrosity, consisting in the extroversion of these viscera from a partial deficiency of the abdominal parietes. Scarpa, in his treatise on hernia, represents a case of umbilical hernia in the human fœtus, in which a considerable portion of the jejunum adhered, doubtless in consequence of previous peritonitis, to the entrance of the hernial sac; in another place he pointed out, also, the "firm adhesion," contracted by the protruded abdominal viscera to the hernial sac, in instances of congenital umbilical hernia, as one of the causes opposing reduction, and leading to the early death of almost all those infants that are born affected with this disease.

In a subsequent essay, Dr. S. remarks that, in reference to peritonitis in the fœtus, there is an interesting and important fact in connection with it, to which he would direct attention, namely: its liability to occur successively in different children of the same mother, and thus sometimes producing a series and succession of prematurely stillborn children.

The subject of intra-uterine smallpox, of which Dr. S. relates two cases, is one replete with interest. The disease has been observed by Mead, Jenner, Hosack, and other pathologists, under the following circumstances:—

"I. In some cases the fœtus was affected with natural smallpox, while the mother was suffering under the modified form of the disease. This was the case in the two instances observed by Dr. S.

"II. Both mother and fœtus sometimes suffered contemporaneously under the natural smallpox. In a case which occurred to Dr. Patterson, of Leith, the disease proved fatal to the mother, and on a *post-mortem* inspection, the child in utero was found covered with the pock.

"III. Occasionally, the child, when thus affected, passes safely, while in utero, through a full course of smallpox, and is, at length, born with the pits of the disease alone remaining. Dr. S. vaccinated repeatedly a person born under these circumstances, and always unsuccessfully.

"IV. In some instances in which the mother has been exposed to the contagion of the smallpox, but herself escapes an attack of the disease, in consequence of previous variolation or vaccination, the fœtus is nevertheless born affected with it. In these last instances, the fœtus in utero being attacked by a disease, to the contagion of which the mother was exposed and yet herself escaped, it is evident,

1st. That we have in this a proof that a morbid contagious matter may be inhaled and introduced into the system without the disease following in the system of that individual, the predisposition to it being destroyed by previous disease.

"2d. That this morbid matter may nevertheless pass into and produce the specific disease in the fœtus, in whom the predisposition to it is present.

"3d. That the morbid matter can only thus pass from the mother to the fœtus through the medium of the circulation, for there is no communication by the nervous system between the economy of the mother and that of the fœtus. And,

"4th. That this affords sure presumptive proof that variolous, and perhaps other contagious febrile matters, affect the body by first entering the vascular system.

Other contagious diseases have affected the fœtus in utero, as dothinenterite, according to Roederer and Wageler; Plague, according to Russell; and numerous instances of congenital measles and scarlatina have been recorded. Morton, Russell, Pauline, etc., have described instances of malarious poison thus also reaching the fœtus, and producing intra-uterine ague."

Two cases are related by Dr. S. of the simultaneous coexistence and progress of smallpox and cow-pox, and, in respect to the mutual influence of the two diseases upon each other, he presents the following general conclusions. As everything in relation to this subject coming from a reliable source is valuable by throwing light upon the true value of vaccination as a prophylaxis of smallpox in subjects exposed to the contagion of the latter disease, we shall make no apology for presenting the following extract:—

"Since the time of Willan, many authors have recorded cases of the simultaneous existence of smallpox and cow-pox. Legendre and Bosquet have, in particular, collected a variety of data on the subject. Here, as elsewhere, in pathology, there are no universal laws; but the principal facts or general laws relative to the mutual effects and influence of these two diseases upon each other in the human economy, may be briefly stated as the following:—

"1. When the smallpox and cow-pox eruptions appear on the skin on the same day, or within one or two days of each other, the two affections usually pass through their natural courses, unaltered in their forms and progress by each other.

"2. If the type of smallpox with which the patient is affected, is originally confluent and virulent, the mere simultaneous coexistence and p [illegible] of cow-pox does not mitigate the severity, or avert the fatality of thgreasiolous disease.

"3. When the specific eruption, however, of one of these diseases distinctly forestalls the other as much as four, five, or six days, the first or earlier disease, whether smallpox or cow-pox, does not undergo any change or curtailment in its own natural phenomena or progress, but the second or latter disease is usually more or less distinctively modified in its intensity, and abridged so much in its course as to arrive at its acme at or near the time of the maturation of the first or prior eruption.

"4. In this last respect, the abortive influence of an already existing smallpox or cow-pox eruption upon a supervening eruption of either disease, is similar to the abortive influence of an already existing smallpox upon a newly inoculated smallpox pustule, or of an already existing cow-pox upon a newly inoculated cow-pox vesicle—and in the latter affection constitutes the so called test-pock of Mr. Bryce.

"5. When fully a week or more has elapsed from the appearance of smallpox or of cow-pox, and more particularly when the variolous or vaccine eruption has already run its full course, the inoculation of, or exposure to the one or to the other disease, is followed by no result or eruption whatever—the constitution being now so changed and protected as to be generally proof for the remainder of life against the poison of either smallpox or cow-pox.

"6. Exceptions, however, occur not unfrequently to this last great general law; persons being sometimes met with, capable of twice taking smallpox, or twice taking cow-pox, or of taking smallpox after cow-pox, or cow-pox after smallpox.

"7. When a second attack of either disease thus occurs subsequently in life, this second attack seems usually not liable to follow till years have elapsed, and commonly the eruption is mild and modified in its character. But I have known a person die of a second attack of smallpox, though pock-pitted by the first, and the late Professor Thomson saw a second and well marked attack of smallpox appear in a student before he had entirely recovered from a previous attack of the same disease."

From the third general law above stated, it will be perceived, as remarked by Dr. Simpson, that it becomes "a matter of great moment to vaccinate always as speedily as possible any unprotected child or adult, who happens to be exposed to the contagion of smallpox—the question of the prevention or modification of the variolous by the vaccine disease being, as a general law, merely a question of relative time and precedence. It is important also to state that numerous recorded facts show that even during the incubating stage of smallpox in the body, artificial vaccination will usually produce a vaccine vesicle, and that this vesicle will protect against or modify the smallpox, provided only the vaccine eruption forestalls the variolous by a sufficient length of time."

The last two hundred and fifty-four pages of the volume before us are occupied with an examination of the propriety and advantages of anæsthesia in surgery and midwifery, more especially the propriety and safety of their employment in the latter.

Dr. Simpson has unquestionably treated the subject with much ability in all its several bearings. He has, it is certain, indulged in not a little special pleading in defence of his views, and some false analogical reasoning in his replies to certain of the objections that have been urged against the employment of anæsthetics merely for the abolition of pain during parturition and the progress of a surgical operation. The subject is one unquestionably of the deepest importance, and the facts and arguments adduced by Dr. S. in reference to it demand a careful study and deliberate consideration. If the pains of parturition can be abolished; if the knife of the surgeon can be made to perform its necessary office without the infliction of suffering, and at the same time, by means that can be proved to subject the patient to no additional risk, either immediate or remote, the practitioner who should refuse to grant to those placed under his professional care the relief from pain and suffering he has it in his power to effect, would be justly chargeable with inhumanity. But, if for the sake of merely avoiding temporary pain or suffering he resorts to the induction of anæsthesia, and thereby adds in any degree to the risk which his patients incur, we cannot hold him entirely guiltless.

Nearly every paper comprised in the volume before us is deserving of a very full notice—they will all be read with interest and profit by American physicians. We have been obliged to confine our attention to but one or two—upon these we may perhaps be accused of dwelling unnecessarily, inasmuch as they are not now made public for the first time. The value of the matters discussed in them, as well as the character and professional character of their author, warrant us in bringing them to the notice of our readers, to many of whom they may perchance prove to be other than "a tale twice told."

D. F. C.

ART. XXVI.—*On the Diseases of Infants and Children.* By FLEETWOOD CHURCHILL, M. D., M. R. I. A., etc. etc. Second American edition, enlarged and revised by the Author. Edited, with additions, by WILLIAM V. KEATING, M. D., A. M., Physician to St. Joseph's Hospital, etc. etc. 8vo., pp. 735. Philadelphia, 1856: Blanchard and Lea.

THE character of Dr. Churchill's treatise, as a full, comprehensive, and accurate exposition of the present state of our knowledge in respect to the pathology and therapeutics of infancy and childhood, has been, on every side, fully appreciated. In the present edition, the work bears evidence of the careful revision to which it has been throughout subjected, and the faithfulness with which every important fact and observation, contributed by recent authorities, has been added to the several chapters to which they respectively appertain.

With a degree of candour and a freedom from prejudice seldom equalled, the author has availed himself of the contributions of all who have, of late years, industriously investigated the etiology and pathology of the maladies peculiar to the early stages of existence, or who have improved and simplified their therapeutic management. From the materials thus derived, and the results of his own observation and experience, he has succeeded in presenting an account of the diseases embraced within the scope of the present treatise, and their mode of treatment—remarkable for its comprehensiveness, perspicoity, and accuracy. Few works devoted to the same subject will be found, in fact, to excel the one before us, in extent of research, copiousness of reference, and fulness and accuracy of detail. It will constitute a valuable and reliable guide to the knowledge of the several morbid conditions incident to infancy and childhood, their causes, semeiology, seats, character, and progress, and the means best adapted for their alleviation and cure, equally suitable to the student, as to the practitioner who would render himself familiar with the lights which recent investigation and discoveries have thrown upon each and all of these particulars.

It might not be uninteresting to examine the manner in which the consideration of the more prominent and least understood of the diseases incident to early life is conducted by Dr. Churchill, and the conclusions at which he has arrived, in respect to their pathological character and therapeutic management. To do this, in a manner that would be just to him and satisfactory to our readers, would, however, extend this notice to an unreasonable extent. Upon every undecided question, the author has presented, with perfect fairness, all the materials that are necessary for a correct understanding of the actual state of medical knowledge in regard to it, irrespective of the judgment he himself offers; and we have little cause to complain of him for having thrown the weight of his authority on the side "where truth doth not, to all appearance, most prevail." D. F. C.

ART. XXVII.—*Obstetric Tables.* By Dr. PAJOT, Agrégé Professor to the Faculty of Medicine, Paris. Translated from the French and arranged by O. A. CRENSHAW, M. D., and J. B. McCAW, M. D., Richmond, Va. With three additional Tables on the Mechanism of Natural, Unnatural, and Complex Labour, by NATHAN P. RICE, M. D., New York. 4to. Richmond, Va. 1856.

THE series of tables before us comprises eight, each one occupying a separate page. 1st. A table of the signs of pregnancy, arranged in methodical order. 2d. Classification of the deformities of the female pelvis in connection with childbirth. 3d. A synopsis of the treatment of hemorrhage. 4th and 5th. Tables of the principal obstetrical operations—namely, the fourth, *version;* the fifth, *application of the forceps.* 6th. Natural labour. 7th. Unnatural labour. 8th. Complex labour, with an addition on post-partum hemorrhage.

These tables are certainly prepared with considerable care and ability, and present a very accurate synopsis of midwifery. The authorities for the leading facts and directions noted in them are given. These are, however, chiefly confined to those of the continent.

Excellent as are these tables in their general outline, simple and methodical as is their arrangement, we can see no advantage the student can acquire from them in his pursuit of obstetrical principles and rules of practice, nor any great assistance the practitioner can gain from consulting them. To the newly admitted members of the obstetrical corps they may perhaps serve as a useful remembrancer of the difficulties of midwifery, the obstacles he may have to encounter, and the method of overcoming them; the character and value of a doubtful symptom, or the actual or probable cause of an unexpected phenomenon—all which instruction he will more effectually obtain, however, and more indelibly impress upon his mind, by keeping up his acquaintance with the teachings of the leading authorities on the theory and the art of obstetrics. It is not, however, by reading, or by oral instruction alone, that the skilful, ever-prepared, and safe obstetrician is to be formed. In no department of his professional ministrations is clinical instruction more imperiously demanded for the acquisition of positive knowledge and skill by the physician than that which relates to the conduct of labour, so as best to insure the safety of mother and child. Without it, however well he may be otherwise prepared, the practitioner enters the parturient chamber as one groping in the dark; and, if he meet with difficulties he has not anticipated, or imagines he has encountered them where they do not actually exist—which is as likely as not to be the case—it is in vain for him to attempt to seek for light to relieve him from his state of uncertainty and to direct him into the course proper for him to pursue by a reference, in the hour of need, to plates, however accurately these may be executed, or to synoptical tables, however excellent and methodical their arrangement. D. F. C.

ART. XXVIII.—*Medical Jurisprudence.* By ALFRED S. TAYLOR, M. D., F. R. S., etc. etc. Fourth American from the fifth and improved London edition. Edited, with additions, by EDWARD HARTSHORNE, M. D., etc. 8vo., pp. 697. Blanchard & Lea: Philadelphia, 1856.

THE work of Dr. Taylor is now recognized by the profession generally as ranking among the best elementary treatises on medical jurisprudence in the English language. We know of none in which the subject may be more profitably studied; no one better adapted for casual reference with the view to refresh the memory in respect to any especial question within the general scope of forensic medicine.

The author has, with admirable judgment, selected from the immense mass of materials at his disposal those best calculated to represent the actual condition of medico-legal knowledge, and has arranged these in a manner calculated to present the requisite information with that clearness and precision so essential in an elementary treatise.

In the edition before us, the work has undergone throughout a careful revision, while many and important additions have been made to it. It may, in consequence, be considered a most faithful exhibition of legal medicine as actually received by our own profession, and confirmed by the latest decisions of the criminal courts.

From the comprehensiveness of the author's text, the labours of the American editor "have been principally confined to a careful revision of the text, the incorporation of the addenda, and the introduction of occasional brief notes of recent cases and decisions, and references to others, as well as to some of the papers and works of interest which have been presented since the date of the author's preface."

The additions and references of the editor are not, however, without value: they render the treatise a more complete exponent of the actual condition of medical jurisprudence. D. F. C.

Art. XXIX.—*Physician's Tabulated Diary, designed to facilitate the Study of Disease at the Bedside.* By a Physician of Virginia. Richmond, Va. J. W. Randolph, 1856.

The keeping of a very full record of the cases that fall under his care should never be neglected by any physician, but more especially by those who have but recently entered upon the duties and responsibilities of the profession. It is only by pursuing this course that the medical man can acquire readily and fully that clinical skill in the detection, diagnosis, and treatment of diseases so essential to his accomplishment as a safe and successful practitioner.

Few, unfortunately, are sufficiently impressed with the importance of recording their cases to be willing to devote to it the necessary time and labour; while even those who do record their observations, seldom do so at the time they are actually made, but at a subsequent period, from memory alone, when important facts may have been forgotten, and those remembered, imperfectly described. Anything, consequently, that may have a tendency to induce physicians to keep a true clinical record of their cases receives our cordial approbation. As a means, therefore, to this end, we feel constrained to recommend the diary before us. It presents for each day eighteen blank spaces. The first being for the date of visit, and the name, age, sex, occupation, etc. of the patient; the second, for the hour of visit, and locality; the third, for the date of attack; the fourth, for the seat of pain; the fifth, for the decubitus and aspect of patient; the sixth, seventh, and eighth, respectively, for state of tongue, skin, brain, and nervous system; the ninth, for gastro-intestinal symptoms; the tenth and eleventh, for the signs and symptoms derived from the respiratory system; the twelfth and thirteenth, for the signs and symptoms derived from the circulatory system; the fourteenth, for the genito-urinary symptoms; the fifteenth, for the name of the disease; the sixteenth, for the state of sleep; the seventeenth, reference to authorities, etc.; and the eighteenth, for treatment.

An appendix is added, for certain records "which are required but once for each patient, or which could not be entered into the diary;" such as thermometrical and barometrical observations, chemical and microscopical observations, previous history of patient, and post-mortem observations.

That a more simple and systematic diary than that of the Virginia Physician could not very easily be prepared we shall not assert; yet we are convinced that even were the one before us used by the generality of practitioners in the different sections of our country, "materials would be accumulated for analysis and generalization," which could not fail "in time, under the auspices of medical associations," or in the hands of some industrious member of the profession, "to greatly elucidate questions of medical topography, etiology, pathology, and therapeutics." D. F. C.

ART. XXX.—*The Causes and Curative Treatment of Sterility, with a Preliminary Statement of the Physiology of Generation. With colored Lithographs and numerous Wood-cut Illustrations.* By AUGUSTUS K. GARDNER, A. M., M. D., etc. etc. etc. 8vo., pp. 170. New York: Dewitt & Davenport, 1856.

THAT Dr. Gardner has presented a very fair exposition of the present state of our knowledge in relation to the physiology of generation, and the causes and treatment of sterility, we very freely admit. Whether, however, the profession was in want of a work of the character of that before us, is a question that will admit of some doubt. We find in it nothing that is original, nothing with which every well-informed physician is not perfectly familiar.

We have a right to presume that the work was intended solely for the professional eye, and yet we are at a loss to conceive what could have induced the author to suppose that the slightest degree of instruction would be communicated to either medical student or practitioner by the coloured lithograph which fronts the title-page, or by one or more of those which follow.

From the manner in which the work is got up, and a certain tone which pervades it, we very much fear that it will attract the attention and be eagerly sought after by a class of readers upon whom it cannot fail to exert a baneful influence. However sound the physiological views it sets forth, however true the facts and statements it details, however sound the curative directions it presents, to the popular reader these will convey but little information from which he can derive any direct practical advantage. To the physician, all that the work contains, whether new or old, was already attainable from sources not easy of access to those who would seek them only to gratify a prurient imagination, and into which the innocent and unconscious would scarcely penetrate.

There is much within the scope of medical science which, while kept within its legitimate limits, is neither offensive to good taste, to delicacy, or to morals, but which, when obtruded before the public eye, with every allurement to attract the observation of the curious and susceptible, may be productive of much and serious evil. D. F. C.

ART. XXXI.—*New Elements of Operative Surgery.* By ALF. A. L. M. VELPEAU, Professor of Surgical Clinique, etc. etc. Carefully revised, entirely remodelled, and augmented with "A Treatise on Minor Surgery." Illustrated by over 200 engravings, incorporated with the text; accompanied with an Atlas, in quarto, of 22 Plates, representing the principal operative processes, surgical instruments, etc. Translated, with additions, by P. S. TOWNSEND, M. D., etc., under the supervision of, and with notes and observations by, VALENTINE MOTT, M. D., etc. Fourth edition, with additions, by GEORGE C. BLACKMAN, M. D., Professor in the Medical College of Ohio, Surgeon to the Commercial Hospital, etc. In 3 vols. 8vo. pp. 970, 911, and 992 respectively. Samuel S. & W. Wood: New York, 1856.

As a matter of course, there is but little to say about a new edition of the American translation of Velpeau's great work on Operative Surgery, except in regard to the additions of the new editor. The previous editions have been long known and appreciated by the profession; and the present one will be equally well received as a decided improvement upon its predecessors, in accordance with the progress of the operative science and art to which its twenty-eight hundred and seventy-three closely printed pages are devoted.

We cannot pretend to undertake an elaborate examination of this mass of printed matter in order to ascertain the amount and character of the labour which has been bestowed upon the work in the very important duty of preparing it for a re-issue in keeping with its previous high standing, and with the nature of its subject. We have seen enough of its pages, however, to be satisfied that Dr. Blackman has performed his laborious and responsible task with adequate fidelity and ability; and that he has well earned the respect, as well as the thanks, of all who desire to possess one of the most voluminous and comprehensive, if not the most authoritative, treatise on the elements of Operative Surgery yet published in the United States.

The object of the new editor, according to his preface, has been to arrange the work "more methodically, and to incorporate the more important contributions made in this department during the past ten years." With this intention we are glad to find that he has introduced a large number of interesting and appropriate notes into different portions of the text of the first and second volumes especially, and that he has also added to the third volume a useful appendix, amounting to one hundred and thirty-five pages, in which many improvements in Operative Surgery are more or less fully glanced at and discussed.

The most copious and satisfactory additions we suspect may be found in the section on "Lesions of the Arterial System," and the treatment of these lesions, in that upon the "Arteries in Particular" (both of vol. i.), and in those upon amputations and upon exsections, in the second volume. The references and statistics presented in these notes are very valuable, and must afford material assistance to the student of the history of the important operations to which they relate, as well as to the already experienced operator and practitioner of surgery.

The articles of the American Appendix are arranged in alphabetical order. They afford a general view, more practical than comprehensive or elaborate, and not always equally full or clear, of a variety of improvements and modifications of operative procedures and apparatus, which have attracted attention since the publication of the previous editien of the work. Between sixty and seventy topics are thus briefly noticed under various heads. Among them may be mentioned anchylosis of the jaw and of the knee-joint; anæsthesia, especially external; artificial anus, imperforate anus, bronchotomy, and tracheotomy, carcinoma, dislocations of the femur (chiefly occupied with Dr. Wm. W. Reid's mode of reduction), empyema (embracing Dr. Bowditch's experience, and statistical investigations), enterotomy and gastrotomy, recto-vaginal fistula, vesico-uterine, vesico-utero-vaginal and vesico-vaginal fistula (Dr. Marion Sims' operation for the last mentioned), fractures of the clavicle, the humerus, the radius, the femur, the patella, and the leg; ununited fractures (Brainard's operation), hernia, lithotomy, lithotrity, œsophagotomy (Dr. John Watson's case), abscess of the rectum (Dr. Sayre's case), spina bifida, imperforate vagina, and many others, for which we take pleasure in referring to the book itself. The volumes are stereotyped, and are altogether very respectably got up under the care of the enterprising publishers. The publication and preparation of a *bonâ fide* revised and enlarged edition of a work of such magnitude and importance surely entitles both publishers and editors to the material as well as cordial thanks of the profession. E. H.

QUARTERLY SUMMARY

OF THE

IMPROVEMENTS AND DISCOVERIES

IN THE

MEDICAL SCIENCES.

ANATOMY AND PHYSIOLOGY.

1. *Minute Anatomy of the Liver.*—Dr. LIONEL S. BEALE has published (*Med. Times and Gaz.*, July 26, 1856) several interesting lectures on this subject. The following is a summary of the most important points brought under notice:—

"The livers of all vertebrate animals are penetrated in every part by two sets of channels, which alternate with each other. One series, *portal canals*, contains a branch of the portal vein, hepatic artery, and hepatic duct, *interlobular;* and the other series, *hepatic venous canals*, is occupied by a single branch of the hepatic vein, *intralobular*.

"The vessels ramifying in the portal canals are ultimately distributed in such a manner that they serve to divide the organ into little masses, and thus map out spaces, or *lobules*, each of which contains all the structural elements of the organ, and may be regarded as an elementary liver.

"In the intervals between the fissures by which the portal vein, artery, and duct are conducted to the lobule, its capillary vessels and its secreting structure are continuous with those of adjacent lobules.

"The size and form of the lobules differ much in different animals; but their essential structure is the same in all, except in the pig, in the Polar bear, according to Müller, and in the Octodon Cummingii (one of the rodents), according to Hyrtl.

"In the pig each lobule is provided with a separate fibrous capsule of its own, and is, therefore, completely isolated from its neighbours. The portal vessels, artery, and duct run between them, and give off branches to contiguous lobules. In the intervals between the fibrous capsules areolar tissue can frequently be demonstrated.

"In all cases, upon a section, the lobule is seen to be bounded externally by branches of the vein, artery, and duct, and in the centre is situated a small branch of the hepatic vein.

"In the liver of the human subject, and in that of vertebrate animals generally, with the exceptions above mentioned, the lobules are not separated from each other by any fibrous partition, and there is no areolar tissue or prolongation of Glisson's capsule between them, or in their interior.

"The vessels at their entrance into the liver, and as they run for some distance in the larger portal canals, are surrounded with much areolar tissue; but the disposition of this texture about the vessels of the liver is very similar to its arrangement about the vessels distributed to other organs.

"The *lobule* itself is composed of a solid capillary network, and of another network composed of a delicate tubular membrane, in which the liver cells are contained.

"These networks mutually intertwine with each other.

"The capillary network is directly continuous with the smallest branches of the portal vein, distributed upon the circumference of the lobule on the one hand, and with the small intralobular vein arising in its centre upon the other. The vessels of the network converge towards the intralobular vein.

"Small branches of the artery open into the venous capillaries of the lobule, near its circumference, and the diameter of these small branches is considerably less than that of the venous capillaries into which they epen; the former not more than the 1-4000th of an inch in diameter, the latter about the 1-1600th.

"In all cases, the blood, enriched with constituents recently absorbed from the intestine, flows with a gradually increasing rapidity from the circumference of the lobule towards its centre, while the bile flows in a precisely opposite direction.

"The cell-containing network is directly continuous with the most minute ducts, which ramify at the circumference of the lobule, and it terminates in the centre by loops, which lie close to the intralobular vein.

"The liver-eells lie within a tubular network of basement membrane, which separates them from the walls of the capillaries. In many cases, however, these thin membranes cannot be separated, and are, no doubt, incorporated with each other.

"The cells are not attached to the basement membrane of the tube, but lie in its cavity. Among them free oil globules and granular matter are often found. Usually, there is only room for one row of cells, but sometimes two or more lie across the tube. In the embryo, in young animals, and in fishes, there is room for several rows to lie transversely across the tubes of the cell-containing network.

"The cells near the margin of the lobule take the most active part in the formation of bile. The secretion passes along the tubes in the slight interstices between the cells and the basement membrane, and coloured fluid can be forced along these same interstices in a direction the opposite to that in which the bile flows during life, and, therefore, at a great disadvantage. The amount of space is in great measure determined by the quantity of blood in the vessels, and it is liable to great alteration.

"The secreting tubes of the network are many times wider than the narrow thin-walled ducts with which they are directly continuous.

"The smallest ducts are lined with a very delicate layer of epithelium, composed of flattened cells of a circular form, contrasting remarkably with the large secreting cells, which are not arranged in any definite manner within the tubes of the network.

"The tubes of the cell-containing network are about the 1-1000th of an inch in diameter, or more, but the finest ducts are not more than 1-3000th, and they are often seen even less.

"The smallest ducts in some animals branch very freely, and the branches communicate with each other at intervals. In others they pursue a long course without branching, and in the pig they form an intimate network upon the surface of the lobule. In fatty livers of the pig, however, this ductal network often contains liver cells loaded with oil globules.

"As the ducts increase in size they are provided with a fibrous coat, and the epithelium in their interior becomes columnar.

"The *interlobular ducts* do not anastomose.

"When the fibrous coat reaches a certain degree of thickness, it contains numerous little cavities or *sacculi*, arranged entirely round the tube in the pig and in most animals, but forming two parallel rows, one on either side of the duct, in the human subject.

"These little sacculi often communicate with each other in the coats of the duct. The smaller branches of the duct also anastomose frequently either in the coats of the duct or just external to them.

"The sacculi appear to serve the purpose of bringing the bile in the thick walled ducts into closer relation with the vessels which surround them, and especially with the branches of the artery which are distributed to their coats.

"In the transverse fissure of the human liver and some others, and in the large portal canals, are found some peculiar branches of the duct, *vasa aberrantia*, with numerous sacculi on their walls, which anastomose with each other and form a network.

"In the same localities in the human subject, and in the gall-bladder, a very peculiar arrangement of the vessels occurs. Both arteries and veins form a network, and each branch of the artery is accompanied with two branches of the vein, one on either side of it.

"The vertebrate liver is to be regarded as a true gland, its secreting structure consisting of a *formative portion* taking the form of a network, and of a system of very narrow *efferent ducts* directly continuous with it. The secreting cells lie within a delicate tubular network of basement membrane, through the thin walls of which they draw from the blood the materials of their secretion, and they are thus brought into closer relation with, and are more nearly surrounded by the blood than the cells of any other secreting gland."

---

2. *The True Spinal Marrow the True Sympathetic.*—Dr. Marshall Hall maintains (*Lancet*, July 12, 1856) that the true spinal marrow is the true great sympathetic, or rather the great dienergetic nerve of the general system, whilst the ganglionic intra and extra-ganglionic system are its branches.

"Since," he says, "the promulgation of the diastaltic nervous system, of which the true and real centre is the spinal marrow and the spinal marrow only, two mistakes have been committed; the first was, to ascribe a similar function to the cerebrum; the second, to ascribe a reflex power to the ganglia. The former error arose from confounding the effect of *emotion* with those of the excitants of diastaltic action; the latter was, I believe, a mistake without foundation of any kind.

"If we see a disgusting object, we experience an emotion which may issue in sickness and vomiting, as other emotions issue in sickness and vomiting. But who does not instantly perceive the difference between this psychological fact and the vomiting induced by the physical excitement of the fauces, for example?

"Of an instance of a reflex action through the medium of the ganglionic system, the spinal centre being intercepted, not a trace has been discovered.

"Is there, in effect, any fact of a physical direct or reflex action, excited from or through the substance of the cerebrum, freed from its membranes; or of any part of the ganglionic system, the spinal centre being removed? I believe not. To speak, then, of reflex actions of the cerebral or of the ganglionic systems, is to confound things essentially distinct, and unwarrantably to extend the use of terms recently introduced and well defined.

"The great experimental question is this: When the cerebral and the spinal centres are removed, is there any possibility of inducing any phenomena such as those which have for ages been denominated *sympathetic?* This question has never been proved or discussed fully and distinctly. It might be resolved in the following manner:—

"The spinal marrow may be partially and even entirely divided in reptiles, the low-feeding and low-breathing fishes, and very young animals. This being accomplished, every means of inducing effects on the remaining functions is to be tried. If such effects be produced, it must be through the ganglionic nerve; if such effects be impossible, it must be because the real centre of reflex action is absent.

"I have destroyed the whole cerebrum and spinal marrow in frogs, carefully avoiding intra-spinal hemorrhage; but I could not afterwards influence the action of the heart, or the phenomena of the circulation, by any means I could devise.

"Still I regard the whole experimental question as requiring to be subjected to new investigation.

"I formerly regarded the diastaltic action as limited to obvious movements; but a multitude of facts show that it has a vastly more extended application.

"We all know the intimate relation between the ovarium, the uterus, and the mammæ. If the new-born infant be put to the nipple, contraction of the uterus is excited. No one doubts that this is a reflex or diastaltic spinal action.

"Pregnancy induces enlargement of the mammæ, and excites the secretion of milk. Is this secretory action less *spinal* than the former one?

"The same derangement of the stomach induces convulsion, cramp, asthma, irregularity of the heart's action, altered secretion of the kidneys. Are they not all and equally diastaltic spinal actions?

"The same pregnancy which affects the mammæ induces nausea and vomiting. The last phenomenon is indubitably diastaltic spinal. Are the others less so?

"Coldness impressed on the skin induces contraction of the rectum and of the bladder, augments the action of the kidneys, stays hemorrhage, and induces various internal inflammations. I know a patient in whom damp feet would induce sneezing instantly, with increased secretion of mucus.

"The whole cutaneous surface is simultaneously contracted or relaxed by the local and partial application of cold or hot water. I knew one patient, a near relative, in whom exposure to damp infallibly produced renal hemorrhage. A similar cause is apt to induce diarrhœa.

"Many other facts of the same kind might be adduced.

"That secretion *is* influenced by diastaltic action through the spinal centre is now placed beyond all doubt by the remarkable experiment of M. Bernard, in which the glycogenic function of the liver is proved to be a diastaltic spinal action. I quote M. Bernard's words:—

"'Le nerf (pneumogastrique) porte au centre cérebro-spinal les sensation (?) internes emanées de sa périphérie; l'excitation qu'il transmet est, dans ce cas, *centripète*, et non pas centrifuge. Et, en effet, après avoir coupé le pneumogastrique, si, au lieu d'agir sur le bout périphérique, ce qui n'a aucun effet sur la sécrétion du sucre, on excite avec le galvanisme l'extrémité qui se rend à la moëlle, la fonction glycogénique non seulement n'est pas interrompue dans le foie, mais elle peut même être exagérée lorsque l'excitation a été poussée assez loin.'[1]

"As it is my present object only to suggest the idea, and to add a suggestion and an observation or two, I conclude this brief communication with one final remark. It is not only obvious that the true spinal marrow is in reality the true sympathetic, but that the diastaltic system has an extension over the animal economy scarcely yet contemplated by the physiologist and the physician. It is in reality, in this latter respect, only second to the circulation of the blood itself. As the blood really describes a *circle*, the diastaltic spinal system describes a *cycloid;* as the blood diffuses its atoms into every minute space of the system, the diastaltic spinal system extends its influence over every one of those atoms! The blood undergoes its changes in the methæmatous, or blood-changing (or capillary) channels placed between the ultimate branches of the arteries and the incipient roots of the veins; to these same points the diastaltic spinal system extends its wondrous influence."

---

3. *On the Antrum Pylori in Man.* By Prof. A. Retzius.—Many writers on anatomy, in the description of the human stomach, comprehend, under the denomination "antrum pylori" (Pförtner Höhle, cul-de-sac pylorique), a portion of the viscus adjoining the pylorus; many do not mention this part; and others allude to it in a very cursory manner. I had been long engaged in dissections of the human body, without paying any special attention to it. Subsequently, I found, in examining the stomach in animals considered to have a single stomach, that the pyloric portion constituted a perfectly distinct part, and that in most vertebrate animals it has a peculiar structure, different from that of the rest of the organ. Many years ago, I investigated and described, in the *Transactions of the Royal Academy of Sciences* (K. Vet. Acad. Handl.) for 1839, the structure of the stomach in some herbivorous Rodentia; subsequently, I have likewise in man, time after time, discovered a certain almost regular ampullæ in this region, as well as, in many cases, a well-defined division, which I had

[1] Leçons de Physiologie, p. 325. Paris, 1855.

no reason to regard as a morbid formation. The denomination "antrum pylori" appeared to me to indicate that its origin was based on observations resembling my own, and I therefore endeavoured to trace the source of the name. I then found that Cruveilhier (*Traité d'Anatomie descr.*, tom. iii. p. 281), who took the same view of the subject as I did, attributes the term to Willis, as also that Haller (*Elementa Physiol.*, tom. vi. lib. xix. sect. i. § 3, "Ventriculi figura") quotes the work and place where Willis employs the name. For his own part, Haller says on this subject, in the section of his work referred to: "Non raro aliqua strictura quasi divisus [here he cites Morgagni, and brings forward several instances of stomachs divided by strictures] maxime posterius, tum paulo cis pylorum, unde tunc *antri* aliqua imago nascitur (Willis), quam aliqui clarissimi viri nimis fecerunt."

Willis's work, where the name "antrum pylori" occurs, and where it seems to have its origin, is his *Pharmaceutices rationalis sive diatribæ de medicamentorum operationibus in corpore humano*, &c., cap. ii., "Partium intra quas medicamenta operari incipiunt, descriptio, usus et affectiones." The most important part, in my opinion, touching the point in question, is that in which the author speaks of the destination of the pylorus, where it is said: "Pylori munus est, non tantum contenta affatim et simul in magna copia ad intestina transmittere (quod quidem in catharsi et diarrhœa frequenter facit), sed potius chylum satis confectum, in *sinum* suum excipere, aliquamdiu continere, et dein paulatim et per minutas portiones excernere. Enim vero hujus *Antrum longum et capax quidam in ventriculo recessus et diverticulum esse videtur*, in quod massæ chylaceæ portio magis elaborata et perfecta accedere, et inibi manere queat, donec alia crudior, et nuperius ingesta in ventriculi fundo plus digeratur," &c. We see from this, as well as from many other passages in the same work, that Willis attached much importance to this division of the stomach.

On a superficial examination, the human stomach appears to be a very simply constructed conical sac, from the form of which anatomy seems not to have much to gain. When, however, we consider the elaborate functions this sac has to perform, both in man and animals, and the numerous divisions and remarkable forms it exhibits in a great number of the latter, with many circumstances, both in health and disease, difficult of explanation, we are soon led to the conviction that very ingenious arrangements must be disposed in this apparently simple structure.

So far as I can recollect, there is not one of the modern writers who has, according to my view, described the pyloric portion of the stomach better than Cruveilhier. After having spoken of the pylorus itself, he says: "It is in the neighbourhood of this constriction (pylorus), at about the distance of an inch, that the stomach, bending strongly on itself, forms on the side of the great curvature a very decided elbow, *coude de l'estomac*, and presents an ampulla corresponding to an internal cavity, designated by Willis by the name of antrum of the pylorus, &c. It is not unusual to see a second ampulla beside the first, and a third, but smaller, at the side of the lesser curvature, in consequence of the bend described by the stomach. These ampullæ, scarcely appreciable in a great number of subjects before insufflation, become very distinct, and even, in some subjects, very considerable, by distention," &c.

According to my experience, this part occurs principally under three forms. The first is that sketched in the description just now quoted from Cruveilhier; the second, in which the part is more elongated, is mentioned by Willis, when he says "Antrum longum et capax;" the third, which may be called the conical variety, is that in which both the ampullæ here referred to by Cruveilhier, and their boundaries, are little marked, while the part itself is more conical.

In the first or shorter form, the part of the pylorus at the base is nearly as broad from the lesser to the greater curvature, as it is long, has two ampullæ at the lesser curve, and most frequently one at the greater, anterior to the great flexure, or *coude de l'estomac*. The first ampulla in the lesser curve is bounded at the thicker end by a deep indentation, which exactly corresponds to the great flexure just mentioned, the *coude de l'estomac*, and at the narrower end by a shallower indentation, separating it from the second ampulla, lying next to the pylorus. The ampulla in the greater curve is separated from the *coude de l'esto-*

mac by a shallow indentation, often amounting only to a depression extending half way round; this ampulla is usually somewhat larger than the corresponding one on the lesser curve, and, like it, reaches to the proper pylorus.

The entire of this part of the stomach is usually provided with a very thick muscular coat. It is particularly the circular layer of the latter which gives the pyloric portion its predominant thickness. The external longitudinal fibres lie here almost as on the colon, collected in bands, one on the anterior, and one on the posterior surface; these bands are not, however, as on the colon, distinctly bounded, but are only denser collections of bundles of muscular fibres, which, both anteriorly and posteriorly, become thinner, and dispersed over all the surrounding parts. This similarity to the tæniæ Valsalvæ on the colon, first observed, as it seems, by Helvetius (*sur la digestion*), gave rise to the now obsolete name, *ligamenta pylori.* Winslow also (*Exposition Anatomique de la Structure du Corps Humain*) directed his attention to them, for he observes: "Along the middle of each lateral surface of the small extremity is a tendinous or ligamentous band, three or four lines in width, and terminating at the pylorus"—*Tr. du Basventre*, § 61. He, however, considers that they lie externally to the muscular coat, in which view he is partly correct, as I shall presently endeavour to show.

Like the colon, the pyloric portion of the stomach is puckered; the ampullæ just now mentioned are formed by the shortness and strength of these longitudinal muscular fibres, resembling the pouches of the colon. As on the colon we very often see, at the sides of the longitudinal bands, the circular muscular fibres pass over the ampullæ in curves, which are closely pressed together in the two situations where the puckering takes place, but towards the bottoms of the ampullæ are further separated, according as the ampullæ are more distended.

In many cases we see these parts shining, like a smooth tendinous aponeurosis, which many authors also have remarked. I have sometimes examined this shining part, and found it composed, as Winslow mentioned, of a thin tendinous tissue in this peritoneal membrane, which is here abundantly provided with fibres of elastic tissue. This tendon-like formation, which in man is so imperfectly developed, and not unfrequently is wanting, acquires a greater importance from the fact that it is found strongly developed in many animals.

By far the thickest portion of the muscular coat is that of the extremity of the stomach bordering on the pylorus; the longitudinal fibres here again form a dense layer, evenly investing the entire part, as on the lower portion of the rectum. This small part of the stomach nearest to the pylorus constitutes, as it were, a little division in itself, and, according to my experience, is that which is least likely to be absent.

In the long form, this division of the stomach looks like an intestine, and is sometimes mistaken for a part of the duodenum; in many stomachs, which have been sent to me for examination, it has even been cut away. It occurs most frequently in women. It has, for the most part, only one ampulla on the lesser arch, but, on the contrary, two on the greater, of which the posterior is the great flexure, separated by a more distinct indentation from the remainder of the stomach.

In the third, or conical form, the great flexure usually appears as if removed nearer to the pylorus, and the greater ampulla in the lessor arch is small. The two other ampullæ, situated next the pylorus, are small, especially that in the lesser arch; and the little division just mentioned, situated next the pylorus, is better marked than in the two preceding forms.

In the new-born child, whose stomach is more rounded, I have not seen these ampullæ or indentations. Still, even in it, the part of the antrum next the pylorus is separately developed into a short cylindrical tube of about one centimetre in length, with thick walls, the thickness of which depends chiefly on a powerful circular, muscular belt. The valve of the pylorus is less developed than is ordinarily the case in adults; the muscular coat is thickest on the side belonging to the greater arch.

In a great number of the Mammalia this part of the stomach forms, as has been already mentioned, a still more decided division than in man, as will be seen by glancing at the representation given even in Cuvier's *Lectures on Com-*

parative Anatomy, and in Meckel's translation, illustrated by a number of figures. Of the animals which are nearest to our hand, the dog and cat tribe exhibit the part in question as a long, slender, bent cone; the horse, as a peculiar, rounded, thick part; in the pig it exhibits two constant ampullæ; in the hare it has, with the ampullæ, a small, reddish, thick, very muscular part next the pylorus: in the porpoise it constitutes a proper stomach, which is by Cuvier called the third stomach. In birds it forms the remarkable muscular stomach, which occurs likewise in many lizards; traces of the same are also found in various serpents.

As to the tendon-like parts, which are comprised in the above-named "ligamenta pylori" (Helvetius and Winslow), they occur considerably developed in a number of Mammalia, as the dog, the bear, the hare, &c.; in a great proportion of birds, especially those which live on seeds and insects, this tendinous formation is so well marked that it must be generally known; as it must be well known that this tendinous formation is found in the muscular stomach of crocodiles, and several Amphibia. Among fishes I have found it in the Siluridæ. From all this it may be inferred that the tendinous formation spoken of deserves special attention, and must, in many cases, play an important part.

In a previous communication I have shown that cases occur in the human subject in which the valve of the pylorus almost disappears. I have, since that communication was written, found that this valve is constantly absent in a great number of Mammalia and other vertebrate animals. On the other hand, there is in general found a broad, thick, circular, muscular formation around the greater part of the antrum pylori, which probably keeps the stomach closed throughout some extent, like the action of the circular muscles in the œsophagus and rectum.

As I have already mentioned, the duodenum likewise has a peculiar cavity, which probably has a special function. I have thought that this part ought to have a particular name, and have called it *antrum*, or *atrium duodeni*. The commencement of this part of the intestine is, in fact, as well in man as in a great number of Mammalia, often separately rounded, wants the valvulæ conniventes on its inner surface, and has small villi, and large Brunnerian and Lieberkuhnian glands. In the porpoise this cavity is, as has just been mentioned, so distinct that it has been regarded as constituting a division of the stomach.—*Dub. Quart. Journ. of Med. Sci.*, Aug. 1856, from *Hygiea*, Dec. 1855.

4. *Evils of Consanguinity in Marriage.*—Dr. Rilliet, of Geneva, communicated to the Academy of Medicine (May 13th) the result of his researches in reference to the influence exercised by consanguinity upon the offspring of marriage. He states that at Geneva a considerable number of marriages take place between relatives; that attention has during many years been attracted to the unhappy consequences resulting from this circumstance, and affecting the health and even the lives of the children. These consequences are, first, absence of conception; 2d, retardation of conception; 3d, imperfect conception (miscarriage); 4th, imperfect offspring (monstrosities); 5th, offspring more specially liable to diseases of the nervous system and in order of frequency: epilepsy, imbecility or idiocy, deaf-mutism, paralysis, various cerebral diseases; 6th, a lymphatic offspring predisposed to the diseases which spring from the scrofulo-tuberculous diathesis; 7th, an offspring which dies at an early age in a larger proportion than children born under other circumstances; 8th, an offspring which, if it passes the first period of infancy, is less capable than others of resisting disease and death. To these rules there are exceptions, due either to the state of health of the progenitors, or to the dynamic conditions in which the parents happen to be at the time of connection. Thus, 1, it is seldom that all the children escape the evil influence; 2, in the same family some are affected, others are spared; 3, those who are affected are almost never similarly circumstanced in the same family—that is to say, one is epileptic, while another is a deaf mute, &c.—*Gazette Méd. de Paris*, May 17, 1856.

5. *Child with two Heads.*—Dr. Budd, of Bristol, read, at the recent Anniversary meeting of the British (formerly Provincial) Medical Association, an account of a most remarkable example of this.

The child was five weeks old, and at the time of the meeting was living in Bristol. The mother was attended in her confinement by Mr. M'Pherson, of that city. The child was the second of a family, the first of which was perfectly well formed, and no known cause for this monstrosity had existed. The case was illustrated with the aid of a photographic engraving. The first head was naturally formed; the second head emerged from it, at the temporal region, on the right side. It was sessile; or, in other words, the two heads had but one neck. The lower jaw of the second or supplementary head was rudimentary, or incomplete; but this head had a mouth and lips, a nose (which was more largely developed than the natural one), eyes, which stood out as globes uncovered by eyelids, and a brain. The roof of the skull was incomplete, and the brain was covered only by a membrane, which for some time after birth had been transparent, and permitted the division of the hemispheres and the convolutions to be seen through it. This membrane had progressively become opaque, as had the corneæ. Shortly after birth, it had been observed that the pupils were well formed, and the iris (in the eyes of the second head) was regular and natural; but it had not been noticed whether the latter was obedient to the stimulus of light, and observation on this was now impossible, owing to the increasing opacity of the cornea. The left ear of the second head is in a state of fusion with the right ear of the first or natural head, and it is difficult to state if all the parts of these two ears exist. A connection of the mouth and nostrils of the second head with those passages in the head proper has not been clearly made out. A regurgitation of milk through them is said to have taken place, but this is doubtful. The child is not likely to survive, for the eyes and hemispheres of the brain in the second head are perishing very fast, and will probably become a source of poison to the system. Except in having a double head, the form of the child is comely. A remarkable fact is that perfectly consensual action takes place between the movements of the natural and of the supplementary face; in the act of sucking the lips of both heads move; in crying, the muscles of both are put into the same action; in sneezing with one head the face of the other is congested, and the child yawns with both mouths at the same time. It is difficult to exaggerate the importance of this phenomenon as connected with reflex and emotional action. In sleep, the closing of the eyes of the second head is lost from the want of eyelids; but I am satisfied (said Dr. Budd) that when the natural head sleeps the other sleeps too, as it then has the passive expression and relaxation of sleep, which ceases when the other head awakes; and when the natural head is asleep you can move or touch the lips of the second head without the notice of the child. We have been unable to ascertain whether consensual emotions may originate in either head. Emotional acts originating in the nervous centre are seen in both. It is difficult to excite reflex acts in the natural head through impressions made on the second one, but easy to excite them in the natural head so as to affect the second. Whatever movement occurs in the eyes of the second head occurs in those of the first, and movements of sucking can be induced in the mouth of the natural head by sucking with the other mouth. Only two analogous cases appear to be recorded. One is that of Rita Christina, the two-headed body described and figured by M. Serres (*Anat. Pathologique*), and another is treated of in the *Cyclopædia of Anatomy;* but both differ from the present case in this, that in each there were two nervous systems united at a lower point in the body, whereas in this it is doubtful whether the junction is at or below the medulla oblongata. Dr. Budd briefly canvassed the question whether this monstrosity had resulted from a fusion of two germs in early uterine life, or whether it were an example of vegetative repetition analogous to the instances of six fingers or toes and similar malformations. He said he had satisfied himself that its origin was of the first-mentioned kind, because vegetative repetition only affected subordinate parts, such as limbs, and not organs of a high and noble character, as the brain and nervous system. He feared that the opportunity to inspect the internal anatomy of the subject would be lost to the profession after the death of the child. What could be done to prevent such a loss to physiology? A short Act of Parliament had before now been passed for less important and useful objects.

In reply to a question asked, Dr. Budd stated that he believed that the tongue of the second head was very rudimentary.

MATERIA MEDICA AND PHARMACY.

6. *Effect of Belladonna in immediately arresting the Secretion of Milk.*—Dr. R. H. Goolden has communicated to the *Lancet* (Aug. 9th, 1856) the two following cases, which seem to show that belladonna possesses the power of arresting the secretion of milk.

E. J., aged 28, was admitted into Anne's Ward, St. Thomas's Hospital, with severe rheumatic fever. She had been ill four days, with a child at the breast four months old. At the time of her admission she had swelling and acute pain in both wrists, right elbow, both knees, and left ankle. The knee-joints were distended with synovia, and erythematous patches were on the skin of the knees, ankles, and wrists. She was bathed in perspiration, and the secretion of milk was abundant. According to the regulation of the hospital, the child was removed; indeed, from her helpless condition, it was necessary, considering the difficulty of attending to an infant in a ward with other patients. Soon after her admission she took eight grains of calomel and a grain and a half of opium, followed by a senna draught; and one scruple of nitrate of potassa, ten grains of bicarbonate of potassa, and half a drachm of spirit of nitric ether, in peppermint water, every four hours. The joints were covered with cotton wool.

On the following day, at two o'clock, I found she had been freely purged; the joints were in nearly the same state. She had had no sleep. The breasts had become tumid, hard, painful, knotty, and extremely tender. The superficial veins were distended. Some milk had been drawn, but the process was attended with great pain, and we could not listen to the heart's sounds on account of the tenderness.

A milk abscess, in complication with rheumatic fever, was of all things to be avoided, and unless the secretion could be at once arrested it appeared inevitable. In this strait I recollected that I had somewhere met with an observation (but I cannot remember whether it was in an English or foreign journal) that atropine applied externally to the breasts would dry up the milk; and, thinking it reasonable, I caused the areola of the breasts to be smeared with extract of belladonna, in the same way that it is used to dilate the pupil of the eye. I likewise ordered the addition of half-drachm doses of colchicum wine, knowing that whenever milch cows eat the meadow saffron in the pasture they immediately become dry; and though I have not much faith in colchicum as a remedy in rheumatic fever uncomplicated with gout, there could be no objection to its use, and it has the sanction of much higher authority than my own.

On my third visit, the following day, the first inquiry was about the breasts. They were all right. But was it the colchicum or belladonna that had relieved them? The extract was used before I left the ward; before the mixture was given the secretion of milk had been arrested and the breasts had become soft. The rest of the case has no further special interest. I will only state that there was no heart affection, and that the fever, though very severe while it lasted, was of short duration, and the patient left the hospital quite well in fourteen days.

The second case that occurred to me was uncomplicated with any disease, and such as would usually fall under the care of the accoucheur rather than the physician.

A lady, the wife of a clergyman, was travelling with her husband, and, in order to accompany him, had weaned her baby (then seven months old). Happening to be at Oxford at the commemoration festival, he came to me in great trouble, telling me that his wife had done a foolish thing in weaning the child, and that they were now arrested in their progress in consequence of the state of her breasts. They were tumid, very tender, painful, and hard, with large superficial veins, and the milk had been drawn with difficulty several times with temporary relief. I recommended the application of the extract of belladonna to the areolæ, desiring them to send for a medical practitioner if the inconvenience did not immediately subside or unless she felt quite well. A few days brought me a letter, giving a very satisfactory account, and thanking me for what she was pleased to call my wonderful prescription. Within two hours she was perfectly relieved, the milk absorbed, and (what is very important) there was no fever or other inconvenience attending the sudden suppression of the milk; and, instead of taking the opening medicine I had prescribed for her, she continued her journey the next morning.

I have not been able to discover that the fact that belladonna is available for the purpose of arresting the milk secretion is at all generally known—certainly it was not to several accoucheurs in large practice of whom I have inquired. The fact is important, if true, for then milk abscesses will become a matter of past history, and probably many diseases of the breast may be rendered less complicated by its use.

The two cases I have detailed are not sufficient to prove that it will always be either successful or safe, but they render it highly probable that it is so.

---

7. *On Coniin.* By Dr. Schroff.—Twenty-seven experiments were made with coniin upon the human subject, three medical gentlemen having each submitted to nine. The doses given varied from 0.003 grammes to 0.085 grammes. The last and strongest dose which was taken corresponded to two drops of newly-prepared coniin taken out of a bottle opened for the first time. Dr. Schroff has found, by observations on rabbits, that exposure to the air weakens the operation of the alkaloid. This dose was dissolved in thirty drops of alcohol. The following account of the symptoms produced embraces those which resulted from the operation of smaller quantities. A very sharp taste, strong burning in the mouth, sense of scraping in the throat, salivation; the epithelium of the tongue was removed in spots; the papillæ were strongly prominent, and the organ lost sensibility, and was as if paralyzed. In about three minutes, the head and face became very warm, accompanied by a sense of fulness, weight, and pressure in the head (symptoms which were not produced by the smaller doses). These head symptoms reached a high degree of intensity; became associated with giddiness, inability to think or to fix the attention on one subjcet, with sleepiness, great general discomfort, and malaise (*Katzenjammer*), which, in a less degree, lasted till next day. The vision was indistinct, objects floating together, and the pupil was dilated; the hearing was obtuse, as if the ears were stopped with cotton; the sense of touch was indistinct, and there was a feeling of formication, and as if the skin were covered with fur; general weakness and prostration, so that the head was with difficulty kept erect; the upper extremities could only be moved with the exertion of much effort; and, on account of the weakness of the lower extremities, the walk was very uncertain and tottering. Even the next day the weakness of the extremities continued, slight trembling being induced by much movement. While going home, the muscular debility was especially great, the walk consisting rather of a throwing forward of the body, so as to bring the muscular action into as little use as possible. On stepping, and, when at home, on pulling off the boots, cramps in the calves of the legs occurred, as well as in other groups of muscles when they were called into action—as, for instance, in the balls of the thumbs when the thumbs were closely bent. This symptom was constantly observed in two of the experimenters when the dose was at least one drop. Under strong effort to move, pain in the muscles and legs occurred. Fresh air diminished the giddiness and fulness in the head, but in one of the experimenters, occasioned temporary pain in the course of the supra-orbitalis and cutaneus malæ nerves. Eructations, abdominal rumbling and distention, nausea, even efforts at vomiting, occurred in all the subjects, even after small doses; in one case, actual vomiting took place. Sometimes there was a tendency to diarrhœa. No effect was produced upon the urine. In all the cases there was dampness of the ends of the fingers; and after large doses, the hands were absolutely moist. The

countenance was sunken and pale; the hands were cold and blue. After the larger doses, the pulse commonly increased in frequency to the extent of a few beats, but subsequently it always lessened; yet this diminution did not bear that relation to the extent of the dose as where aconite was given. Respiration was often yawning, but otherwise no constant anomaly presented itself. The sleep was good, and mostly very sound.—*Brit. and For. Med.-Chirurg. Rev.*, July, 1856, from *Vierteljahrsch. für die Praktische Heilkunde*, 1855.

8. *Ergot of Wheat.*—Dr. Jobert makes the following statements respecting this substance: 1. The medical and obstetrical property of this ergot is as incontestable as of ergot of rye, and its effects are as prompt, as direct, and as great. 2. Its hæmostatic action appears certain. Dr. Jobert has administered it several times against abundant discharges of blood, and immediately after labour it has almost constantly and fully succeeded. 3. In the dose of one or two grammes, according to urgency, in cases of uterine hemorrhage, during any period of pregnancy, it has frequently succeeded in lessening, if not in completely arresting, the hemorrhage; and this without appearing to produce any stimulant action on the uterus.—*Gaz. des Hôpitaux*, March, 1855.

9. *A New Solution of Iodine in various Skin Diseases.* By Dr. Max Richter.—The solution is made thus: Half an ounce of iodine is to be dissolved in an ounce of glycerine, and subsequently half an ounce of iodine is to be added, which completely dissolves in a few hours. In the experiments made with this solution, it was applied to the surface by means of a hair pencil; the part was then covered with gutta percha paper, fixed at the edges with strips of plaster, so as to prevent the volatilization of the iodine. This was removed after twenty-four hours; and for a similar time, cold pledgets were applied. Burning pain, more or less intense, but rarely of more than two hours' duration, was produced. The repetition of the painting depends on the appearance of the part and the amount of disease. The conclusions of the author are—1. That the iodine thus applied acts as a caustic. 2. That while it possesses considerable curative powers in respect of scrofulous and syphilitic affections, it is especially useful in lupus. 3. That the solution dissipates even deeply-seated tubercles of lupus, and may be applied for this purpose to the most tender surface without fear of eroding it. 4. That when the solution was applied only to a part of a diseased surface, the remainder was, nevertheless, influenced. 5. That it is particularly serviceable to large and superficial sores. 6. That after a series of paintings, and when the sore was almost healed, the local pains greatly increased in intensity.—*Wochenblatt der Zeitschrift der k. k. Gesellsch. der Aerzte zu Wien*, 1855.

10. *Caustic Collodion.*—Dr. Macke (of Sorau) has for some years successfully used a solution of four parts of deutochloride of mercury in thirty of collodion, to destroy nævi materni. There is no better caustic when it is desired to cause them to disappear quickly and certainly, in those cases in which the use of a cutting instrument is objected to, or where excision is not very practicable, as on the cartilages of the ear; it is especially useful with very petulant children, when other caustics cannot be retained in their place, or when they are likely to be soiled by urine or fecal matters.

The application of this caustic is easy, and is performed with a fine camel's hair brush; its sphere of action may be perfectly determined, and it dries so quickly that it is impossible that it should extend to any neighbouring healthy part, or be removed in any way by the patient.

If much inflammation supervenes, cold applications are useful; the eschar is solid, one or two lines in thickness, according to whether the caustic is applied once, or more frequently; it separates from three to six days after, and leaves but a trifling cicatrix.

The pain is seldom intense and soon passes over. The author, who has found great success in many cases with caustic collodion, is quite certain that there is no fear of poisoning, and recommends its use to the profession as being as certain in its results as it is easy of application.—*Dublin Hosp. Gaz.*, July 1, 1856, from *Journal de Chimie Médicale.*

11. *Preparation of Caustic with Gutta Percha.*—M. Richard has recently brought this before the Paris Society of Surgery. Gutta percha in powder is intimately mixed with pulverized caustic in proportions according to the strength required, as, *e. g.*, two parts of chloride of zinc to one of gutta percha. The mixture is to be gently heated in a tube or porcelain capsule, over a spirit lamp. The gutta percha softens, and becomes thoroughly impregnated with the caustic, so that on cooling a gutta percha porte-caustic is formed. By its properties the gutta percha possesses the advantages of not altering the tissues, of preserving its consistence and flexibility, of insinuating itself by its suppleness into either natural or abnormal canals, however tortuous, of assuming any desired form under the fingers of the surgeon, and of allowing, by reason of the porosity of its molecules, the exudation and unimpeded action of the caustic it contains.—*Med. Times and Gaz.*, Aug. 2, from *Journ. de Chimie Médicale*, 1856.

MEDICAL PATHOLOGY AND THERAPEUTICS, AND PRACTICAL MEDICINE.

12. *Typhus in the Crimea.*—M. Baudens, Surgeon-in-Chief of the French army, has addressed a letter from Constantinople to the President of the Academy of Medicine of Paris, wherein he states that the typhus which reigned amongst the French troops is not identical with typhoid fever, notwithstanding a certain amount of analogy as to cause, periods, and sequelæ.

Typhus, as lately observed in the Crimea, is engendered by want, and crowding, either in prisons, hospitals, or on board vessels; the disease may, indeed, be called forth and removed at will. This is not the case with typhoid fever and other epidemics, as cholera, which, in spite of all precautions, break out suddenly and disappear without any appreciable cause. Typhus is propagated both by infection and contagion; the latter mode of transmission, which is doubted by some as to typhoid fever, is quite evident as to the Crimean typhus.

The difference between typhus and the generality of epidemics is, that the latter reign only temporarily, according to the duration of certain atmospheric influences, whilst typhus continues until the causes of infection have been removed. The Crimean typhus has presented less regularity and uniformity in the accession of symptoms than the ordinary typhus described by Hildenbrand. This irregularity may be ascribed to various causes, amongst which should especially be noted scurvy, dysentery, and the intermittents, which were excited by the marshes of the valley of the Tchernaya. There were mostly no premonitory symptoms, as lassitude, sleeplessness, lumbar pains, horripilatio, tension in the head, and vertigo, so common in typhoid fever. The Crimean typhus began at once by shivering, frontal cephalalgia, stupor, muttering or violent delirium, total prostration, more or less discharge from the eyes, the nares, or bronchi, intense thirst, and a foul state of the alimentary canal. The burning skin was covered in two or three days with an exanthematous eruption, different from that which is seen in typhoid fever, and presenting irregular groups of round spots of a dull red, smaller than a split pea, and not disappearing upon pressure with the finger. There were generally neither petechia nor sudamina. The fever proved continuous, with from 100 to 130 beats in a minute, but was interrupted by one, or sometimes two, regular paroxysms in the twenty-four hours, somewhat similar to fits of ague, which circumstance has given the Crimean fever a peculiar character. The abdomen was generally soft, painless, and without either tympanitis or that gurgling in the iliac fossa pecular to typhoid fever. Instead of the diarrhœa which generally accompanies the latter affection, constipation was present in the Crimean fever, except in those cases where dysentery existed before the attack. The inflammatory period lasted five or six days, and was followed by cerebral symptoms of the ataxic and adynamic character. The latter lasted only four or five days, and were slight in the cases which recovered.

The short duration of this fever contrasts strikingly with the length of time during which typhoid fever generally lasts. Death has often occurred on the third day, sometimes on the second, and even on the first. The latter were fearful cases. The fever continued rarely beyond the twelfth or fifteenth day, save when complications occurred, such as congestion of the viscera of any of the three splanchnic cavities. Convalescence almost always took place within the first ten days, the patient passing at once, as it were, from death to life. Coma and delirium left him as by magic, but sleep continued heavy, and there remained deafness, weakness of sight, and some loss of memory. No falling of hair, as happens after typhoid fever, was noticed. The favourable changes were often preceded by epistaxis, diaphoresis, critical urine, and sometimes mumps. Convalescence, which advances so slowly in typhoid fever, is rapid in typhus, and errors of diet have no unpleasant results. This is owing to the absence of inflammation of the intestinal follicles, and the non-congestive state of the mesenteric glands, the reverse being one of the principal characteristics of typhoid fever.

The liver and the spleen, in the Crimean typhus, were often found gorged with blood, and softened; the lungs, when congested, were either clogged or hepatized; the meninges injected; opaline effusion in the arachnoid, sometimes with pseudo-membranous patches; cerebral surface dotted, softened, or presenting on its surface a layer of pus.

Treatment.—First, by pure air and powerful ventilation; non-interference with the inflammatory stage, as being an effort of nature to throw off the morbid poison by an exanthematous eruption; no bleeding, except in very robust subjects, and when cerebral apoplexy is threatening; leeches to the mastoid processes, or cupping between the shoulders, preferable to venesection; to have recourse to the same means when the smallness of the pulse points to an oppression of vital forces, which latter rise again after moderate depletion? to stop the intermittences which sometimes occur by quinine, in order to recall the continuity of the fever, which generally then gives way, when it is not kept up by an accidental organic lesion. At the outset, an emeto-cathartic is advantageous, when the primæ viæ are out of order; mucilaginous and acidulated drinks, and even wine-and-water. In the comatose stage, such remedies as are usually employed in adynamia and the ataxic state. In the latter circumstances, tonics and port or Malaga have proved very beneficial. The above treatment has been the most successful in the East, and the most experienced medical men have employed it with excellent results.

—

13. *Softening of the Brain in a Child, with the Absence of the ordinary Symptoms.*—Dr. F. Churchill read to the College of Physicians of Ireland, June 4, 1856, the following interesting observations on, and detailed the following history of, a case of softening of the brain in a child, aged nine years and a half.

Dr. Churchill first alluded to a case of ramollissement of the cerebellum, which he brought before the Association in the session 1852–3, and in which "the only marked symptoms were headache in paroxysms, vomiting terminating these paroxysms, and slow but perfectly regular pulse; and, besides these, two others which only occurred once, and speedily passed away, viz: double vision, and a kind of spasmodic action of both arms, but there never were either convulsions, coma, squinting, delirium, or paralysis."

The case he now wished to draw attention to was one of softening of some of the central portions of the cerebrum, in which the absence of the ordinary symptoms was even more striking. "Such cases," he continued, "occurring in children, appear to be rather rare. MM. Rilliet and Barthez quote them, but none appear to have occurred within their own experience except as secondary to other diseases, or as consecutive to ancient lesions of the brain.[1] Genuine cases, however, have been repeatedly recorded by Abercrombie, Duparcque, and others, to which I shall presently refer.

[1] Maladies des Enfants, vol. i. p. 150.

"As to the disease itself, Dr. Abercrombie's description partakes of his usual clear precision. He divides the cases into two classes, one in which the disease attacks persons advanced in years, and which has been so ably investigated by M. Rostan; in the other, the disease was found chiefly 'in the dense central parts of the brain, the funix, septum lucidum, and corpus callosum, or in the cerebral matter immediately surrounding the ventricles, and occurred in persons of various ages, but chiefly in young persons and children.' He remarks subsequently: 'I am still disposed to contend that the ramollissement of young persons, occurring in acute affections, and seated chiefly in the central parts, is one of the terminations of inflammation in that particular structure.'[1] As regards the symptoms, he considers that they exhibit no uniformity, but 'the cases which terminate by ramollissement seem in general to be characterized by convulsions more or less extensive, followed by paralysis and coma, the convulsion ceasing some time before death; but in case 27 the convulsions continued with the utmost violence till the very time of death. In case 29, on the other hand, there was no convulsion, but a sudden attack of palsy, exactly resembling the ordinary attack of hemiplegia from other causes. In some of the subsequent cases, again, we find most extensive destruction of the cerebral substance without either paralysis or convulsion, and even without coma. In one remarkable case, to be afterwards described—viz: the last case under tubercular disease—we shall find destruction of the cerebral substance to as great an extent, perhaps, as is upon record; while the patient went to bed in the state of health in which she had been for many months before, and was found dead in the morning.'[2] With the exception of this observation, I find nothing in this author to lead us to suppose that the disease may exist with an absence of the usual symptoms of convulsions, paralysis, or coma.

"Dr. Rowland, in his essay, enumerates all the symptoms of the disease which have ever been recorded, and gives us a comparative estimate of their value. For example, he speaks of headache being one of the earliest symptoms, but accompanied by confusion of thought, restlessness, excitement, and delirium; sometimes with a convulsive paroxysm, and afterwards with threatenings of paralysis. He remarks that the 'character of the headache is not usually acute; but occasionally it is shooting and lancinating, like neuralgia. The nature of the malady might, therefore, be overlooked, especially as the headache occurs in paroxysms, sometimes even with distinct intermissions. A careful examination will, even under these circumstances, detect the lurking evil; obtuseness of intellect, or delirium, or some feeling of weakness, or tingling in the limbs, an anxious expression of countenance, or other sign, will be observed.'[3] Nevertheless, I do not find any intimation given that cases occasionally occur in which almost all the usual symptoms are absent.

"Dr. Russell Reynolds, in his valuable work on the *Differential Diagnosis of Diseases of the Brain*, gives a concise summary of the distinctive symptoms of cerebritis and ramollissement. He carefully points out intense pain, which often accompanies the former, and also the obscuration of the mental faculties, but he states that the stage is ushered in with convulsions. Partial cerebritis, he remarks, 'resembles more the non-febrile than the febrile affections;' and, so far, this is in accordance with the case I shall presently submit.

"MM. Rilliet and Barthez consider ramollissement of the brain to be extremely rare in children, unless where it is an accompaniment, or perhaps a consequence, of another disease, as hydrocephalus, for example; in which case they regard it as an œdematous softening, or when it is consecutive to ancient cerebral disease. They, however, quote two cases from authors, but in both convulsions and other marked cerebral symptoms occurred.

"But by far the most satisfactory account that I have met with of this affection is contained in a paper on the subject, by M. Duparcque,[4] which I did not

[1] On Diseases of the Brain and Spinal Marrow, p. 24–25.
[2] Ibid., p. 108.
[3] P. 35.
[4] Archives Générales de Médecine, vol. xxviii. p. 151. 1852.

read until this paper was written out. He regards white softening of the brain as a primary affection, not inflammatory, but dependent upon disordered vital action. From the five cases he has recorded, he has drawn the following general description: '*Predisposing and determining causes*—precocious or developed intelligence, intellectual fatigue, profound or vivid moral emotions. *Positive symptoms*—headache, with somnolence; integrity of the intellectual functions; exaltation of the special senses, and of the general sensibility; apyrexia, and even slowness of the general circulation. *Negative symptoms*—absence of delirium, of convulsions, of contractions; absence of stupor, of loss of intellect, of paralysis.'

"This summary evidently refers to a class of cases in which we may include the one I am about to relate, and it differs remarkably from every other description of the disease I have read. One of M. Duparcque's cases, however, has such a striking resemblance to mine, that I hope I may be excused for giving a short abstract of it. The patient was a boy, aged 13, very intelligent, and at that time studying hard for a prize: he complained first of fatigue, restlessness at night, headache, which was relieved by vomiting. He returned to school, but was obliged to leave from headache and sleepiness, which continued the next day. He complained of headache, increasing in paroxysms; his intelligence was perfect; he was pained by light and sound, and sensitive to the touch generally, but there were neither convulsions nor paralysis. The skin was dry, warm; countenance calm; pulse sixty; urine scanty; tongue clean; bowels free. Considering the probable cause of the disease, and the symptoms which were referable to the brain, M. Duparcque satisfied the family that the child had cerebral fever (fièvre cérébral); but, as he candidly tells us, reserving to a later period the decision as to whether it was a case of 'cerebritis or of meningitis, simple or tubercular.' For some days the symptoms continued much the same, no new ones being developed. The pulse had diminished in frequency in the morning, and there was a slight exacerbation in the afternoon; 'little fever, little assoupissement, slight somnolence, neither contractions, convulsions, delirium, nor paralysis.' Under these doubtful circumstances, Dr. Blache was called in, and, reasoning '*par voie d'exclusion*,' he rejected the supposition of its being either cerebritis, meningitis, hydrocephalus, or typhoid fever, and decided in favour of 'nervous fever,' or 'nevrose cérébrale.'

"On the fourteenth day there was a sub-delirium, stupor, agitation. It was difficult to make him speak, but he answered correctly. The eyes were turned up, the eyelids half open; the extremities became cold; the face changed; and in the night the respiration became embarrassed, sighing, and rattling; the head was thrown back convulsively, and he died.

"The *post-mortem* examination exhibited no marks of inflammation of either the membranes or the substance of the brain, but white ramollissement of both anterior lobes of the cerebrum, particularly of the left. The limits were not defined, but the solution was greater in the centre and in front. Every other part of the brain was healthy. There were two or three spoonfuls of fluid in the ventricles, but not enough to distend them.

"From even the foregoing slight sketch of what is laid down in books, we may infer, I think—1. That inflammation and softening of the cerebral substance is somewhat rare in children. 2. That it is generally said to be accompanied with pain, obscuration of the intellect, disorder of the senses, convulsions, or paralysis, or all of these symptoms, according to the severity and duration of the attack. 3. That, however rare, cases have been recorded in which few or none of these symptoms were present, and yet the patient died of ramollissement—whether inflammatory or not, may be disputed, but in which the disease appeared as a primary affection. 4. That such cases, from their rarity and the difficulty of diagnosis, possess great practical interest; and that it is only by the collection of individual cases that we can hope to arrive at any positive conclusions.

"CASE.—On Tuesday, the 21st March, I first saw A. B., aged 9½, a little girl, of a slight, delicate appearance, with very fair skin and red hair, and of unusual intellectual activity, a member of a family rather obnoxious to head affections; first complained of severe headache on Monday, March 17, 1856. We have since found reason to believe, however, that she had been unwell for more than a week, but, as she was anxious to compete in some school examination, she concealed her illness from her mother. On the Monday, however, the pain was too violent to be longer hidden, and it continued without intermission, though with aggravated paroxysms, until I saw her. During this time she slept well, and had some appetite, but no fever. She insisted upon going to school on Wednesday, and was sent home, much the worse for the exertion and excitement.

"I found her in bed, complaining of severe pain and throbbing in the head (especially at the top), which increased occasionally to an almost intolerable degree. There was neither intolerance of light nor sound at that time. Her intellect was as active and clear as usual; she spoke freely, nor did she dream when asleep. There were neither startings, convulsions, nor stupor. The pulse was 74; neither full nor feeble, but slightly irregular. She had vomited once or twice, but, upon inquiry, I found that it was always after taking food or medicine; however, she took many things without vomiting; she complained of no nausea; the tongue was loaded, but furred and moist: the bowels were quite regular. The sensitive and motive powers were perfectly natural.

"These were the symptoms which presented themselves; and, judging by them, I found it no easy matter to come to any decided conclusion as to the nature of the affection.

"1. Of the reality and intensity of the headache there could be no doubt, and the case might be one of meningitis, tubercular or simple; or it might be a mass of tubercular matter in the brain, or of inflammation of the cerebral substance. But, if so, how account for the absence of disorder of the senses—of startings, convulsions, or stupor—of fever and delirium, or paralysis?

"2. If the case were the result of gastric disturbance, or were the beginning of infantile remittent, which would be consistent with the headache and state of the tongue, age of the patient, and absence of nervous symptoms, startings, convulsions, &c., still, there was no accounting for the quiet pulse, and the absence of remissions and exacerbations. Moreover, though there had been vomiting, it had only occurred a few times, and when provoked, and generally the stomach was little disturbed. There was no abdominal distension, and no disorder of the bowels.

"Could it be neuralgia? The age of the child was against the supposition; and the only argument in its favour was the deficiency of symptoms characteristic of either of the diseases just mentioned.

"I found it impossible to come to any positive conclusion; and, if I have clearly described the case, it will be probably conceded to me that the wisest thing I could do was to suspend my judgment until the course of the disease should elucidate its nature. Meantime I treated the case very cautiously, so as to meet the possibility of its being inflammation of the brain or its membranes. Leeches were applied, and the legs were fomented; a brisk purgative was given, followed by hydrargyrum cum creta and James's powder at short intervals.

"Whether the course of the disorder did elucidate its nature, remains to be determined; but, omitting *daily* reports, I shall state merely the changes in the symptoms throughout, in a more connected though cursory manner, premising that the patient died on Wednesday, April 2—the sixteenth day of her illness.

"The headache continued as bad as ever throughout the entire illness, unless, perhaps, the last two days, increasing in paroxysms, and accompanied by moaning. Still, she slept very well at night, from which I infer that the pain must have remitted; but she almost always woke with it. The sleep, for the most part, was sound and natural, but one or two nights it was so deep as to resemble stupor while it lasted. Her intellect was clear throughout; there never was anything like delirium. At first she spoke freely; but, as the disease advanced, she either could not or would not make the effort to speak—I rather think the latter, as she occasionally spoke a few words, quite intelligibly, up to the last day; up to within an hour of her death she evidently recognized those around her. She never had either startings, squinting, the least convulsion, or loss of power. Occasionally, but not frequently, she yawned. The vomiting ceased entirely the day after I first saw her, and never returned. There was no thirst up to the twelfth day, and no appetite; the bowels required, at first, a little medicine, but afterwards she was troubled with mercurial diarrhœa. The urine was secreted in the natural quantity, and of the usual appearance; but towards the end she had twice some delay or difficulty in passing it, which speedily disappeared.

"The senses at first seemed more acute, both light and noise annoyed her; but after a few days this diminished; a strong light seemed disagreeable; and throughout, although the pupils answered to the light, I should say that, considering the position of her bed, facing the window, they were ordinarily more dilated than one would have expected.

"The pulse, I have mentioned, was at first about 72, and slightly irregular; but this irregularity disappeared after two days, and never returned; when asleep, it was below 70. This continued up to the twelfth day, when suddenly, in the afternoon, a smart outburst of fever occurred; the skin became hot (having been quite natural previously), the pulse rose to 120, and there was great thirst. I do not think the headache was worse, and no nervous symptoms were developed. This attack lasted five or six hours, and then subsided, without perspiration. She fell asleep, and in the morning I found a complete remission. The same attack was repeated on the thirteenth, fourteenth, and fifteenth days, but rather less severely each day; so that on the day she died the prospect seemed rather less dark than previously; although the exact nature of the disease seemed, if anything, rather more obscure.

"Thus, on April 2, at 9 o'clock, of the sixteenth day, she took beef-tea, swallowed well, recognized those around her, and seemed unusually free from headache and fever. At 10 o'clock she suddenly became insensible, but not convulsed; the breathing became laborious and rattling; the pulse quick and weak; lips blue; countenance livid; and at 11 o'clock she died, quite calmly.

"However puzzled I might be to explain satisfactorily the nature of the attack, it was quite clear that there were grounds for very serious apprehension, and that the wiser plan would be to treat the case as disease of the brain, with such modifications as the symptoms called for; and in this view I was fortunate to have the concurrence of Sir H. Marsh, who saw the patient with me soon after the commencement of my attendance, and up to the day but one before she died. We applied leeches to the head and feet; blisters, constantly renewed, to the neck and head; ice to the head; mustard cataplasms to the legs; gave hydrargyrum cum creta, subsequently calomel and James's powder, until diarrhœa had set in, and afterwards James's powder alone, and mercurial frictions; but I cannot say that even temporary relief appeared to result from any of these measures.

"Having obtained permission to examine the head, Dr. M. Collis was good enough to make the *post-mortem* dissection, about twenty-four hours after death. There was no congestion of the scalp, but, on raising the skull, we found the superficial vessels of the brain were somewhat fuller than usual; there was no opacity of the arachnoid, no tubercular deposition, and no effusion. The substance of the brain was natural to a considerable depth, but we found the posterior portion of the great commissure of the brain, the fornix, and septum lucidum so much softened as to be semifluid. It was of much the usual colour, neither yellowish nor reddish. A superficial layer of the corpus striatum was also softened. The ventricles contained a considerable quantity of opaline serum; and there was more beneath the arachnoid of the cerebellum, and at the base of the brain, but nowhere did the membrane exhibit marks of inflammation.

"Thus we see that we may have fatal softening and effusion, with an absence of almost all the symptoms which are usually attendant on these affections; for the only permanent symptom in this case, and, I may add, aspect of serious disease, was the headache. Neither fever (at first) nor disorder of the senses or intellect; no starting, convulsion, nor paralysis; no continued vomiting, nor obstinate constipation, marked the disease. Towards the end, indeed, a change took place, and then the aspect of the complaint rather resembled remittent fever than anything else.

"There is, however, a very important question remaining for consideration, viz: the relation, in point of time at least, of the softening and the effusion.

Was the case one of inflammation of the brain running on into softening, followed by effusion; or was it a case of arachnitis, in which the softening was a secondary consequence, as noticed by Rilliet and Barthez? So far as we may venture to draw an inference from the history of the case, I think it is in favour of the softening being the primary disease, for we know, as in the case to which I alluded in the commencement of this notice, that ramollissement of the central nervous structure may exist with but few symptoms; whereas I believe it to be extremely rare, if it ever occurs, that meningitis should run a course of sixteen days at least, with such an utter absence of the ordinary characteristic symptoms.

"My own impression is, that the primary affection was inflammation of the central portions of the brain, and that the membranes participated in the morbid action, about the time when the febrile action set in; but that the effusion did not occur until the morning of the day on which she died, and that it was the immediate cause of death."—*Dublin Quart. Journ. of Med. Sci.*, Aug., 1856.

14. *On Alteration of the Capillary Vessels predisposing to Apoplexy.*—M. Ch. Robin gives the following as the conclusions of his researches on this subject:—

1st. The pathological anatomy of the capillary vessels in individuals who have had cerebral hemorrhages discloses a constant and peculiar alteration of the proper walls of these vessels.

2d. This alteration, commencing in the finest capillaries, gradually extends to the larger tubes, and especially to the arteries, advancing from the internal towards the external face of the walls.

3d. This alteration in apoplectics is of the same order as that observed in the capillaries of all old men, and even of many adults; but it constitutes a more advanced phase, becoming, sooner or later, according to the individuals, the cause of the rupture of the vessels.

4th. When these morbid accidents manifest themselves, the alteration has already existed for a shorter or longer period, but in a degree still insufficient to deprive the vessels of their natural power of resistance.

5th. This lesion consists in the production of fatty granulations or drops in the substance of the walls of the tubes, so as gradually to replace a continuous, homogeneous, transparent, and tenacious substance by an assemblage of little fatty and simply contiguous corpuscles, which offer so much less resistance as they are accumulated in greater number.

6th. The anatomico-pathological examination of the vessels in apoplexy enables us to establish a very accurate and highly important practical connection between the normal state of the vessels and their gradual modifications in proportion to the advance of age, by which they attain, sooner or later, according to its rapidity, the condition which deserves the designation of morbid lesion. Now, the knowledge of this gradation between the normal and the pathological states is one of the constant results of the anatomico-pathological study of all the tissues of the economy which best enables us to connect the symptom with the corresponding lesion.—*Dub. Med. Press*, May 28, from *Gaz. Méd. de Paris*, May 17, 1856.

15. *Pneumonia, Asthenic or Passive Form of; Treatment by Quinine.*—Dr. Corrigan, in an interesting clinical lecture (*Dublin Hospital Gazette*, July 15, 1856), makes the following practical remarks:—

"I have two objects in view in this lecture; first, to impress on your minds, gentlemen, this position, which you ought never to forget, viz., that the name of a disease is not a sufficient guide either as to the nature or treatment of a case; and, secondly, to draw your attention to the treatment of certain forms and stages of pneumonia by quinine, both on account of the importance of this treatment, and of the cases before us forming a good illustration of the first point.

"Medical students are very apt to fall into the same mistake as is occasionally fallen into by botanists, florists, and conchologists, viz., fancying that when they have acquired a knowledge of names they have acquired a knowledge of the nature of the objects of their studies; but the mere knowledge of the name of a plant, or a shell, or a flower, gives no more acquaintance with their respective natures than was possessed previously. You must avoid such a mistake in medicine, for its consequences would be too serious; and yet I am sorry to say that this error prevails very generally among our students, and it is because I see it prevail so generally that I feel myself called upon, even in the middle of a session, to notice it, and to warn you against it. I know it prevails, because I see the great tendency there is to substitute book-reading and knowledge of names of diseases merely, for the more troublesome task of reading disease in nature's book at the bed-side. The mere acquaintance with names, and the rules for treatment, will enable you to pass a very creditable examination, and even to win examination prizes, but it will not make you practitioners; and you should ever bear in mind that the passing of an examination with credit, and the obtaining a degree, are not to be your main objects. They are only the means to an end; that end is station in your profession, and its result competency; and believe me the only way to acquire both is to acquire a knowledge, not of the names, but of the intimate nature of the objects of your study.

"Let us now proceed with the illustration of our first point, that *the name of a disease is not an index to its nature or its treatment.* With the name of "pneumonia" you generally and properly associate the ideas of sthenic vascular action of the capillaries, of throbbing of the arteries, increased action in frequency and strength of the heart, and with the accompanying symptoms of flushed face, pink lips, hot breath, burning heat of skin, high-coloured and scanty urine, and orange-coloured viscid sputa. With these there will be naturally associated, as to treatment, bleeding and tartar emetic, those remedies that possess such power over high inflammatory action and over pneumonia, as we have sketched it; but if you were to imagine that the name "pneumonia" always indicated the same nature in the disease going under its name, you would fall into a very grievous error in knowledge and in practice. Pneumonia occasionally means a state of disease the very opposite in character to the picture first drawn, and requiring a very opposite treatment. It is this knowledge, so as to recognize the altered character of the disease, which you can only learn in clinical study.

"To make my observations as simple and as easily intelligible as possible to you, I will confine my observations to what is usually called the first stage of pneumonia, that is the state in which, if a patient die, the lung will be found dark-coloured, from the great quantity of blood contained in it, its capillaries congested, distended frequently beyond their natural caliber, its smaller air-tubes loaded with effused fluid, and the whole lung pitting on pressure and much heavier than natural. Bear in mind next, the peculiar structure of the lung, resembling, as it were, two large sponges, made up nearly altogether of a great congeries of vascular capillaries, the capillaries of the pulmonary artery, loaded with venous blood, and those of the pulmonary veins with arterial blood.

"Now let me recall to your mind one of your earliest physiological lessons. If the capillary vessels of the web of a frog's foot be stimulated, the effect of the stimulation is very soon to cause a distension of the capillary, and a more rapid movement in the contained blood. This, along with the momentary preceding contraction is its sthenic state, for all that is necessary to enable it to return to its healthy state, is to withdraw the stimulant, and the capillary contracts of itself. But if the distension and stimulation be continued another phase occurs: the blood becomes darker, the circulation becomes slower, the capillary has lost its power of contracting, and, to enable it to return to its healthy contractile state, the application of some stimulant is required, when under its influence the capillary regains its lost power, and it again returns to its previously healthy state.

"Now, this simple experiment is really the key to the sthenic and asthenic states of the vascular system, and is the foundation on which we rest our principles as to the treatment of pneumonia, which I bring before you in this lecture.

"Carry your mind's eye from the experiment on the frog's foot to what goes on in some forms and types of pneumonia, and you can no more doubt of what is taking place in the lung within the interior of the chest, than you can doubt your ocular evidence of what you see in the experiment. In the first stage of an attack of pneumonia, in a healthy constitution, with the whole capillary system, including, of course, that of the lungs in possession of its ordinary vigour, the capillaries become distended, but still preserve their sthenic state. In such a case the line of treatment is at once indicated; venesection, to relieve their over-distension, and tartar emetic, to act both upon them and upon the whole vascular system, including heart and arterial and capillary system, are the great means of treatment upon which we rely. But if, from the state of constitution, or from the epidemic type of disease at the time, the capillaries do not retain their sthenic tone, they pass into the state exemplified in the experiment on the frog's foot, they lose their contractile power, and we have then to deal with quite a different state—with an immense mesh of pulmonic tissue, formed nearly altogether of capillaries that have lost their contractile power, and in which further depletion will be not only useless but injurious, for while its effect in lessening the distension would at best be doubtful, it would tend still further to aggravate that asthenic character which they now present; and extension of the disease, increasing debility, exhaustion, and death will follow. It is to meet the supervention of this second or asthenic stage that you have seen me exhibit quinine in large doses; the result has been satisfactory, and it is the more satisfactory to know that its employment has not been a mere empirical experiment, but has arisen from considering the physiological state of the capillaries in the lungs, as illustrated by a physiological experiment, and revealed to us by an analysis of the symptoms. I will now shortly notice some of the cases.

"The first case that suggested the treatment occurred in private practice. The patient was a man of about 35 years of age. He was attacked by pneumonia of right lung; he was a man of rather full habit, and flabby texture. The physical signs were the ordinary ones of the first stage. The constitutional symptoms did not indicate any very high degree of vascular action, and the treatment was of the usual kind, cupping, blistering, and calomel and opium. About the fifth day there was every symptom discouraging in this case. He became slightly jaundiced, or rather assumed a yellowish, sallow cast of countenance, the pulse became very full, very soft, and very yielding, and the expectoration presented the appearance of softened down dissolved blood. The lung had not passed into the second stage of the disease. He appeared now to be rapidly sinking, and it then occurred to me to administer quinine, guided by the principles that I have already explained. He got five grains of quinine every three hours, and the alteration in twenty-four hours was very marked indeed. The same treatment was continued for the next day, and within three days more he was out of danger. I never treated a case in which I was more satisfied of the efficacy of the medicine.

"In this case the disease set in presenting a moderate degree of the sthenic form, but the capillaries speedily lost their contractile power, and then the asthenic form rapidly succeeded. Quinine appears to possess the same power in giving contractile action to the capillaries of the lungs, which we know it possesses in so marked a degree over the capillaries and venous radicles in the spleen, and it may further support this view to recollect that both in lungs and spleen the capillaries are in a very large proportion venous.

"This asthenic form of pneumonia may, however, exist from the very commencement of the attack, that is, either from type of disease, from nature of constitution, or from long-continued action of depressing influence, the capillaries of the lungs may lose their sthenic power from the very onset, and thus we may have asthenic pneumonia either as the second stage of sthenic pneumonia, or we may have it as the primary disease.

"James Hayes, ætat. 21, previously a healthy man, was admitted into the Hardwicke Hospital on the 24th of March, 1856, complaining of pain in the right side, and of great dyspnœa. On examination, double pneumonia was discovered, both lungs were extensively engaged, but the disease had not gone beyond the first stage; there was extensive crepitation with bronchial respiration. The pulse was extremely rapid and small. The debility was extreme, and the surface of the body was pale and rather cool. He presented very much the appearance of a dying man. He was a boatman, constantly exposed to wet and cold, and for four days had been suffering under his illness, and all this time had lain in a canal luggage boat, on its way to Dublin, in extremely inclement and cold weather.

"In the night the dyspnœa became so urgent that he seemed on the point of suffocating; from this he was somewhat relieved by draughts of ether and by wine. A blister was applied to his chest. The next day he was ordered five grains of sulphate of quinine every three hours, and the quinine was continued. On the 29th he was so much improved that the quinine was diminished to a dose three times a day, and his convalescence then set in. I merely give you these cases in illustration of the disease and of its treatment; you have seen a great many cases of a similar kind treated here on the same principle during the past winter and spring, and I will now briefly sum up in propositions what I wish to impress on you in this lecture.

"1. That the name of a disease is not an index to its treatment; but that on the contrary, under the one name, the pathological conditions of the organ affected may change so much, as to require the most varying or even opposite mode of treatment.

"2. That pneumonia presents an illustration of this principle, as it may be of a sthenic or an asthenic form.

"3. That the asthenic form may be consequent on, or be the second stage of the sthenic form; or that the primary attack of pneumonia may be of the asthenic form from the commencement.

"4. That quinine in large doses is a remedy of great power over the asthenic form of pneumonia, whether it be primary or secondary.

"I have only to add, that these observations as to the pathology and treatment of this form of pneumonia have reference to the disease in the stage of extreme congestion, or what is commonly called the first stage of pneumonia."

---

16. *Obliteration of the Thoracic Aorta.*—At a meeting of the Medical Society of Vienna, held on the 19th October, 1855, Professor Skoda introduced a man affected with obliteration of the thoracic aorta. In illustration of the lesion, the Professor exhibited preparations of a five months' fœtus and of a new-born child, in which he indicated the point at which alone this anomaly can take place or has hitherto been observed. It is the point at which the ductus botalli communicates with the aorta and the short space intervening between this point and the origin of the left subclavian artery. During fœtal life, this portion is commonly narrower than the remainder of the aorta, and only acquires the same calibre after birth.

The individual in question was a man, aged forty-seven; a jeweller, of normal complexion and throughout well nourished. On the whole, he enjoys good health, and has only come under clinical observation owing to his having, for three years past, suffered from some dyspnœa in making violent exertion. This is due to an insufficiency of the tricuspid valve, which has only been established for three years.

The following are the grounds upon which Professor Skoda has diagnosed a co-existing obliteration of the aorta: In addition to the blowing murmur coincident with the impulse, and which indicates the above-mentioned insufficiency, a "peculiar vibration or whirring (schwirren) is to be perceived over the greater part of the thorax, partly by palpitation, partly, as in the course of the intercostal arteries, by auscultation; it follows the impulse, and for that reason has its seat in the arteries. The vibration of the arteries of the thorax is due to their dilatation, as may be shown by touching the superficial epigastric arteries, which are much dilated and very tortuous. The beat of the crural arteries at the groin is very feeble, and no pulsation can be felt in the abdominal aorta."

These are the indications characteristic of obliteration of the thoracic aorta; the collateral circulation is carried on by the branches of the subclavian arteries, which must therefore be dilated. A large volume of blood passes from the anterior intercostals to the posterior intercostal, and by centripetal movement reaches the descending aorta, which is thus filled with blood sufficient to supply the arteries of the intestines, but not sufficient to produce distinct pulsations. The inferior extremities probably also receive a supply by the anastomosis of the superior and inferior epigastric arteries. No cyanosis is observed, because nowhere venous blood is introduced into the arterial system.

In connection with this case, Professor Skoda made the following remarks: 1. That in examining the heart, we occasionally perceive murmurs which give rise to the assumption of valvular disease, while the heart is afterwards found healthy; and that the murmur was produced in the coronary arteries or in other arteries, in the vicinity of the heart. Such errors can only be avoided by carefully attending, as in the case detailed, to the coincidence or non-coincidence of the murmur with the movements of the heart. 2. The circumstance that the nutrition of the individual was unimpaired, although the circulation in most of the organs must be, doubtless, slackened, proves that the deranged nutrition, so frequently coinciding with impediments in the circulation, does not depend solely upon the latter.

Professor Skoda was of opinion that the obliteration of the aorta was due either to a complete obliteration or absence of the corresponding portion of aorta in the fœtus, or to the contraction of the latter coincidently with the ductus botalli, owing to the exceptional extension of the tissue of this channel into the coats of the aorta. Professor Skoda maintained that the obliteration could not be set down to inflammation, as arteritis led, not to obliteration, but to aneurism. He referred to an analogous case which had occurred in his wards some years previously, where no disturbance of function was manifested until, accidentally, endocarditis supervened. Death occurred later from pneumonia; and the obliterated aorta has been preserved in the anatomical museum of Vienna.—*Brit. and For. Med.-Chirurg. Rev.*, April, 1856, from *Wochenblatt der Zeitschrift der k. k. Gesellschaft der Aerzte zu Wien*, Nov. 5, 1855.

—

17. *Bronzed Skin and Disease of the Supra-renal Capsules.*—In our previous number (p. 233 *et seq.*) we gave a tabulated report of twenty-seven cases of bronzed skin with disease of the supra-renal capsules drawn up by Mr. HUTCHINSON. We now give an analysis of these cases by Mr. H.

"Of the twenty-seven cases included in the table, in twelve both supra-renal capsules were proved by post-mortem examination to be destroyed by chronic disease, and in every one of these the change in colour of the skin was marked and positive, and the death had been attended by peculiar symptoms of debility. In seven others no post-mortem was obtained, but the kind of cachexia and mode of death had very closely indeed resembled those in which, after death, the theory was confirmed. In one, the patient is still living, the symptoms quite corresponding with those usually met with, and appearing to be irremediable. In one both organs were affected by recent suppuration, and in this only a yellowish brown tint was noticed, the disease having probably not existed long enough to produce the characteristic pigmentary change of hue. In four the disease affected but one of the organs, the other remaining healthy, and in these only a slight (but yet positive) degree of the bronzing had been observed. It cannot be necessary to stop to point out that the but partial extent to which the change in tint of the skin had proceeded in the latter cases, so far from constituting any exception to Dr. Addison's opinion, strongly confirms it. Just in proportion to the extent to which the supra-renal organs are structurally disorganized, and to the length of time which they have been so, appears to be the intensity of the cutaneous discoloration. From this it seems fair to argue, that they probably stand to each other as cause and effect, and are not coincident effects of some other cause. Thus, then, of the whole number recorded (twenty-eight), we have twenty-five, the evidence of which is more or less in favour of the theory under discussion. Let us now glance for a moment at the three

Seemingly Exceptional Cases.—In case No. 26 the patient recovered, and, after lasting somewhat more than a month, the peculiar "dirty-brown tinge" of the skin disappeared. Now, there is every reason for believing, that, in this instance, no pigmentary change had taken place, and that the state described was rather a diffused muddiness than a real bronzing. The reason for believing so is, that the change took place suddenly, and was complete in the course of a day or two. Possibly it was of hepatic origin; at any rate it may be presumed to have had a different cause from that of the change which in all the other cases was very slowly progressive, and requiring several months for its development. In the second exceptional case, a woman who died of cancer had shown no alteration in the colour of the skin, and yet malignant deposit was found in both supra-renal bodies. Here, however, a considerable degree of functional vigour may have been retained, since neither organ was wholly involved, and in one, only a few small nodules existed. It is very possible that the portions remaining healthy may have sufficed for the wants of a body which had been reduced to extreme emaciation by long existing disease. Case 21 of the Table supplies us with what is more like a real exception than any other. It is, however, to be remarked, that no mottling of the skin had been observed, only a diffused muddy condition, and that some doubts had been expressed during life as to its being an example of true bronzing. The patient, moreover, had not been seen by the reporter for some months prior to death, and no note was made as to the state of the skin at the date of that event. On account of these circumstances of doubt, we may, perhaps, fairly hold this case as not proving anything, and, if so, the whole of the seeming exceptions are disposed of.

Having regard, then, to the large amount of evidence in support, and the very doubtful character of what little might at first sight seem to range itself on the opposite side, we may perhaps be permitted from this point to assume that the theory is well grounded, and proceed to examine as to the nature of the

Symptoms attending Diseases of the Supra-renal Capsules. 1. *Change of Colour of the Skin.*—The term "bronzing" probably conveys as good an idea of the exact character of the appearance assumed by the skin in this disease as could well be given. It resembles strikingly the colour of a bronzed statue from which the gloss has been rubbed off. Pressure has no effect in causing its diminution. It seems as a rule to commence first in patches with ill-defined borders, on those parts most exposed to the sun and to friction, the neck, the backs of the hands, the fronts of the thighs, the arms, &c. Around the nipple, and in other parts where pigment naturally abounds, it is generally well-marked, while others, possessing little or no pigment originally, as the palms of the hands, the ungual matrices, &c., remain as pale as ever. This tendency to show itself in patches, is strongly in support of the belief that the change is really one of deposit of pigment; which derives further confirmation from the circumstance, that in not a few cases the punctate, or even patchy deposit of black matter was observed in the mucous membrane of the mouth, and in the serous investment of the abdominal viscera. The conjunctiva usually remains pale and pearly, a condition which well distinguishes true bronzing from the various states of jaundice. The changed colour of skin, although most important for purposes of diagnosis, is probably of very minor consequence among the other departures from health which attend renal capsular disease.

2. *Debility.*—Next to the bronzing of the integument the extreme and peculiar feebleness manifested appears to be the most striking of the symptoms. Without any evidence of thoracic disease, without any great loss of flesh, the patient becomes liable to faintings, loses energy, is unable to exert either body or mind, and, in short, appears to be on the point of death from sheer weakness. In almost all the cases comprised in the Table this state of things was very well marked. In cases 14 and 15, however, the loss of strength had not proceeded *pari passu* with the change in the tint of the skin, and appears to have attracted attention only a few days prior to the fatal event.

3. *Emaciation.*—That there has generally been observed a want of correspondence between the extreme debility and the degree of emaciation coincident with it, seems evident. Several of the patients are described as having remained muscular and fat up to the very last. In almost all, however, there had been

some loss of flesh, and in many it had even been considerable. Dr. Addison's observation, that flabbiness of the solids rather than actual wasting is characteristic of the condition, seems true of the majority of cases.

4. *Anæmia.*—In almost all cases, there would seem to have been present great depravation of the coloured constituents of the blood, as manifested by the pallor of those parts not involved in the bronzing, the general flabbiness of the muscles, the pearly state of the conjunctiva, &c. In two only (cases 3 and 13) was the blood examined with the microscope, and in both those it was found to be loaded with white corpuscles. To the impoverished state of the blood is, no doubt, to be referred the breathlessness on exertion, the debility, the feebleness of the heart's action, and perhaps also the irritability of the stomach.

5. *The Pulse.*—With a few exceptions, in which it became rapid, the pulse has generally been of but average frequency, and peculiar only in its extreme softness and compressibility.

6. *The Tongue.*—It does not appear that any state of the tongue other than that common to most conditions of debility has been observed in connection with this disease.

7. *Dyspepsia.*—In almost all cases prior to death, and in many for protracted periods, great irritability of the stomach was present. In most there was loss of appetite, more or less persistent nausea, and occasional vomiting, with pain and sense of sinking at the epigastrium. In the majority, it would seem that the bowels have been costive rather than otherwise, while, in a few, attacks of diarrhœa had occurred. In several instances the patients had been liable to "biliousness." Much more detailed observations as to the symptoms of indigestion present are desirable.

8. *The Urine.*—The urine was tested for albumen in many of the cases, and in some for sugar; but in no instance was any important departure from its normal constitution observed.

9. *Lumbar Pain.*—Aching, more or less severe, in the back or loins, was a symptom present in a considerable proportion of the cases. In two of these there was, however, disease of the vertebræ, by which it might have been occasioned; and the evidence respecting it is not such as to induce us to attach much importance to its signification.

10. *Nervous Symptoms, Convulsions, &c.*—Symptoms referable to disorder of the cerebro-spinal functions occurred in several of the cases. In three, epileptiform convulsions preceded death. In one, failure of memory, and remarkable change in temper was observed; and in a second, numbness of the fingers, legs, and the tip of the tongue, had been present. In one, the man had suffered from tic douloureux.

11. *Odour of the Body.*—In two cases, both under care at the Brighton Hospital, it was noticed that a peculiarly disagreeable odour was exhaled from the patient's body. In one this was present for a few weeks, and in the other only for a few days prior to death. The phenomenon is not mentioned in the reports of any other case in the series, and Dr. Addison informs us that it was not noticed in any case under his observation.

Such, then, appear to be the more important of the train of symptoms observed in connection with this disease. It is, necessarily, as yet, from the paucity of facts, meagre and inexact, but the general features of the group are, nevertheless, well characterized, and would seem to have been present with tolerable uniformity.

Mode of Death.—In only a small proportion of the cases included in our series has the exact mode of death been recorded. In several the death is stated to have been that of exhaustion. In some, a peculiar form of collapse, without obvious cause, preceded it, while, in two or three others, this collapse followed very slight, and usually inefficient causes, such, for instance, as the action of an aperient dose. In one the collapse was so extreme, and had supervened so suddenly, that poisoning was suspected. In one the patient died of pericarditis with pneumonia; and in another a torpid condition, resembling that of typhus, preceded death. In three, convulsions had been present. Speaking generally, we may say that the phenomena attending death are those of utter prostration of the vital powers, not unfrequently complicated by disturbance of the nervous functions.

Diagnosis.—The combination of a bronzed state of the skin with great systemic debility may be held indicative of disease of the supra-renal capsules; and the more marked these conditions are, the more positively may the opinion be formed. A differential diagnosis may sometimes be requisite, however, as regards the following diseases: 1. *Jaundice.*—In some states of chronic jaundice the skin may be brown rather than yellow, and great vital depression may exist. Here, however, the conjunctiva and the matrices of the nails would, by their discoloured state, prevent the possibility of deception. The tint in jaundice is also a diffused one, and does not occur in patches, as in true bronzing. 2. *Browning from exposure to Sun, &c.*—In these, the examination of parts protected by the clothes would generally be sufficient to prevent error. 3. *Pityriasis versicolor.*—The patches of pityriasis versicolor sometimes remarkably resemble those of the bronzed skin. Their limitation to the abdomen and chest, their defined outline, their furfuraceous surface, the slight itching which attends them, their contagious character, and, above all, the microscopic examination of the cuticle, furnish, however, abundant means by which to distinguish between the two. 4. *The diffused brown muddiness of some other cachexiæ.*—The dark areola round the eye, so often seen in states of disordered menstruation, is in rarer cases found coincident with a loss of healthy tint in the skin generally, which assumes a dirty, sallow, brownish appearance. This, in exaggerated instances, might be mistaken for bronzing; and, indeed, we are not sure that cases 21 and 26 in the series are not examples of this mistake having been committed. It would be premature, indeed, to assert that this state may not have something to do with functional, and perhaps transitory, disorders of the organs, upon structural disease of which the states of more extreme discoloration are found to depend. We have, however, no positive evidence that it does so. In the meantime, it should be borne in mind that in all cases in which bronzing is to be held as positively indicative of diseased capsules there ought to be traces of patching and mottling in some parts; and that in proportion as the tint is equally diffused over the whole body is the diagnosis doubtful.

Prognosis and Treatment.—We have as yet no reason for believing that in cases of true bronzing of the skin, the physician can do other than give the most unfavourable prognosis. No recovery has yet been recorded, nor, indeed, has even temporary improvement under treatment been very marked in any case. After such an avowal it may, perhaps, seem superfluous to speak of treatment, since in our search for principles to guide us in it, we can avail ourselves only of that very delusive light which pathology furnishes. There seems, however, reason for believing, that the morbid changes to which the supra-renal bodies are liable are most of them more or less closely allied to inflammation; and from this fact one might, perhaps, be justified in selecting remedies from the class of drugs known to possess influence over that process. The exhibition of a course of mercury (in very small doses), or the use of the iodide of potassium, the patient's strength being meanwhile supported by a nutritious but non-stimulating diet, would probably be the most rational practice which could be suggested for a case of bronzed skin. As the change in colour is, however, only produced, in all probability, after the organic disease has considerably advanced, there would not, it is to be feared, be much to be hoped for in the way of restoration of function.

Morbid Anatomy.—The cases recorded show examples of the following conditions of disease in the supra-renal bodies. A remarkable symmetry of disease appears to have existed in all excepting the cases of cancer.

1. Acute and recent inflammation ending in abscess (case 17). 2. Atrophy with fibro-calcareous concretions. This condition appears to have been present in seven cases. In some of them cysts existed, and in several a fluid matter resembling pus was contained in the cysts, and bathed the solid fibro-calcareous concretions. These changes probably result from inflammation of chronic character. The complete disorganization of the viscus is usually effected, and in all the cases recorded both glands were involved (cases 2, 4, 7,

12, 13, 14, and 16). 3. The conversion of the viscus into a sort of fibroid structure, with great enlargement and induration. This occurred in cases 1 and 6, and in both all trace of healthy tissue was lost. 4. The deposit of tubercle. In three instances (cases 3, 5, and 9), masses of deposit resembling tubercle were observed, and coincidently, great enlargement of the organ and loss of normal texture. In two the deposit existed in both organs, and in one there was no tubercle in other viscera. It may be doubted whether the deposit is not really more nearly allied to some form of fibrinous effusion, the result of inflammation, than to true tubercle. 5. *Cancer.*—In six[1] cases (cases 7, 8, 10, and 11), the deposit of cancer has been observed. In all it was secondary to the same disease in other organs. In four it affected but one organ, and in two both were involved. In but one was complete disorganization of both effected.

Theory of the Disease.—The observations of Dr. Addison, although they may not as yet have resulted in discovery of the function of the supra-renal bodies, have certainly proved them to possess some very important one. We see their destruction followed in every case by extreme constitutional disorder, loss of strength, depravation of the blood, failure of digestive power, a peculiar tendency to pigmentary deposit, and, finally, by the death of the patient, in spite of all measures for his relief. By whatever morbid change that destruction has been effected, whether cancer, tubercle, or inflammation, the same sequences appear to result, and it would seem that we are fairly authorized in classing them as consequences on it, and not as mere coincident effects of some other cause. Taking these facts in connection with the observations of anatomists as to the very large supply of nerves received by the supra-renal bodies, and the great similarity of certain of their so-called "gland cells," to those of nerve-ganglia, the conjecture that these viscera are in some way very closely associated with the organic nervous system, seems to have much in its favour. Supposing them to exercise a presiding influence over the functional efficiency of some of the viscera of the abdomen, it is easy to see how fatal lesions of health might ensue on their destruction. Dr. Gull has pointed out the close resemblance between the pineal gland and the supra-renal bodies in minute anatomy and also in liability to calcareous deposit, and the idea seems to well merit attention.

We shall venture to conclude this report by a few words on what appear to us as

Desiderata in the further Prosecution of the Inquiry.—1. With regard to the cases of *bronzed skin.* It is desirable that in all cases in which any approach to bronzing is observed, that detailed notes should be preserved, having especial reference to the following points: *a.* The degree of discoloration, the parts affected by it, the parts retaining their healthy hue, the state of the mouth, conjunctiva, &c. *b.* The history of the alteration in colour, when it first occurred, &c. c. The patient's previous state of health. *d.* The patient's present health, as to emaciation, debility, dyspepsia, symptoms of nervous disorder, &c. *e.* The condition of the excreta. The urine should be carefully examined, and the feces inspected from time to time. *f* The state of the blood, both by microscope and chemical analysis. *g.* The presence or absence of any peculiar odour from the patient's body. *h.* The abdomen and thorax should, of course, be submitted to physical exploration, and the exact order of sequence of the various symptoms should be carefully examined into.

2. With regard to the *supra-renal capsules.* It is desirable that henceforth it should become the practice of pathologists to inspect these organs in all post-mortems, without regard to the cause of death. If appearances suspicious of disease are found they should be minutely described, regard being especially had to the extent to which the natural structure of the viscus has been destroyed. As yet so little familiarity with the very different appearances which the capsules may present in a state of health prevails even among experienced morbid anatomists, that great caution will be necessary to prevent mistakes. Whenever doubt is felt, the specimens should be submitted to the inspection of

[1] Two of these are not included in the table. For one, see Dr. Addison's work, page 8; and for the other Mr. Sibley. Report, *Medical Times and Gazette*, page 189.

some more practised observer—an end which, we may suggest, would be well obtained by bringing them before a meeting of the Pathological Society.

3. In the publishing of cases, it is desirable that much more of detail should be given than has been done in most of those hitherto recorded. More facts are wanted, but these facts must have the stamp of accuracy and exactitude, or they will be comparatively valueless. That the important field of investigation, to which Dr. Addison has attracted the attention of the profession, will be cultivated with zeal, we cannot doubt. Great care, however, as well as zeal, will be requisite. The success of the investigation will be greatly served, if all of us who may take part in it are careful always to bear in mind the motto of the philosophic Cavendish—*παντα μετρω, και αριθμω, και σταθμω*.—*Med. Times and Gaz.*, March 22, 1856.

18. *Disease of the Supra-renal Capsules.*—Dr. W. H. Ranking makes (*Assoc. Med. Journ.*, Aug. 9, 1856) some interesting remarks on this new form of disease, founded upon an instance which has recently proved fatal in his practice.

"For the earliest notice of this peculiar disease," he observes, "we are, I believe, indebted to Dr. Addison, of Guy's Hospital; or, at all events, he has been the first to call attention to it in a special publication (*On the Constitutional and Local Effects of Disease of the Supra-renal Capsules*). It appears that a form of anæmia, which doubtless has not really been of rare occurrence, attracted his attention, as differing in many respects from those varieties of cachexia with which we are more familiar as constituting the chlorotic state, the cancerous habit, and the results of direct abstraction of blood. The cases in question almost invariably proved fatal; but the eyes of the pathologist, confidently bent upon the finding of a lesion of some of those important organs to which we are accustomed to look for the causes of death, failed to be gratified, and the disorder remained for some time longer a mystery. It then followed that, accidentally (for he speaks of 'having stumbled upon the curious facts' which he makes known to the profession), Dr. Addison was led to examine into the condition of a class of organs hitherto treated with great *nonchalance* by pathologists, viz., the supra-renal capsules; and he discovered in them a morbid condition, which his acute mind did not fail at once to grasp as a clue to the elucidation of the mystery. These organs, so long neglected, were found in these cases to offer the chief indications of disease; and, however difficult it may be to explain the real association of their lesions with the symptoms during life, the constant presence of such lesions, to the exclusion of lesions of other organs, left no room for doubt that they were associated in the relations of cause and effect.

"Then came the question, *How* does disease of organs, hitherto considered so unimportant that they were even not looked at in nine *post-mortems* out of ten, produce such a train of symptoms as, in all well-marked cases, have invariably resulted in death? This question is still unsolved: Dr. Addison does not attempt an explanation: neither does the reporter in the *Medical Times*, who has collated all the recorded cases with the utmost caution and accuracy.

"The reason of our ignorance on this point is patent. Before we can draw legitimate conclusions on the pathology of an organ, we must know its physiology; and here we are bound to confess our ignorance. Let us consult any or all the works on physiology within our reach, and we shall find little to enlighten us. According to some, the supra-renal capsules form one of a series of blood-perfecting organs, such as the spleen, the thyroid, and the thymus—blood-glands without ducts, which are supposed to elaborate a something necessary to the due constitution of the vital fluid, which is at once reabsorbed. Among other and older writers there seems to be a vague idea, but perhaps the truer one, that they are intimately associated with the nervous system, through the agency of the solar plexuses. But which, if either, is the correct view, we must at present leave in abeyance, satisfied simply with the fact, which is, I think, sufficiently established, that there is a disease marked by a certain train of symptoms during life, which, after death, exhibits a disease of the supra-renal capsules as the special lesion, to the exclusion of any disease of other organs which may not be accounted for by collateral morbid phenomena. And more than this has been ascertained, viz., that, in a large series of *post-mortem* examinations instituted with reference to this very point, no disease has been found in these organs, where the peculiar train of symptoms in question has not existed.

"What these symptoms are I will now briefly state, premising that they may occur in either sex, though generally, but not universally, after the middle period of life. These symptoms (I draw my description from a well-marked instance) are, a gradual and almost imperceptible failure of strength, a gradual but not an extreme loss of flesh, a feeling of sinking in the epigastrium, constant nausea and indisposition to take food, depression of spirits, and failure in power without quickening of the circulation. At some indefinite period, the *pathognomonic sign* makes its appearance, in a peculiar discoloration of the skin, most marked on the exposed surfaces. This is unlike any other discoloration with which I am acquainted. It is not the pallor of chlorosis, the dirty sallow colour of the cancerous diathesis, or the yellow of jaundice; it is something *sui generis*. Once seen, it cannot fail to be recognized, and by this sign alone, perhaps some here present may call to mind cases which have previously been inexplicable to them. The colour is a peculiar dark coppery or bronzy hue, such as is seen in some oriental nations, very marked in the face and hands, less so on the body, and here varying in intensity, so as to give a patchy appearance. This symptom increases *pari passi* with the disease, as does also the inscrutable debility which resists every form of tonic and stimulant treatment. Pains in the joints resembling rheumatism are after a time superadded, and the patient gradually sinks; the liver, kidneys, and other emunctories, discharging their duties fully, until at last the patient becomes delirious or comatose, from sheer exhaustion, and dies.

"But I cannot give a better idea of this disease than by the detail of the case to which I have alluded.

"CASE.—The subject was a lady, aged 58 years, of remarkably tall and robust frame, and of great obesity previously to the commencement of her fatal illness. Her habits of life were peculiar, especially in her partiality for fatty matters, and her abstinence from farinaceous diet. She was also a considerable consumer of porter and wine. When she first consulted me, in August, 1855, I was struck with the diminution of her bulk, and her great general prostration. Her chief complaint was of debility. Her appetite was bad, and she suffered from constant nausea and sinking at the pit of the stomach. She also incidentally called my attention to her colour, being particularly dissatisfied with the appearance of her hands, which resembled those of a creole. I confess that, on this occasion, I paid no attention to this apparently unimportant symptom, being interested only in the endeavour to discover a cause for the emaciation and exhaustion. I examined the heart, the lungs, and, on a subsequent occasion, the urine, without finding any such disease as could explain the nature of the case. The heart's action was feeble, and its sounds sharp; and the only conclusion I could come to at the time was, that I had a case of general decadence of the digestive powers from over-stimulation, together with fatty degeneration of the heart. The latter suspicion was borne out by the results of the *post-mortem* examination.

"She paid me several visits, but made no satisfactory progress; and the discoloration of the skin gradually deepened, perplexing me as much as it annoyed the patient. At this time I noticed the first of a series of cases publishing in the *Medical Times*, and I at once saw a clue to the enigma. I published the case at the time, and at once informed the friends of the peculiarity of the disease, and my conviction of its ultimate fatality. To be brief, the pregress was, with some fluctuations, daily for the worse; and, in the month of March, there were the additional symptoms of pains in the joints, neck, and limbs, which continued to the time of her death. In the latter two months of her life, she emaciated rapidly; and, in the final days, she had alternations of delirium and coma, the kidneys and bowels, however, acting naturally to the very last.

"The *post-mortem* examination exhibited the following appearances: The body was emaciated. The integuments, especially the face and hands, were of a deep bronzy colour. The eyes were sunken; the conjunctivæ pearly white. The subcutaneous fat, as well as that in the omentum and other internal parts, was firm, and of a deep chrome yellow. The head was not examined. The thoracic organs were healthy, with the exception of the heart, which was dilated, and in a state of fatty degeneration. The liver was softened, but otherwise healthy. The stomach was dilated, and its coats atrophied and destitute of rugæ. The spleen was of natural size and consistence. The intestines were healthy. The kidneys were congested and flabby. The *supra-renal capsules* were both enlarged, nodulated externally, and, when divided, were seen to be filled with tubercular deposit of various consistency, some portions being almost cartilaginous, others of the fluidity of scrofulous pus.

"I have but little to add to this interesting case, further than to remark, that it offers one of the most perfect specimens of the disease yet placed on record. I do not venture on an opinion as to its true pathology. Whether the disease in the supra-renal capsules is the *fons et origo mali*, or only the chief local manifestation of a new and general cachexia, remains yet to be proved. All that can be affirmed at present is, that the two facts are coincident, and that their conjunction is manifested by a train of symptoms against which medicine is inoperative."

---

19. *Treatment of Diabetes.*—Dr. JOSEPH BELL has furnished to the *Glasgow Med. Journal* (July, 1856) some interesting remarks on the treatment of the cases of diabetes admitted into the Glasgow Royal Infirmary from Nov. 1854 till April, 1856.

The following are his conclusions:—

"1. Opium has a most powerful effect in diminishing the quantity of urine, but does not cure the disease.

"2. Ammonia seems to possess, at least in some cases, the power of reducing the amount of urine, the specific gravity, and quantity of sugar.

"3. Opium and ammonia combined have a most beneficial effect.

"4. Cod-liver oil alone is beneficial; it improves the general condition of the patient, reduces the quantity of urine, and lessens its specific gravity.

"5. Cod-liver oil, combined with opium, rapidly improves the strength of the patient and reduces the urine.

"6. The combined use of cod-liver oil, opium, and ammonia, effects the most prompt and permanent benefit.

"7. Blisters to the hepatic region are useful.

"8. The restriction of diet is rather baneful than beneficial. A mixed generous diet is the best.

"9. In the present state of our knowledge we can only expect to improve the general condition of the patient, restrain the waste of tissues, maintain the vigour, and reduce the amount of urine. In this way we can mitigate the disease and protract the life of the patient. We are bound to confess that we have no cure for diabetes. It is not the only disease which defies the efforts of our art. In many other affections we can only palliate suffering and prolong existence. These objects we can very satisfactorily accomplish in diabetes by the judicious use of cod-liver oil, opium, and ammonia.

"But it may be asked how are we to explain the instances of reported cures that from time to time are published, ever and anon exciting our hope that an agent has been placed in our power by which we can secure an easy victory over the disease? My answer is twofold: 1st, That such cases may have been of a mere temporary nature, a character under which diabetes is sometimes presented. 2dly, That in many of the published cures an erroneous diagnosis may have been made in consequence of the use of Moore's or Trommer's tests, both of which are deceptive, a brown precipitate being produced by the presence of other organic matters as well as by sugar. I would admit no case as genuine diabetes unless the yeast test had been employed. I do not speak from conjecture on this point, but from experience. Indeed, I fell into this very mistake some years ago in consequence of this brown deposit. The fallacy was pointed out to me by the late Dr. M'Gregor. I have reason to suspect that many of the cases that have been published regarding the presence of sugar in the urine of old persons, especially when labouring under disease of the lungs, the deoxidation of the copper is effected by some other organic matter and not by sugar. I have often, in such cases, been able to produce a brown sediment, but I have always failed to effect fermentation."

20. *Drowning successfully treated by Dr. Hall's Method of Inflating the Lungs.*—Dr. David Hadden records an interesting example of this. "The case was that of a boy, about thirteen years of age, who, when bathing, got a cramp in the right leg, and, after struggling for a considerable period, sank exhausted. He remained under water for nearly twenty minutes, and when brought to land appeared quite dead.

"I happened to be passing at the time, and immediately put your plan into operation, and, after continuing it for more than a quarter of an hour, he begun to show some symptoms of returning animation.

"His recovery is the most remarkable I have ever witnessed, and must have been impossible if treated according to the methods heretofore in use."—*Lancet*, Aug. 9th, 1856.

21. *Cinnamon in Metrorrhagia.*—M. Chomier, after adverting to the eulogiums, often exaggerated, passed upon this substance by some of the German writers, observes that, so far as he knows, M. Gendrin alone has laid down the indications for its employment. That author states he has employed it with remarkably good effect in chronic metrorrhagia, as also in the acute form, when the first symptoms have been subdued by bloodletting; and he has often been surprised at the rapidity of the results produced. The form that most promptly yielded to its influence was that occurring some days after delivery, unaccompanied by plethora. The author has observed it employed most beneficially by M. Teissier, of Lyons, and it is upon his cases the present memoir is based.

Metrorrhagia is very rarely primary, being most commonly connected with a general affection, of which it is merely an epiphenomenon, or dependent upon a local affection of the uterus and its appendages; and it is only in certain cases that the cinnamon can be usefully given: 1. *Metrorrhagia due to the chlorotic condition.* This, both in its manifestation and recurrence, seems closely connected with the regular return of the menses, whence, indeed, its name "menorrhagia." Iron, properly administered in the intervals, will often rapidly modify the chlorotic condition; but, even when well supported, it often proves powerless against menorrhagia, and, when we resort to the hæmostatic power of alum, tannin, or ergotine, gastralgia or other disorders of the stomach often oblige us to renounce their employment. It is in such cases M. Teissier has found cinnamon, given a few days prior to the period, so useful. It is only palliative and fugacious in its effects; and, in order to operate upon the chlorosis itself, M. Teissier combines iron filings with it. 2. *Metrorrhagia symptomatic of cancer.* According to M. Teissier's observations, ergotine and tincture of cinnamon are the best means for treating the hemorrhage of the advanced period of cancer; but the former, while possessing a remarkable power over the hemorrhage, produces such an aggravation of pain as to compel its rejection. The tincture of cinnamon exerts a similar power over the discharge, without this inconvenience.

Given in doses of 2 to 4 grammes, it suppresses the metrorrhagia, often in a very short time. In all cases, by its prolonged employment, we are able very sensibly to diminish those daily losses of blood which take place in almost all women in the second stage of cancer of the cervix, and we often succeed in suspending all discharge for more or less time. The cinnamon also exerts a beneficial effect on the economy. The strength and digestion are improved; and when we allay the pain also by anodynes, so great an improvement occurs in some cases as to lead the patient to hope for a speedy cure. 3. *Puerperal metrorrhagia.* Lymphatic, feeble, cachectic women, with lax tissues and languid circulation, and liable to irregular menstruation or chronic leucorrhœa, are often seized with hemorrhage during pregnancy, which in the end may lead to abortion. Here a tonic treatment, as by iron and bitters, is clearly indicated, and cinnamon exerts the same useful effect as in chlorotic patients with too abundant menstruation. Such women are also very liable to hemorrhage from inertia of the uterus after delivery, and constitute the cases in which ergot is so beneficially given just prior to the expulsion of the child. From facts he has observed, however, M. Teissier is convinced that the ergot is mischievous to the child; and for such women he prescribes, hour by hour from the commencement of labour, a draught containing 4 grammes (ʒj) of the tincture of cinnamon; and in the limited number of such cases that have occurred to him, with the best effect. Such women are liable to repeated hemorrhage during the puerperal state, and although the discharge may not be abundant, it becomes important by its persistence and the alarming degree of chloro-anæmia it may rapidly induce. The cinnamon here is of surprising efficacy. Six of the cases observed in M. Teissier's wards are given.—*Med. Times and Gaz.*, June 7, 1856, from *Rev. Méd. Chirurg.*, tom. xviii.

---

22. *Chorea treated by Inhalations of Chloroform.*—According to Dr. Gery, chloroform inhalations have been used with advantage at the Hôp. des Enfans in severe cases where the violence of the movements have been beyond the control of opium or belladonna. It has been found at once to calm the movements and produce sleep, and in this way time has been gained for the employment of other remedies. On the first application of the vapour, the intensity of the movements is often greatly increased, but a calm succeeds as the inhalation is continued. Sound sleep thus induced lasts in children for ten or fifteen minutes, or even half an hour, and no ill effects have been observed to follow. The usual precautions, however, which are taken in the instance of adults, are necessary to be observed, such as insuring that the stomach be empty, removing all obstacles to the respiratory movements, and watching the respiration and pulse, &c. The usual quantity administered has been ten to twenty grammes.

Dr. Bouchard relates a case of a girl in which severe chorea had lasted twenty-one days. She was subjected to the influence of chloroform twenty-seven times in fourteen days, at first twice, then three times, and lastly once a day, at the end of which time she was cured.—*Brit. and For. Med.-Chir. Rev.*, July, 1856, from *Bull. Gén. de Thérap.*, March, 1855.

---

23. *Chloroform in Lead Colic.*—M. Aran, after using chloroform in lead colic, both externally and internally, for four years, now repeats an opinion formerly expressed of its superiority over all other methods of treatment. At the same time he modifies some of his former statements. He regards the internal use of the medicine as the basis of the treatment, whilst he considers the application of it externally as only indispensable during the first days, and in the most severe cases. His observations have also taught him that it is impossible to lay down precisely the maximum dose, which must depend on the intensity of the pain, &c. It may be necessary to give as much as 100 or 300 drops (four to twelve grammes) in twenty-four hours, while 60 drops may suffice in slight cases. As the effects of chloroform rapidly pass away, the patient must be kept continually under its influence for a certain number of days by repeated small doses, given by the mouth or by enema. He applies the chloroform topically by dropping it on a fine and dry compress, to an amount varying with the degree of pain (*e. g.*, two to four grammes), and after placing this upon the abdomen, it is covered with some dry compresses. It produces its effect in from one to five minutes. He gives the chloroform internally suspended in water by tragacanth. The lavement contains from 30 to 50 drops, similarly suspended. The topical application is rarely of any use beyond the second day. Reducing the dose, he continues the medicine in lavement, as a precaution, when the case has been severe, up to the eighth or twelfth day. He founds his recommendation on the results of 21 cases.—*Ibid.*, from *L'Union Médicale*, Jan., 1855.

SURGICAL PATHOLOGY AND THERAPEUTICS, AND OPERATIVE SURGERY.

24. *The Microscope* versus *Common Experience in the Diagnosis of Cancer of the Breast.*—The diagnosis of cancer by the cancer-cell is not infallible. It cannot be repeated too often, perhaps, as the result of what is seen every year in hospitals, that cancer is the result of a cachexia which steals unawares on the patient, at first unaccompanied by pain; and that, if we could detect it at the onset, more perhaps might be done in saving life. Cancer is more frequent in females than males, in proportion of ten to three; mental distress and a cacheotic habit of system, induced by mental distress, leading, perhaps, even more than temperament or hereditariness, to cancer. A tumour once formed, there is too much reason to fear, becomes a medium as it were for the multiplication of analogous growths; but inoculation of cancer only shows that this plan fails, and a constitutional diathesis is necessary for the disease.

A very remarkable tumour of the breast in a woman was removed by Mr. Lawrence on the 14th inst. It seemed one of those growths, as we might say, in a transition stage to become cancerous. The woman was 52 years of age. A hard growth was detected in the left mammary region. There was, however, no retraction of the nipple; nor were there enlarged glands. The woman could give no history of the case; but though some microscopic observers deemed, under an inspection, it was not scirrhus, Mr. Lawrence was not so sure it was not malignant and constitutional, the age of the patient unfortunately turning the balance against her.—*Association Med. Journal*, June 21, 1856.

25. *Value of the Microscope in Cancer and Adenoid of the Breast: Psychological Effect of Pain and Ulceration.*—Mr. Hilton, at Guy's, removed a scirrhous tumour of the breast a few days ago, not with any intention of curing it, but as a temporary expedient gratifying to the patient. It seems now very generally understood that cancer, more especially of the breast, is a substitution of a peculiar cell-growth of remarkable reproductive vitality, but of deficient stability, for the natural tissues of the breast—a growth early prone to degenerate into fat, the lowest perhaps of the animal constituents, and quite incapable of resisting inflammatory changes; and that possibly some good may arise in taking cancer out of the way, and thus calming the patient's mind, or, at all events, directing her attention from it. It is not impossible (and all good therapeutics tend in this direction), it is rather quite in analogy with all we now know of the effects of cod-liver oil and other agents in tubercle, that we may yet arrive at some means of checking cancer. All good surgeons yet look to the hopeful side, and yet trust in something which shall not stop at merely staying the ravages of this fell disease, but may prevent this imperfect kind of nutrition and growth, or, as in diabetes, stop the supply of elements which go to make up fresh cancer.

Lebert and Velpeau have recently shown that there is no confidence to be placed in the so-called "cancer-cell" as a test of the incurability of growths termed cancerous; and they would place the fibro-plastic cell in the same category as the epithelial. They show that a tumour of the testis may cause the removal of this part, from its striking resemblance to cancer—may be followed by what is termed secondary cancer in the abdomen—and yet, whether as the result of treatment or otherwise, the latter tumours in the abdomen are destitute of cancer-cells, and merely exhibit fibro-plastic elements; and the disease, though the microscope says the opposite, has never been cancer at all, from first to last.

At Guy's, Sir Astley Cooper, in 1815, first described adenoid tumours as "chronic mammary," which Velpeau rediscovered in 1824. These growths are now, by the still later researches of Mr. Birkett, easily distinguished from cancer; but it is not so clear that, after the grand climacteric in a woman's life, this very tendency to adenoid and fibro-plastic disease may not glide insensibly into a cancerous diathesis. Mr. Hilton, in the present case, looked rather in a psychological way at the operation, as relieving the woman's *mind* of much misery and apprehension, leading to dyspepsia, etc., this dyspepsia aggravating the cachexia already so liable to increase.—*Assoc. Med. Journ.*, June 14, 1856.

26. *Tumours of the Upper Maxilla, malignant and non-malignant.*—Mr. Fergusson removed a tumour of the upper jaw on the 21st ult., of the "compact osseous" character, by an operation we have often seen. The tumour had been growing for twelve months, and had pushed the inferior turbinated bone inwards, so as to make a projection in the nostril. Mr. Fergusson divides the lip in the mesial line, thus happily making a "virtue of necessity," and converting what might be an ugly scar into a linear wound of little moment. This, in an operation of *convenance*, as the French term it, is a matter of no small anxiety; but the mechanical aptitude of the Surgeon of King's College Hospital is so well known that we did not fear for the result. Mr. Fergusson divided the lip, as we said, in the median line, and then dissected, in the usual familiar manner, the tissues of the cheek off the tumour. There was nothing, however, in the operation that our provincial brethren are not conversant with. The disease was simple hypertrophy of the osseous structure, fortunately not malignant.

A tumour of a still more interesting character was removed by Mr. Curling, April 25th, at the London Hospital. Here the tumour was situated above the alveolar processes of the molar teeth, on the right side, expanding the bone in the mode so familiar to hospital surgeons. The common directions followed by Mr. Fergusson, of making the first incision in the mesial line, did not answer; and Mr. Curling wisely preferred not to cut uselessly through parts not diseased, as a matter of *convenance* and credit for the operator, but, in the first place, to consult what was best for the patient, even at the risk of a little deformity. Mr. Curling's incision, accordingly, as he found he could not obtain space to work in by the mesial incision, was made ingeniously through a dimple in the cheek. From a long familiarity with Mr. Curling's excellent operations, we do not know but that in specific instances one would give a preference to his operation, especially in men, where the beard will cover over the scar; but in females, the plan of incision in the mesial line at some little risk of injuring vital parts may be adhered to. The tumour in Mr. Curling's case was examined by Dr. Andrew Clark, when it proved to be one of the familiar —we had almost said endless—varieties of growths, so often met in hospitals, which Mr. Paget would class perhaps under myeloid tumours, the Middlesex Hospital school under the class of "colloid growth," but which Dr. Andrew Clark showed to be made up of both, together with epithelial cells in various shapes, and fat-globules—a tumour, in a word, which abstract histological data would rather surround with mystery, and experience alone decide as to malignancy.—*Assoc. Med. Journ.*, May 2, 1856.

27. *On Gangrene from Arteritis.*—The following are some of the conclusions arrived at by Prof. Porta, from the observation of thirty-one cases of his own, and the consideration of those published by others:—

Although the tunics of arteries consist of tissues little disposed to inflammation, yet are they not exempt from liability to it; and external violence, the extension of phlegmasia from other tissues, rheumatism or metastasis may induce an arteritis that may lead to gangrene of subjacent parts. Among all these causes, metastasis is pre-eminent, so that eighteen out of the thirty-one cases are referable to it. Not unfrequently, on the decline or disappearance of some serious internal malady, a reverberation is directed to the arteries of the limbs, the original disease either then disappearing, or remaining as a complication of the newly-developed arteritis. The large external arteries, such as the axillary, humeral, femoral, or popliteal, are usually the subjects of such reverberation, but it has not as yet been met with in the carotid. Exceptionally, smaller arteries are attacked, such as the radial, ulnar, or tibial.

The end to which arteritis tends is the closure of the artery, all the manifestations observed subsequent to the cessation of its pulsation being but the sequelæ of that. Strictly speaking, however, such cessation of pulsation is not pathognomonic of obliteration, as sometimes a minute stream continues to pass, which excites so feeble an oscillation of the vessel as not to be perceptible to the touch. The obstruction of the artery does not necessarily give rise to gangrene, for not only may it be incomplete, but even when complete, it may have been formed with sufficient slowness to allow the development of the lateral anastomoses; the amount of the obliteration, indeed, exerting less influence than the rapidity with which the coagulum is formed. This local condition is not the sole cause of the gangrene, for the production of this may be favoured by a disordered state of the general circulation, or a temporary enfeeblement of the cardiac impulse. There is, however, no lesion of the function of the capillaries operating, as the minute vessels are found healthy and empty in the midst of the gangrened parts, just as they are in mortifications that supervene upon ligature. Gangrene from arteritis presents a great analogy to senile gangrene, which may take place slowly or rapidly, according to the amount of ossific deposit, and the other conditions of the subject.

There is nothing constant observed as regards the form, extension, or duration of this result of arteritis. Sometimes the patient dies during the prodromic stage, in consequence of the rapid exhaustion of his powers before the limb has mortified. In other cases, there are eschars, limited to the skin, or the gangrene may attack only one or more toes. Frequently, however, it extends to the foot and leg, or the hand and forearm, until the power of the lateral circulation restores the equilibrium, if it succeed in so doing. If even it is arrested, there is a disposition to relapse; and a paresis, and temporary or permanent atrophy of the limb, remains. Danger to life, however, is not alone dependent upon the degree of extension of the gangrene, but also upon the general state; this allowing us sometimes to hope for recovery in even extensive gangrene, while at others it renders a limited gangrene a most grave circumstance. So dangerous an affection is it, that few succeed in escaping from its effects.

Besides the internal changes that may exist as the effects of the malady which has also caused the arteritis, we often find in the artery supposed to be affected but slight traces of lesions. In bad cases, however, a sero-gelatinous fluid is found external to the artery, the cellular coat is finely injected, and the proper tunics are adherent to each other, and fragile. Sometimes there is thickening of the cellular tunic, and exudation of puriform matter or plastic lymph, externally to the vessel, affixing it to neighbouring parts. All these lesions are not of frequent occurrence in arteritis; and except in the case of violence, all the coats of the vessel may present a normal appearance, and they would be so pronounced, were it not for the obstruction caused by the product of inflammation. This consists of a solid coagulum of plastic lymph, varying in size, length, and degree of adhesion to the vessel. Sometimes small coagula are observed obstructing the artery at intervals; but more commonly it is a single coagulum, one or more inches in length, converting the vessel into a cord. Sometimes, however, the coagulum assumes the form of a canal, or presents here and there small lacunæ, containing a milky or semi-fluid reddish matter, which may also cover the whole surface of the coagulum, or almost constitute its entire substance. Maisonneuve and Cruveilhier have found even the smallest vessels corresponding to the gangrened part obliterated; but, for the most part, the closure will be found only in the vessels above the gangrened part, those corresponding to this remaining open—showing that the coagulum has preceded the gangrene.

The principal veins of the limb sometimes participate in the inflammatory condition, and exhibit the signs of this more plainly than do the arteries. Their coats become thickened, and rich in vasa vasorum; while their cavity is filled with lymph, or, oftener still, by puriform matter combined with cruor. In ordinary cases, however, the principal veins remain free, contain a small quantity of blood, in part fluid and in part coagulated, or, without exhibiting any signs of phlegmasia, are obstructed by a sanguineous coagulum.

As the arteritis is unpreceded by any prodrome, no prophylactic can be employed; but in order to prevent or circumscribe the formation of coagula, the arteritis itself must be actively combated by antiphlogistic means, general or local, according to the amount of reaction and the condition of the patient. These must, however, be employed with due caution; for while we combat the inflammatory action, we have to favour the lateral circulation. As soon as the more urgent symptoms are mitigated, aromatic fomentations or warm applications should be made to the part, improving the patient's diet, and even exhibiting stimuli, if not specially contra-indicated. If the pain is violent, opium is here, too, of great use. These means are, however, often of no avail; for the arteritis, especially when metastatic, appears suddenly, gives rise to the exudation, and at once disappears; gangrene following if the lateral circulation cannot resist, and leaving to the practitioner only the office of administering palliatives. So, too, all attempts at dissipating the coagulum are useless, this remaining even in the case of recovery; and all that can be done is to endeavour to limit it by favouring the lateral circulation. Even in the case of recovery, until the circulation is completely re-established, there is great danger of relapse.—*B. and F. Med.-Chirurg. Rev.*, from *Omodei Annali di Med.*, Feb., 1856.

28. *New Mode of Reducing Strangulated Hernia.*—Baron Seutin declares, that with his mode of reducing strangulated hernia, which he has now practised for twenty years, he hardly ever, in his large practice, finds it necessary to have recourse to an operation.

The patient is laid upon his back, with the pelvis raised much higher than the shoulders, in order that the intestinal mass may exert traction upon the herniated portion. The knees are flexed, and the body is slightly turned to the opposite side to that on which the hernia exists. The surgeon ascertains that the hernia, habitually reducible, cannot be returned by continuous and moderate taxis. He next seeks with his index finger for the aperture that has given issue to the hernia, pushing up the skin sufficiently from below, in order not to be arrested by its resistance. The extremity of the finger is passed slowly in between the viscera and the herniary orifice, depressing the intestine or omentum with the pulp of the finger. This stage of the procedure demands perseverance, for at first it seems impossible to succeed. The finger is next to be curved as a hook, and sufficient traction exerted on the ring to rupture some of the fibres, giving rise to a cracking very sensible to the finger, and sometimes to the ear. When this characteristic crack is not produced, the fibres must be submitted to a continuous forced extension, which, by distending them beyond the agency of their natural elasticity, generally terminates the strangulation. This mode of procedure is more applicable to Gimbernat's ligament, the hooking and tearing of which are more difficult than in the case of the inguinal ring. Considerable strength has sometimes to be exerted, and the index finger becomes much fatigued. When, in consequence of the narrowness of the ring, the finger does not at once penetrate, it is to be pressed firmly against the fibrous edge, and inclined toward the hernia. After a time the fibres yield and the finger passes. When the finger becomes fatigued it is not to be withdrawn, but it should be supported by the fingers of an intelligent assistant, who seconds the action it is desired to produce. In inguinal hernia, the traction should not be exerted with the finger upon Poupart's ligament, but in a direction from within outwards, and from below upwards, by which the aponeurotic layers between the two ligamentous pillars constituting the inguinal aperture are easily torn through.

The ring is then enlarged by this tearing, just as if it had been divided by a cutting instrument, or largely dilated, and reduction takes place easily, by performing the taxis in a suitable direction. The mobility of the skin, its laxity in parts where hernia prevails, and its extensibility, greater in proportion to its thinness and to the absence of a lining of fatty cellular tissue—by allowing the sliding and the thrusting of this membrane in front of the finger it cushions, affords protection to the intestine from all immediate contusion. When the strangulation is induced by the issue of a considerable mass of intestine, or an accumulation of fecal matters, it is desirable first to disengage one of the extremities of the noose, and to seek to expel the gas or fecal matters by moderate pressure, in order to facilitate the reduction of the tumour. In the few cases in which the finger cannot be introduced, a small incision may be practised in the skin, and the handle of a spatula or any blunt instrument may be passed in by separating the cellular tissue. Pressing this against the border of the ring, while avoiding the intestine, this orifice may be eroded or dilated without danger. The greater the resistance offered by the aponeurotic fibres, the greater will be their tension, and the more easily will their laceration be produced.

As a general conclusion, it may be laid down, that the facility and promptitude of this procedure, and the immunity that attends it, ought to diminish the gravity of the prognosis of strangulated hernia, by rendering the circumstances under which recourse need be had to an operation quite exceptional. Such exceptional cases will be found (1) in old, irreducible herniæ. (2.) When the strangulation in inguinal hernia occurs at the internal ring. Generally the external ring and inguinal canal are large, and allow of the easy penetration of the finger; and then the new method is applicable, and the rupturing or dilatation of the internal ring should be attempted, and the manœuvre is rendered the easier by the fact, that in these cases the canal is much shortened, and the two rings much approximated. If, however, the external ring is too narrow to admit the finger, an operation is required. (3.) When there are general symptoms of a gangrenous state of the intestine.—*Bull. de Thérapeut.*

29. *Expiratory Method of Performing the Taxis to effect the Reduction of Hernia.*—This method, introduced by Dr. ANDREW BUCHANAN, Prof. Inst. Med. Univ. of Glasgow, is a modification of the ordinary manual operation for reduction of hernia by taxis. The patient is placed in the position usually recommended, or which may be deemed most suitable in the various forms of hernia, and the compressing force is applied in the usual way. The peculiarity of the method consists in this, that just before the force is applied the patient is directed to make a very full expiration, and thereafter to refrain as long as possible from making a fresh inspiration; or, as it is more intelligibly expressed to the uninitiated, he is directed to blow as much air out of his mouth as he possibly can, and to continue thereafter as long as he can without drawing a fresh breath. While this is going on, the operator, having made all necessary preliminary arrangements, attempts to return the hernia, beginning as soon as the expiration is a little advanced, and continuing his efforts gently but steadily during the whole period of suspended respiration. When the patient is at length compelled to draw a fresh breath, the pressure should be relaxed, so as not to oppose the force of the muscles of inspiration; but it should not be altogether given up, and as soon as the patient is a little recruited from his exhaustion, he is made to perform another expiration, and so the operation is continued as long as may be required. The first indication of success, consisting in a slight internal motion or gurgling noise in the tumour, almost universally occurs during the suspension of the breathing; and it is during the same period that the complete return of the hernia is usually effected.

There are some important minor details in the operation which depend on the intelligence and strength of mind of the patient. If he possess both those mental qualities in a sufficient degree, he will be able, after making the full expiration, to refrain from inspiring by a voluntary effort. Such cases are the most favourable for the success of the operation. In other cases, and these cases occur more especially among females, the patient understands and acts more fully upon the direction of blowing out the breath, but wants strength of mind for the subsequent control over the inspiratory muscles. In all such cases it is indispensable to have an assistant, whose duty it is, as soon as the expiration is completed, to apply his hands over the mouth and nose of the patient, so as to prevent inspiration for as long a period as may be deemed safe and advisable. If, however, the lungs can be sufficiently emptied, such cases are little less favourable than the former. Last of all, there are persons who, whether from natural stupidity or from fright and confusion of mind arising from the condition in which they are placed, cannot be made to comprehend and follow out the directions given them. In those cases the lungs are never emptied to the necessary degree, and the success of the operation is proportionally uncertain.

The theory of this operation is simple. In the first place, it disassociates the diaphragm from the abdominal muscles, and, by preventing them from acting in concert, removes the chief obstacle to the reduction of hernia. Secondly, it weakens the muscular power of the body, and diverts it from the act of resistance.

It is the simultaneous contraction of the diaphragm and abdominal muscles which enables the patient to press down and resist the efforts made to return the hernia. This is one of the most important combinations of muscular action in the whole animal economy. It constitutes the *nixus* of physiologists. Acting in its natural way, it forces out the contents of the bowels, of the urinary bladder, and of the uterus, according to the direction given to it; and, when misdirected, it becomes the principal cause of the production of hernia, forcing out the bowels themselves where the walls of the abdomen are least able to resist the pressure; while it becomes also, after the disease has been once produced, the force which opposes the return of the hernia into the cavity of the abdomen. Now, it is quite indispensable to the existence of this force that the diaphragm act as well as the abdominal muscles, and the moment the diaphragm is relaxed the force is necessarily destroyed. The intention of the instructions given to the patient before proceeding to the taxis will therefore be at once apparent. Expressed in other terms, those instructions just amount to this—"Relax your diaphragm, and keep it in a state of relaxation;" for there is no mode of relaxing the diaphragm but by making an expiration, nor any mode of keeping the diaphragm relaxed but by refraining thereafter from breathing.

In so far as the general muscular system is concerned, the mode of proceeding here recommended is not confined to the application made of it, but might be successfully employed in facilitating the reduction of dislocations, or counteracting any other muscular resistance. The state of expiration and the suspended breathing which follows it produce rapidly an overwhelming sense of debility over the whole body, which paralyzes all muscular exertion. These conditions of the respiratory organs not only produce a positive, but also a negative effect of a useful kind, for they prevent full inspiration, and the *nixus* of which it constitutes a part. Now that act, by giving fixity to the trunk of the body, and a firm point of support to the muscles thence arising, is an indispensable preliminary to every vigorous muscular effort, and of course to every act of resistance. Last of all, there is no feeling more absorbing than that produced by a want of breath, whether kept up voluntarily or enforced, and the diversion of the patient's mind from the hernia so produced operates just like the well-known expedients employed in cases of dislocation to facilitate reduction.

It is now four-and-thirty years since I first reduced a hernia in the way described above, while I was a clerk residing in the Royal Infirmary of Glasgow. I have since employed the same method in every case of hernia that came into my hands, both in private and in hospital practice, and my confidence in it has increased with every year's experience of its efficacy. I have taught it to numerous pupils, many of whom, I know, esteem it as not one of the least valuable of the practical lessons which they learned at the clinical school of this city. I have shown it to various professional friends, who have adopted it; and among these I have the pleasure of mentioning the Professor of Surgery in our University here, who has not only long employed it in practice but recommends it every year to his students, both on account of its efficiency and the readiness of its application. Lastly, I have had many opportunities of testing its relative value; for in cases which I have seen in consultation, I have frequently found it succeed when the simple taxis and other methods had been tried in vain. I mention only a single case of this kind, because it is fresh in my recollection, and because I can appeal in confirmation of my statements to two of my colleagues in the University, Dr. Lawrie and Dr. Easton. Having met with these gentlemen in consultation on a case of strangulated hernia, we found that the simple taxis, and the taxis under chloroform, had been fully tried to no purpose. We resolved, although everything was in readiness for the operation, to give a trial to the method here recommended. The tumour yielded under the fingers during the third or fourth expiration, and was completely reduced during the following one.—*Glasgow Med. Journ.*, July, 1856.

30. *Operation for Radical Cure of Hernia.*—M. de ROUBAIX has described, in the *Presse Médicale Belge*, a new operation devised by him for the radical cure of hernia.

The hernia having been reduced, and the integument being pushed into the orifice, the operator seizes that portion of the skin which lies immediately over the spermatic cord and femoral vessels, so as to form a vertical or slightly oblique fold; this fold is raised as much as possible, its base is transfixed with a straight bistoury, and it is cut through from behind forwards. From the extremities of this incision two others are made, of a semilunar form, with their concavities looking towards each other, and approaching each other towards the upper part of the hernial orifice, leaving a sufficient space for the nutrition of the flap. The flap is introduced into the orifice so as to form a plug.

The edges of the ring and of the skin have now to be united. To effect this, M. de Roubaix draws firmly together the edges of the incisions and the neighbouring skin; then, the left index finger or a small gorget having been introduced into the transverse aperture, the integuments and the aponeurosis are connected by means of a small trocar. He then introduces through the canula a piece of platinum wire fitted to receive a small screw at each end. If convenient, a second platinum wire may be introduced. An oval piece of gutta-percha, with a small hole in the centre, is passed on each side over the wire, so as to come in contact with the skin. The pieces of gutta-percha are then drawn together by means of the screws. In this way, a longitudinal wound is obtained, the edges of which are brought into apposition by the twisted suture, care being taken to leave the lower part free for the escape of pus.

The advantages of this procedure, according to the author, are:—

1. The hernial sac being untouched, and the lesion of continuity affecting only the skin and aponeurosis, there is no danger of peritonitis.
2. There is no danger of injury to the spermatic cord and femoral vessels.
3. The cutaneous flap, having its pedicle upwards, is not liable to be drawn downwards either by the weight of the scrotum and testis, or by the movements of the thigh.
4. The hernial orifice is narrowed and partially obliterated, and in front of it is placed a powerful obstacle which adheres to and fortifies it.
5. In front of the vessels and cord there is a firm cicatrix, which, by its connection with the plug and the adjacent parts, forms an impassable barrier to the viscera.

M. de Roubaix has performed this operation successfully on a female aged 61, who had suffered for twelve years from a large femoral hernia, which descended as far as the patella.—*Assoc. Med. Journ.*, Jan. 19th, 1856, from *Gaz. Méd. de Paris*, Sept. 29th, 1855.

31. *Unusual Cause of Strangulation in Inguinal Hernia; Advantages and Disadvantages of Opening the Sac; Danger of Purgatives after Operation.*—Mr. STANLEY operated in a case of hernia on the 31st ult., on J. P., aged 42. The case has exhibited the fact, that the chief injury, in many cases of herniotomy, arises rather from the previous bruising of the intestine from prolonged efforts at the taxis, joined to the excessive use of purgatives both before and after operation, than from the operation itself.

The case was one of large scrotal hernia, which had come down two days previously (July 29th), and had been followed by all the distressing symptoms so common in strangulated hernia, and so well described recently by Mr. Baker, of the Birmingham Hospital. The herniary sac was tense and large, of fully the size of two closed fists; what the nature of the stricture was did not so well appear; the sickness and vomiting were intense; the pulse was irregular; the scrotum had a thickened distended feel. The taxis and ordinary treatment by purgatives were tried out of doors; but on the admission of the patient to hospital, he was placed in a warm bath, then ice was tried, and, finally, chloroform, with no amelioration whatever of the symptoms.

As the sickness continued (though there was no other very pressing symptom to call for operative interference, as Mr. Stanley observed to his class), he decided to operate, as it is always better, he said, to operate too early rather than too late. Every kind and modification of the taxis had failed. Mr. Lawrence agreed with Mr. Stanley in the propriety of operation, as a last resource; Mr. Paget also seemed to be of entirely the same opinion as his colleagues.

The case, as to the seat of stricture, was somewhat doubtful. But if, under the effect of chloroform, the gut did not go back, Mr. Stanley proposed to cut down on the seat of stricture without opening the sac. An incision, accordingly, an inch and a half long, was made, without opening the sac, over the abdominal ring. The operation is, perhaps, thus far an illustration of the fact which is seen every week in hospitals, that there is really no mathematical rule in hernia, as well pointed out especially by Mr. Ward, at the London Hospital, as to opening the sac, or not opening the sac; and that even though we sometimes do not open the sac, one may do mischief by working in the dark; we may thus, for instance, return a portion of sphacelated omentum, or even a bowel on the point of bursting, or, as in this case, be cutting a stricture where really none existed.

In the present case, after this usual operation by incision, so as not to open the sac, Mr. Stanley found he could still make no impression on the hernia. He then, as it would not go up, opened the sac, when the cause of the strangulation was apparent in the shape of a quantity of fluid, fully ten ounces, in the sac, joined to a merely thickened neck to the sac, the latter preventing the fluid getting back into the abdomen, and causing constriction of the intestine, or a sort of hydrostatic pressure, equal all round.

Could this fluid have been diagnosed early, it might have been a question how it should be evacuated. The intestine, however, was healthy, which is a very cardinal point in all such operations, and as such, it was easily and satisfactorily reduced. The man had large doses of purgatives out of doors, which did not act, of course, but which, it was feared, would act now with considerable force.

Mr. Stanley and Mr. Lawrence have seen, perhaps, as many cases of hernia as any other two surgeons in Europe. We were, accordingly, very much interested in some bedside observations incidentally made by Mr. Stanley in this case, more especially as to the use of purgatives after operation. The general result, he thinks, is a curious instance of the success of arguing from false premises, or arguing in a circle, but some accident breaking up the magic ring. Mr. Stanley recollects the times of Mr. Abernethy, when a series of discussions of a grave nature arose as to the best character of purgative to be administered after hernia operation; manna, senna and salts, colocynth, croton oil, had each its doughty champion. "I have bushels of such cases," said Mr. Stanley, "where the fatal peritonitis may be traced to the drastic purge. There were regular pitched battles for the cause of Glauber's salt, elaterium, or croton oil, as the case might be, till it began to appear that the manna and magnesia men, the weak aperients, carried the day. Some one then suggested *no purgative at all:* that, I need not say now, is the right treatment. Purgative medicine is almost sure to do mischief if prescribed before the fourth day, and even then it must be a mild warm water enema."

Aug. 6th. With the exception of some cough, he progresses very favourably. —*Assoc. Med. Journ.*, Aug. 9, 1856.

32. *Successful Operation for the relief of Internal Strangulation.*—The following case is quoted from the *Gazzetta Medica Italiana* in the *Gazette Médicale* for Dec. 1, 1855.

A robust countryman, aged 40, had congenital inguinal hernia on the left side. On September 7, 1854, he was attacked with borborygmi, which were usually premonitory of the descent of the hernia. In a short time, the hernia descended, and was attended with vomiting and violent pain. He was seen by a medical man, who found the following symptoms: repeated vomiting, violent thirst, fever, tumefaction of the abdomen, and a small tumour in the left groin. Two bloodlettings, castor oil (which was rejected), poultices, ice, enemata, and purgatives, were all tried without effect. On Sept. 9th the symptoms continued, and he was bled again. On Sept. 12th, the vomitings continued; there was no alvine evacuation; the skin was nearly cold, and the pulse low; the countenance and spirits were depressed; the abdomen was extremely tense, the swollen intestines forming irregular projections. The left inguinal region was perfectly free and painless; the finger passed easily into the external ring. Along the left iliac fossa there was a little puffiness, but altogether less than in many other parts of the abdomen. The patient stated that, after the first two bleedings, the hernia had receded spontaneously, and that he had felt no more pain in the part. The existence of an internal strangulation was suspected; and croton oil was rubbed over the abdomen, and given internally, without any effect. In the evening, an operation was determined on.

The patient having been placed under the influence of chloroform, M. Borelli made, at the level of the left iliac fossa, a large transverse incision, at the height of about ten *centimètres* (four inches). A mass of small intestine escaped from the wound; but in this there was found no obstruction. M. Borelli then introduced nearly his whole hand into the abdomen by the side of the umbilicus, and discovered the strangulation, in the form of a very firm and tight ring encircling the intestine. This was divided by a bistoury, the intestines were replaced, and the wound in the abdomen was closed by sutures.

The operation was followed by relief from the vomiting. The distension and pain of the abdomen continued two days, during which there was no alvine evacuation. Enemata, poultices, mercurial inunction, calomel and jalap, were employed, with the result of obtaining motions. On Sept. 15th, the patient was bled twice. On Sept. 16th, the abdomen was greatly distended, and the patient's strength was much prostrated. Enemata, with castor oil, produced evacuations, which were followed by improvement in the symptoms. The patient had a relapse, which was suspected to be due to indigestion; he had also an attack of intermittent fever. He recovered from these, however, and was able to leave his bed early in October.—*Assoc. Med. Journ.*, Jan. 19th, 1856.

33. *Prolapsus Ani.* By Prof. Syme.—About three years ago Dr. Dick, of Mid-Calder, called upon me with a gentleman suffering from an enormous protrusion of the rectum, which he had been led to regard as irremediable, and which at first sight certainly appeared to be so. A slight expulsive effort brought into view the tumour, which in size and form resembled a large cocoa-nut. It had a firm consistence, rough irregular surface, dark brown colour, and coating of bloody mucus, so as to be more like a malignant growth than a simple descent of the bowel. Nevertheless, being satisfied from the history of the case that the disease was of the latter kind, I held out the prospect of beneficial treatment, and the patient readily promised submission to whatever I should propose.

The integuments round the anus being greatly relaxed and thickened, so as to constitute a number of pendulous folds, I removed all this redundant texture by repeated applications of the scissors, not in a circular direction, but pointed from the circumference towards the centre of the orifice. This would have been a painful operation if performed on a conscious patient, but, being executed under the influence of chloroform, was accomplished without suffering, and also the difficulties attendant upon involuntary straining. I then enjoined the necessity of strictly maintaining the horizontal posture, and of abstaining from food beyond what was absolutely requisite. The bowels were not disturbed for several days, and at the end of this time were evacuated without any protrusion or difficulty, in consequence, no doubt, of the intestinal coats regaining their natural condition, while the sphincter was no longer impeded in the discharge of its duty. In the course of a few weeks, the patient felt able to resume his service in an office of the government in London, where he has ever since been employed, and felt so well as to enter into the matrimonial state. He lately sent me the following account of his case, which contains some details that may prove instructive as well as interesting.

"My earliest recollection of having prolapsus ani is that after every stool the nurse had to push up the rectum. I remember that I always used to throw myself forward on my knees, with my face almost touching the floor, and while in this attitude she pushed in what I (as a child) then called 'the bone,' having an idea that a bone always came out when I went to stool. I am told that the origin of my misfortune was caused by my receiving a severe blow on the back, after which I ran to the nursery, and on attempting to go to stool the gut immediately fell. This must have occurred between the age of three and four. I have no recollection of it whatever, but I believe that from that time I never evacuated the bowels without the gut coming down.

"At the age of six I was able to replace it myself, and having at that time left home and entered a boarding-school, I was of course obliged to make the best of it. Then, and afterwards, I thought it a matter of course that I should suffer as I did. I always felt very keenly the difference betwixt myself and other boys. I could neither jump, run, nor play in any way like them, and was a poor hand at most games, from a strong fear of 'receiving a blow on the back.' I have frequently been struck on the back with a handball, after which I felt overcome for the rest of the day. I always felt ashamed to speak to any one about the gut, and spent my years at school in silent suffering. Many a time have I felt cut to the heart by the boys calling me 'heavy bottom!' knowing that justly I did not deserve the name, but that my want of agility was caused by what I then began to call 'my weakness in the back.' I was quite uncared for at school, with respect to this weakness, and the teachers have frequently joined in the laugh against 'poor heavy bottom!' During my first two or three years at school, this hurt me very much, and my spirits, already overcome by my complaint, were increasingly depressed by frequent shedding of tears in secret. I mention this merely to show what a poor child may suffer when neglected.

"After the age of nine, I had sufficient sense to refrain from joining in any but very quiet games, where there was no running, pushing about, or any danger of rough movements. Being obliged always to accompany the other boys, I used to sit a solitary spectator of their games; and I well remember that, when any boy happened to come rushing near me, I had a standing cry of terror —'I'm not playing! I'm not playing!'

"I always considered myself a most unfortunate boy as I advanced in years, and I had no one to whom I could communicate my feelings, excepting during my yearly holidays of five or six weeks, which I spent at home. On these occasions both my father and mother were always very anxious about me, and tried to get me to do many things with a view to effect a cure; but I was then too glad to enjoy the short opportunity I had of joining in all the pleasures of home, and used to tell them that 'I did not mind it.' The only thing they got me to do was to sit in water which had been boiled with oak bark.

"On my return to school matters always went on as usual, and thus I passed my early years. I never could undergo the same amount of fatigue as others of my own age and apparent strength. In severe cold weather I was generally in a state of shivering, except when leaning over a fire—skating being almost the only exercise at which I could get thoroughly warm.

"In December, 1845, I sailed from this country for Ceylon, and during the voyage was more troubled than I had ever been before with indigestion and constipation, which caused great straining of the bowels.

"In April, 1846, I arrived at Ceylon, and was for a long time under a strong impression that the climate suited me well. Towards the end of my first year's stay in the island the bowels became more slackened than usual, and the gut protruded further than formerly, but I did not take any particular notice of this at the time. Towards the end of 1848 I was obliged to go more frequently to the water-closet, and the straining became more and more severe, so much so that I had often to stay half an hour, and sometimes longer, before I could push up the rectum.

"In the beginning of 1849 blood and mucus began to pass so freely that I took medical advice. Simple diet and the use of the enema were recommended, but the malady increased. In the month of March my medical friend told me that my only chance of recovery was to return to England.

"Up to this time the anus retained its usual natural appearance; but I now found an excrescence on the sphincter like a long wart, the top of which was open, and discharged a sticky waxy sort of matter. To this I was advised to apply caustic, which I did; but one trial was quite enough—I never touched it a second time.

"During former years the appearance of the rectum was a healthy red, but it now began to look dark and inflamed, and towards its outer edge was covered with little growths like the top of a cockscomb.

"In the month of May I sailed for England. The first circumstance which alarmed me in connection with my illness occurred on the morning I left the island. On getting out of bed, I had hardly stood upright when a quantity of stuff fell from me (without my feeling anything of it); it was a jelly-like substance, and looked very much like prepared arrowroot coloured with port wine. During my voyage I was constantly passing this bloody mucus; and, as I lived almost entirely on arrowroot and sago, I passed but little feces.

"The discharging excrescences on the anus, like the one above described, increased in number, and I was tortured by the sea doctor with an application of strong pepper to the affected parts. Like the caustic, however, I never applied it a second time.

"Several times during the voyage I almost lost entire control over the rectum, and felt as if it would fall out and remain so in spite of me.

"I reached London in the end of June in a state of great exhaustion. I was almost as helpless as a child, and had it not been for the kindness of some of my fellow passengers and the strangers who took care of my luggage and found lodgings for me, etc., I know not what I should have done.

"After a short stay at Richmond my strength began to increase so that I could walk without assistance, and was soon able to undertake the journey, by sea, to the North of Scotland, without a protector.

"During the winter of 1849-50 I had kind medical advice, but the rectum and anus continued in an inflamed and shattered state, and my life was still a misery and burden. Constant running to the water-closet, continued straining, rectum bleeding, and the constant flow of discharge made me think that I was to remain for life unfit for any of its duties.

"In 1851 I was placed under the care of Dr. Macleod, of Benrhydding. The use of the sitz-bath and spouting water on the lower part of the back were the principal items of treatment, with occasional slipper and such like baths. This treatment was the first from which I derived benefit; the rectum and its vicinity resumed a healthy red appearance, the straining was not so great, the discharge and bleeding lessened, my strength greatly increased, I could often walk a mile without much inconvenience, the stomach and digestive powers restored to action (indeed, they seemed entirely renewed), and the whole system changed from a diseased to a healthy condition.

"The prolapsus still remained, and, during a residence in London, with sedentary employment and confinement in 1852 and beginning of 1853, it became very much worse. Its size increased, and it bled very profusely. I had more difficulty in replacing it, and frequently could not do so until I had soaked it for fifteen or twenty minutes in a basin of water. I have had this to do three, four, and five times a day. The attitude in which I had to place myself over the basin was so awkward that it aided in exhausting my strength, and I had invariably to lie down for half an hour or longer after having succeeded in pushing up the rectum.

"Since the beginning of 1849 I had always bled more or less when straining with the rectum, but the flow of blood was now greater than ever. It often ran in a perfect jet, as if a vein had been opened with a lancet; and when occasionally I have raised the rectum out of the basin, in the act of straining, the blood has spirted six or seven feet across the floor.

"One other feature of the case I will mention, which made me very miserable. I do not know that I can describe it correctly, but I will try. When the large ball of the rectum came down the heart or centre of it was frequently filled with feces, and so distended it that in this state it was impossible to replace it. Occasionally it would empty itself slowly, after I had soaked the rectum for some time in warm water; but I frequently had to introduce my finger and take them out piece by piece before it could be pushed up, and then it was always accomplished with difficulty.

"In February, 1853, I had a severe attack of diarrhoea, which reduced me very much in strength and increased the diseased state of the rectum. In the month following, I visited Mid-Calder with a view to recover my strength, and there met my kind friend Dr. Dick, through whose friendly interest, in the month of April, I received from your hands that act of kindness which relieved me from the troubles of the prolapsus, and which I ever remember with a sense of the deepest gratitude."

There is no better illustration of the evils which may result from the improper naming of a disease than in the case of prolapsus ani. This title being understood to comprehend all protrusions beyond the orifice of the bowel, includes conditions entirely different in regard to their nature and remedy. It also suggests the idea of weakness in the sphincter, and leads this to be regarded as the cause of derangement, when, in truth, it hardly ever is so. Under the erroneous impression thus produced, mechanical support has been most improperly employed; and, if the frequency of advertisements in respect to contrivances for this purpose may be taken as a measure of the extent to which they are used, the amount of suffering thus unnecessarily endured must be very great.

In nearly all the cases of what is called prolapsus ani there is no displacement of the bowel, and merely a protrusion of its lining membrane in the thickened vascular condition which constitutes internal hemorrhoids. When pain or bleeding is the predominant symptom of this disease it generally retains its proper designation; but when the patient is chiefly annoyed by descent of the tumour, through the effect of exertion in the erect posture, the morbid state of the texture concerned is apt to be overlooked, so that the evil is attributed solely to relaxation of the sphincter. Many unhappy people pass through life in perpetual misery from this source, to which peculiarities of conduct and manner might often be more correctly ascribed than to original disposition. A well known and much respected member of the medical profession in Edinburgh, whose writings are extensively read by the public, accidentally discovered, through comparing his own case with one for which he had requested my assistance, that a distressing annoyance of this kind, from which he had suffered and endeavoured to palliate by bandages for twenty years, admitted of effectual remedy by means no less easy than safe; and, while writing these remarks, I have under my care a citizen of this place who during the same period of time has been similarly afflicted without obtaining the relief which might have been so readily afforded. If such things happen in the very centre of metropolitan science and skill, the state of matters existing in less favourable circumstances may be readily imagined.

Whatever may be the symptoms proceeding from them, the treatment of internal hemorrhoids should be always the same; and this I established thirty years ago, at a time when very vague and unsatisfactory opinions existed upon the subject. I say *opinions*, since such was the dread of interference with the disease in those days that it rarely became the subject of operation. The principles conducive to safety and efficiency then laid down were, 1st. That the whole of the existing enlargement within the sphincter should be removed by ligatures; 2d. That each of the tumours of which it is composed should be transfixed at its root by a double ligature; 3d. That the ligatures should be tied with the utmost possible tightness; and 4th. That any enlargement exterior to the sphincter should be removed by scissors. Morbid growths, whether within or without the anus, being thus taken away, the sphincter is allowed to resume its proper action, and the patient is relieved from prolapsus no less effectually than from pain and bleeding.

But in other cases, comparatively rare, the coats of the rectum descend so as to constitute a tumour independently of any morbid growth beyond mere thickening or engorgement of their texture. In children, this usually depends on the straining caused by irritation, as that of a stone in the bladder, and in old people it may proceed from a paralytic state of the sphincter. It may also, as in the case just related, depend upon a condition of the anus remediable through proper management. For this purpose it is requisite that the whole of the pendulous folds of skin should be removed by incisions radiating from the centre of the orifice, that the patient should be confined to the horizontal posture for several weeks, even when the bowels are evacuated, and that the diet should be restricted so as to prevent distension by feculent matters.—*Edinb. Med. Journ.*, August, 1856.

34. *Vaginal Cystocele removed by Operation; Specific Treatment of such Cases.* —One of a class of cases of very practical importance, for which St. Mary's Hospital has been for some time remarkable, was operated on by Mr. Baker Brown, on the 16th instant—a case of vaginal cystocele, caused by relaxation of the parts from ruptured perineum. The condition of prolapse of the vagina, as met in hospitals, occurs under three very distressing forms, according as it affects the anterior or posterior wall, or the entire circumference of the canal; the yielding of the anterior parietes, as in the case operated on the 16th inst., draws down the bladder; and, when the poor young woman was placed on the operating table, one saw the collapsed bladder hanging through the external opening of the vulva, giving a painful but vivid idea of the condition of things when the bladder became filled. The ruptured perineum, by removing the natural support of the pelvic viscera, seems sufficient cause for the accident. Nor is this all; for, as was well observed by Mr. Baker Brown to his class, the relaxation of the vagina in front causes an alteration in the position of the bladder itself and its meatus, so as to cause something very like constant retention of urine; this again leading to imperfect action of this viscus, and excessive accumulation, by the weight of which the vagina is stretched even more, and thrust forwards and downwards. Thus one accident, by remaining uncured, causes several others to follow in its train, rendering the life of the woman one scene of wretchedness and misery.

As might be expected, patients such as this woman, though not anxious to tell their complaints, are in the habit of speaking of dragging sensations in the lower part of the abdomen, pain in walking, and horrible dysuria. In some instances, the woman is obliged to push back the viscus into its normal position before she can evacuate the urine. The bladder also becomes a focus of irritation, inside and outside, very singular in itself. The extruded part is liable to injury, and becomes the seat of ulceration; while a very distressing irritability is also set up in the interior, arising from the fact of a small portion of urine always remaining in the cavity, which becomes decomposed, giving rise to much fetid and ropy mucus.

This is the state of things which Mr. Baker Brown proposes to cure; and we do not say too much when we affirm that we know no operation that has met such opposition, and none which has proved to be such a blessing to these poor patients. In milder cases of this disease, and occurring in young females, the treatment is usually confined to frequent catheterism, the recumbent posture, astringent injections, tonics internally, and attention to keep the bladder free from accumulations of urine, by a bent metallic catheter, with an elastic bag attached, and a sponge-tent in the vagina to uphold the bladder. Various means of producing contraction, it need hardly be said, have also been tried, such as the actual cautery, or removing a triangular slip of mucous membrane, the base towards the orifice of the vagina, and then bringing the edges together by suture.

We observed, on the 16th inst., that Mr. I. B. Brown, after the usual horseshoe section of the vaginal mucous membrane, had recourse to the still more formidable proceeding of removing a flap of mucous membrane from the thick central portion of the protruded bladder itself, on its vaginal aspect—a new adaptation of plastic surgery, of a delicate if not dangerous character.

We have seen this operation of Mr. Baker Brown's now so often, that it is only a matter of duty to say that his success with his cases has been most remarkable, almost unexpected. One sees poor women every month, from all parts of the country, many prenounced incurable, whose lives have been a burden to themselves and all about them, either with cystocele or rectocele, prolapse of the uterus of the very worst kind, or some other grave malady, yet who return home to the country quite cured, the strong muscular arch of the perineum quite renewed, and all the pelvic organs restored to their normal position.

The object of the operation on the 16th, was contraction of the caliber of the vagina generally. By the first step, now so well known, the contraction of the vagina *laterally* is secured, while the posterior horseshoe incision completed the operation *posteriorly*. We noticed two deep sutures, which are usually removed on the third day, the interrupted sutures on the fifth day; a bent catheter being secured in the bladder, attached to an India-rubber bag. Much care is observed to keep the woman under the effects of opium, so that the parts shall not be disturbed by the bowels acting.—*Assoc. Med. Journ.*, July 26, 1856.

35. *On the Treatment of Hydrocele of Children.* By Dr. LINHART.—In hydrocele, met with immediately after birth, there is usually a wide communication with the abdominal cavity; and as there is frequently a fold of gut at the upper part of the tumour, it sometimes occurs that hernia and hydrocele alternate—so that two practitioners, called at different times, may give different opinions respecting the case. This form scarcely requires any special treatment, since the serum returns, during the horizontal position, into the cavity of the abdomen, where it is easily resorbed. The only treatment likely to be of any use would be the keeping the neck of the processus vaginalis compressed by a bandage.

It is otherwise when the hernia occurs later after birth, when it is tense, and the communication with the abdomen is either very small or absent, the processus vaginalis being closed above. In the first case, the fluid will often return slowly into the abdomen, although it may occupy six or eight days in so doing; and such cases deceive the attendants of the child into the belief that the means employed have produced the resorption of the fluid. The deception is the more likely, as, in very great narrowing of the upper mouth of the processus vaginalis, which is often more than an inch long, reposition cannot be induced by the taxis. This difficulty of returning the fluid is often mistaken for an impossibility, and unnecessary operations resorted to. Indeed, the diagnosis of complete closure is very difficult. When such closure does exist, the case does not differ from one of ordinary hydrocele of the tunica vaginalis.

The indications of treatment are, the removal of the fluid and the closure of the processus vaginalis. With regard to the first, resorption frequently occurs spontaneously, but it can rarely be influenced by the practitioner. The various stimulants employed for this purpose are inoperative, or may be even hurtful by irritating the scrotal skin. When they seem to have been of avail, an aperture has, in fact, existed. The resorption, however, is remarkably facilitated by a subcutaneous incision of the processus vaginalis, which allows the fluid to become effused into the scrotum, where it is rapidly absorbed. A fold of the scrotum should be raised, and a concave tenotomy knife passed in flat between the scrotal skin and the serous sac, so as to make an incision of from one to one and a half inches in length in the processus vaginalis. Dr. Linhart prefers this to seeking to obliterate the vaginal process by means of pressure applied to its neck, which is either ineffectual or cannot be borne, or to the employment of injections, which at this age are not without danger.—*Ibid.*, from Froriep's *Notizen*, 1856.

36. *Reduction of a Dislocated Femur by Manipular Movements only, three weeks after the Accident—Diagnosis of Dislocations of the Femur.*—R. E., aged 44, a tall and muscular man, by trade a painter, consulted Mr. Wormald, at his own residence, on July 15. He had that morning walked from his own home, a distance of nearly a mile. He stated that three weeks before he had fallen off a wall a height of fifteen feet, and had been lame in his hip ever since. At the time of the accident, he was quite unable to stand, and was carried home to

bed, where his hip was examined by a surgeon, who assured him that it was only sprained. He laid in bed ten days, with the exception of getting up each day to have his bed made. On the eleventh day he got up, and, with the help of a stick, walked down stairs and up again. Since then he had been up daily, and had walked about, but still continued lame. Under these circumstances, he now sought further advice. Having had him stripped, Mr. Wormald examined the part, and at once detected a dislocation into the thyroid foramen, the symptoms of which were very well marked. He advised the man to go into the hospital. On the following day (the twenty-fifth after the accident), reduction was effected in the following manner: The patient, under the influence of chloroform, was laid on his back on a table, a towel for counter-extension being passed round the inside of the hip. The operator then, standing in front of the patient, placed the front of the knee of the affected limb in his own axilla, passing the right arm under the thigh, from within outwards. With the left hand he then grasped firmly the upper part of the displaced bone, at the same time taking his left wrist in his right hand. In this manner, the thigh was firmly held, easily managed, and great force in rotating it and directing its movements could be applied.[1] Mr. Wormald now, bending the thigh on the pelvis, accomplished a rotatory movement outwards. The first few attempts had the effect only of breaking down adhesions, and loosening the bone. Complete reduction was, however, after a short time (about ten minutes) effected, the slipping the head of the bone into its socket being attended by a snap distinctly felt by the operator. The symmetry of the two sides was perfectly restored.

In commenting on this case, Mr. Wormald mentioned one treated by himself some years ago, in which, after a failure in the attempt to reduce by pulleys, he succeeded by the plan just described. The patient was a very muscular man, aged 22, and the bone had been out of place six weeks. The dislocation had originally been on the ilium, but, in the attempt with pulleys, the head of the bone had been thrown into the ischiatic notch, from which all the force that could be applied by them had failed to remove it.

In the case above given, Mr. Wormald pointed out to the students present a sign of dislocation of which no mention is, we believe, made in books. On looking at the limb from the side, the front outline of the thigh (the belly of the rectus) was seen to present a concavity instead of the curved prominence natural to it. The explanation was of course easy, in the circumstance that the bone was thrown backwards, carrying with it the muscles of the thigh.

In a case which occurred some few months ago under his care at Guy's, Mr. Hilton drew attention to a condition which was extremely well marked, respecting which he observed, that although rarely attended to, he believed it to be one of the most useful diagnostic signs in difficult cases. It consisted in the loss of support from behind to the vessels. On pressing the finger on the latter, the existence of a hollow behind them, and the deficiency of that firm support which they naturally possess, was most readily appreciated. This sign would be of great value in those cases in which the difficulty in diagnosis lay between dislocation of the bone and fracture of its neck or shaft high up.—*Med. Times and Gaz.*, August 16, 1856.

37. *Unusual Case of Injury of the Hip; Fracture with Modified or Muffled Crepitus; Detected under the Effect of Chloroform.*—Mr. Skey has had a somewhat remarkable case of fracture in one of his wards, which seemed very puzzling at first, but which is now progressing very favourably. The accident

[1] We have been thus precise in describing the manner of holding the limb, because it is a point to which Mr. Wormald attaches much importance. We believe also with him, that it is the method in which the greatest amount of motor and directing force can be applied with least of inconvenience to the operator. It is not difficult, however, to succeed in the reduction of these dislocations by manipular movements, without attending to any precise rules on this head, the requisite degree of force being easily obtained. Many cases which we have previously recorded have proved this.—J. H.

was so peculiar, yet of such an eminently practical and suggestive kind, that we deem it worthy of notice.

The case is that of a boy, otherwise healthy, admitted into Harley ward, with a singular condition of the left hip joint, and the following history. It seemed that he had been riding in a cart and fell over, pitching heavily on the ground, but he was taken up, placed in the cart again, sitting up, and taken home. He hobbled about for six or seven days, but then fell again, and observed something to give way in the neighbourhood of the hip-joint. He still made nothing of the accident, but walked with a stick for not less than three weeks more in this state. He was ultimately forced to give up, and come to the hospital. Mr. Skey saw him very soon after admission, and, on making a careful examination of the case, he found the left leg to be half an inch shorter than the right, everted, and the great trochanter obviously turned backwards. Much excitement was now caused as to its being an undetected dislocation, whereas Mr. Skey had been assured there was no dislocation of any kind. Several surgeons saw the case; some considered it to be a fracture of the ossa pubis, others a dislocation of some kind. Mr. Skey had the boy placed carefully under chloroform, so that he could make a thorough examination of the parts; when, in addition to the points just noticed, eversion of the foot, shortening, and turning of the trochanter backwards, he noticed that there was evidently no fracture of the acetabulum, that, under the influence of the anæsthetic, the eversion ceased, the shortening was removed, and, by a particular movement or shaking of the parts, a muffled or soft crepitation was perceived. Mr. Skey observed to his class that it is unwise to be going half way to meet difficulties that only exist in our patient's imagination, or our own craving for novelties. This case appeared neither fracture of ossa pubis nor dislocation, but fracture of the femur at the neck, only with the thick fibrous capsule or periosteum not torn. This accident, after the original injury in the cart, having been followed by inflammation, effusion, and softening, which eased the pain, the boy hobbled about as described, but the parts ultimately yielding and breaking right off when he was brought to the hospital. Mr. Skey said the feel was quite different from the crackling of egg-shells sort of sound in the crepitus of old patients with this accident.

June 20. The boy has gone on very well, with a graduated screw to the splint and perineal bandage. The patella is normal; the eversion is gone; crepitus gone.

While in consultation on the preceding case, some practical observations were made by Mr. Stanley, Mr. Lawrence, Mr. Skey, etc., on the general treatment of fractures of the thigh.[1] Mr. Lawrence referred to a case a little while before, which we had an opportunity also of seeing, where the condition of the fracture was precisely as imagined by Mr. Skey; the two ends of the broken neck of the femur being held in close apposition by the strong ligamentous bands which embrace the acetabulum superiorly, the patient apparently "hobbling about" with a stick for some time, and throwing the weight of the body on the sound hip. There is even an accessory band of ligamentous structure, which descends from the anterior inferior spinous process of the ilium to the base of the neck of the femur, strengthening the anterior portion of the capsular ligament amazingly. This question, it need scarcely be said, is one of immense importance, as the surgeon who first saw the case of this boy under the care of Mr. Skey, pronounced it not dislocation; and if Mr. Skey pronounced even the word dislocation, the friends would have had an action at law, and, we believe, threatened it.—*Assoc. Med. Journ.*, July 26, 1856.

---

38. *Amputation at the Hip-joint.*—Mr. Curling performed this important operation in the London Hospital, in March last, on a woman about forty years of age, in weak health, who had a large tumour imbedded in the muscles of the right thigh, and reaching nearly to the pubes. Chloroform having been ad-

[1] Some substitute for the long splint and the confinement it causes was eagerly wished for; but at Guy's Hospital the use of sand-bags, and at University College Hospital stiff starched bandages, are found to meet almost every requirement.

ministered, the main artery was compressed at the pubes, and the thigh acutely flexed. Mr. Curling then made a large posterior flap, cutting rapidly from without inwards. Two of the chief branches of the gluteal artery having been secured, and a large sponge applied to the flap, the thigh was depressed, and, an anterior flap being made, the bone was disarticulated. This mode of proceeding was adopted to prevent the loss of blood, and not more than four or five ounces were lost in the amputation. After the bleeding vessels had been tied, the two flaps were brought together with numerous sutures, and the surfaces were kept in close contact by a large quantity of cotton wool applied on the outside, covered with lint, and well secured with strapping. The stump healed favourably, and at the end of two months the patient was sent to the sea-side for the improvement of her general health. The tumour was situated beneath the vastus externus muscle, and rested on the outer part of the femur, extending close to the bone as high as the great trochanter. It consisted of masses of brain-like matter, large coagula, and numerous imperfect cysts. The surface of the femur in contact with the tumour was abraded and very vascular. The morbid growth exhibited the microscopic characters of encephaloid cancer. Her health is improving, and, up to the present date, there have been no symptoms of a recurrence of the disease.—*Assoc. Med. Journ.*, July 26, 1856.

39. *Amputation through the Knee-joint.* By GEO. H. B. MACLEOD, M. D., Surgeon to the Civil Hospital at Smyrna, &c. &c.—Amputation through the knee-joint has been performed in this army seven times. Four patients died, two were sent home previous to the 31st of December, and the remaining one went to England, recovered, in January. In at least four of the seven cases in which the operation was performed, it can hardly be said to have been applicable, as the end of the femur was more or less destroyed in each of them. The French have, very properly, had recourse to this mode of operating only in those cases —frequent enough in their occurrence—in which the head of the bones of the leg are fractured into the articulation, but in which the injury has not extended to the femur, and I am led to understand that the result of the operation has been very satisfactory in their hands. In the four cases above referred to, the operation performed was not strictly that known as amputation through the knee-joint, but more nearly the low amputation recommended by Mr. Syme in disease of the articulation.

So far as I have had means of judging, the practical advantages of this operation are no less in its favour than those theoretical ones which its advocates claim for it; and they would seem to recommend its more general adoption in any future campaign.

The obtaining of a longer and firmer stump, and one to which a false limb can be more easily attached, than when amputation in the continuity of the bone has been performed, is in itself no small advantage presented by this operation. Few now participate in Liston's opinion of a long thigh stump. The rectus, with its point of insertion remaining entire, is a matter of vast importance to the power of progression. The non-interference with the medullary canal obviates many of the dangers of amputation, according to Cruveilhier; while the extremity of the femur, which is largely supplied with bloodvessels, being retained, there is less risk of exfoliation than when the dense substance of the bone has been opened by the saw. There is little fear but that the flaps will adhere over the cártilaginous extremity of the bone. It is much to be regretted, then, that the operation has not been more largely tried during the war than it has been, when so many cases fitted for it have p[illegible] themselves. Two-thirds of the cases recorded by Chelius recovered; and, in the French ambulances, it is reported to have been at least as successful as amputation of the lower third of the thigh. When much of the end of the femur has to be removed, as it was in several of the cases operated on in our hospitals, many of the advantages secured by the correct operation are, of course, lost. Baudens' operation has been that followed by the French; while in five cases, operated on in this hospital, that method was modified, in so far as that the posterior flap was made from within outwards, in place of the reverse, as practised by that distinguished surgeon, and the anterior flap, too, was made not quite so long. Of the five cases which occurred in this hospital, one died on the forty-third day, of phagedenic sloughing; another, a soldier of the 62d, died on the sixty-seventh day, of enteritis, the stump being healed to a point; a third sank on the ninth day after operation, of exhaustion; a fourth, who was a Russian, never fairly recovered from the shock, and died very soon; while the fifth and last case completely recovered. The successful case was operated on by Dr. George Scott, civil surgeon. The patient, a soldier in the Buffs, was struck by a ball on the right knee-joint, when inside of the Redan, on the 8th of September. He thought himself very slightly injured, as the only thing he observed wrong with the joint was his inability to flex it, on account of "something catching in it." A small opening was found in the middle of the popliteal space, slightly external to the middle line, from which a good deal of blood flowed. This opening was found to lead into the cavity of the articulation, and spiculæ of bone were felt within. A part of the end of the femur was removed, but the patella left. A round ball had, it was found, pierced the external condyle and lodged. The posterior flap eventually sloughed, and exposed the end of the femur, but the bone became subsequently covered, once with granulations, and, though the patient's progress towards recovery was much impeded by the formation of an abscess among the muscles of the thigh, which required extensive incisions, he went to England in perfect health in January. His stump was strong and firm, and over its movements he had much power. The patella could be felt on the upper surface, to which position it had been gradually retracted. In several of the cases which I have seen in the French hospitals, where sloughing of the flaps had taken place and exposed the extremity of the femur, the cartilages were alone thrown off, but not a scale of bone.

Of the many ways of performing this operation which have been proposed and practised, none appear so good as the old one of Hain; it seems to fulfil more of the "desirabilities" than any other. If cases were selected for the performance of the operation, in which the femur remaining intact, and the leg bones being destroyed, a sufficiency of flap could be got from the calf; and if the amputation was performed early, I firmly believe, with Malgaigne, that it is "Encore une de ces operations trop légèrement condamnées, et qui lorsqu'on a le choix mérite toute préférénce sur l'amputation de la cuisse dans la continuité."—*Edinburgh Med. Journ.*, July, 1856.

---

40. *On the Comparative Value of Amputation at the Knee-Joint and of the Thigh.*—M. Baudens states, in a recent communication to the Academy of Sciences, that the above question is one of those that have engaged his attention during his directorship of the French army in the East. He found that the opinions of all the medical officers whom he consulted, whether in the Crimea, at Constantinople, or the military hospitals at Marseilles and Toulon, were in favour of disarticulation of the knee whenever the amputation of the extremity could not be performed below the patella. And, in fact, the disarticulation of the knee has succeeded in a given number of cases oftener than the amputation of the thigh, even when performed at the lower third. But the disarticulation is only to be preferred upon one express condition—viz: that it be performed immediately after the receipt of the injury. Consecutively, amputation of the thigh should be preferred. This second statement agrees in every respect with all that he has observed, written, and taught during the ten years he has been at the head of the Val-de-Grâce. The excellent results of disarticulation of the knee, especially recorded in his Clinical Observations upon Gunshot Wounds, were obtained in soldiers who had just been wounded on the field of battle. This difference in the results derivable from immediate and secondary amputation at the knee-joint, depends upon the fact that even in a state of health the size of the bones is not in complete accord with the amount of soft parts—a disproportion that becomes still greater when the patient has lost flesh during prolonged suffering and abundant suppuration.

In another communication, M. Baudens observes that, although the surgeons of the Sardinian army in the Crimea hesitated to employ chloroform, those of the French army have used it in twenty-five thousand cases without any accident resulting. It was always administered with great care, so as not to go beyond the production of insensibility.—*Comptes Rendus*, t. xli.

41. *Statistics of Amputations in the Crimea.* By Geo. H. B. Macleod, M. D., &c.—The leg has been amputated 149 times;[1] 35 have died here; 14 have been discharged cured; 95 sent to other stations; 1 readmitted for other disease, and 4 remained in hospital on 31st December. Supposing that a fourth of those transferred and remaining died, the mortality in amputations of the leg will be thus 40.2 per cent. The preservation of as much of the limb as possible has, I think, been the rule followed.

At the ankle-joint, there have been 20 amputations; no deaths in the Crimea, but 16 cases were transferred and 1 remained, while 3 were discharged cured. Perogoff, in Sebastopol, is said to have performed many amputations at the joint, according to his own method, during the siege. Roux's mode of operating has not been so much adopted as it seems to merit. I hear that M. Baudens (who is here at present) strongly advocates a modification of the procedure of Roux, by which the flap is taken from the external surface of the foot, in those cases in which the inside and heel flaps are destroyed, rather than have recourse to an amputation of the leg. Chopart's operation has been performed 12 times; 1 was discharged cured and 11 transferred. Lisfranc's amputation of the metatarsal bones has been practised 8 times, of which number 1 was discharged cured, and 7 transferred to other stations.

The upper extremity has been removed at the shoulder 60 times; 19 have died in the Crimea, 11 were discharged cured, 29 transferred, and 1 remained. This, on the same calculation as has been followed in the case of other amputations, gives a mortality of 43.3 per cent. In at least two cases, the scapula was so much destroyed that it was removed, piece by piece, at the same time that the arm was amputated. My friend, Dep. Inspector Gordon, C. B., was the operator in both of these cases, of which one recovered. The shock, in such a case, was necessarily very great. Mr. Howard, of the 20th Regiment, removed successfully the right arm of one man and the left of another, at the joint, in close succession, the injury to both patients having been occasioned by the same round shot. The ball struck fairly between the men as they were marching in close column to the trenches. No case has fallen under my notice in which the limb was fairly torn from the body, as sometimes happens from machinery; it has always remained attached, though fearfully mangled.

The upper arm has been amputated 158 times; 29 died here; 23 were discharged cured; 100 were transferred, and 1 was readmitted. This gives a mortality of 35.2 per cent., allowing a fourth of those transferred to have died, which, perhaps, in this instance, is too large a calculation. The forearm has been amputated 73 times; 3 died in the Crimea, 11 were discharged cured, 54 sent to other stations, 1 readmitted, and 4 remained. As in the instance of the upper arm, probably a fourth of the cases transferred did not die; but, if we presume they did, the resulting mortality from amputation of the forearm has been 23.2 per cent. As no distinction is made in the returns between primary and secondary operations, I cannot, of course, show what was the relative success of amputation performed early or late on the above parts. It may, however, be said that amputation of the upper extremity, performed during the secondary period, has been sufficiently successful in its results, to warrant an attempt being made, in almost all cases, to save the limb in the first instance. In military surgery, secondary amputations are hopeful only when practised on the upper extremity.

Serious secondary hemorrhage has not been common after amputation. Cases in which the main vessel has been ligatured, in consequence of such acci-

[1] The return from which the figures in these papers have been taken, was made up at the head-quarters of the army, and a copy was furnished to the Army Medico-Chirurgical Society by its respected president. Since the completion of that return, I understand that some errors have been discovered in it, but they chiefly occur in the summing up of the different details. I believe the *relative* proportion of the different items to remain unchanged, though in various points the numbers given are not *absolutely* correct. There are no errors in the case of operations. I have not seen a copy of the corrected return, or I would have substituted its figures for those given in this paper, in such instances as there was any call to do so.

dents, have been, I believe, singularly fortunate. Well applied pressure along the course of the principal vessel, adapted to diminish the circulation through it, has sufficed, in some most threatening cases, to arrest finally bleedings which had recurred frequently. Take the following case as an example. The state of the vessel, as discovered after death, also lends an interest to the case. Hemorrhage took place to a slight extent, from a thigh stump, on the ninth day after operation, and was repeated on the following morning. A tourniquet, applied over the course of the femoral, so as to moderate the flow of blood through it, was applied. On the fourteenth day, the bleeding returned, and the tourniquet was tightened for four hours, so as almost to arrest the current of blood in the great vessel, and then, though loosened, was still left so tight as to restrain the free flow of the blood through the main artery. On the sixteenth day, the bleeding returned, and the same treatment was followed, the position of the compressing force being carefully shifted from time to time. From this period, the hemorrhage never reappeared. The patient subsequently died of pyæmia; when it was found that an abscess had formed around the great vessels, extending from the end of the stump upwards, for a couple of inches; that the artery was fairly opened by ulceration, to the extent of an inch from its termination, but beyond that distance a dense clot occupied its caliber for an inch and a quarter. The vein contained much pus. Purulent matter was freely deposited in the lungs. Here the ulceration of the end of the artery allowed the bleeding to take place, while the subsequent formation of a clot above arrested it.—*Edinburgh Med. Journ.*, July, 1856.

42. *Use of Chloroform in Military Practice.*—Dr. Mouat, C. B., Deputy Inspector-General, read, at a meeting of the Crimean Medical and Surgical Society (April 19, 1856), the following observations on some points connected with the use of chloroform in military practice. The author commenced by stating, "The subject of the administration of chloroform in the well-known shock or depression following severe gunshot injuries, is one, from its nature and the peculiar interest it possesses at the present time, that requires no apology for its introduction, and appears to me to be a fit and proper one for discussion in this society. The profession at home naturally look to the medical officers of the army to contribute their mite of practical experience towards the settlement of this important and disputed question; but I much fear they will be somewhat disappointed in the results and conclusions arrived at. Great and grave doubts are beginning to arise in the minds of some unprejudiced practical surgeons and thinking observers at home and abroad, as to the indiscriminate use of this powerful anæsthetic; so tempting to the sufferer, yet at times so fraught with danger and uncertain in its results, that I defy the most strenuous advocates for its employment to say, *à priori*, what its results may prove in any given case; in other words, to say distinctly what fixed laws it invariably follows, if any. The fatal cases, unfortunately, from the simple extraction of a tooth, or removal of a finger, to the more formidable amputation at the hip-joint, leaves no doubt as to its occasional melancholy result. Dr. Simpson's cases are in a great measure confined to its administration in parturition—a simple process of nature; therefore, his great experience does not apply strictly to the subject now under consideration. Dr. Snow's practice—at least a very large proportion of it—I have been informed, has occurred in dental surgery; at all events, not in gunshot wounds; and no one, I am sure, will attempt to compare the shock of the extraction of a tooth, or ordinary surgical operation, to the amputation of a limb close to the trunk. The first case in which I saw chloroform administered in this war, was one peculiarly adapted to test this question. It was on the day of the memorable and bloody battle of Inkermann, and the patient was an officer, 29 years of age. The injury was a compound comminuted fracture of the femur near its neck, with injury to the bloodvessels and nerves; much blood had been lost on the field. I need hardly say, after this explanation, what the operation was. Several hours were allowed to elapse after the receipt of the wound, and reaction, with the aid of stimulants, had taken place. The patient was in great pain, most anxious and urgent that the operation should be performed, and earnestly stipulated for the administration

of chloroform. At the request of the operator, and after a deliberate consultation had been held, I administered the chloroform, which was measured and amounted to about two drachms. He was rapidly and easily affected, and was neither sick nor convulsed. The operation was performed by Mr. Wyatt, with great skill, and the loss of blood was inconsiderable; but, I regret to say, the sufferer died somewhat suddenly after, notwithstanding all attempts at artificial respiration, the cold douche, etc. Some persons present entertained the opinion that he perished from the effects of chloroform. My own opinion was, that he died under the combined influence of shock and the depressing effects of the chloroform inhalation. It is worthy of remark, that the patient had previously been put slightly under the influence of chloroform, in order to examine the extent of injury, as he would not submit without, and no harm resulted. This is case No. 1, and cannot, therefore, be explained under the convenient term of idiosyncrasy. Great weight is, undoubtedly, due to the opinion of so experienced and talented an operator as Professor Syme; but I much doubt if even this distinguished surgeon has had any experience in injuries of the peculiar nature we are now about to discuss (notwithstanding the opinion of most civil surgeons as to there being no essential difference between gunshot and railway injuries). I am fully aware that I am standing on dangerous ground in provoking many antagonists, to say nothing of public opinion, for this appears to have become a popular as well as a professional subject. No one can yet have forgotten the storm of abuse, indignation, and misrepresentation with which a certain memorable departmental order on this subject was received. Even the Sebastopol Committee, in their anxiety to saddle somebody with something, actually went out of their way in their endeavour to cast unmerited odium on the medical department of the army on this very subject; and yet what did this famous order, after all, amount to? A wise and humane caution from an old and experienced officer in the field to his younger professional brethren, most of them entering for the first time on new and trying duties, requiring all the resources of our art, backed by the wisdom of experience; for, after all, experience must be our schoolmaster. We were bound to respect such an opinion, coming from such a source. I am not about to enter into the question as to whether that caution might not have been more carefully and judiciously worded; for, no doubt, it would have been differently expressed, if intended for the perusal of a popular, instead of a professional public. The introduction of chloroform was, no doubt, one of the proudest discoveries and greatest blessings of the age. It has often contributed to sustain the fortitude of many a brave warrior, and given confidence to many a timid operating surgeon; and anything calculated, in the remotest degree, to lessen the horrors or soften the terrors of war, cannot but be considered a boon to suffering humanity; hence, chloroform must claim almost universal approbation. It does not, however, follow that such an agent should be used indiscriminately, or as a matter of routine, as is too frequently done; but its employment should be withheld when it can be dispensed with, and whenever it is intended to be employed, too much caution and care cannot be exercised in its administration. Most of the fatal cases have, doubtless, been sought out, and brought before the public. A reference to statistics is here not in my power, but I have been informed by one medical gentleman, Dr. Rooke, that, for some time, about four years ago, he kept an account of fatal cases, and in a short period collected no less than forty. The statistics of this subject are very imperfect. Many cases may have been hushed up, but by far the larger number have sunk silently into their graves. It is that peculiar state of nausea and depression following its use, in which perfect reaction is never thoroughly established, the desire for food never returns, and the patient sinks, as it were, stealthily, and dies from exhaustion in from twelve to twenty-four hours. These cases are far more numerous than is generally supposed, and many of them may fairly be termed 'deaths from chloroform,' but are never so returned. I can at this moment bring two or three such to my recollection. Medical men are naturally anxious to avoid the kind of publicity which must attach to fatal cases of operation under chloroform, and, therefore, only return such as actually die on the table. If the patient survives only half an hour, it is very easy to say he died from the effects of the operation. This obvious source of fallacy ought candidly to be taken into consideration, and I think will go some way in accounting for the uniform success of certain practitioners.

"To continue the illustration of this subject from the actual cases occurring in the surgery of this war, the next instance to which I shall refer was a case of destructive injury to the bone and soft parts of the thigh. The left leg of a soldier was carried away by a round shot during the second bombardment; the knee-joint was smashed, and the femur fractured high up. The muscles and integuments of the opposite thigh were likewise lacerated. The patient was a remarkably fine, muscular young man, and in perfect health. The shock had been great, from the extensive injuries and loss of blood, and perfect reaction had been established. He was calm, collected, and anxious for the operation under the influence of chloroform, which was administered carefully, and in the usual manner, by Dr. Bleckly, of the 14th Regiment, and he was easily influenced. I then proceeded to amputate the thigh at its upper third, by the flap operation. About the average quantity of blood was lost, and it was necessary to apply the saw pretty close to the trochanter. The patient regained his senses for a short time, complained of præcordial oppression and abdominal pain, with great restlessness. He never rallied fairly, and died within an hour, never having been removed from the table; this is case No. 2. I was kindly assisted in this operation by Deputy Inspector-General Taylor, who compressed the femoral artery at the groin, and who, I think it fair to state, considers that the chloroform enabled the patient to go through the operation. For his opinion, founded, as it is, on the experience of two previous campaigns, I entertain the highest respect; but it appears to me to be a fair illustration of the shock of a severe gunshot injury, in which the depressing after-effects of the chloroform were not rallied from. As an instance of what may be done in such cases without chloroform, I may here state that Dr. Gordon, Deputy Inspector-General of 2d Division, successfully removed the thigh by amputation at its middle third, and the arm at the shoulder-joint on the same subject in succession: and I have the authority of Deputy Inspectors-General Taylor and Gordon (both officers of great practical experience in India) for stating that, in the campaign on the Sutlej, amputations of the thigh proved more successful without chloroform than they have done in this campaign under its influence. Dr. Taylor, however, is of opinion that this result may be due to other causes. With regard to the stimulating effects of chloroform upon patients about to sink from the exhaustion of disease, as above quoted, this is a totally different state from the shock occasioned by severe gunshot injury, with or without loss of blood. But I can adduce an instance of secondary amputation of the thigh, in which the patient was much exhausted after twenty-four days' suffering from a wound implicating the knee-joint. In this instance, there was an unsuccessful attempt at conservative surgery, at the earnest solicitation of the patient, who nearly lost his life from the inhalation of half a drachm of chloroform administered by myself. The operation was ultimately performed without chloroform, and with but little suffering. As this case (Sergeant Bennett, of the 30th Regiment) was seen by several medical officers here, I shall not enter into any further detail. Let me, however, here at once inform the Society, that it is not the intention of this paper to treat on the merits of chloroform generally; they are admitted; and, to quote the words of a public commentator on this subject, 'Chloroform is so priceless a boon to mankind, that we should all endeavor to ascertain with the utmost watchfulness, the nature of the difficulties and dangers which beset its use.' It is only to such that I refer; and I will, therefore, repeat the real question at issue:—

"1. Is the administration of chloroform, in the severe depression consequent on large gunshot injuries, fraught with danger?

"2. Are we justified, in a moral point of view, in giving a dangerous remedy for such trifling operations as the removal of a finger or toe, or the extraction of teeth, or bullets lying near the surface?

"I think any candid, conscientious observer, who has had the misfortune to meet with such a case as that of Private Martin Humphrey, 62d Regiment (to recur to the surgery of the war), who died suddenly while under the influence of chloroform for the amputation of a finger, will unhesitatingly answer: 'We are scarcely justified in trifling, or, in unimportant injuries, in resorting to an anæsthetic that may so suddenly deprive a fellow-creature of life, while we possess so simple, so ready, and so efficient a means of producing local anæsthesia as that described by Dr. James Arnott in the *Medical Times and Gazette* for July, August, and September, 1854.' Whatever objections may be urged against this simple and humane means of producing anæsthesia, no fatal result can occur from its use. In all superficial operations, says Dr. Arnott, which constitute the immense majority, cold is superior to chloroform in the circumstances of safety, ease of application, and the saving of time and trouble, certainty of producing anæsthesia, and, lastly, of preventing subsequent inflammation. Anæsthesia will, no doubt, be henceforth a required element of every operation; but chloroform, fortunately, is not the only mode of producing it; and I trust there is a time coming when we may be able to restrict its use to such cases as cannot be affected by other means. The propriety of using an anæsthetic which occasionally destroys life in simple cases is questionable, while we possess one free from danger, easy of application, requiring no assistance, and, what is invaluable in military practice, 'saving of time.' Anæsthesia from cold may be complete in a minute. There is yet another agent of great power and efficacy in a certain class of cases, which it has been the custom of the profession to sneer at, but which Dr. Esdaile's reports and returns place beyond a doubt. I allude to mesmerism. It is not, however, applicable to military practice.

"One more case in illustration of the occasional ill effects of chloroform in the shock following loss of blood. Stephen Newing, a private of the 97th Regiment, aged 21, was wounded, on the 8th of September, in the attack on the Redan, by a musket-ball through the left forearm, producing compound fracture of the ulna. He had likewise a flesh wound of the right thigh, and a graze of the belly, both by musket-balls. He experienced a slight attack of diarrhœa on the 25th, up to which period he had been doing well; this was of no great severity. On the 30th, he had slight bilious vomiting, shortly after which it was discovered that hemorrhage had taken place to a considerable extent from the ulnar artery, in all probability induced by the exertion of vomiting. He had lost about two pounds of blood before it was discovered. Upon a careful examination of the limb, it was discovered that about three inches of the ulna were dead, and the wrist-joint appeared to be involved. Amputation was therefore decided on, and was performed in about two hours after the discovery of the hemorrhage; so that the man might, in a certain sense, be said to be under shock. Chloroform to the extent of one drachm only was administered, the operation was rapidly executed, and an unusually small quantity of blood lost. He did not, however, rally from the effects of the chloroform, vomited a fluid of the appearance of coffee-grounds, and gradually sank. Artificial respiration, the cold douche, etc., failed to restore animation. Staff-Surgeon Matthews remarks, that he never at any time recovered from the effects of the chloroform insensibility; and, although the immediate cause of death was, doubtless, by loss of blood, or the direct action of chloroform on the brain, or asphyxia, still he is strongly inclined to believe that, had chloroform not been employed, he would not have lost the man. In such cases, the ebbing powers of life are just as likely to be suddenly arrested, as stimulated to fresh vitality; for chloroform does not prevent syncope; indeed, it is one of the modes in which it destroys life. I have not seen that supporting power attributed to it; and here I differ from Dr. Snow, who thinks accidents from chloroform are to be prevented by care in the administration, not in the selection of cases.

"In confirmation of Dr. Matthews's view of the case, a precisely similar one happened to me in 1849, in which I had to amputate the forearm for secondary hemorrhage after gunshot injury, implicating the wrist-joint. The patient in this instance, Private Hugh Swift, of the 13th Light Dragoons, shot himself through the wrist, while in a fit of intoxication. An attempt was made to save the limb. Secondary hemorrhage suddenly took place on the eighth day after the receipt of the injury, at midnight; and, before it was discovered, he had lost a considerable quantity of blood. A tourniquet was immediately applied, but, such was his state of exhaustion, that the propriety of amputation was questionable. He had, however, rallied sufficiently in about two hours, under powerful stimulants, and the amputation was performed without chloroform, and apparently without pain; but such was his condition that he could not be removed from the table for some hours. He ultimately recovered. Chloroform, I think, under these circumstances would have killed him. In conclusion, I may state that I was present at every operation under chloroform performed at the General Hospital in camp during the siege, and several in the 3d Division; that in many instances I administered the chloroform myself, generally on a piece of lint, the patient always being in a recumbent position, and in no instance was organic disease detected, and I most reluctantly come to the conclusion: 1. That there are states of shock, or depression from loss of blood, following extensive injury—such as the loss of a thigh high up, or the arm at the axilla—in which chloroform may destroy life in various ways. 2. There are likewise cases in which, as I have stated, the patient never fairly rallies, but sinks gradually without any effort at reaction; these cases are never returned as deaths from chloroform. 3. I cannot subscribe to the kind of argument sometimes used to justify its indiscriminate use, viz.: that the invariable absence of pain to the patient and advantage to the surgeon, fully counterbalance the risk of an occasional fatal termination. In trifling injuries, life is too precious to be thus trifled with; it is opposed to all moral laws, nor can the opinion of hosts of authors, dead or living, make it right in such cases."—*Med. Times and Gaz.*, August 30, 1856.

43. *Injection of Balsam of Copaiba in Gonorrhœa.*—M. Dallas, of Odessa, states, in confirmation of the observations already published by Taddei, Marchal, and others, that the injection of balsam of copaiba is the most efficacious mode of treating gonorrhœa. In sixteen cases he has so employed it, using no internal remedy, either in recent or old gonorrhœa, with complete success. His formula is copaib. five drachms; one yelk of egg; gummy extract of opium, one grain; water, seven ounces. The injection should be used several times a day.—*Brit. and For. Med.-Chirurg. Rev.*, July, 1856, from *L'Union Médicale*, No. 2, 1856.

44. *Lupulin in Spermatorrhœa.*—Dr. Pescheck has employed lupulin for several years in a great number of cases in which spermatorrhœa seemed to depend upon no mechanical cause. At first, he used to give two grains night and morning; but finding such doses of no avail, he prescribed from ten to fifteen grains to be taken just before bedtime, prohibiting the drinking of water after it. From such doses, even continued for a long time, he has found no inconvenience to arise, while they have acted beneficially on the disease. In some cases he combined with it one or two grains of pulv. digitalis. A valuable peculiarity in the operation of lupulin, is the beneficial action it exerts upon the digestive process, which so often suffers in these cases. It is also very useful in mitigating the urethral irritation and discharges consequent on former excesses, and in many cases more so than iron or quinine. Its especial utility in the chordee of gonorrhœa, Dr. Pescheck has had many opportunities of witnessing. It is best administered without any additions that might diminish its bitterness, as its effects are very proportionate to the intensity of this property. Old lupulin deprived of its oil and bitter taste is almost always useless.—*Ibid.*, from *Buchner's Repert. für Pharm.*, No. 1, 1856.

45. *Large Doses of Opium in Obstinate Chancre.*—M. Rodet observes that the general conclusions to be drawn from the observations of writers on syphilis are: 1. That opium, conjoined with mercury, in the treatment of bad chancres, acts as a powerful auxiliary. 2. That it often cures ulcers of this description that have not yielded to mercury. 3. That it may ameliorate, but not cure, such ulcers, when given alone, and without having been preceded by mercury. 4. That it is well suited for assuaging the inflammation which complicates syphilitic accidents.

After considerable employment of it in such cases, he has himself come to the conclusion that it is an error to regard it as a mere succedaneum of mercury; it acting, in fact, most efficaciously in just those cases in which mercury is of least use, and *vice versâ*. Thus, in constitutional syphilis, it acts as a mere corrective of the powerful specifics with which it is conjoined, and should only be given in very small doses. Here, as also in the case of indurated chancre, given alone and in large doses, it not only would do no good, but might do great mischief. When, however, the chancre manifests any tendency to phagedena, or is irritable and painful, mercury should be rigidly forbidden, while opium is always useful in assuaging the pain, diminishing the irritability, and modifying the suppurative process. But the case in which truly remarkable effects are produced by opium, and in which it acts almost as a specific, is that of *phagedenic, serpiginous ulcers*. These are fortunately rare. All those met with by the author have succeeded to a virulent bubo, which empties itself of a sanious discharge. The bottom of the ulcer is grayish, pultaceous, and irregular. Its edges are raised, very jagged, and deeply detached, so that the ulcer is always much larger than it appears to be at first sight. If the edges are raised up, we may observe, at several points, anfractuous cavities, irregularly disposed, and filled with sanies and organic debris. These result from a chancerous erosion, which seems to act by destroying the tissues circularly around several partial centres. The general progress of the ulcer consists in its extension from the centre to the circumference, its edges being formed by partial, semicircular ulcerations, each having its particular centre, and extending from this to the circumference. Those partial ulcers do not extend uniformly, some progressing much more rapidly than others, giving always an irregular form to the principal ulcer. Not only do they destroy the subcutaneous tissues, but they also gnaw away the deeper surface of the skin, rendering it more and more thin, until at last it disappears. Sometimes it is the free edge of the skin that first disappears, and, at others, the portion corresponding to the small *cul-de-sac* of the little ulcer, so that we then see around the circumference of the principal sore one or several little ulcers, with notched and everted edges, which look like chancrous pustules accidentally developed around this ulcer. Once formed, these little sores continue to enlarge until the skin separating them from the large one is completely destroyed. But, as these small ulcers become confounded with the original ulceration, other partial ulcerations are produced in the same way. To these others succeed, and so on, for an indefinite period. Ulcerations of this kind may persist for years, laying waste vast regions, extending from the inguinal region along the upper part of the thigh, the hypogastrium, the scrotum, perineum, or the buttock. The irregularity of their form is usually greater in proportion to their extent, and is shown in advancing and retreating angles, and sinuous and irregular lines, which cannot be more accurately compared than with the lines of certain shores as depicted on geographical maps. The sore progressively cicatrizes over as it extends, fresh ulcerations simultaneously breaking out, so that an actual displacement from its original locality has taken place. Sometimes, the cicatrices are only partial, forming a kind of islets; but such cicatrices are sometimes destroyed by the ulceration taking a retrograde course. Generally, the surface of the ulcers is violaceous, and formed of softened tissue devoid of vitality. The edges are always more irritable than the centre, bleeding easily, sensitive to the slightest touch, and the seat of incessant pain of varying degrees of severity. These ulcers never give rise to constitutional symptoms, whatever their extent or duration, but the patient becomes gradually enfeebled, and falls into a state of marasmus, his spirits being at the same time much depressed. The appetite and digestion are feeble, sleep is interrupted, the skin becomes dry, and the countenance assumes a leaden, roughened aspect.

No form of syphilis resists the action of remedies with such tenacity as do these phagedenic serpiginous ulcerations. M. Rodet, prior to resorting to large doses of opium, treated them by a great variety of means, without any satisfactory result. The cyanide of potassium, although incapable of healing them, effected considerable amendment in their appearance. The iodide of potassium was found to be of no avail; and those who believe in its efficacy have confounded these primary ulcers with other serpiginous ulcerations, which much resemble them in appearance, but which appear during the tertiary period of syphilis. As to mercury, not only is it useless, but mischievous, and should be rejected. When the ulcers decidedly manifest the appearances above described, opium exerts a most beneficial effect upon them. In less well-marked cases, it is also useful, but its efficacy is not so complete. For this remedy to succeed, therefore, it is necessary that the case be properly chosen, and that it be administered with certain rules and precautions. M. Rodet prefers the gummy extract to any other preparation, and always commences with small quantities (as five or ten centigrammes),[1] in order to ascertain whether the patient will bear the remedy well. This quantity must be increased gradually, and somewhat rapidly, as every second or third day; for, when the increase is made too slowly, the effect is far less satisfactory. Not only must the dose be increased at short intervals, but also somewhat suddenly, as the economy has not then time to become habituated to the action of the remedy, which then exerts upon it more rapid and more complete modifications. Such increase must be continued until the therapeutical effect is produced. When the ulcers are covered with granulations, and tend to cicatrization on every side, further increase is uncalled for; and, when the sore has taken on the aspect of a simple ulcer, we pursue a retrograde course, diminishing the quantity more or less rapidly until complete cicatrization is obtained, when the opium must be left off.

If some obstacle impedes the progress of cicatrization, the opium does not operate against this, which has to be removed by other means; and the neglect of this precaution may lead to the loss of much time, and to the taking of large unnecessary quantities of opium. The opium must not be given in too divided doses, as, if the stomach be kept too constantly under its action, digestion is interfered with. The entire daily quantity should be taken at two doses, morning and evening, leaving a sufficient space of time after meals to secure the completion of the digestive process before administering it. If this is not attended to, indigestion, accompanied by nausea, vomiting, diarrhœa, sweating, prostration, or cephalalgia, &c., comes on; compelling a temporary cessation of the remedy, and reacting unfavourably on the ulcer. Sometimes, notwithstanding this precaution, the stomach becomes fatigued, and digestion is indolent and accompanied by nausea. This inconvenience is easily avoided by recommending the patient to take light wines with their meals, proportionate to the quantity of opium employed. Thus, suppose the quantity of opium taken daily amounts to fifteen grains or thereabouts, from a pint to a quart of wine should be allowed. The wine not only corroborates the functions of the stomach, but exerts analogous effects on other organs. Thus, constipation, so common a consequence of taking opium, is almost certainly obviated by this means, and an excess of sleep is quite exceptional. The wine is, indeed, an indispensable corrective of opium when given in large doses. If, in spite of all precautions, the head becomes heavy or painful, the conjunctiva injected, or other signs of cerebral congestion appear, the opium must be at once left off, mustard poultices applied to the limbs, and the question of leeching the anus or of general bleeding taken into consideration. If diarrhœa occurs, which is rare when wine is given with the opium, it is usually obstinate, but, refusing to yield to astringents, it does so to ipecacuanha given in emetic but divided doses.

As under the employment of the opium in these cases the general health becomes rapidly meliorated, it is evident that it exerts a powerful action upon the entire economy. M. Rodet furnishes the details of two of his cases. In the first of these, the daily quantity of 10 centigrammes of opium began with on November 9, was gradually augmented to 80 on December 6, and to 90 on January 22, thence descending again to 60 on February 3. In the other, the quantity of 10 centigrammes, began with on January 19, was raised to 80 on March 21, and then diminished by 5 centigrammes every 5 days; but relapse occurred in this patient, and we find him taking from 40 to 60 centigrammes during November.—*Med. Times and Gaz.*, August 16, 1856, from *Bull. de Thérap.*, xlix.

[1] A centigramme is one-seventh of a grain.

46. *Perchloride of Iron as an Hæmostatic.*—A correspondent of the *Moniteur des Hôpitaux* (No. 24, 1856), states that one of the principal elements of his success in the difficult and dangerous operations M. Maissonneuve is famous for undertaking, is the remarkable use he makes of hæmostatics during their performance. He cites a recent case, occurring in a lad of sixteen, of fungous tumour of the dura mater, the growth of which, after having been temporarily arrested by ligature of the carotid, took on enormous proportions, and was accompanied by exhausting hemorrhages. M. Maissonneuve determined upon its removal, but the tumour bled on the slightest contact, and the patient would not be able to bear the slightest loss of blood. The line of incision extended from the anterior parts of the ear to the summit of the head, and descending along the nose, was carried backwards, and then upwards to the base of the jaw, and its point of departure. A great number of arteries were thus divided, five or six of which, by reason of their anastomotic enlargements, had acquired almost the size of the radial artery. Intelligent assistants immediately compressed them with the finger, but it was impossible to thus continue the dissection without exposing the patient to the danger of death from syncope. M. Maissonneuve therefore applied to each vessel a little pledget of charpie soaked in perchloride of iron, which was allowed to attach itself to the wound. At every stroke of the bistoury or scissors he applied a new plug, so that during the operation the patient scarcely lost a spoonful of blood; and when the tumour had been entirely removed, the entire surface of the wound was found completely dried and tanned, and was at once dressed, without the necessity of the application of a single ligature. The brown eschar which covered the wound was detached about the 20th day, without giving rise to any hemorrhage; and although the cure can scarcely be expected to prove radical, the patient for the present is perfectly well.—*Ibid.*

47. *On the Influence of Phosphate of Lime in the Production of Callus.* By M. A. Milne-Edwards.—The question of aiding the formation of callus by the administration of phosphate of lime has recently been revived in Paris, and the author of this paper alludes to some experiments tried by M. Gosselin at the Hôpital Cochin, especially in cases of fracture of the arm, which are sometimes so long in uniting. In the six cases observed by him the result seemed satisfactory, inasmuch as the apparatus could be removed in from twenty-seven to thirty days, the fracture appearing quite consolidated. As, however, in these cases, the condition of the callus could not be verified, M. Edwards undertook a series of comparative experiments on animals. Fractures as nearly as possible alike were executed upon dogs and rabbits of the same size and strength, to some only of which the lime was administered. The phosphate employed was prepared by the calcination of bones, and consequently was combined with carbonate. The results were decidedly favourable; and the author believes that the phosphate may be usefully employed as an adjuvant, expediting the union in ordinary fractures, and tending to prevent the non-consolidation of others.

From another communication,[1] it appears that in one of M. Gosselin's cases of fracture of the lower third of the humerus, complete consolidation occurred in thirty days. He administers as a minimum dose half a gramme per diem.—*Ibid.*, from *Comptes Rendus*, xlii.

OPHTHALMOLOGY.

48. *Difference between Coloration of the Lens, Incidental to Old Age, and Cataract.*—Mr. Haynes Walton, in a paper read before the Harveian Society (June 5th, 1856).

Coloration of the lens, Mr. W. states, is not a disease, not a progressive affection, that destroys sight, but a slight natural change, incidental to age;

[1] Gazette des Hôpitaux, No. 150. 1855.

while cataract is a degeneration, a decay that progresses; and he gives the following interesting microscopical investigations of Mr. R. Taylor in conformation of that view:—

"In elderly people, without an exception, so far as I have observed, the lens assumes an amber colour, more or less deep. The age at which this change commences varies exceedingly. I have seen it distinctly present at 30, and very strongly marked at 35, while, again, it has been but slight in a person of 60. Generally speaking, it will be found at the age of 40; I have never failed to find it at 45. It appears to be more easily developed in the coloured races, and in persons with any admixture of black blood; but my opportunities of observation on this point have been very limited. The colour pervades the whole of the lens, but is most intense in the nucleus, and fades off gradually in the cortical layers. When the 'coloration' is very intense, it impedes the transmission of light, so as to impair the sight, though the lens remains perfectly clear and free from opacity. Such persons are best in a bright light, and are frequently benefited by convex glasses, which concentrate the light. Notwithstanding the depth of colour, I have never heard any complaint of a yellow hue being thrown over objects, as is the case in looking through a piece of yellow glass, nor is there any difficulty in distinguishing different shades, even of blue and green. The colouring matter, which is said to be iron, is in solution. There are not any pigment cells or granules; which last, as it is said, are found in black cataracts. The coloration does not appear to interfere in any way with the healthy condition of the lens; in the oldest which I have examined, from a woman, 93 years of age, the lens tubes, both nuclear and cortical, were perfectly healthy; though they, as well as the superficial cells, were tinged of a bright amber colour. In cataract, on the contrary, the lens is disorganized; the superficial layers are softened and broken up, so as, in advanced cases, to be reduced almost to the condition of a pulp, which renders the drop of water, in which it is examined, turbid and milky. The opacity is due chiefly to a quantity of fine molecular matter, the result of the coagulation of the albuminous blastema of the lens, which is found partly aggregated in masses, and partly studding the exterior, perhaps also the interior of the tubes, as well as, in many instances, filling the large globular cells which lie immediately within the capsule. Occasionally, in cases of long duration, crystals of cholesterine are found interspersed among the lenticular *débris*. The nucleus also undergoes a very remarkable change, becoming hard and dry to an extent very far from anything that is ever seen in the healthy lens of the oldest persons. The tubes are withered, atrophied, and brittle, and fall asunder and in fragments on the slightest touch of the dissecting needle. Their outlines are disfigured by deep, transverse, and longitudinal cracks and fissures, and by irregular nodules, probably of coagulated albumen, and in many instances they show a tendency to split into minute fibrillæ. It is evident, therefore, that on the recognition of these data, and the practical application of them, much error may be avoided, and the absence or existence of cataract rendered more certain, not to speak of the assistance that they offer in unravelling other ophthalmic disease; for lenticular 'coloration' has been described as an objective symptom of other affections, 'amaurosis' being one of these. It would answer no good purpose to tell of any of the many cases of 'coloration' and impaired vision, not due to opacity of the lens, that have been sent to me by surgeons for operation, under the supposition that cataract existed, nor of other mistakes connected with the subject that have come under my notice, such as the extraction of lenses, not cataractous, but merely coloured. I may say that mistakes are frequently made. In the case that I have detailed, it is easy to understand that had there been defective sight in the left eye, from disease at the posterior part of the eyeball, how readily it might have been supposed that cataract was present. It may be received as a rule, that, if a person can see to read the smallest type with or without glasses, and discern distant objects clearly, the pupil being undilated, no matter how clouded the lenses may appear, cataract does not exist. After this is understood, the only point on which there can be difficulty is to pronounce whether, in any given case of defective sight, cataract is present or absent; and the solution of which, so far as it can be told, depends on the proper discrimination of physical appearances, the distinction between 'coloration' and lenticular degeneration, rather than on any subjective symptoms, although these may greatly assist. With undilated pupils it is difficult, if not often impossible, to recognize the difference. I have known surgeons of the first eminence in this metropolis err respecting it; hence the necessity, whenever doubt exists, for dilatation. Then, in the expanded pupil, the presence of striæ or opaque bundles of fibres, which so commonly exist in the early stage of cataract, at the circumference of the lens, can at once be detected. 'Coloration' is more central and browner, the light penetrates the lens, and the concentration of it is perceptible in the direction in which it falls. The opacity of cataract is more diffused and opaque, and reflects the light. In the first, vision is made worse by dilatation of the pupil, while in the other it is almost always improved, certainly always when the opacity is marked. Indeed, when the pupil is dilated, it is seldom that a correct conclusion cannot be arrived at. The exception is this: When the lenticular degeneration is yet slight, and has commenced in the centre, it may be impossible to detect it, that is, to be able to say with certainty that cataract is present, and the lapse of time only can decide. The late Mr. Dalrymple treated a gentleman for amaurosis. He had prescribed an arsenical preparation for some time without benefit. I was then consulted, and, after a long investigation, I decided that cataract was present, at least in one eye. This disease soon became palpable, and in time I operated on both eyes with the best success. There has never appeared the slightest amaurotic symptom. Can I afford a stronger proof that there may be uncertainty in the matter? When vision is much affected by loss of transparency in the lens, the opacity must be palpable; therefore, when this is not readily detected, any material loss of visual power must be attributed to some other cause, and this applies especially to defective vision in the very aged, in whom the 'coloration' is most marked, and when the eye, in obedience to the laws of mortality, which allows an exception, perhaps, only in the prostate gland, is apt to get shrunken, and also becomes, so to speak, vitally impaired. Several times, under these circumstances, I have prevented the performance of a needless operation, and proved that a feeble retina was the defective cause. I have not found the ophthalmoscope of any service in this matter."—*Med. Times and Gaz.*, June 28, 1856.

49. *Statistics of Myopia.*—M. Devot states that of 3,295,202 young men examined in France for military service, during 19 years, from 1831 to 1849, 13,007 were exempted for myopia.—*Gazette Méd. de Paris*, May 17, 1856.

50. *Tincture of Iodine as a Collyrium in Hypopyon.*—M. Rivaud-Laudran recommends (*L'Union Médicale*, April 6) the tincture of iodine, four or five drops to six drachms of water as a collyrium to produce absorption in hypopyon.

MIDWIFERY.

51. *Triplet Birth.*—Dr. Geo. Montgomery detailed to the Dublin Obstetrical Society (April 4, 1856) the following history of a triplet birth, which recently occurred in the Dublin Lying-in Hospital. One of the children was born alive, after having undergone the process commonly called "spontaneous evolution." All did well.

"As cases of *triple births* are of extreme infrequency, occurring in this country only once in about 5,000 deliveries, I have thought that the history of a case which happened recently in our hospital would not be uninteresting; more particularly as it was attended by some unusual circumstances, which I think of considerable practical importance.

"The subject of these observations is Jane Toole, a delicate-looking woman, of about twenty-eight years of age; her husband is a shoemaker, and she resides at 48 Golden Lane, in this city.

"Jane Toole was admitted into the Rotundo Lying-in Hospital on Tuesday, the 1st of April, 1856, at 11 o'clock A.M., in labour, as she said, of her fifth child.

"She stated that, for several months past, her health had been 'wretchedly bad,' and her stomach so irritable that every species of food was rejected; her attenuated frame, and great debility, sufficiently attested the truth of this statement. She complained, also, that her bowels were, in general, obstinately constipated; and stated that she had enjoyed excellent health in all her previous pregnancies. She was not positive as to the exact date of the last catamenia, but says it was either towards the end of July, or the beginning of August, 1855.

"The abdomen appeared very large, and there was œdema of her feet and legs. Labour set in before 9 o'clock on the morning of her admission, when the os was found dilated to the size of half a crown, soft and flaccid, the head presenting, and the membranes unruptured; but the pains were weak and inefficient. At about 3 o'clock in the day, the pains still continuing the same, another examination was made, and it was found that labour had not progressed. She appeared to be very weak, and was ordered some beef-tea. At 4 o'clock the pains were somewhat increased, and the os was then found rather more dilated. Strong pains now occurred, and before twenty minutes had elapsed the membranes were found protruding externally; they were ruptured, and in a quarter of an hour more she gave birth to a healthy boy.

"The hand over the abdomen now detected that it was very little diminished in size, and an examination confirmed our suspicions that there was a second child in utero. In about five minutes the second membranes ruptured, and, the right hand and arm coming down, presented externally, the aspect of the palm being anterior.

"During the minute or two that elapsed whilst I sent down stairs for the Master, who was in the house at the time, the arm and side of the thorax rapidly descended under the frequent and strong contractions of the uterus; so that, by the time that Dr. M'Clintock entered the ward, the *entire* arm was expelled beyond the vulva, and the right and rather posterior part of the thorax was actually pressing on the perineum.

"Turning was out of the question, and it was apparent to all that the child would soon be expelled by the unaided efforts of nature; in fact, the breech was actually beginning to descend into the hollow of the sacrum, and we surmised that '*spontaneous evolution* of the fœtus,' as described by the late Dr. Douglas, would take place, which really did happen, as will be presently seen.

"At this stage of the process we felt curious to know whether the child was still alive; and on placing the end of the stethoscope between the labiæ, against the thorax of the child, a feeble cardiac pulsation was distinguishable.

"To expedite the delivery of the child, a finger was hooked in the flexure of the nearest thigh, when the next pain expelled the breech; the extraction of the *left* arm and head was easily effected, and though the child seemed weakly when born, yet very little exertion was required to establish respiration in a satisfactory manner; this child was also a boy.

"The uterus still remaining above the umbilicus, another internal examination was made, and a third child was detected presenting with the *breech;* the membranes were at once ruptured, and she was soon delivered of a third boy, which was alive and strong.

"The woman was much exhausted after the completion of the labour, and the pulse extremely weak, beating but thirty strokes in the minute; she was, consequently, allowed a few ounces of brandy, in addition to some wine which had been previously given immediately after the birth of the second child.

"The uterus contracted tolerably well, and in about ten or fifteen minutes the placentæ were expelled, accompanied with some hemorrhagic discharge.

"Two of the placentæ were united into one mass, and the other was perfectly distinct; each fœtus was inclosed in a separate bag of membranes.

"With a view to maintaining uterine contraction, so as to prevent the occurrence of any further hemorrhage, the effects of which were much to be dreaded in her then exhausted state; half a drachm of the powdered ergot of rye was administered in some brandy; this, with the steady application of the hand over the uterus, had the desired effect.

"About three-quarters of an hour after delivery there was a return of weakness. She became restless, and vomited a large quantity of fluid; and, in addition to these symptoms, there was a state of slight general spasm, bordering on convulsions, with grinding of the teeth, but without any loss of consciousness. She was ordered a small quantity of burnt brandy, forty drops of the solution of the acetate of morphia, and half a drachm of Hoffmann's anodyne.

"The children were carefully weighed and measured, immediately after birth. The weight of the first born was 5 lbs. 6 oz., that of the second 4 lbs. 10 oz., and of the third 4 lbs. 14 oz., making an aggregate weight of 14 lbs. 14 oz. avoirdupois. The length of the first was 18¼ inches, and that of the second and third 18 inches each; the mother and children are all going on well, at the moment I now speak.

"Perhaps the most interesting point of a practical nature connected with this case, is the mode of delivery of the second child, which, we shall presently show, corresponded in every particular with Dr. Douglas's description of '*spontaneous* evolution of the fœtus.'"

Dr. Montgomery then quoted Dr. Douglas's description of the mechanism of spontaneous evolution, and proved satisfactorily to the Society, that the mode of delivery of the second child, in the case just detailed to the Society, was precisely in accordance with Dr. Douglas's description. He concluded his paper as follows:—

"In all the examples of *spontaneous evolution* recorded by Dr. Douglas, the child was stillborn; and though very many observers, of large experience, have also published cases of the same mode of delivery, yet, after some research, I am not able to find more than two instances where the child was expelled alive, as above described; one recorded by Dr. Read in the *Medical Gazette*, and the other by Dr. Mitchell in Hays's *American Journal of the Medical Sciences.* Hence, then, we may fairly infer that the preservation of the child, under this mode of delivery, is a circumstance of extreme rarity.

"It is a curious coincidence that the first case seen by Dr. Douglas occurred in the same ward of our hospital (No. 3) as the one I have just read. Dr. Douglas says: 'The first time I had an opportunity of witnessing the process of the evolution of the fœtus was in the Lying-in Hospital of this city, in the year 1810, at which time I was resident of that establishment; the case occurred in ward No. 3.'"[1]—*Dublin Quarterly Journal of Medical Science*, August, 1856.

52. *Labour with Ruptured Uterus.*—Dr. W. H. Sandham communicated the following example of this to the County and City of Cork Medical and Surgical Society, May 14, 1856:—

"Mrs. C., aged 40, twice married, stout and healthy, had three children at the full time, stillborn, with each of which she had bad confinements, and was told by her last attendant, the late Dr. Kehoe, that, should she have another, she could not survive it. She took her labour on Sunday evening, April 20, and on Monday, according to the midwife's account, the membranes were ruptured. At 3 o'clock A. M. on the following Wednesday, I was sent for. I found her strong, and her circulation good, but in evident dread of the result, as she almost immediately begged of me, as she knew she could not be delivered in the natural way, to open the side and remove the child. What put this in her

[1] Dr. Montgomery has since informed the secretary that the woman and children, the subjects of this case, did well, and were all discharged in a healthy state. The mother's health improved considerably during her sojourn in the hospital, which was prolonged much beyond the usual term, on account of her previous delicacy. The secretary has also been directed to state that the children were christened by the following names, in the order of their seniority: Francis Alma, Edward Inkerman, and James Sebastopol. It may be gratifying to know that a list was immediately formed, and a sum of money collected for the benefit of the poor woman, and that at the head of the subscribers are our most gracious Queen and her much respected Viceroy.

head I cannot tell, unless the prophetic language of her late attendant. On examination per vaginam, I found the os uteri fully dilated, and the elongated scalp presenting very little below the pelvic circle; the side of the occiput rested firmly on the crest of the pubes. She had pains at regular intervals, but they at once struck me as being of that suppressed character indicating some obstruction. I still more minutely examined, and reached the ear, and at the same time discovered a more than natural projection of the promontory of the sacrum, which I considered as the probable impediment to delivery. The nurse assuring me that the fœtus occupied the same position from the day before, I at once endeavoured to deliver her with the long forceps; with very little difficulty I succeeded in passing in and locking the blades, but no effort of mine could succeed in disturbing the head from its position. The abdomen was exceedingly tense, and hung forwards over the pubes in a remarkable manner. After taking considerable pains to deliver her, I determined, if possible, to suspend the uterine action, and procure her some repose. I administered a full dose of laudanum, and left her at 6½ o'clock, requesting the husband to inform me when she awoke. At 11 o'clock I again saw her; the opiate failed to procure sleep, but the pains were not so distressing. On examination, the head still occupied the same positiou; I again, with ease, introduced the forceps, and, after using considerable force, could not stir it in the least. I then called for another to assist, and at 3 o'clock P. M. my friend, Dr. M'Evers, and I visited her, and, on examination, satisfied himself of the difficulties present. We agreed to wait until 5, and in the mean time endeavoured to procure her rest; an anodyne was accordingly given. When we returned to deliver her at 5, the moment we approached the bedside we saw she was dying; she was retching, and the pallor of death on her face, very restless, and pulse sinking rapidly; we could not, under such circumstances, do anything to relieve her, and in less than an hour she died. As I was anxious to find out the cause of death so sudden, I represented to the husband and mother that it was usual, in such cases, to remove the child, and next morning they called on me and requested I would do so.

"*Autopsy, eighteen hours after death.*—On examination of the abdomen externally, previous to section, I felt one large, hard tumour hanging over the edge of the pubes, and another immediately above the umbilicus, close to the diaphragm, leading me to suppose she had twins. I made an incision a little to the right of the medial line, extending from the edge of the rib to the crest of the pubes. On the edges of the incision being drawn apart, the first thing that presented itself was a vast clot of extravasated blood, concealing all below; this at once revealed the cause of death. On carefully removing this, things were as follows: Superiorly lay the breech and back of the thighs, with the scrotum hanging forwards between them, the legs crossed one over the other; below this was a large detached portion of the placenta; lying transversely, still lower down, was the uterus, the walls very much thickened, contracted, and bloodless, and hanging over the pubes. I first caught the fœtus by the legs, and gradually raised it out of the abdomen; but when the head came to be removed, it required some little force to take it from its position. The child was a very large male child, the head very large, and the scalp elongated, and was marked in the usual way by the forceps, and showed the good position the blades occupied. The head measured round the occiput and chin 18 inches, round the parietals 16½ inches; breadth of shoulders 7½ inches, and 22½ inches in height. I next removed the placenta, but first cut the uterus, which I now found ruptured to a considerable extent, so as to enable me to peel off the attached portion; on now viewing the empty uterus *in situ*, it lay as before described, tilted forwards, but it was torn transversely for about three-fourths of its circumference, at the point where the neck and body united, and appeared to be that part which was pressed between the promontory of the sacrum and parietal protuberance of the child, which circumstances have led me to conclude that this pressure, exercised for so long a time on one particular spot of the uterus, with the efforts of the uterus itself, was the cause of the rupture. In order to remove it from the abdomen, I simply completed, by incision, the laceration already described. I also now satisfied myself of the contracted state of the antero-posterior diameter of the pelvis.

"At 2 o'clock, the hour Dr. M'Evers and I saw her, rupture certainly had not taken place, for at this hour I examined her and felt the uterine contraction, and the woman pulled hard beside; both considered that she had a good and strong circulation. Concluding there must have been some sudden hemorrhage, I inquired of the nurse whether there was any since we last saw her, and being told she had none, and that she made no complaints of any sudden internal feeling, I then considered that death was caused by fright, as she feared very much for her safety when she saw two doctors necessary, and a serious operation about to be performed. The moment we entered and got to the bedside we saw she was dying, so exsanguined was the countenance; the pulse could not be felt, and she died in less than an hour.

"There are two questions in this case I think worthy of discussion, as they are of great consequence, not only to the parties immediately concerned, but to the public at large. In a former paper I advocated the early evacuation of the waters, and the present case, with very many others, have convinced me that we should not trust nature too much, but, at the proper time, without hesitation, bring in the aid of art, and, if possible, relieve the patient of her sufferings, and save the infant's life. First, then, I would ask, what is the proper moment for instrumental interference? Next, in a case such as the one now brought forward, where the death of the parent is inevitable, what should be the practitioner's conduct with reference to the infant, he supposing it still alive? My own opinion is, that he should watch the moment of the parent's demise, and then save the child by the Cæsarean section. In a case I had some time since, of a young woman, who, after carrying a heavy load on the head at her full time, fell down suddenly and expired, I at once proposed saving the child, but the husband had some little delay in searching for and getting the consent of the sister. I opened the side and delivered the child, a fine healthy female, which I am satisfied might have been saved alive were not time lost. And this, and the case now related, have made such an impression on my mind, that I intend strenuously advocating such practice.

"These questions are of such importance, that, could we arrive at a unanimous opinion, the sufferers and the public, no doubt, would be gainers."

On exhibiting the ruptured uterus, the lacerated edges were seen rugged and very thin, compared to the part in the centre cut by the scalpel; the torn edges were the only part where red blood was visible; the part cut to enable Dr. Sandham to detach the placenta, having a cheesy granulated appearance, and very firm from contraction.—*Dublin Quart. Journ. of Med. Sci.*, Aug., 1856.

53. *Metastatic After-pains.*—Dr. Noegerath, of Bonn, relates the following case: A woman, æt. thirty-four, experienced no after-pains on her being delivered of her second child, but in their stead she suffered from violent pain in the lower part of the right thigh, which continued for about five days. The author attended her in her third confinement, which was short and easy, and took place at half-past 10 P. M. The uterus remained large and soft after the expulsion of the placenta, but neither after-pains nor hemorrhage occurred. At seven o'clock next morning, the patient was suddenly seized with violent pain in the lower part of the right thigh, which was most intense from there down to the foot, along the outside of the limb. The uterus was still flaccid and uncontracted. The author immediately administered a large dose—a heaped teaspoonful—of secale cornutum, and in ten minutes thereafter there was a discharge of blood from the vagina; the pain left the foot, and, after a second dose, the pain was so much abated that the patient could turn over on her other side, and could bend the hitherto powerless knee-joint. After the third dose of the ergot, the uterus became fully contracted, and the pains in the bones quite disappeared. From this period, her recovery went on uninterruptedly.

Dr. Noegerath remarks, that in this case there was a true metastasis of the after-pains—the deep-lying parts supplied with nerves from the lumbar portion of the spinal cord having been affected with pain, instead of the uterus. Acting on this conviction, he administered ergot to re-establish the normal contractile pains, and, this having been effected, the local distress disappeared instantly.—*Edinburgh Med. Journ.*, July, 1856, from *Deutsche Klinik.*

54. *Cases of Placenta Prævia.* By Thomas Radford, M. D.—We continue from our last number, page 279, these cases.

Case XXIV.—November 29, 1819. I was desired by Mrs. Blakeley to visit a hospital patient residing in Shudehill, who was flooding. I found her in labour of her sixth child. The pains were strong and forcing; and the hemorrhage, which had existed only slightly for several hours, had now become very profuse. She was pale, and her pulse was frequent and feeble. The os uteri was dilated rather more than the size of a crown-piece: it was soft and dilatable. The placenta (which must have been centrally fixed here) was felt occupying, and, as it were, protruding through the uterine orifice. The head of the child was felt above. The flow of blood was at this time very alarming.

Having had a bandage and compress applied, I passed my hand, and, as quickly as possible, *completely detached* the placenta, and afterwards ruptured the membranes. The bleeding immediately ceased. The pains continued very effective, so that the head rapidly descended, pushing before it the placenta, and in about an hour and a half the child was (still) born. The bandage was tightened, and a drachm of tincture of opium administered. There was no further discharge, and she recovered without the least interruption.

Remarks.—The effectual and immediate suppression of the hemorrhage *after the complete detachment* of the placenta was decidedly demonstrated in this case. Although I had recourse to this plan from (what I have chosen to call) necessity, still the important fact was conspicuously clear to my mind.

Case XXV.—May 20, 1820. I was called by Mrs. Bradley, Sen., to visit a hospital patient residing in Back Bridge Street, who had flooded. I found her very low and faint, from the great loss of blood which had taken place. She was very pallid; her pulse was very frequent and weak. The placenta had been brought away an hour before I arrived. There was now scarcely any discharge; a bandage was placed on, and tightened as required. Some brandy and water was administered. The pains continued to force down the child, and in about an hour it was born dead. A compress was placed on, and the bandage tightened and fixed. There was not more than an ordinary discharge. A drachm and a half of tincture of opium was administered.

Remarks.—The midwife stated that she found a very large portion of the placenta hanging down into the vagina, and therefore, as she thought it would impede the descent of the head of the child, she drew it (the placenta) away. This case is, however, an additional evidence of the cessation of bleeding after the complete detachment of the placenta.

Case XXVI.—March 26, 1821. Mrs. Capper desired me to visit a hospital patient residing in Hulme, who was in labour, and had flooding. She was very low, from the large discharge which had taken place. She was in the ninth month of her third pregnancy. During the seventh and eighth months, slight hemorrhage happened; but at both these periods it was readily arrested by rest and cold external applications. When her labour first commenced, the discharge was very trifling, and continued so for a long time, during which the pains were frequent and feeble; but as they became stronger the discharge increased. The midwife stated that she found the placenta protruding through the os uteri into the vagina; and, as the pains were strong, she unhesitatingly drew away this organ, which she considered was loose; but, on strict inquiry, I found she had used more force than would have been required if it had been completely separated. The hemorrhage had now (three hours after the extraction of the placenta) ceased. The pains had entirely subsided. I found the os uteri dilated, and the head of the child presenting. Some brandy and water was ordered, a drachm and a half of tincture of opium given, and a bandage applied. I decided to immediately deliver her by means of the long forceps, which was easily accomplished. There was no further flooding; and although the woman was considerably reduced, she was quite as well as could possibly be expected. Some brandy in gruel, and a drachm of tincture of opium, were ordered.

On the day following, she was not quite so well; she felt some uneasiness in the belly, but still not amounting to pain; the lochia were less in quantity than usual; and she was restless. A draught with pulv. ipecac. co. gr. xij was prescribed, and an anodyne stimulant liniment and hot poultices were ordered to be applied to the belly. During the night she had a severe shivering, which was succeeded by heat and thirst. Pain in the abdomen, increased on pressure, now came on, and which extended downwards to the left groin; she felt a stiffness in the thigh and leg of that side. Salines, doses of Dover's powder, and suitable aperients, were administered. Leeches, turpentine, hot poultices, and a large blister, were successively applied to the belly. Notwithstanding all these means were carefully carried out, she died. A *post-mortem* examination could not be obtained.

Remarks.—This case affords another example of the arrest of bleeding by the entire separation of the placenta, and also of phlebitis, which is not an unfrequent contingent on cases of placenta prævia. The delivery was readily and safely completed by the long forceps; but the operation was unnecessarily performed, as the flooding had ceased. Saving of time (a most unjustifiable motive), and unwillingness to leave the woman undelivered, induced me to adopt this measure. If such a case happened to me now, galvanism would be the means I should employ.

Cases XXVII., XXVIII., XXIX.—Three other cases, in which the placenta had been forcibly extracted by midwives, have occurred within my observation; they are briefly cited in the *Lancet.* In all of these the hemorrhage ceased.

Case XXX.—The following memoranda were given to me by my esteemed friend and neighbour, Mr. Barton:—

"An athletic woman, the wife of a labourer, residing at Didsbury, having had several children, and falling in labour, was disappointed of the surgeon, and sent for the village midwife.

"I was informed that the labour proceeded naturally, and at 4 o'clock a full-grown child was born dead. A second child presented with the arm. The midwife attempted to deliver this child by forcibly pulling at the presenting arm. About 8 o'clock, four hours after the delivery of the first child, I saw her; the pains were incessant and excruciating; it was at this time impossible to pass the finger beyond the shoulder, and every moment I expected a rupture of the uterus. I bled the woman until she fainted. During this interval, I turned and delivered the child.

"There had been little or no hemorrhage after the delivery of the first child. The second was also dead; and, looking for the funis, it appeared to have been torn from the umbilicus of this child in dragging away the placenta, to which two cords were attached after the birth of the first. The woman recovered without any troublesome symptoms. Both children were full grown."

Remarks.—Although the foregoing statement does not belong to a case of placenta prævia, yet I thought it would be interesting, as the result showed the great conservative normal power against such mischievous practice; more especially in the prevention of hemorrhage after the extraction of the double placenta, immediately after the birth of one twin, whilst the other remained in the uterus. The malpractice of this ignorant woman is one amongst numerous instances, which loudly call for legislative enactment, to secure the poorer part of the community against these horrible murders.

I am indebted to my nephew and colleague, Mr. Henry Winterbottom, for the following four cases. They are cited in his words:—

"Case XXXI.—On the 14th day of March, 1850, I was summoned by Mrs. Mather, midwife, to visit a poor woman residing in a court out of Deansgate, who was stated to be in labour of her first child. Upon my arrival at the house, immediately afterwards, I found her almost *in articulo mortis*, apparently from hemorrhage (as she had the appearance of being thoroughly drained), which I ascertained had been going on for some time; and, upon making an examination, I found the placenta centrally situated over the os uteri, which was considerably dilated and dilatable. In consequence of her extreme state of exhaustion, the uterine action had entirely ceased, and her dissolution seemed rapidly approaching. Not wishing her to die undelivered, which event seemed inevitable unless this operation was instantly performed, and not having time to obtain the necessary apparatus for applying galvanism, which would have been peculiarly applicable in this case, I at once administered the only stimulant which I had at hand—viz: brandy—in order to raise the vital powers a little, if possible, so that she might not die under the operation. I then introduced my hand into the vagina, ruptured the membranes, and turned the child by bringing down one foot; its extraction was speedily accomplished, as well as that of the placenta. The child was, of course, dead. She never rallied, but sank in about two hours afterwards.

"After very mature consideration, I feel convinced it would have been better if I had not acted upon the received dogma, 'not to allow a woman to die undelivered;' for, although the exhaustion from the flooding was very great, I have no doubt that this unfavourable condition was increased by the operation. The plan I should adopt, if a precisely similar case again occurred, would be, in the first place, to send a messenger for the galvanic apparatus, as by so doing I should not be prevented from adopting other required measures in the mean time. After having duly and effectually applied a bandage, and placed a compress under it, I should completely detach the placenta, and endeavour, by every means in my power, to raise and support the vital powers; and, as soon as the galvanic apparatus arrived, I should have currents carried through the different axes of the uterus, with the object of exciting that organ, as well as acting as a general stimulant.

"CASE XXXII.—During the night of the 11th of December, 1851, I was requested to visit a lady, a private patient, who was stated to be at the end of pregnancy, and flooding. Upon my arrival, I found very profuse hemorrhage; she had no pains; the os uteri was closed. I therefore effectually plugged the vagina; I also ordered perfect rest in the horizontal position, with an acid mixture, the free admission of air, and cool drinks. On the following morning I was again desired to see her, and found that uterine pains had set in (probably excited by the sponges used as plugs, which I had introduced, and forcibly placed against the os uteri). I at once removed them, and found the os uteri partially dilated, and the placenta centrally situated over it. Feeling a degree of anxiety about the case, I sent for my friend and partner, Mr. Clayton, who kindly gave his immediate attendance; and, as the case was very urgent, we agreed at once to detach the placenta entirely. I proceeded to do this, and the hemorrhage, which had up to this time been very considerable, immediately ceased. We afterwards administered a couple of doses of secale cornutum at intervals of about a quarter of an hour; and as she seemed faintish from her loss, we gave a little brandy and water. After waiting for a recurrence of the pains (which had entirely ceased) for about two hours, and as she seemed much rallied, we deemed it better to deliver her without further delay. I therefore passed my hand, and withdrew the placenta, and afterwards carried it into the uterus, and brought down one foot. The extraction was soon accomplished, and she recovered without a bad symptom. The child was dead.

"In reviewing this case (although the woman's life was spared), I must acknowledge that I should not again have recourse immediately to artificial delivery, but should rather wait and endeavour to rouse the energies of the uterus by the application of galvanism, etc. The secale cornutum failed to produce any effect. After the complete detachment of the placenta, the flooding immediately ceased, and therefore there could be no necessity for turning and extracting the child.

"CASE XXXIII.—In the early part of September, 1853, I was requested to visit a female residing in Salford, who had previously bespoken my services to attend her in confinement. Upon my arrival at the house, I found her suffering from uterine hemorrhage, which she stated had occurred at intervals for several days. As she did not appear to be much affected from her loss, I merely enjoined perfect rest in bed, and ordered her to take an acid mixture and cool beverages, and to avoid everything stimulating. On the following morning, upon my calling to see her, I found her complaining of slight pains, which she stated she had felt several hours. The discharge continued, and was increased on the recurrence of each pain. Upon making an examination, I found the os uteri about half dilated, soft and dilatable, and the placenta situated over it. As the hemorrhage was profuse, I considered further delay would place my patient in a worse position. I therefore concluded to completely detach the placenta; and, in doing so, I ruptured the membranes. The hemorrhage entirely ceased, and did not again recur. I then administered about half a drachm of the secale cornutum, and a little cold brandy and water. The pains continuing with increased severity, the placenta was first expelled, and the child's head immediately descended; and in about an hour from the time of the detachment it (the child) was stillborn. She continued to do very well for several days; but afterwards she had an attack of phlebitis in the leg and thigh, which considerably retarded her convalescence.

"This appears another example of the complete suppression of hemorrhage by the entire detachment of the placenta. Fortunately, the vital powers were not so entirely lowered in this case as in the one before cited, and therefore I considered it warrantable to give the secale cornutum, which had the effect of rousing the uterus to more active contraction, by which first the placenta, and afterwards the child, were expelled.

"Case XXXIV.—On the 23d of January, in the present year, I was requested to visit Mrs. M., who had engaged my services to attend her in confinement, and whom I had twice previously attended. I found her suffering from uterine hemorrhage, which she stated had first made its appearance that morning, and which she attributed to having walked a long distance the day before. I was told she had lost a considerable quantity of blood, but it had much abated on my arrival. As there was no symptom of labour present, I ordered her an acid mixture, with cool drinks and perfect rest in bed, as well as the application of a good firm binder. I continued to see her at intervals, until the 9th of February. During the whole of that time the hemorrhage occurred to a greater or less extent. On the evening of the latter day I was again sent for, when I found that labour had commenced. The os uteri was very much dilated, and the placenta was partially placed over it. The child's head presented. As the hemorrhage still continued, I at once ruptured the membranes, and gave a full dose of ergot, after which the pains became more frequent and stronger. The hemorrhage was now completely arrested. In a very short time the head of the child descended, and passed by (pushing aside) the placenta; and in about an hour the child was expelled by the natural efforts. The infant, a female, was apparently stillborn; but after a very long continued use of artificial respiration, strong mustard baths, and a large mustard plaster over the whole of the chest, slight symptoms of animation showed themselves, at first only by a few gasps, but afterwards perfect respiration was established. My patient continued to do well for a few days, but afterwards she had an attack of phlegmasia dolens, under which she is now suffering.

"After rupturing the membranes, the hemorrhage entirely ceased; and it was very fortunate that the uterus acted so immediately and powerfully after the administration of the ergot; for if the birth had been longer delayed, most likely the child would have been lost.

"We have here another example of phlebitis contingent on placenta prævia."

55. *Cases Illustrating Different Methods of Treating Placenta Prævia.* By Henry Oldham, Obstetric Physican and Lecturer on Midwifery, &c., at Guy's Hospital.—The following cases are selected from those which have occurred to me in practice, to illustrate the principal methods of managing placenta prævia, under different circumstances:—

Case 1.—*Placenta Prævia; Labour terminated by natural efforts, the Placenta being detached, and passing down with the head into the Vagina; Recovery.*—In August, 1847, I saw a poor woman, residing in Spitalfields, and engaged in the market, who was suddenly seized with hemorrhage between the seventh and eighth month of her fifth pregnancy, which subsided spontaneously. In eleven days after it had ceased, it again came on profusely, and was followed by a coloured discharge; notwithstanding which, she had gone out as usual. Labour came on about a fortnight short of term, with a large loss of blood; and the assistant of a neighbouring medical man saw her, but left her after ordering some medicine, without examining her. The bleeding returned; and, in alarm, I was asked to see her. She had evidently lost a large quantity of blood, and was in a very feeble state; but there had been some faint labour pains. On examination, I found the head low down in the vagina, with the placenta pressed between it and the back wall of the vagina, the edge, however, coming far forward over the head, but not directly below it. While examining, an expulsive pain was excited; and the head rapidly descended, and was expelled before the placenta, which followed with the body of the child. It had been completely separated, and during the short time I was present, and for some time before, hemorrhage had ceased. The child (a male) was stillborn. The poor woman, though seriously exhausted, recovered.

Case 2.—*Partial Placenta Presentation; Rupture of Membranes; Recovery.*—I was summoned to Mrs. P., residing a few miles from town, who was seized with hemorrhage suddenly within a fortnight of term with her fifth pregnancy, in December, 1852. She was a stout, florid person, of good general health, and her former labours had been favourable. She lost a large quantity of blood very rapidly at 5 P. M., and had become faint; on recovering from which, she had vomited a good deal, and some clots were occasionally discharged. Stimulants had been given, but generally were rejected, and some ice had been applied to the lower abdomen and vulva. I found this lady pale, with a feeble pulse and cold surface, and very apprehensive of dying. The vagina was filled with clots, on displacing which the os was found open and flaccid enough readily to admit the finger, and the placenta was felt passing from the anterior lip to the posterior, and there, by a stretch of the finger, the edge could be felt and the membranes beyond. Attempts were made to rupture the membranes by the finger; but they gave too much, and this was accomplished with the stilette of a catheter, after which a free flow of liq. amnii took place. An enema of the decoction of secale (℥ij to the ounce), with a tablespoonful of brandy, was administered per rectum, cooled down by a few lumps of ice; a bandage placed round the abdomen; a blanket interposed between the body and the wet clothes; warm clothing over the body; and she was encouraged with the assurance of doing well. Hemorrhage entirely ceased; labour pains soon came on, and she was confined of a dead child in three hours after the membranes had been ruptured, and recovered favourably. The portion of placenta which had presented was marked by a darker hue, and was broken; and at its edge, when floated out in water, were the thin broken edges of some large utero-placental veins.

Case 3.—*Partial Placenta Prævia; Rupture of Membranes; Version.*—June 16, 1846.—I met the late Mr. Quekett, of Wellclose-square, in the case of a female who had had seven children and two abortions, and was expecting labour in a fortnight. When advanced six months and a half, after lifting a weight, hemorrhage came on, which ceased spontaneously, and recurred five weeks after. Again it came on suddenly and in considerable quantity, accompanied with some slight pain, which was suspended from the faintness which ensued. The os was found dilatable, but not open beyond the circle of a shilling; and on removing a clot the placenta was felt over the os; but its edge could be detected, and the membranes beyond. I ruptured the latter with the finger, and the liq. amnii escaped freely. The fœtal heart was heard to beat. In three hours I saw her again, and found that pains had been scarcely perceptible and some coagula had escaped, and that blood was then dribbling away more than I quite liked. The hand was introduced, the os steadily opened without difficulty, a knee brought down, and version performed. She recovered well. Child alive.

Case 4.—*Complete Placenta Prævia; Version; Child alive.*—I was engaged to attend a lady in her fourth confinement, whose former labours had been favourable, in July, 1851. Three weeks before term she was alarmed, in attempting to pass water, at finding a large quantity of blood flow away from the uterus, without pain. Under the influence of rest in the recumbent posture, acid drinks, &c., it passed off, and did not recur until a week before her expected time, when a copious gush of hemorrhage took place, soon after which I saw her. On examination, I found the os but slightly open, but its structure soft and yielding, and covered over with placenta. Without difficulty the hand was passed into the vagina; the os yielded to steady pressure; the placenta was separated by the advancing hand, the membranes ruptured, and a foot seized and brought down, and a living male child extracted with facility. The placenta was completely over the lower segment of the uterus. This lady has had two natural labours since.

Case 5.—*Placenta Prævia; Difficult Version; Craniotomy.*—In the summer of 1855 I was requested to see a lady at Clapham with Dr. Young. Her second labour, at term, had been ushered in with hemorrhage, which was ascertained to depend on the placenta being over the os uteri. The amount of bleeding had not been great. I found the placenta completely over the os uteri, which was already opened to the size of half a crown, and yielding. I introduced my left hand, and seized a foot, which was brought down, and a tape fixed over it. Traction was made at first steadily; the power of it increasing with an unusual resistance. The body of the uterus, however, so firmly grasped the fœtus, that no power I could exercise, aided even with efforts to raise the head, would make it revolve on its axis. Fearing rupture, which appeared to me imminent, I was obliged to perforate the child's head, after which version was completed. This lady recovered, and, Dr. Young writes me, is now three months advanced in another pregnancy. Out of numerous instances, and a large variety of cases, in which it has fallen to my lot to perform the operation of turning, I have never encountered so much difficulty when once the foot had been seized as in this instance.

Case 6.—*Partial Placenta Prævia; Rupture of Membranes; Arm Presentation; Version; Laceration of Cervix; Death.*—A poor woman, residing in the Borough, began to bleed at the onset of labour, when the medical man who saw her, feeling an edge of the placenta within the disk of the os, ruptured the membranes. After this the arm descended, and I was summoned to attend her. The os uteri was by this time moderately dilated, and dilatable, and the patient in good condition. Version was performed by the gentleman without any undue effort, and a dead child delivered. The placenta was readily removed, and the uterus contracted well. I was struck, however, with a considerable and continuous flow of blood afterwards, of a florid hue, and that, too, in spite of a well sustained contraction of the body of the uterus. Laceration of the cervix was anticipated, and a sponge was applied to this part, a bandage to the abdomen, and brandy and arrowroot administered. After three hours' watching the bleeding desisted. An opiate, with saline medicine, was given, and the strictest rest enjoined. I did not see this patient again, but I learned that, in spite of all attempts to control the bleeding, it again and again recurred, and she sank exhausted fifty hours after delivery.

The expectation of the cervix having been torn in the act of version, was verified after death, there being an open rent, to the extent of an inch, on one side of the cervix. The gentleman who performed the operation was a powerful man, with a large hand and arm.

Case 7.—Another instance of laceration of the cervix, with fatal hemorrhage, has occurred in my experience, where delivery was forced by the accoucheur, in consequence of a sudden bleeding in a complete placenta prævia. The lady, the mother of several children, had lost a great deal of blood by repeated bleedings in the last month of pregnancy, in one of which I saw her. She had been warned to keep strictly at rest, and the usual precautionary treatment against hemorrhage had been prescribed. Feeling herself revived, she determined to stand up to dress her hair, and, in the act of doing so, had a return of hemorrhage. The nearest medical man was sent for, who proceeded at once to turn the child, which he accomplished, after overcoming, with considerable difficulty, the resistance of the os uteri. The uterus contracted well after delivery, but bleeding continued, and she died in two hours. The cervix was found to be torn in two places; one but slightly, but the other formed an oblique rent, nearly an inch in extent.

Case 8.—*Placenta Prævia; Plug; Natural Delivery; Metrophlebitis; Death.*—A poor, feeble woman, about 40 years of age, a patient of the Lying-in Charity of Guy's Hospital, had lost blood for three weeks at intervals, without applying for assistance, when a more copious hemorrhage, with some amount of pain, induced her to send. When I saw her she was seriously exhausted, and the placenta was found completely covering the os, which, notwithstanding the loss, was still rigid. The vagina was filled with sponge, and a large pad of cotton wool was pressed against the perineum externally, so as to bear freely on the sponge within the vagina, and with a T bandage formed an effectual plug. Brandy and beef-tea were provided, and freely given. This was at 2 P. M. At 9 P. M. I was informed that, in about an hour after leaving her, when she had rallied from her exhaustion, pains came on, and increased in severity. The student in attendance removed the plug, and at 6 P. M. she was delivered naturally, a part of the placenta being pressed out into the upper and back part of the vagina, and the head passing out before it. There was but little bleeding during this process, but she remained very feeble and exsanguine. The child did not exceed seven months, and was dead. On the third day after delivery she had a rigor, followed by signs of metrophlebitis, of which she died.

In this instance the plug appeared to have been of great service—not only controlling the bleeding, but stimulating the uterus to labour-action. In other cases, it has not in my experience proved so serviceable.

Case 9.—*Placenta Prævia; Rigid Os Uteri; attempt to separate Placenta; Version without the introduction of the hand.*—On Good Friday, 1852, I saw Mrs. ——, with Dr. S. Ward. She was in bad health from cardiac disease, and was nearly advanced to the seventh month of her fifth pregnancy, when she was suddenly seized with bleeding, and lost a large quantity of blood in a short time. When Dr. Ward visited her, he discovered the placenta completely over the os uteri, which was slightly open. He introduced a plug, and gave her support. When I saw her she had rallied from the loss of blood; but was pale, with a feeble pulse. Slight labour pains had set in, and the os was opening; but its structure was rigid and undilatable. Fearing a recurrence of the hemorrhage I tried to separate the placenta from the uterus; but only partially succeeded, as it appeared to be unusually diffused and adherent. During this time bleeding was going on; and, finding that the hand could not be passed through the os uteri, I ruptured the membranes, and with two fingers stretched within the cavity of the uterus, and hand pressure from above, I had the good fortune to catch a knee, which I brought down and secured. With traction by this limb the os uteri was dilated, and she was slowly delivered of a dead male fœtus. I was obliged afterwards to introduce the hand to remove one portion of the placenta, which was very firmly adherent. The patient recovered.

Case 10.—*Placenta Prævia; complete Artificial Detachment of Placenta; Arrest of Hemorrhage; Natural Labor; Recovery.*—At 4.45 A. M., on March 9, 1850, I was requested by Mr. Blenkarne, of Dowgate-hill, to see Mrs. W., who had been seized at midnight with violent bleeding after an attack of coughing. She was 43 years of age; of feeble constitution and delicate health; in whom the effects of hemorrhage were likely to be very perilous. On examination, Mr. Blenkarne found a placenta prævia. At the time of seeing her she was in a weak, low state, with a rapid pulse, and complained of some feeble labour pains. I found the os sufficiently patent to allow the introduction of two fingers, and the placenta was implanted completely over the disk. I fully expected that the os would yield to the dilating pressure of the hand in an attempt to turn; but in this I was disappointed, for when put on the stretch, its firm, dense tissue would not yield to such force as could prudently be used. By stretching the fingers freely into the uterus I was enabled to separate a portion of the placenta and reach its edge, and after a great deal of trouble to rupture the membranes. I then detached a larger portion of the placenta, and tried to gain the extreme edge by lifting off the placenta from it. During this time some bleeding was going on; but I had reason to hope that the placenta was completely detached. A sponge was placed in the vagina, and she was left lying on her side.

At 9.30 she appeared to be more comfortable. No hemorrhage had trickled through the plug. No pain.

At 2 P. M. I found her in active labour, the os being fully dilated, and the head descending; both the placenta and the sponge being pressed between it and the posterior wall of the vagina, with a coil of funis down. I removed the sponge and a large portion of the placenta during the pause between the pains, and shortly the head was expelled. I do not think an ounce of blood had been lost between the separation of the placenta and the birth of the child. The child was stillborn. The mother recovered.

The two following cases are related to show the difficulty which would arise in some cases to this operation, from the placenta being widely diffused and adherent.

Case 11.—On the 27th June, 1847, I was sent for by Mr. Linnecar to see a poor woman in the neighbourhood of Charterhouse-square, who had reached the full period of pregnancy when she was seized with severe hemorrhage (a gallon was said to have passed). This was on the 25th. Mr. Linnecar found her on the 26th much exhausted, and detected the placenta completely over the os uteri, which was but slightly open; and there was no evidence of labour. Ergot was given, and the vagina plugged. At 5.30 on the 27th I first saw her, and learned that blood had been draining through the plug, and that in this way a great deal had been lost. Brandy and opium had been given. She was in a very feeble state, but had revived under the influence of the stimulants which had just been administered. On removing the plug, and some clots with it, I found the os open to about the size of a half crown, but soft and yielding; and I at once passed the hand gradually through it, raising the placenta with unusual difficulty from the anterior lip of the uterus; and perforating the membranes, I brought down a foot, and delivered her of a dead child. During this time she was freely supplied with brandy, but there was no uterine action until the breech was distending the vulva. In attempting to remove the placenta the cord gave way; and, on introducing my hand, I found it universally adherent; and it took some time to separate, as it was diffused over a very large space. The uterus contracted well, but the patient was much exhausted; aggravated by the tedious operation of detaching the adherent placenta. Thirty drops of laudanum were given, and as much nourishment in the shape of beef-tea, brandy, and arrowroot as could be taken. Warmth to the feet and over the body, and perfect rest, were enjoined. She was, however, in so exhausted a state that we despaired of her recovery; and I was informed that she died. The placenta was thin, and extended over a larger surface than I ever witnessed. There was but little liq. amnii; and it appeared as though, during the process of growth, there had been a force directed on it to press it out. The attached decidual surface was thick and opaque; and a portion somewhat larger than the hand was broken and of a purple colour, indicating the presenting portion which had to be separated in the attempt to turn. It appears to me very probable that adhesion and diffusion of the placenta in a case of placenta prævia may be produced by such a preponderance of the solid contents of the ovum over the fluid, as to prevent the mobility of the fœtus; and thereby keep a certain pressure over the lower segment of the uterus during the latter months of gestation.

Case 12.—On September 29th, 1855, I saw Mrs. F., with Mr. Tuckey, of Bermondsey. She was far advanced in her seventh confinement, when she was seized, on the morning of the 29th, with copious flooding, followed by syncope, for which Mr. Tuckey was summoned to her. She had previously bled a fortnight before, and a placenta prævia was anticipated, which Mr. Tuckey detected. When I saw her she had quite recovered from the immediate loss, which had not seriously exhausted her. I found the os uteri covered over by placenta, but yielding enough to allow of turning, which was at once accomplished, and a live male child extracted. On removing the placenta it proved to be bilobed, and very largely extended, so as almost to complete a zone. Between the two lobes the separated veins were quite distinct, with their thin coats and large orifices. In both these cases it would have been physically impossible to have detached the placenta without the introduction of the entire hand. No sweeping of the fingers within the os, or any other mode of digital manipulation, could have accomplished its complete separation.

The observations which flow from these and other cases which have occurred to me may be thus summarily expressed:—

1. There are two kinds of bleeding in placenta prævia: the bleedings before labour, and the bleedings at the onset of labour and during the first stage—the

former occurring at intervals between the sixth and ninth months, and sometimes not at all; the latter unavoidable.

2. The cause of the bleedings during pregnancy arises, not from what is called the development of the cervix—if by that term is meant the expansion of its cavity into the cavity of the body of the uterus—but from the general softening of its tissue, making it more yielding, and from the walls of its cavity being more widely separated by the accumulation of mucus within; and then, again, by the augmented volume of the utero-placental circulation. It is this latter—but feebly supported at the os uteri—which is liable, under any disturbing cause, to break through the decidua and lining membrane of the placental cell-texture, and so occasion a maternal placental bleeding. It is checked for a time by the coagulation of blood in the cell-texture, favoured by its temporary collapse, again to break forth, if not carefully guarded against by rest, diet, and general precautions.

3. The bleeding during labour is the result of the same form of laceration, combined with separation of the placenta from the uterus, and the consequent regurgitating hemorrhage from the uterine veins, and slightly from the torn arteries; the flooding from these sources being so copious and so exhausting, as rarely to allow the patient to survive delivery by the natural efforts. Occasionally, however, it does so, as in Case 1.

4. The opening of the os uteri in placenta prævia is generally retarded, first, by the exhaustion from the profuse bleeding which accompanies the very first pains, and for the time weakens, and often suspends labour; and, secondly, because the labour force has to overcome the additional resistance which the implantation of the placenta over the os uteri occasions; and hence, this part is commonly found to be correspondingly more dilatable than dilated.

5. In cases of partial placenta prævia, great confidence may be placed in rupturing the membranes and draining the ovum, with such stimulants to uterine action as are afforded by liberal support with stimulants, an abdominal bandage, and it may be ergot of rye, either by enema or by the stomach; but should a draining of blood go on, version should be performed.

6. In a larger or central placenta prævia, there is one method of treatment which excels all others for prompt and efficient relief, and to which all others ought to be subordinate, as rare and peculiar deviations from a general rule; and that is, to make a way to the membranes by introducing the hand within the uterus, separating the intermediate portion of placenta, and, at the same time, dilating the os uteri, bursting the membranes, seizing one foot, and turning by it. In selecting the time when version may be performed, the great thing to distinguish is the yielding or dilatable character of the os uteri; and, if this be present, the size of the disk itself, whether it be that of a shilling or a crown piece, is comparatively of little moment. It is too often a fatal delay, and a serious error in practice, to make the rule for the time of version depend on the extent of dilatation which the os has acquired.

7. In forced delivery, it requires great care that the dilating force be steadily applied, and evenly distributed, by the intelligent adaptation of the hand, so as to diminish the shock of forced delivery, and to guard the cervix from laceration, which may prove fatal from hemorrhage. The operation of version, when a foot is grasped, is generally easy; but in one case it was attended with remarkable difficulty.

8. Version is sometimes prohibited, from the immediate exhaustion of hemorrhage, or from rigidity of the os uteri, in spite of hemorrhage. In the former case, a good vaginal plug, aided in its action by a large perineal pad, and the free exhibition of stimulants, is a good temporary, but not always a permanent, resource—version being sometimes required when reaction has succeeded. In the latter case, there is the valuable alternative of separating the entire placenta, so as to destroy the utero-placental circulation, rupturing the membranes, and exciting uterine action. This operation is difficult to perform completely, and sometimes impossible, from the wide diffusion of the placenta, or from morbid adhesion, or from both these conditions combined.

9. Occasionally, when the ovum is small, and the os uteri rigid, a knee or foot may be seized, without the introduction of the entire hand into the uterus,

and the os be dilated by the pressure of the body and head of the child in the act of extraction, as practised by Dr. Robert Lee.—*Med. Times and Gaz.*, July 12, 1856.

56. *Dropsy of Pregnancy.* By M. Becquerel.—Four forms of dropsy are observed in pregnant women, which are far from being of the same importance.

1. *Mechanical Dropsies*, perhaps the most common, are due to the pressure exerted by the gravid uterus, their production being favoured by the lesser density of the blood in pregnant women, and the slight diminution of albumen that exists in its serum. These dropsies are confined to the lower extremities, are of no importance beyond their inconvenience, and disappear after delivery.

2. *Dropsies due to Changes in the Blood, but unaccompanied by Albuminuria.*—The change in the blood which induces these dropsies consists in a diminution in the amount of the albumen of the serum, a diminution that is sometimes considerable, and for which we can assign no other cause than the fact of the pregnancy and its influence on the various immediate principles of the blood. This description of dropsy, like the two next, tends to become general. It is of importance to distinguish it from the two others, and especially the 4th, for it does not predispose to eclampsia. It is by analysis of the blood alone that we can establish its existence. It disappears also after pregnancy, but far more slowly. It has been observed that women suffering from it remain feeble for a long period, their "getting up" being slow and difficult.

3. *Dropsies with Changes in the Blood and Albuminuria, but without Bright's Disease, properly so called.*—These dropsies are the consequence of the diminution of the albumen of the blood, produced by its deperdition through the kidney. Until lately, it was supposed that such loss might take place without material lesion of the kidney; but from the investigations made by M. Robin and the author, it results that this albuminuria is due to a special modification taking place in the epithelial cells of the tubuli, a modification consisting in the infiltration of the cells and tubuli by numerous granules of a proteric nature. This infiltration is analogous to that which M. Robin had already found in choleraic albuminuria, and like it is susceptible of cure. The absolute diagnosis during life of this disease from Bright's affection is very difficult, and yet it is highly important, as the prognosis must be entirely based upon it. It is in women who are the subjects of these dropsies that we have to fear eclampsia, and the predisposition to puerperal peritonitis. Eclampsia is not, however, a necessary consequence; and when we find general dropsy, change in the blood, and albuminuria coexisting, we still cannot affirm that this terrible accident will follow. On the other hand, whenever we find eclampsia we are certain of finding, not always dropsy, but albuminous urine, and change in the blood. In respect to the termination of this form of dropsy, it may be observed that, if eclampsia does not supervene, a cure is almost certain; while, in the case of its occurring, the result is dependent upon that of the eclampsia.

4. *Dropsies due to Bright's Disease.*—It is very important to establish the diagnosis of this form. We may lay stress upon the somewhat larger quantity of albumen, the presence of fragments of the tubuli, of fibrinous filaments, and fatty globules. When eclampsia complicates this form it is invariably fatal; and even when eclampsia does not occur, the disease is not arrested after delivery. The dropsy continues to increase, the termination proving, after a certain period, fatal.—*Med. Times and Gaz.*, July 5, 1856, from *Rev. Medico-Chirurg.*, tome xviii.

57. *Contagiousness of Puerperal Fever.*—Dr. Credé in a report on puerperal fever (*Verhandl. der Ges. für Geb.*, 1855), confirms the conclusions arrived at in Vienna, as to the contagiousness of that disease. He relates that for nearly two years puerperal fever had raged with but little intermission in the Charité Hospital in Berlin. He refers to a statistical account by Dr. Quincke, to show that of about 650 women delivered there in the last year, 139 had been removed for illness to the inner station; all of these, with the exception of 15, were affected by puerperal fever, and 68 died. All the apartments used for the labour patients were twice changed, and once every utensil and all the attend-

ants were changed. All had little or no influence. In the new rooms, as in the old, puerperal fever continued. Upon this the physicians of the outer station made the observation that the contagion of hospital-gangrene and of pyæmia, which also had not ceased within that time, was in close relationship with the puerperal fever contagion. It was therefore weighed by the committee whether it would not be desirable to remove the lying-in institution altogether from the Charité. Dr. Credé added, that it appeared manifest that wherever hospitals were connected with lying-in wards, puerperal fever contagion assumed far greater development and intensity, as in Vienna, Prague, Stuttgard.—*Brit. and For. Med.-Chirurg. Rev.*, April, 1856.

58. *Case of Injurious Effect of Prolapsus Uteri upon the Urinary Organs.* By Prof. Retzius, of Stockholm.—On a previous occasion, a case was communicated by Prof. Düben, where, in an individual suffering from prolapsus uteri, one of the kidneys was found atrophied, with dilatation of its pelvis and ureter, in consequence of pressure by the tumefied lower portion of the uterus. Shortly afterwards, Prof. Retzius had an opportunity, in the anatomical rooms, of examining a subject affected with an extensive prolapsus. He found here both kidneys atrophied, forming, as it were, thin caps over the greatly dilated pelvis; the calyces and the papillæ renales being obliterated. The ureters were also dilated, and lengthened to more than twice the normal dimension. They lay flattened, of the breadth of half an inch, and presented many windings. The urinary bladder was also remarkably large, and its lower part considerably thickened. The place where the ureters enter into the posterior wall of the bladder was pushed down into the lower opening of the pelvis. The under portion of the bladder was thrust forward, between the arch of the pubis and the prolapsed and swollen uterus. The urethra, which in its natural condition has a straight direction between the vagina and the arch of the pubis, through the fascia profunda of the pelvis, was here compressed towards the arch, by the prolapsus, and had a greatly bent course upwards, around and beneath the arch, almost in the form of a loop. The canal was at the same time widened and lengthened; and from its orifice depended a flat, lancet-shaped flap, a prolongation of the mucous membrane.

It is obvious that the prolapsus had proved here a source of pressure, as well posteriorly on the corpus trigonum, into which the ureters open, as towards the arch of the pubis, and upon the prolonged and thickened neck of the bladder itself. Hence ensued an obstruction of the flow of the urine, which had evidently, as the case of Professor Düben had already demonstrated, led to the atrophy of the kidneys, and to the lengthening and distension of the urinary passages; which again, in their turn, must have conduced to a deleterious influence upon the condition of the blood, and upon the whole organism.—*Edinburgh Med. Journ.*, July, 1856, from *Anat. iakttagelser.*

59. *Polypiform Prolongation of the Os Uteri.* By Dr. Szukits.—The subject of this paper is a remarkable case, considered indeed by the author, when taken in all its bearings, as unique. It is an example of polypiform prolongation of the anterior lip of the os uteri becoming developed towards the end of pregnancy, and disappearing spontaneously some time after delivery. Such prolongations are usually congenital, or come on at, or soon after, puberty, and they are rarely confined to one lip. It is not very rare to meet with hypertrophy of the vaginal portion of the uterus, as a consequence of injury done to the cervix in labour, the anterior lip usually being the part that suffers most, and sometimes the only part affected. Still more frequent are cases in which we meet with prolongation during the first days of the puerperal state, induced by inflammatory or œdematous swelling. This is easily distinguished by the œdema of the surrounding parts; but even after the involution of the uterus has become completed, the part does not diminish to its former volume. The few cases of polypiform prolongation of one or both lips, that have hitherto been recorded, have required amputation.

This case occurred in the person of a primipara aged 29, who had menstruated regularly since she was 19. During the latter months of her pregnancy, she had observed something pressing from the genitals, but coition was not impeded; and three weeks prior to delivery (which took place at the eighth month), she perceived a tumour projecting from the vagina, which was declared to be a prolapsus uteri. Examined the day after her confinement, a dark-red, smooth, almond-shaped tumour, was found projecting about half an inch beyond the external parts, and consisting in a prolongation of the anterior lip of the os uteri, the posterior one being of its normal size. The swelling was painless, and the vagina was in a normal condition. The consistence of the tumour was hard and knotty, resembling swollen glands. The condition of the patient, suffering from high fever with delirium, forbade amputation of the part; and during a severe endometritis that ensued all that was done as regards the tumour was to observe the strictest cleanliness. Nevertheless it gradually diminished in size, so that by June 19 (she having been admitted May 15), the two lips of the os were equal, no trace of hypertrophy remaining.

Such prolongations of chronic origin, and only removable by surgical operation, are not so rare. The author gives a brief account of two cases, and refers to *Virchow's Archiv.* for two more.—*Med. Times and Gaz.*, Jan. 26, 1856, from *Wein Wochensch*, 1855, No. xxxiii.

60. *On Carbonic Acid as a Local Anæsthetic in Uterine Diseases, &c.*—Prof. SIMPSON made some remarks on this, at a recent meeting of the Obstetrical Society of Edinburgh. He said that he had used carbonic acid successfully, as a local anæsthetic, in neuralgia of the vagina and uterus, and in various morbid states and displacements of the pelvic organs accompanied with pain and spasms. He had found it also sometimes of use in irritable states of the neighbouring organs. Two years ago, he had under his care, from Canada, the wife of a medical gentleman, who was suffering much from that most distressing disease—dysuria and irritability of the bladder. Many modes of treatment had been tried in vain. The injection of carbonic acid gas into the vaginal canal several times a-day, at once produced relief, and ultimately effected a perfect cure. She has remained well since her return to America, and lately became a mother. Occasionally, relief follows immediately. In two or three instances, he stated he had seen the use of the gas continued daily for months, and that he had notes of one case where the patient was invalided, and almost entirely kept to the supine posture, for years, from feelings of pain and bearing down in the uterus and neighbouring parts, particularly on attempting to sit or walk. Many modes of treatment were tried by himself and others, with little or no benefit. She has, however, at last regained in a great measure the power of progression, and freedom from suffering in the erect posture—a result which she herself ascribes to the local application of carbonic acid gas.

In practice, he generally used a common wine bottle for the formation of the carbonic acid gas, and formed the gas by mixing in the bottle six drachms of crystallized tartaric acid with a solution of eight drachms of bicarbonate of soda, in six or seven ounces of water. A long, flexible caoutchouc tube conducts the gas from the bottle into the vagina. The cork fixing this tube into the mouth of the bottle should be adapted so as to prevent any escape of the gas by its sides. With this view, the cork should be perforated by a metallic tube, and covered externally with a layer of caoutchouc. In a case in which the two preceding children were both lost, he had successfully brought on premature labour at the eighth month, by the repeated application of carbonic acid gas to the vaginal canal with this apparatus—the carbonic acid not acting directly as a specific oxytocic or excitor of uterine contraction, but indirectly only by distending greatly and mechanically (as examination with the finger proved it to do) the vaginal canal, and ultimately separating, like the injection of water, the membranes from the cervix uteri.

The application of carbonic acid as a local anæsthetic to the uterine mucous surfaces, and to other parts of the body, is not a discovery of late times. He had found that in this, as in many other examples, that what appeared at first novel, was, when fully investigated, a practice known previously in its essence, and perhaps in its more minute details also. Besides, here as elsewhere, when once a principle is detected, such as the anæsthetic power of carbonic acid gas when applied topically, we can explain by it the good effects of modes of practice which previously, perhaps, we were inclined to ridicule and reject. The fact that carbonic acid, when locally applied to a mucous surface, acts as a sedative or anæsthetic, explains a practice common among the ancients, viz., Hippocrates, Paulus Ægineta, Rueff, Paré, etc., all of whom used to burn herbs, aromatic and medicinal, and convey the fumes, by means of tubes and appropriate apparatus, to the interior of the vagina; and, such vapour being loaded with carbonic acid, it is more than probable that if such treatment was effectual, it was through the anæsthetic properties of the gas here alluded to. Again, there is a modern practice much in vogue on the Continent, of injecting the vagina, etc., with the German waters of Nuheim, Marienbad, etc.; the utility of the practice, which Dr. S. has been assured by his friend, Dr. Funck, of Frankfort, is most marked in some diseased states, will find its true explanation in the local anæsthetic effect of carbonic acid, as these waters contain a large quantity of the gas. A knowledge of the topical effects of carbonic acid serves, perhaps, also to afford an explanation of other points in common therapeutics; as, for example, its action in subduing gastric and intestinal irritatien. Hence the use of effervescing draughts, aerated waters, etc., in gastric irritability and nausea; perhaps the antacid action of the alkali may have some effect, but most likely it is the anæsthetic properties of the carbonic acid gas. The sedative and curative effects of injections into the rectum of carbonic acid gas in dysentery have a similar explanation, and serve to corroborate this view of its action. As an example of its use as a local anæsthetic to a cutaneous surface, Dr. S. alluded to the *cataplasma cerevisiæ*, or yeast poultice, which exhales from its surface a quantity of the gas. It was commonly applied to irritable and sloughing sores, and its soothing, healing, and antiseptic properties were doubtless owing to the carbonic acid gas. As an anæsthetic application to cancerous ulcers, the effects of carbonic acid gas are excellent. Dr. Ewart, of Bath, says "he has kept a person in ease and comfort, who, for so great a length of time before, had known only agony and torture." "What," he elsewhere observes, "strikes us in the two preceding cases with the greatest astonishment, is the *almost instantaneous relief of pain* which *never failed to follow the application of the gas.*" In reference to the effects of carbonic acid upon raw surfaces and wounds, Dr. Ingenhouz mentioned to Beddoes the following experiment: "Blister your finger, so as to lay bare the naked and sensible skin. The contact of air will produce pain; put your finger into vital air (oxygene), and this will produce more pain; introduce it into fixed or azotic air (carbonic acid or nitrogen), and the pain will diminish or cease." In relation to this statement, Dr. Beddoes informs us that he made the following experiments on three different persons: *First.* The raised epidermis of a blistered finger, after all action from the cantharides had ceased, was cut away in carbonic acid gas. No pain was felt. *Secondly.* A second blister being opened in common air, smarting pain came on. In a bladder of fixed air, this pain soon went off. *Thirdly.* After opening a third blister, the finger was instantly plunged into oxygene. It felt as when salt is sprinkled on a cut. In carbonic acid gas, the pain, in two minutes, quite subsided; but returned when the denuded skin was again exposed to the atmosphere. If there be no source of fallacy in these experiments, they certainly point to one kind of improvement in the treatment of some painful burns, wounds, etc.; for they appear to suggest the possibility of the suffering which is attendant on such injuries being controlled and cancelled by keeping the pained parts in contact with carbonic acid, or with some other gas or fluid capable of acting as a local anæsthetic. If the reports of Ewart, Beddoes, and Fourcroy are correct, we ought, also, indeed, to find carbonic acid an excellent application even as far as the mere healing and cicatrization of the broken surfaces are concerned.—*Edinburgh Med. Journ.*, July, 1856.

HYGIENE.

61. *Unwholesome Meat in London.*—We make the following extract from a report made by a committee appointed by the Metropolitan Association of Medical Officers of Health to inquire into the subject of unwholesome meat:—

"*Sale of Bad Meat.*—In the first place, your committee consider the fact to be fully proved, that large quantities of unwholesome meat are constantly on sale to the lower orders in London. At their first meeting, on the 21st of June, Dr. Challice produced several specimens which had been exposed for sale at butchers' shops in Southwark, and which had been either purchased by him or seized under his directions on the same day. For example, there was a sheep's liver which had been seized. It was dark, soft, and ill-smelling, and the veins contained fibrinous coagula. There was a shoulder of mutton, purchased at 7*d.* per lb.; the fat of a dirty yellow, the muscle emaciated, and of a peculiar light colour and sour smell. There was part of a sirloin, purchased at 6*d.* in Bermondsey, not ill-looking, but wonderfully thin and quite destitute of fat. There were also specimens of veal and beef of nauseous appearance; and side by side with these Dr. Challice exhibited a piece of the boiled flesh of a healthy horse, accidentally killed, which looked and smelled quite wholesome, and a leg of mutton, plump, firm, and of pure white fat, which was destined for the pauper's dinner at Bermondsey workhouse on the next day. The contrast between the mutton provided by the board of guardians for the paupers and that which was offered for sale to the industrious classes was palpable enough.

"At a subsequent meeting, Mr. Fisher and Mr. Pocklinton were good enough to bring and exhibit portions of beef and lamb which had been seized, on that day, in Newgate market. The beef was thoroughly wet and soft; the lamb, wet, soft, utterly devoid of fat in the areolar tissue and within and around the kidney; pus was found in the areolar tissue of the pelvis by Dr. Gibbon, and the smell of both specimens was incredibly nauseous.

"Your committee have also the evidence of Mr. Fisher, that he often sees meat exposed for sale in the suburbs which he should seize if within his own jurisdiction in the city; and of Dr. Gibbon, who has caused unwholesome meat to be seized in the Holborn district.

"*Great Quantity Sold.*—The fact, then, that such meat is habitually offered for sale is indisputable. As to the quantity of it, your committee can only refer to a return with which they have been favoured by Mr. Daw, of the City Sewers' Office, showing the quantity seized in the city of London during the year 1855. By this it appears that 26 live animals, 612 entire carcasses, 696 quarters, 8 sides, and 227 joints of beef, mutton, veal, and lamb were seized in that year, besides an immense quantity of poultry, game, and fish, which probably was condemned because putrid. But it must be borne in mind that the city of London is a privileged place, that the inspection of meat and slaughter-houses is there carried on systematically, and that, as Mr. Fisher declares, much meat which could not be exposed in the city is sold openly in the suburbs.

"*How to Detect Bad Meats.*—In order to give a useful and practical turn to their labours, your committee, on one occasion, invited the inspectors of nuisances out of their several districts to meet Mr. Fisher and Mr. Pocklington at Dr. Dundas Thompson's rooms, in St. Thomas's Hospital, in order that the appearances and characters of diseased meat might be explained to them from actual specimens, and that thus they might be prepared for the more efficient discharge of their duties.

"Your committee then endeavoured to draw up a short summary of the marks by which unwholesome meat may be known, in plain, unprofessional language, for the use of inspectors of nuisances, as follows:—

"The chief marks which show that meat is unwholesome are, in the first place, its colour, which is generally either dingy or too bright.

"Secondly, there is the smell, which is peculiarly sour and sickening, even when such meat is fresh, and very different from the smell of good meat when tainted through overkeeping.

"In the next place, there is a sign which is considered of more value than any other. It is a peculiar and decided wetness of the meat, which is also soft, flabby, and not set.

"Moreover, it should be noticed that there is often a large quantity of blood in the veins, which has curdled there, and not run out as it does when sound beasts are killed. Or, if there are no clots of blood, there will be very likely shreds and flakes of white matter in the larger veins, particularly in the liver.

"Then, there is a whole set of signs which show that an animal, before being killed, was greatly out of condition; such as a pale, bloodless eye, a paleness of the 'bark' of sheep, and unnatural whiteness of the flesh, which are often seen in sheep which have the rot. Want of fat, and especially of the suet about the kidneys, in place of which a watery flabby stuff is sometimes found, wasting of the fleshy part of the meat, and a watery jelly-like state of the tissue which lies between the muscles, insomuch that drops of water may run out when it is cut across, are other decided signs. It is to be remarked, that drovers are said sometimes to strike heavy blows on the eye to hide the pale look which arises from wasting disease.

"Again, there are some signs of special disease. Thus, when cattle have died of pleuro-pneumonia, or lung disease, the insides of the ribs will usually be found to be furred up with a quantity of white curdy matter (pleuritic adhesions); and the same is found inside the flanks when beasts have died of inflammation of the bowels. In these cases, the natural smooth glistening surface of the membrane which lines the ribs and flanks is lost.

"One thing to be specially looked for is the little bladders among the flesh of pigs, which constitute the disease known as measles; and similar things in the liver of sheep which have the rot.

"Experienced butchers are said to know by the smell of meat whether the beast had certain medicines given to it before being killed.

"The above are the chief signs of unwholesome meat. Of course, they will vary with circumstances; for one animal may be killed at the very beginning of an acute disease, another after it has undergone considerable wasting, and a third may have been merely killed for appearance sake, just before it would have died of itself.

"*Doubtful Meat.*—Your committee must observe that, in speaking of unwholesome meat, they refer to the flesh of animals in a state of disease, and not to meat which has become putrid from having been overkept, nor yet to meat of second-rate quality. The flesh of old bulls, cows, ewes, and rams, for example, is not first-rate, but has nothing unwholesome in it. Moreover, all traces of previously existing but now extinct disease, such as old pleuritic adhesions, need not be regarded; for, as Mr. Fisher observes, if all marks of former disease were considered cause of seizure, the market would sometimes be entirely cleared. The presence of animalcules in the liver, if the sheep is not yet out of condition, is not considered sufficient cause of seizure by the inspectors, but your committee are not prepared to sanction the exemption.

"There are several other cases in which, according to the inspectors, doubt may exist whether meat ought to be seized or not; as in the case of a healthy animal dying by accident; and of cows which are just beginning to suffer from confinement in cowsheds; and of cows which die in calving, the fore quarters of which exhibit no traces of mischief. But your committee think that it is better to err on the safe side. Slipped calves are always seized, but the market is full of calves very little different, which are killed when very few days old, and sent up in abundance from the dairy districts of Somerset and Wilts.

"It is quite certain that very much of this doubtful meat, together with large quantities of that which is certainly unwholesome, and especially slipped calves and measly pork, is made into sausages, and daily consumed by the public. Your committee have reason to believe that the flesh of horses (except the tongue) is not used, certainly not extensively used, for human food, simply because it fetches such a good price as cats' and dogs' meat.

"Your committee have learned that most of the diseased meat supplied to the metropolis is brought from the country, that is to say, that very few diseased animals are brought into or slaughtered in London, but that they are killed in the country by persons who make this a regular business. More unsound meat, according to the inspectors, is found in Newgate than in any other market, solely because more country meat is sent there. But there are persons well known in the London trade, who make it their business to dispose privately of meat which could not be exposed openly in any market.

"As for the distribution of this meat, there is no doubt that it is purchased after regular market hours, by tradesmen who retail it to the labouring classes late in the evening, in the suburbs of what are called low neighbourhoods. Much meat is sold by gaslight which could scarcely be exposed in broad daylight.

"*Illness produced by it.*—We must now touch upon the important subject of the ill-effects of unsound meat. These are twofold. In the first place, the consumer is robbed of his fair share of nourishment; for it is notorious that second-rate and unsound meat cannot stand the fire, and wastes in cooking to an extraordinary degree. Thus it is the most extravagant kind of food, and furnishes one example among the many, that the poorest people always pay most dearly for everything.

"In the next place, there can be no doubt but that the use of diseased meat may be a specific cause of illness. We need scarcely remind you that the eating of measly pork, and of ill-cooked animal food in general, is notoriously a cause of tapeworm, and of various forms of hydatid that infest the human subject. Instances have come under the notice of Dr. Gibbon, Dr. Challice, and other members of the committee, of symptoms of poisoning arising from the use of unsound meat partially cooked. It appears to be almost established that, in most cases, prolonged boiling deprives it of any active poisonous properties; and it is said that the flesh of glandered horses, after being boiled, can be handled and eaten with impunity; but roasting and frying are far less efficient means of subjecting flesh thoroughly to the purifying influence of heat.

"We may allude in passing to the overfed condition in which cattle are commonly killed at Christmas. Dr. Druitt has seen several instances of illness from eating that kind of meat, but it is matter of gratification that excessive and unnatural fatness seems now to be less cultivated by breeders of cattle.

"Your committee may observe that, although it may be difficult to prove it by actual cases, they have no doubt that unwholesome meat is one cause among many, of the debility and cachexies, the poverty of blood and intractable maladies of the poor who flock to the dispensaries and parochial medical officers, and especially of diarrhœa during hot weather.

"But your committee feel that it is a question which must be argued on far higher ground than that of special ill consequences. They believe that public decency demands that a stop be put, as far as possible, to the sale of the flesh of diseased animals, and of those which have died a natural death. They appeal to that highest and best sanitary code contained in the law of Moses (Leviticus, xi. 39, and xviii. 15), which they would willingly see observed at the present day."—*Med. Times and Gaz.*, Aug. 30, 1856.

MEDICAL JURISPRUDENCE AND TOXICOLOGY.

62. *Case of Poisoning by Chloroform taken internally.* By JAMES SPENCE, Esq.—On the 19th of May last, at a quarter past ten P. M., I was called to see A. B——, aged twenty-one, one of the female servants of this hospital, who, I was informed, had twenty minutes previously swallowed two ounces of pure chloroform. I found her lying in bed, half dressed, in a state of perfect unconsciousness (apparently in a profound sleep), from which she could not be roused. Her breath did not smell of chloroform. Pupils very much contracted; conjunctiva quite insensible; body of normal temperature; respiration tranquil and regular; pulse 78, soft and tolerably full; no congestion of face. I immediately ordered sinapisms to be applied to the extremities and over the epigastrium, and,

having secured the able assistance of my colleague, Dr. Thorburn, proceeded to evacuate the stomach by the stomach-pump, it being impossible to make her swallow an emetic. A delay of nearly ten minutes occurred before the stomach-pump was procured. When it was applied, the matters evacuated had not the slightest odour of chloroform, nor of opium, which was suspected from the excessively contracted state of the pupils. About half an ounce of mustard was introduced into the stomach, which was again emptied, and then a drachm of aromatic spirit of ammonia, with one ounce of brandy, administered by means of the stomach-pump. Some feeble attempts at vomiting ensued, and the pupils became fully dilated, and continued so for some minutes, but still continued quite immovable when exposed to a strong light. At the same time the beats of the pulse and number of respirations slightly increased in frequency, but shortly after fell below their previous standard. A powerfully stimulating enema was now administered, and, after the lapse of ten minutes, respiration becoming slow and stertorous, the pulse at the same time sensibly flagging, and the face becoming livid and congested, galvanism was resorted to, a free circulation of air being kept up around the patient, and her tongue held forward by a pair of catch forceps to prevent closure of the glottis. The number of respirations, however, continued to decrease, falling so low as seven in the minute, and, accordingly, an additional pair of plates were added to the galvanic battery, greatly increasing its strength and efficiency, while enemata of beef-tea and brandy were administered frequently. Dr. William Gairdner, one of the visiting physicians to the hospital, had been sent for, and arrived about twenty minutes past eleven, P. M. He recommended the administration of a large black draught, which was done by means of the stomach-pump. This produced severe retching and attempts to vomit, during which the patient was repeatedly almost asphyxiated. Keeping up artificial respiration with the aid of galvanism was now evidently our only resource, and this was continued, with occasional short intermissions, for nearly two hours. Stimulating enemata were given every half hour, and warmth applied to the extremities, which became excessively cold. Everything, however, appeared of no avail, and respiration fell to two per minute; the pulse at the wrist became imperceptible, while the face and neck were perfectly livid. At one time, indeed, breathing ceased altogether for nearly two minutes, and the jaw fell. The remedial measures were, however, persevered in, and in about half an hour we had the gratification of perceiving some signs of amendment. Her pulse gradually gained in strength, while her breathing became less embarrassed, *her breath now smelling strongly of chloroform.*—Half-past two P. M. Pupils became widely dilated, the sensibility of the conjunctiva returning, and the lividity of the face disappeared. Galvanism was now desisted from, although the patient still remained unconscious, all attempts to rouse her being unavailing.—Three A. M. Bowels very freely purged; pulse 94, gaining strength; respiration 28 per minute; the extremities have recovered their natural temperature.—Half-past three A. M: Consciousness slowly returning.—Four A. M. For the first time the patient answered when addressed, and of her own accord opened her eyes. The white of egg beat up with mucilage and warm milk was now cautiously administered, and attendants were directed to watch her carefully.

May 20th.—Ten A. M. Perfectly sensible; pulse 100, soft; respiration unembarrassed, and not hurried in any marked degree; complains of general pain in abdomen, of thirst, and great nausea; tongue moist, but is considerably swollen and very painful. Hot fomentations applied over abdomen, and she was ordered to have five minims of tincture of opium, every three hours, in half an ounce of mucilage. Has not passed any urine since last night; bladder empty.—Evening. Tongue moist, and still extremely painful; pulse 120, soft and regular; general pain over abdomen; has been severely purged, and a considerable quantity of blood passed by stool; urine passed freely; complains of a dull aching pain across the loins. To continue the fomentations, have a starch enema containing half a drachm of tincture of opium, and to swallow pieces of ice occasionally.

21st.—No return of the diarrhœa; slept a little during the night; pulse 132, soft; tongue furred; thirst excessive; pain is now entirely referred to the epigastrium, and is increased by pressure, which also induced a tendency to vomit; feels drowsy, and pupils are slightly contracted; urine passed abundantly. To apply twelve leeches to the epigastrium and a sinapism along the spine.—Evening. Much relieved; pulse 130; tongue moist; less drowsy, and free from nausea; diarrhœa has recurred, but not severely. To repeat the starch and opium enema.

22*d.*—Greatly better; pulse 100; complains merely of a general feeling of soreness; has taken a little beef-tea, which was retained in the stomach.

23*d.*—Doing well; pulse 90, soft.

25*th.*—Is able to sit up, and the following day returned to her work.

I have communicated the particulars of this case from its great interest, being, as far as I am aware, the only one on record of poisoning by chloroform administered internally. The only other case I know of its occurrence happened also in this hospital, some years ago, when a patient, having surreptitiously got possession of a bottle of chloroform, swallowed (if I remember rightly) the enormous quantity of six ounces. The man recovered from the immediate effects of the poison under the use of stimuli and galvanism, but died in great agony, within forty-eight hours, with symptoms of acute gastritis. When first called to the present case, I should certainly have thought it a case of poisoning from opium had I not been shown the bottle which had contained the chloroform, the contracted state of the pupils, coupled with the patient's complete insensibility, strongly resembling the effects produced by the former drug. The diminution of the frequency of respiration, however, was not proportionate to the amount of stupor. The indications for treatment were evidently to sustain the flagging vital power by stimulants and galvanism; but I am doubtful of the propriety in such cases of administering alcoholic stimuli, which might tend to aggravate the symptoms; and, should I ever meet with a similar case, I should trust more to the preparations of ammonia, as we are, I think, justified in supposing that chloroform, to a certain extent at least, acts by causing an excess of carbon in the blood, which would be still further increased by the administration of any form of alcohol. In fact, the patient's condition was precisely that of extreme drunkenness. It is worthy of notice that, although certainly not more than forty minutes elapsed from the time the chloroform was swallowed till the stomach was evacuated by the stomach-pump, no smell of chloroform was appreciable in the contents of the stomach. This could have arisen only from extremely rapid absorption of the poison, or from its having quickly passed into the small intestines, and been thence absorbed more gradually. The latter supposition is favoured by the fact that a strong odour of chloroform was perceived in the patient's breath when she began to rally from its effects, nearly four hours subsequently to its administration, although it could not be detected before. It was from a consideration of this kind that Dr. Gairdner prescribed an active cathartic, in hopes of emptying the intestines of their noxious contents. It is still a disputed point whether the action of chloroform on the nervous centres affects primarily the respiratory or circulatory systems. The former is maintained by Mr. Bickersteth, of Liverpool, who has supported his arguments by several interesting and carefully conducted experiments, while, in the case of death from inhalation of chloroform recorded by Dr. Dunsmure, the heart appeared to cease to beat before the respiratory movements were suspended; and a similar observation was made in the case lately published by Dr. Mackenzie, of Kelso. In the case before us, the heart and lungs seemed to flag *pari passu*—certainly the radial pulse disappeared before respiration was entirely arrested, but unfortunately at the moment it was not observed if the heart had likewise stopped.

The successful result of this case may serve to encourage medical men to persevere, even against hope, under similar circumstances, in continuing their exertions. Mr. Lowe, two or three years ago, published a case of inhalation in which respiration and the heart's action were arrested for fully four minutes when under continued artificial respiration; the *pulse first* slowly reappeared, followed by a return of the natural respiratory movements.

In cases, however, where chloroform has been swallowed, it is not only the immediate effects of the drug that we have to fear, and this is well exemplified in the instance of the patient already quoted, who died from the subsequent inflammation set up. Fortunately, in the present case, the symptoms of the secondary danger were never very severe, and were easily controlled by mild remedies.—*Lancet*, Aug. 9th, 1856.

63. *Symptoms and Post-mortem appearances produced by Poisonous Doses of Strychnia.*—Drs. LAWRIE and COWAN read before the Medico-Chirurgical Society of Glasgow (June 10th, 1856) a very interesting account of a case of poisoning by strychnia, and the results of experiments which they had made on inferior animals, with a view of determining the symptoms and post-mortem appearances produced by poisonous doses of that drug. (See *Glasgow Medical Journal*, July, 1856, p. 162.)

As the subject is one which has lately given rise to much discussion, we shall give from the report of the proceedings of the meeting (*Glasgow Med. Journ.*, July, 1856, p. 233 *et seq.*) the principal points of interest in the paper, with some of the remarks of the various speakers.

Dr. Lawrie stated that although the chemical detection of strychnine formed no part of their inquiry, that department of the subject had not been altogether neglected. They had sent two dogs to Dr. Anderson and one to Dr. Penny, each poisoned with a quarter of a grain of strychnine, and, in all of the stomachs, the most unequivocal evidence of the presence of strychnine was afforded by all of the tests employed. Dr. Anderson found traces of it in three of the livers.[1] Dr. Easton had kindly examined urine voided by one of the dogs while under the influence of chloroform, and had, with the greatest care and certainty, discovered the presence of strychnine. This was a most important fact in several points of view; it showed the great advantage to be derived from examining this excretion in all cases of poisoning by strychnine. It farther showed the most probable manner in which chloroform arrests the action of strychnine. It occurred to us that this interesting fact might depend on the inhalation of chloroform suspending the absorption of the strychnine, and, if so, it would not be found in the excretions. Dr. Easton's experiment upsets this theory, and makes it probable that the effects of the two poisons are physiologically antagonistic, and that the action of chloroform, being the more powerful, keeps the strychnine at bay so long as the effects of the inhalation continue. It also encourages the hope that if the inhalation were persisted in for a sufficiently long period, the strychnine might be entirely eliminated without exhibiting even its mildest physiological effects.

The diagnosis of strychnine poisoning and tetanus is a subject of great importance. Before the present inquiry was commenced, he (Dr. L.) had little doubt that the state of the jaw would be in a great measure diagnostic. The results of their experiments had confirmed this suspicion; for although it was true that, during the violence of the paroxysm, the jaw is spasmodically, even firmly closed, the moment relaxation occurs it can be easily and widely opened. Indeed, the animal generally lies with it open. This is not the case with tetanus. The horse that got 58 grains of strychnine illustrated this fact admirably. After 48 grains had been exhibited, and while he was powerfully under their influence, his mouth was widely opened, his tongue laid hold of, and ten grains in solution were, with the greatest ease, poured over his throat from a common beer bottle. In no case of tetanus that he had seen could this have possibly been done. It so happened that he had that day seen two cases which illustrated still further this subject. The one was a case of traumatic tetanus in a man aged fifty, the other of idiopathic opisthotonos in an infant. His mind being full of the subject, he had carefully made the following observations. The muscles of the jaw, neck, and upper part of the back of the tetanic patient were, as they have always in his experience been found in tetanus, while those of the limbs were perfectly quiescent and obedient to the will. A sudden touch on the face or any part of the body produced no spasm. The risus sar-

[1] Since the meeting of the society, Dr. Penny has most kindly examined for me, with great care, the brain and spine of a dog poisoned with strychnine, and has failed to discover the poison.—*J. A. L.*

donicus was absent. There was no excitement; on the contrary, there was that uncomplaining endurance of suffering and calm mental composure which he had always found so characteristic of this disease, even in its most acute forms. There was one peculiarity which he had never seen before in acute traumatic tetanus. The patient could not lie, but sat constantly day and night in an armed chair, with his body bent forwards and his forehead resting on a high stool placed before him. At the first glance, he thought that he had at last seen a case of emprosthotonos; but it was not so—the patient's posture was every now and again disturbed by a spasm, during which his head and neck were thrown back as in ordinary opisthotonos. The moment the paroxysm passed off he resumed his former position. No two conditions could be more markedly different than that of this man and Dr. Z., or an animal under the influence of strychnine. His pulse was quick, and although some circumstances and symptoms were favourable, he gave a very unfavourable prognosis.[1]

The opisthotonos of the child seemed to depend on chronic meningitis, with effusion of serum. The spine was permanently and more completely bent than he had ever seen it, and any attempt to straighten it, or even move the little patient, gave great pain. There were no convulsive paroxysms, no closure of the jaw, and no risus sardonicus. In no respect, except the opisthotonos, did the case resemble either tetanus or strychnine poisoning.

Great attention had been paid to the state of the heart in their experiments. So far as he knew, sufficient attention had not been paid by other experimenters to the effects of the rigor mortis on the heart. He believed the fact was as follows: If an animal's heart is examined *immediately* after death by strychnine, it will be found flaccid, and its four cavities filled with dark blood, sometimes (as in one of the hearts on the table) to enormous, almost incredible, over-distension; without one single exception, this was the case in all their experiments. There was not the shadow of evidence that death had been caused by spasm of the heart, and it would very greatly surprise him if reliable proof in the affirmative were ever adduced. It was far more probable, if the condition of the heart were the immediate cause of death, that it was one of paralysis. Soon after death, indeed, so far as they had observed, cotemporaneously with the setting in of the rigor mortis, the left side of the heart begins to contract, and by degrees becomes firm, and, in doing so, probably empties itself.[2] In no case, however firm and small, had they found it empty. It generally contained dark coagula. On Palmer's trial, much was said on the state of the heart, and the bulk of the evidence went to show that in man it was empty after poisoning by strychnine. It would very much surprise him if subsequent observations did not prove that this was a fallacy. He had no manner of doubt that the same law would be found to hold good in man as in the horse and dog, and *that* law he believed they had correctly ascertained. Now, could the alleged discrepancy be reconciled? It appeared to him very easily, by presuming that the post-mortem examinations hitherto made on the human subject had not been conducted with special reference to this point, and to the quantity of blood in the other organs. The autopsy should be made as soon after death as the case permits. The pericardium must be the first cavity examined, and in doing so great care must be taken that *no* large vessels be opened. The heart should be carefully observed "in situ" undisturbed; a ligature must then be passed round the root of each lung, and two ligatures around the ascending and descending large vessels. These vessels should be cut between the ligatures, and the heart and lungs removed together. Each cavity of the heart should be opened separately, the blood taken out and weighed; and he would almost stake any little professional

[1] The patient died in two days, but unfortunately I had not an opportunity of examining the body.—*J. A. L.*

[2] In proof of this, Dr. Buchanan has since suggested and assisted in making the following experiment: Into the abdominal aorta of a dog a tube was inserted and tied immediately. After death by strychnine, the pericardium was opened, and the heart *watched*. As the carcass cooled, the left ventricle contracted, and blood flowed from the tube in the aorta.

reputation he might possess on the statement, that the right side of the heart will *always* be full, and the left side *never* empty. If the heart be removed in the manner generally followed, when our sole object is to ascertain the existence of structural disease, it will be *impossible* to give a correct statement of the quantity of blood it had contained. The rigor mortis has been pretty fully discussed in the paper you have heard read. He would ask how many of us have practically attended to the subject? He doubted very much if there was an individual in this crowded room who had made a single reliable observation on the human subject; and knowing this, he had read with pain the loose unguarded statements made on Palmer's trial, and he could not, without fear and trembling, contemplate the importance which had, seemingly, been attached to opinions so vague, that the bench ought not to have allowed them to be recorded.

Before sitting down, Dr. Lawrie begged to say a very few words on the practical use of chloroform inhalations in strychnine poisoning. There is a dog in this room to which a poisonous dose of strychnine was given twelve hours ago; that dog has been kept continually under chloroform during that period, and hitherto no symptom of its having swallowed strychnine has shown itself; we hope that we may keep it alive until the kidneys shall eliminate the whole strychnine.[1] But, even should we be disappointed in this, we must not conclude that it is useless as a remedy; on the contrary, by suspending the action of the poison and prolonging life, it will give time for the use of the stomach-pump and the exhibition of emetics, and enable us to sustain the strength by enemata. Further, if an antidote should ever be discovered, chloroform may be found to suspend the action of the poison until the antidote shall altogether neutralize it.[2]

Dr. Easton remarked, that the most important fact which had been ascertained by the essayists, was the power of chloroform to suspend the characteristic action of strychnia. These experiments Dr. Easton had been privileged to witness; and though, from the comparatively few trials which had yet been made, it could scarcely be maintained, that it had been completely established that chloroform was an antidote to strychnia, yet all the observations hitherto made were undoubtedly leading to that conclusion. By antidote, it was not meant that chloroform acted as a *chemical* antidote to strychnia, converting it into a new and innocuous substance, such as took place, for example, on the union of albumen with corrosive sublimate, or of chalk with oxalic acid; but that it raised in the system a physiological action antagonistic to that of strychnia, counteracting the spasms produced by the latter, and thereby keeping the animal alive until the poison had been eliminated by the usual channels. Chloroform merely kept the animal from dying, and thus gave nature the opportunity of working out her own recovery. Referring to the much controverted point, whether strychnia could be detected in the excretions, Dr. Easton stated that he had found no difficulty in detecting it in the urine of two of the dogs, to which Drs. Lawrie and Cowan had given respectively half a grain and one grain of the poison. Two processes were instituted for this purpose, in the conducting of which Dr. Easton had been ably assisted by Mr. William Hutton, of the chemical laboratory of Anderson's University. One of these consisted in digesting the urine, after considerable concentration, in animal

[1] In this we were disappointed; it died at 12 P. M., sixteen hours after swallowing the strychnine.

[2] Since the above, it occurred to me to make the following experiments:—

1. To try the effect of sulphuric ether by inhalation, in suspending the action of strychnine—it entirely failed.

2. A quarter of a grain of strychnine dissolved in ʒi chloroform, was given to a full-sized terrier; tetanic spasms came on before the animal could be untied, and he died almost instantaneously.

3. One drachm chloroform was given to a small terrier bitch, she died instantaneously.

A temporary absence has suspended our experiments; should they be resumed, the results will be communicated.—*J. A L.*

charcoal, and agitating the whole for several hours. Thereafter, the animal charcoal, separated by filtration, and containing the strychnia in its interior, was boiled in alcohol, so as to dissolve out the alkaloid which had been absorbed. To the evaporated alcoholic solution, bichromate of potash and sulphuric acid were added, and the characteristic appearances of strychnia, when so treated, were immediately displayed. The other process was a little more complex. The urine was first acidulated with acetic acid and then boiled. By this means a soluble acetate of strychnia was obtained. Caustic potash and animal charcoal were then added; the potash to decompose the acetate, the charcoal to absorb the liberated strychnia. The strychnia was boiled out by alcohol from the charcoal, the filtered alcoholic solution evaporated as before, bichromate of potash and sulphuric acid were added, and with a similar result. In conclusion, Dr. Easton was of opinion that medical jurists might derive an important practical lesson, hitherto too much overlooked, from these and similar experiments. If strychnia could be detected thus readily in the urine, might not those other vegetable poisons, which were recognizable by tests, be detected in that excretion also? In particular, should we not test that fluid in cases of poisoning by opium? In cases of poisoning by that narcotic, we have hitherto been satisfied with a chemical examination of the contents of the stomach alone, and failing to find opium there, further search was deemed unnecessary, because unavailing. Now, every one who had had any experience in medico-legal investigations was aware how rapidly opium passed into the blood, and that it was impossible, if a few hours only had intervened between administration and death, for even the most expert analyst to find that poison in the stomach. If, then, there were any urine in the bladder of a person supposed to have been poisoned by that narcotic, or even by any other vegetable peison, for the discovery of which, chemistry had supplied the means, Dr. Easton was of opinion, that henceforth we should fail in our duty if we neglected to submit the excretions—nay, even the blood itself and the tissues—to the requisite chemical examination.

64. *Special Points of Similarity and Dissimilarity between the Effects on the Human Body of an Overdose of Strychnia and the Symptoms of ordinary Tetanus.*—Dr. R. ADAMS records (*Med. Times and Gaz.*, Aug. 16, 1856) an interesting case of poisoning by strychnia, and offers some interesting observations on the similarity and dissimilarity between the effects of strychnia and the symptoms of ordinary tetanus.

The diagnosis between ordinary tetanus and that form produced by strychnia, Dr. R. thinks, will be found "by looking to the expression of the countenance, rather than to any other single phenomenon. This expression is admitted by all to be most peculiar, and that once looked upon with attention it cannot be forgotten. The forehead is wrinkled transversely and in the perpendicular direction, the eyebrows being drawn in a remarkable manner towards each other; the eyes are not fully opened; the nostrils are more or less dilated; the angles of the mouth are drawn backwards and a little upwards. These characteristic marks become momentarily exaggerated at every paroxysm."

It does not appear, he says, that the true tetanic expression has been noticed in any of the cases of strychnia tetanus.

The following are Dr. A.'s conclusions:—

"1. Strychnia tetanus resembles ordinary tetanus in its spasms, particularly when they assume, as they frequently do, the form of opisthotonos.

"2. A rigid condition of the muscles exists in both cases, not only during the actual paroxysms, but also during the intervals between them.

"3. Strychnia tetanus, in its progress to a fatal result, is much more rapid in its course than ordinary tetanus.

"4. The commencement of this last is silent, and the expression of the countenance is peculiar and characteristic.

"5. The beginning of the former is announced by loud and repeated screams and moanings.

"6. The hands in strychnia tetanus are early and severely affected; in ordinary tetanus the hands are the part, of all others, the last and least affected."

AMERICAN INTELLIGENCE.

ORIGINAL COMMUNICATIONS.

On the Digestion of Starch in the Intestinal Canal. By JOHN C. DALTON, Jr., M. D., Professor of Physiology and Microscopic Anatomy in the College of Physicians and Surgeons, New York.

In the *American Journal of the Medical Sciences* for October, 1854, in an article on the *Gastric Juice and its Office on Digestion*, I stated, as the result of a considerable number of experiments, that starchy substances were not digested in the stomach. This statement was in accordance with the opinion of Bernard, but in opposition to that of Lehmann, who asserted, partly on his own authority and partly on that of Jacubowitsch and Bidder and Schmidt, that after an animal, with gastric fistula, had been fed with starch, glucose could be detected in the fluids drawn from the stomach. Lehmann, however, in his third edition, retracts this opinion and embraces the opposite one. "Bidder and Schmidt,"[1] he says, "under whose superintendence the experiments of Jacubowitsch were instituted, have convinced themselves, by later experiments, that the saliva loses its action on boiled starch in the stomach of the living animal. * * * We are, consequently, led, by the earlier observations of Bernard, as well as by the more recent investigations of Bidder and Schmidt, to the conclusion that notwithstanding its energetic action on starch, and notwithstanding its abundant supply, the saliva takes no very important part in the digestion of the amylacea." So far as regards the lower animals, therefore, it seems to be quite generally acknowledged that starch is not converted into glucose in the cavity of the stomach.

In a pamphlet recently published by Dr. Francis G. Smith,[2] of the Medical Department of Pennsylvania College, some very interesting experiments are detailed which were performed by the author on Dr. Beaumont's old patient, Alexis St. Martin, during his recent visit to this section of the country. Their results lead Dr. Smith to the belief that my own observations, in this respect, as well as those of Bernard, were erroneous, or at least not applicable to the human subject; and he concludes that "starchy materials are digested in the human stomach; that human gastric juice does not prevent the conversion of starch into grape sugar, and that this conversion may take place in the stomach, independently of the action of the saliva."

The two experiments upon which these conclusions were based were the following, in which the "amylaceous materials" were "represented by wheaten bread."

"*Experiment* 11. On the 6th of May, a portion of wheaten bread was given to St. Martin while fasting, which he masticated deliberately and swallowed. In two hours and a half afterward a portion of the contents of the stomach was removed for examination. The reaction of this fluid was acid, and the microscopic appearances have been detailed already. Suffice it to

[1] Physiological Chemistry, English translation. Philad. edit., vol. i. pp. 434–5, 1855.

[2] Experiments upon Digestion. Philad., 1856.

say, that, in addition to epithelial and mucous cells, starch granules, some whole, some broken, were distinctly recognizable.

"After allowing the fluid to stand until it had settled, a portion of the supernatant fluid was tested with iodide of potassium and nitric acid with the effect of manifesting decided evidence of the presence of starch by the production of the characteristic blue colour. The same reaction was produced with the tincture of iodine.

"Another portion of the same fluid was subjected to Trommer's test (solution of sulphate of copper and liquor potassæ); the result showed the brick-dust red precipitate from a reduction of the oxide of copper in very considerable quantity." (The above fluid was also filtered through animal charcoal, and afterwards acted in the same way with Trommer's test.)

"*Experiment* 12. In order to ascertain, if possible, what effect the saliva might have had in producing the glycogenic change in the bread masticated, a portion of bread moistened with water was introduced through the fistulous orifice, and St. Martin was requested to swallow as little saliva as possible, which, as he used tobacco, he had little difficulty in complying with. In an hour and a half afterwards, the contents of the stomach were withdrawn. The same acid reaction was manifest; the same microscopic appearances, and the same solution of the materials were present, although not to the same degree as when the bread was masticated.

"The fluid was carried through the same tests with a like result, viz: faint evidences of starch and decided evidences of glucose."

I cannot think that the above experiments really indicate that the amylaceous matters were digested in the stomach. On the contrary, it is extremely probable, to say the least, that the glucose which was detected in the gastric fluids, was not formed during the process of digestion, but *existed beforehand in the bread used as food.* When I first commenced to investigate the subject of the digestion of starch, and the place of its conversion into sugar, the plan adopted was to feed the animals (rabbits and dogs) with bread or biscuit, kill them after a short time, and then examine the contents of the stomach and intestine. It was very soon found, however, that this method would not answer the purpose—for the reason that nearly every kind of bread and biscuit contains a certain quantity of glucose; and when this substance was found in the fluids of the alimentary canal after the death of the animal, it was impossible to determine whether it had been produced by digestion or taken in with the food. The only sure mode of experimenting is to feed the animal with a recently prepared emulsion of starch, mixed with meat, the mixture being tested beforehand to make sure that it contains no sugar. This was the mode finally adopted; and it led to perfectly satisfactory results.

I have recently examined fifteen different specimens of wheaten bread, procured at random from ten different establishments, and found glucose to be present, in larger or smaller quantity, in all of them. In twelve specimens the glucose was sufficiently abundant to reduce the oxide of copper in Trommer's test promptly and copiously; in the remaining three instances, the traces of glucose were slight, though distinctly present. The bread is simply rubbed up with a little distilled water, allowed to soak a few minutes, filtered, and the filtrate tested in the usual manner for the presence of sugar. In some kinds of crackers, or hard biscuit, there is also a considerable quantity of sugar; in others it is not present. Sometimes one biscuit will furnish evidences of the presence of sugar, while another, taken from the same lot, will fail to do so.

Most of the glucose which is found in ordinary bread is derived directly from the flour, in which it exists in considerable quantity. During the process of fermentation, or "rising," a part of it is converted into alcohol and carbonic acid, but a certain portion escapes decomposition, and remains unaltered. It is probable, also, that some of the starch of the flour becomes converted into glucose, either during fermentation, or in the process of baking. Whenever milk is used as an ingredient of bread or biscuit, it supplies, of course, an additional quantity of sugar. It is certain, at all events, that bread is quite unfit to be used as the material for experiments on the digestion of starchy substances.

The method adopted in my experiments on dogs, as already mentioned, was to administer to the animal, after a twelve or twenty-four hours' fast, boiled starch mixed with meat. The experiments were first performed on animals with gastric fistulæ, the fluids being withdrawn from the stomach at various intervals after the meal. It was found that in the fluids so extracted starch was easily recognized, by its reaction with iodine, ten, fifteen, and thirty minutes after the ingestion of the food. In forty-five minutes it had diminished in quantity, and in an hour had almost invariably disappeared; but no glucose was present at any time. It was thus ascertained that the starch disappeared from the stomach without undergoing any appreciable conversion into sugar; but the manner and place of its final digestion was still uncertain. A second set of experiments were then performed on healthy animals, which were fed in the same way, then killed, and the contents of the alimentary canal examined. In this way it was definitely ascertained that during digestion starchy matters pass unchanged from the stomach into the duodenum, and that they there meet with the mixed intestinal fluids, by which they are at once converted into glucose. The intestinal fluids taken from the duodenum of a recently killed dog exert this transforming action on starch with equal promptitude outside the body, if the two substances be mixed in a test-tube and kept at the temperature of 100° Fahr. The following experiment, which I have often repeated, shows that the same conversion occurs in ordinary digestion: If a dog be fed with a mixture of meat and boiled starch, and killed a short time afterwards, the stomach contains starch, but no glucose; while in the duodenum there is abundance of glucose, but little or even no starch. The experimenter may, however, fail to discover sugar in the intestine under these circumstances, if the examination be too long delayed; for it is remarkable how rapidly starchy substances, if in a fluid form, and disintegrated by boiling, are disposed of in digestion. If the animal be fed, as above, with boiled starch and meat, while much of the meat remains in the stomach for eight, nine, or ten hours, the starch immediately begins to pass out of it into the intestine, where it is at once converted into glucose, and then as rapidly absorbed. The whole of the starch may be converted into glucose and absorbed in an hour's time. I have even found, at the end of three-quarters of an hour, that all trace of both starch and sugar had disappeared from both stomach and intestine. The promptitude with which this passage of starch into the intestine takes place, as well as its subsequent digestion and absorption, varies to some extent in different animals, according to the activity of the digestive apparatus; but it is always a comparatively rapid process.

Some caution requires to be used in examining the gastric and intestinal fluids for sugar, owing to the peculiar property of gastric juice in modifying the action of Trommer's test on a solution of glucose. If much gastric juice be present on adding the sulphate of copper and potassa, a fine purple colour is produced instead of the ordinary blue tinge; on boiling, the colour changes to yellow, but no deposit of copper takes place. If the quantity of sugar be very small, and only a little sulphate of copper used in the test, no change of colour may occur on boiling, and the mixture may remain purple. This singular property was first described in an article, already alluded to, published in the number of this Journal for October, 1854. At that time I was unable to ascertain on what ingredient of the gastric fluids this peculiar action depended. Subsequently, however, the same thing was noticed by M. Longet, of Paris, and described by him in the *Gazette Hebdomadaire* for April 9, 1855.[1] He ascribes this modifying influence on Trommer's test to the presence, in the gastric fluids, of digested albuminose. I have since found that this opinion is correct. Pure, colourless gastric juice, taken from the stomach of the fasting animal by irritation with a metallic catheter, does not interfere with the usual action of Trommer's test. But if it be artificially digested for some hours with finely chopped meat, at the temperature of 100° Fahr., and then filtered, it will be found to have acquired the property in a marked degree. As the fluids of the stomach, while digestion of meat is going on, always contain more or less albuminose in solution, they will modify accordingly the action of Trommer's test. If care be taken, however, this need not produce any great uncertainty in its use; for the albuminose acts only to a limited extent, and in proportion to its relative quantity. In other words, a certain quantity of albuminose will only prevent the reduction of a certain quantity of copper. Thus, if we have a specimen of gastric juice containing both albuminose and grape sugar in solution, if we add a small quantity of sulphate of copper (one drop of the solution, for example, to one drachm of gastric juice), on making the mixture alkaline by the addition of potass, it takes a purple colour, and no deposit occurs on boiling; but if we add a larger quantity of copper (four drops to the drachm), the colour of the mixture is blue, and the copper is partly precipitated on boiling. As a general thing, whenever sufficient sulphate of copper is added to make the mixture blue instead of purple, some of it is thrown down on boiling if glucose be present.

Another precaution is necessary in the examination of the animal fluids for starch. Since both the gastric and intestinal fluids interfere in a marked degree with the mutual reaction of starch and iodine, it is necessary, in searching for starch, to employ the iodine in excess; since a small quantity would be altogether held in check by the organic matters, and would fail to detect the starch which might be present.

The Patella torn away by a Circular Saw, with other Serious Injuries; Recovery. By Wm. J. Alexander, M. D., of Salem, Va.

On the 6th day of April, 1855, I was called to visit Mr. John Eller, a Dunkard preacher, aged 60 years, and of a bilious temperament, residing five miles distant in the country, who after having shut the water from a seventeen foot wheel, by which the saw was propelled, turned around quickly and in attempting to remove a piece of scantling which lay upon the carriage, the end came in contact with the saw, and Mr. Eller was instantly drawn towards it; falling on the left side of the saw, he received four severe wounds before it ceased its motion. When I arrived and examined my patient, I found the pulse at the wrist scarcely perceptible under the fingers; a cold perspiration pervaded the whole system. After the system had fully reacted from large and repeated draughts of brandy which had been given, I proceeded to examine the injuries which he had sustained, and found that

[1] *Nouvelles Recherches relatives à l'Action du Suc gastrique sur les Substances Albuminoïdes.*

the entire patella on the left knee had been torn into small pieces and removed; together with at least a quarter of an inch of the condyles of the femur, leaving a perfectly flat surface. The saw did not pass entirely through, but left the flap still adhering to about an inch and a half of skin and ligament upon the inside of the knee, &c. The radius and ulna of the left arm were broken in two places, and the soft parts bruised from the wrist to the elbow. The right arm also came in contact with the saw about two inches above the wrist, making a considerable wound across the arm and injuring the tendons somewhat, but not seriously. The next wound was upon the right leg about four inches above the ankle, where the saw passed entirely through the tibia, and about one-third through the fibula, leaving a very extensive flesh wound. The bones scaled when the teeth of the saw came in contact with them, leaving a space between the upper and lower ends of the bones at least half an inch. This was the extent of the injury received. I next proceeded to dress his wounds, and first the knee. Several fragments of broken bone were still adhering to torn portions of ligament, which were all removed by a pair of scissors. After having sponged the parts with tepid water, the flap was immediately closed down and held "in situ" by ten sutures, and several adhesive strips passed across the flap. The leg was then laid in a box and confined in a straight position. The arm and other leg were treated in the same way as in cases of compound fracture. The knee was examined, and all the sutures removed on the seventh day, and union by the first intention had completely taken place over the whole extent of the wound. The patient suffered but little pain at this time, but complained of considerable tenderness upon pressure being made over the joint; this, however, soon subsided by the use of the camphorated soap liniment At the expiration of about seven weeks from the time of the accident, I directed that flexion and extension of the limb should be practised each day, as the patient might be able to bear it. At first it was exceedingly painful in consequence of the joint being stiff and the recently united portions being tender, but this did not continue long; the pain diminished more and more every day, and at the same time the joint offering less resistance until the leg could be flexed back against the thigh.

The patient improved rapidly, and has entirely recovered; he walks very well, frequently without the use of a stick, complains of some weakness of the joint, and in travelling upon an inclined plane requires some effort to prevent the knee from springing forward; otherwise he suffers no inconvenience. As the patella forms a very important part in the structure of the joint, my impression at the time was, that my patient would have a stiff joint.

SALEM, Roanoke County, Virginia.

Iodine in Chronic Ulcers. By B. ROEMER, M. D., of Va.—Hannah, a negro woman, about 45 years old, and of strong and regular formation, was attacked three years ago with an indolent ulcer on the right thumb, which degenerated in consequence of irritating frictions in washing, since a year, into an irritable chronic ulcer. The thumb and index were both involved; the carpo-metacarpal bone presented through the surrounding excavations a caries-like appearance; the opponens and flexor brevis pollicis bearing the signs of high and irritable inflammation combined with sloughing on the edges, and a deep-seated sinus communicated with the abductor pollicis. There existed also arthropyosis in the joint of the first and second phalanges of the thumb, which (we could not determine the direction of this sinus) seemed either to connect co-ordinately with a canal seated between the tendons of the extens. carp. rad. l. and the extens. polli. tertius, or was only the prolongation of the same. The system was much debilitated through the continuance of sloughing ulceration, and at times one ounce of blood escaped from the irritated surface on slight contact.

Treatment.—A seton was placed over the extralateral fascia of the biceps muscle, the tinct. iod. comp. administered internally (25 drops gradually increased to f℥ss) twice daily, and the tinct. iod. simplex applied externally over the inflamed surface by means of a glass brush once every morning. At the end of the second week the irritable character of the ulcer subsided, while the edges suppurated to a greater extent. The seton acted but imperfectly. In the fourth week the patient felt slight nausea, which left her in two days, when an acute pain was experienced in the right mamma. In the fifth week the papilla of the same contracted and sank; and in the sixth week the right breast was absorbed to half its original size. No other symptom of iodine occurred. Iodine was detected in the urine and in the blood, which at times escaped from the ulcer, the bichloride of palladium reacting out of the alcoholic extracts, evaporated and resolved in water as dark brown iodide of palladium. The pus was destitute of iodine on testing it with starch and bichloride of palladium. In the eighth week the ulceration began to dry up; both the sinuses were closed without rendering their former situation tender. With the tenth week all traces of the former ulcer were obliterated and new membranes had formed. A slight anchylosis remained in the phalanx joint of the thumb in consequence of arthropyosis. The breast begins slowly to fill. An arthritic swelling on the right knee seems to stand in an idiosyncratic relation to iodism, and the urine is destitute of its proportional quantity of uric acid. Should urate of soda, phosphate of lime, etc., become deposited in consequence of a predisposing affinity of iodine to their respective solvents?

DOMESTIC SUMMARY.

Acetate of Lead in Yellow Fever.—Prof. Geo. B. Wood made some interesting practical remarks at a meeting of the College of Physicians of Philadelphia (Nov. 7, 1855), on the use of acetate of lead in yellow fever. He said that the recent prevalence of yellow fever in Norfolk, and many parts of the South, had called general attention to that disease; and any suggestion in relation to its treatment might be considered at present as peculiarly appropriate. There was one point in the therapeutics of the affection to which, he thought, scarcely so much attention had been directed as it merited. It was well known that the first stage of the disease usually consisted of one long, continuous, febrile paroxysm, which, after a duration of one, two, or three days, rather suddenly subsided into a period of apparent remission, in which, however, though the febrile excitement was diminished, there was no decrease of the danger. This, indeed, was the period of greatest danger; the patient, in bad cases, being much prostrated, and often throwing up large quantities either of pure blood, or of altered blood in the form of black vomit. He knew well that, in a great many cases, all remedial efforts were of no avail; the blood being irreparably poisoned by the violent action of the cause. But there were others in which the chances were about evenly balanced between life and death, and in which the occurrence of gastric hemorrhage might turn the scale against life, by increasing a debility already as great as the vital forces were adequate to struggle through. In such cases, it appeared to him that there was a strong indication to prevent this exhausting hemorrhage.

Besides, in the same stage, there is a species of inflammation of the gastric mucous membrane, as indicated by the exquisite epigastric tenderness during life, and the appearances presented upon examination after death. This strongly tends to a disorganization of the tissue, and to that effusion of altered blood, so well known and so much dreaded under the name of black vomit. Dr. Wood believed that this discharge was not attributable solely to the state of the blood, but somewhat also to the condition of the mucous membrane. Here then was another indication; namely, to obviate the phlogosed condition of the membrane, to empty, as far as possible, the inflamed vessels of the blood that was distending them, and thus give them some opportunity of resuming their healthy functions.

Now he knew no medicine so well calculated to meet these two indications as the acetate of lead, at the same time an energetic astringent and a decided sedative. This remedy had, so long since as the year 1820, been recommended and employed by Dr. Irvine, of Charleston, S. C., who wrote a pamphlet on the subject, the substance of which may be seen in the *Eclectic Repertory* of the same year (vol. x. page 519). Having perused this pamphlet, Dr. Wood had an opportunity of trying the remedy in a severe case, which occurred towards the close of the epidemic that appeared in Philadelphia in 1820; and he was much pleased with its apparent effects. In this case, the patient had, at the beginning of the second stage, begun to throw up a darkish flocculent matter, which appeared as if it might be the result of a commencing effort to form black vomit. The acetate of lead was given, as recommended by Dr. Irvine; and the patient ultimately recovered. This was the only case of the disease he had under his charge on that occasion, after reading Dr. Irvine's account of the remedy. Two others had since occurred to him; one some years since in the person of a seaman from the South, in the Pennsylvania Hospital; and the other recently, in that of a student of medicine who had come to Philadelphia to attend the medical lectures, and on the way had passed through two towns in which the fever was prevailing at the time. He had the characteristic phenomena of a fever of two days' duration, and a remission of the febrile symptoms at the end of that time, with intense tenderness in the epigastrium, and deep yellowness of the skin. Both of these cases recovered under the use of acetate of lead. He did not pretend that the three cases mentioned were at all decisive as to the efficacy of the remedy under the circumstances mentioned; but they were certainly sufficient to justify a further attention to the subject, and a more ample trial.

Dr. Wood had sought in vain among the medical journals of late, for testimony in relation to the use of the acetate. Such testimony may have been given; but it had not fallen under his notice. He had heard that, in a particular locality, the remedy had been tried, and not been found to answer. But it may not have been employed at precisely the right juncture, or in sufficient quantity, or in a sufficient number of cases, to justify a determination of its value on this score. Before it can be pronounced to be worthless, it must have undergone a much more extensive trial, and under a variety of circumstances. He did not suppose that it would cure all cases. He should despair of a cure from it after black vomit had fairly taken place. But, with his present views, he considered it as probably having the power of preserving life in some cases, and as deserving of the notice of the profession.

Attention is necessary to the period and circumstances of its administration. It should be commenced with at the earliest signs of the approach of the second stage. This was highly important, as, after this, it would probably be too late. It should be given in doses of two grains every two hours, without the accompaniment or simultaneous use of any other substance that might serve to decompose it; and should be continued steadily until thirty-six grains have been taken. The use of this remedy does not preclude the application of leeches or a blister to the epigastrium, one or both of which Dr. Wood had employed in all the three cases referred to.—*Summary of the Trans. of the Coll. of Phys. of Philadelphia*, vol. ii., N. S., No. X.

Origin and Propagation of Yellow Fever.—The No. of the *Southern Med. and Surg. Journ.* for September contains an interesting paper by Dr. RICHARD D. ARNOLD, Professor of the Theory and Practice of Medicine in Savannah Medical College, and a practitioner of very extensive experience and highly cultivated mind, "Upon the relations of Bilious and Yellow Fever"—prepared at the request of, and read before, the Medical Society of the State of Georgia, at its session held at Macon on the 9th of April, 1856.

Dr. Arnold discusses the two opinions—1st. Is yellow fever only a higher grade of bilious fever? 2d. Is yellow fever a disease *sui generis?* Dr. A. expresses his conviction of the truth of the latter. And in this belief Dr. A. accords with those who have had most experience, and have most faithfully studied the two diseases.

In regard to the origin and propagation of yellow fever, Dr. Arnold says: "I can bear my decided testimony that in no instance has there ever been the shadow of the shade of proof, that it ever was imported into Savannah from abroad. On the contrary, the proof is positive that its first victims had had no communication, direct or indirect, with any source of infection. Moreover, when the British steamer Conway, which ran to the West Indies, touched at this port, I attended two cases of yellow fever from her, both of which died in the city, and yet no disease was propagated from them. In March, 1841 (as will be seen by my article quoted before) I brought a case from a ship from Demerara, and placed it in the hospital where the patient died. It is said that it can be propagated from abroad in a city, although most give up the point as to its contagion in the country. The whole experience of 1820 and 1854, when our citizens fled by hundreds into the country, and into neighbouring villages, towns, and cities, does not afford a single instance where the disease was spread by the fugitives. If, then, it is not propagated into the country, and into other cities by land routes, why is it supposed to be so fatal when it comes by sea? If one case can originate in a place, why not ten or twenty? Case upon case occurred in 1854, in which the patients had not been near a deceased subject. Isolation was no protection. The poison, whatever it may be, spread like a pall over the whole city, and covered in its embrace all who stayed, or entered its precincts; but a quarter of a mile beyond its limits the poison became innocuous. Such is fact. Let those who appeal to fancy, disprove it, or theorize upon it.

"Again: facts prove that yellow fever is a city disease. Exposure to swamp malaria, staying on a rice plantation in the summer, and in the fall before a frost, will produce a malignant and most fatal congestive bilious fever; but *never*, no, *never* yellow fever.

Appearance and Progress of Yellow Fever in the Port of New York in 1856.—Dr. H. D. BUCKLEY gives (*New York Medical Times*, Sept., 1856) the following interesting account of the appearance and progress of yellow fever in New York during the present year, up to the 29th of August, derived from documents furnished by Dr. E. Harris, Physician to the Marine Hospital at Staten Island, and Dr. A. B. Whiting, formerly health officer at Quarantine:—

"Up to the 25th of August of the present year, there had been admitted to the Marine Hospital at Quarantine, one hundred and thirty-three cases of yellow fever, and in addition to this number, eighteen cases had occurred among the permanent residents within the Quarantine inclosure.

"One case of the disease was received from Havana in the month of April; but no other cases were seen until June 18, when the bark Julia M. Hallock, from St. Jago de Cuba, arrived, with captain, first mate, and a passenger sick with the fever. On the 21st of the same month, the ship Jane H. Gliddon, from Havana, arrived, having a passenger and four seamen dangerously ill with it; and from the same vessel three other cases were subsequently received. These were all of a strongly-marked character; and some of them occurring many days after the ship's arrival, an infected condition of the vessel was naturally inferred, and the spread of the infection anticipated. From this ship the infection did spread, until at least twenty of the stevedores and lightermen who were engaged in unloading her, contracted the disease.

"On the 2d of July, one case of yellow fever was received from the Lilias; on the third, one from the Eliza Jane; and on the sixth the ship Lady Franklin arrived from Matanzas, having eight cases of it, and one seaman dead with it. Thus the prevalence of this malady seemed fairly inaugurated for the season.

"The infected vessels were principally freighted with sugar; though the Jane H. Gliddon had a portion of a cargo of rags, about thirty bales of which were subsequently stored in an open shed upon the U. S. Government Dock at Quarantine.

"On the 14th of July, a stevedore, who had been engaged in unloading these rags from the Gliddon, was admitted to the Marine Hospital, with black vomit. From this date, the fever rapidly spread among the labourers employed in unloading the infected vessels, whose cargoes were being lightered to the Atlantic Docks, Brooklyn. Thirty of these men, sick with the fever, have been conveyed to the Marine Hospital from the city, and from various parts of Staten Island.

"Cases of yellow fever have already been received from as many as thirty different vessels, arriving from the various West Indian ports. Besides these, a considerable number of cases have been admitted from the city, in which the source of the infection could not be completely made out, owing to the moribund or delirious condition of the patients; but in all cases, it has been ascertained that these persons had been freely exposed near the waterside in the lower wards of the city.

"As regards the special cause, or causes, which are believed to have introduced an endemic of yellow fever within the Quarantine inclosure, it seems highly probable that the infected goods which were landed upon the Government Dock, together with the close proximity of highly infected vessels lying at anchor in the stream, produced an infected state of the atmosphere in a narrow zone by the waterside. The physician of the Marine Hospital reports that this endemic appears to have ceased; and it is worthy of remark that the infected goods referred to, and the vessels near by, were long since removed.

"That our readers may see how the present compares with past years of the prevalence of yellow fever at the Quarantine establishment, we append the following statistical table, which has been prepared for another purpose by Dr. Harris, the physician of the Marine Hospital, and which he has kindly placed at our disposal:—

"*A Tabular View of the Statistics of Yellow Fever as it has prevailed in the Port of New York, at the Marine Hospital, from* 1799 *to* 1856.

	1799	1800	1801	1802	1803	1804	1805	1806	1807	1808	1809	1810	1815	1816	1817	1818	1819	1820	1821	1822	1823	1824
Admitted	163	38	35	5	141	8	43	2	3	1	2	1	19	2	5	7	26	2	26	105	8	28
Discharged	87	17	19	3	72	3	18	2	...	...	...	...	12	2	1	3	7	...	10	58	3	20
Died	76	21	16	2	69	5	25	...	3	1	2	1	7	...	4	4	19	2	16	47	5	8

	1825	1826	1827	1828	1829	1830	1832	1833	1834	1835	1838	1839	1843	1844	1845	1846	1847	1848	1849	1850	1851	1852	1853	1854	1855
Admitted	2	2	6	1	4	2	1	12	3	2	26	4	18	9	...	2	1	26	...	...	...	1	44	45	12
Discharg'd	1	...	2	1	4	1	...	10	2	...	18	...	15	7	...	2	1	14	...	...	...	...	30	25	7
Died	1	2	4	...	...	1	1	2	1	2	8	4	3	2	...	...	...	12	...	...	...	1	14	20	5

"The average mortality at this hospital will be found to have been about 35 per cent.

"The disease has also appeared this year on the southern end of Long Island, in that portion of King's County lying along the Narrows from Red Hook to

Fort Hamilton, the first case having appeared at Fort Hamilton, in the latter part of July, in the practice of Dr. Bailey, Surgeon of the Fort. It then appeared in the village of Fort Hamilton, and soon after at Yellow Hook and Gowanus, and finally at Red Hook; the latter place being in the confines of Brooklyn. According to the statistics by Dr. Whiting, which appear to have been collected with care, 73 cases and 35 deaths had occurred in this region up to the 22d of August, when the disease seemed to be decidedly on the decline. Dr. W. has not the least doubt that the disease is wholly and purely yellow fever, notwithstanding the doubts on this point which have been expressed by some. Most of the cases have occurred within a few rods of the shore, and none at a distance of more than fifty rods, a fact which seems fully to warrant the opinion that the disease owes its origin to infected vessels at Quarantine and Gravesend Bay. In no case has it been communicated to a person living out of this immediate locality. These vessels have been removed, and the disease has now almost ceased. Another account (newspaper) states that the disease first appeared on a bluff overlooking Gravesend Bay, where infected vessels were lying at anchor, and gives 58 as the number of deaths at Fort Hamilton and Yellow Hook. All accounts agree as to the origin of the disease from infected vessels at Quarantine.

"The weather during the last two weeks of July was very hot and dry, the mean average of the thermometer having been 85° and 81°. In the early part of August, there was a very heavy fall of rain, after which the heat was somewhat moderated; and during the last half of August, the weather was unusually cool, for the season, the mean average of the thermometer during the last two weeks having been 71° and 69°."

Report of the Cases of Yellow Fever which have occurred in Charleston and on shipboard in the Harbour during the Summer of 1856.—Dr. J. L. Dawson gives (*Charleston Medical Journal*, September, 1856), the following report of the cases of yellow fever which have occurred during the summer of 1856, up to the 25th of August, in the city of Charleston, and on shipboard in the harbour:—

"The first case of yellow fever reported this season occurred on the 14th of July, on board of the schooner Exchange, at Palmetto Wharf; the febrile paroxysm was short and the patient speedily recovered.

"On the 26th of July, Collens, ten days from Savannah, was seized with the usual symptoms of yellow fever; the fever lasted four days, with constant vomiting. He recovered slowly, and has had no return of fever up to this date (25th August). I have ascertained since his recovery that he passed a night on a farm, in the neighbourhood of the city, a few days before his attack. This being a malarial district may possibly have caused the fever; but as the fevers of this locality are generally of a remittent or intermittent type, and are apt to return without active treatment with quinine, which practice was not pursued in this case, I am inclined to the opinion that it should be recorded as a case of yellow fever. The patient resided at the west end of Tradd Street, and worked at the Standard office on East Bay.

"On the same day (26th) I was requested by the attending physician to visit Abbot, an Irishman, residing on King Street near Broad, he stating that he regarded it as a case of yellow fever. I concurred in his opinion, and advised the Mayor to have the case removed to the Lazaretto, which was done early the next morning. Abbott had passed through the severe epidemic of 1854. For a week before his attack he had been engaged loading the brig St. Andrew, from West Indies, then undergoing quarantine. The brig had no sickness on board, but had lost one or more of her men with yellow fever during her stay at Havana. Abbott recovered.

"On the 31st of July, Denner, residing at 125 East Bay (near Pinckney street), was taken with fever and sent to the Roper Hospital; it being ascertained that he had been loading the bark Industria, at quarantine, from West Indies, he was ordered to the Lazaretto by the Mayor, and died with black vomit on the 7th of August.

"The bark Baldur, at Brown's Wharf, arrived on the 22d of July from Bordeaux, after a passage of sixty days. On the 30th, three of her seamen were taken with fever, which was pronounced by the attending physician to be bilious catarrhal. One of these died on the fifth day; the other two recovered. [These cases are not included in the enumeration.]

"On the 25th of July, a young man from Tennessee, but ten days in the city, and residing on King Street, between Hasell and Wentworth streets, was taken with fever. His physician states that it was a strongly-marked case; he recovered.

"The bark Jasper arrived on the 21st of July, from New York; lay at Accommodation Wharf. On the 1st of August, one of her seamen, Joseph Diola, an Italian, was taken with fever, and admitted into the Marine Hospital on the 2d; he died on the 10th, after excessive hemorrhage from gums and bowels.

"The schooner George Harris arrived on the 21st of July, from Baltimore, after a passage of eight days; lay at Central Wharf, next above Accommodation. On the 3d of August, Pettighon, one of her crew, complained of being unwell, and was sent into the Marine Hospital on the next day, and died on the 8th with black vomit.

"Crowell, another of the same crew, entered hospital on same day and recovered.

"On the 5th of August, Nelson, an inmate of Marine Hospital for four months (with fractured leg), was taken with the fever, and died on the 10th, with slight hemorrhage from the tongue.

"Mrs. Molona, twenty months in Charleston from Ireland, and residing in Weems' Court, near the southern end of King Street, was attacked on the 5th of August. After a very severe illness she recovered. Upon inquiry, it was found that her habits were good; that she visited the market every Saturday; that on the day of her attack had visited Vendue Range to make some purchase; had never been on any of the wharves, or visited any one whose business called them there; her husband had been working for several months in the western part of the city.

"The ship Royal Victoria arrived from England on the 8th of July, and lay at Union Wharf; on the 4th of August went round to the Ashley River and lay in the stream a short distance from Chisolm's Mill; on the 7th, one of the mates entered the Marine Hospital with yellow fever—he recovered.

"On the 5th of August, an Irishman, named Matthews, residing on Mazyck Street, but recently removed from the corner of Elizabeth and Washington streets, was attacked with fever, and after a few days sent to the Roper Hospital. He had an attack of fever during the epidemic of 1852, and had never been out of the city since. He was employed on the new custom house, and had been drinking hard for two weeks. The attending physician regards it as a case of fever—recovered.

"On the 6th, an Irishwoman, who had been residing in same house on Elizabeth Street, but recently removed to Laurens Street, was attacked and recovered.

"On the 7th of August, Mr. Chamberlain, of New York, a resident of the city for seven months, and residing on Society Street, near Meeting, was violently attacked, and died on the 10th, having had hemorrhage from the bowels. The history of this case has been closely investigated, and the disease cannot be traced to any imprudence or contact with infected person or vessel.

"On the 9th of August, Captain Crowhurst, of the Royal Victoria, was attacked, and is now recovering. (The history of this ship has been given above.)

"On the 9th of August, Mrs. Kegan, residing in same yard with Mrs. Molona, in Weems' Court, was attacked with fever. Had not been out of her house for two months, and had not seen Mrs. Molona, although residing in the same yard. The attack was rather mild, and she recovered.

"The bark Carolina, from New York, arrived, on the 24th of July, at Accommodation Wharf; on the 4th of August one of her crew was lodged in jail as a witness; was attacked with fever on the 10th, and recovered.

"On the 11th of August, two seamen from the Royal Victoria, still in the Ashley River, entered the Marine Hospital. One died on the 15th, with black vomit; the other recovered.

"On the 11th of August, Richard Clark, from bark Helois, in dry dock, was sent into Marine Hospital with fever, and recovered.

"On the 11th of August, Thomas Lawson was admitted into Marine Hospital from schooner G. Tittle. The schooner was from Philadelphia; had been three weeks at Central Wharf, and eight days in Ashley River, before Lawson was attacked—he recovered.

"J. H. Frederick, from schooner G. Harris, entered the Marine Hospital on the 12th of August, and died on the 15th.

"Dunbar and Painter, from schooner Tittle, entered Marine Hospital on the 14th of August; were removed to the Lazaretto on the 15th; the first recovered; the latter died with black vomit on the 19th.

"The steamer George's Creek arrived from Baltimore on the 11th of August; on the 8th, during her voyage, two seamen were taken sick; on the 13th, they were sent to the Lazaretto, where one died on the 15th with black vomit; the other recovered.

"On the 15th of August, an unacclimated slave, residing in Legaré Street, near South Bay, was attacked; had hemorrhage from gums and uterus; regarded by the physician in attendance as a very severe case—recovered.

"Hansler, a seaman from schooner Webster, and residing in Marine Hospital since 2d of August (in venereal ward), was attacked severely with fever on 15th —is now recovering. His nurse, from Maine, in hospital about three months, has also been attacked, and died this evening, 25th.

"Mrs. L———, from Philadelphia, in Charleston one year, and residing in Queen Street near Rutledge, was attacked on the 15th; has had black vomit, but is now recovering.

"Thomas Kegan (a son of Mrs. Kegan, in Weems' Court, before mentioned), was attacked with fever on the 15th; has had black vomit—recovered.

"On the 16th of August, Douglass and his wife, eight weeks in the city, and residing at 125 East Bay, near Pinckney Street, were attacked with fever—both have recovered.

"Ann and Bridget Burns, aged 6 and 17 years, twelve months from Ireland, residing in Pinckney Street, near the last mentioned cases, were attacked on the 17th and 18th of August. Both had black vomit; the elder died on the 23d; the younger is recovering.

"A German girl, residing in Queen Street, near Mrs. L———, was attacked on the 17th; has had black vomit; is recovering.

"Elizabeth Graham, from Ireland, four years in Charleston, was seen by a physician for the first time on the 21st; died same day with black vomit. Resided in Cromwell's Court, immediately opposite Marine Hospital.

"Two other sons of Mrs. Kegan, in Weems' Court, were attacked, the one on the 19th, the other on the 21st of August. They are now under treatment, and likely to recover.

"A German girl, five months in Charleston, was admitted into the Roper Hospital on the 23d; presumed to be sick five or six days; had resided on Vendue Range; died same night with black vomit.

"On the 23d, an Irishman was admitted into the Roper Hospital from Queen Street, near State. Also, an inmate of the hospital (with sore leg) since 24th of July, was attacked. Both still under treatment.

"I have heard of new cases in the past two days in the following localities, but have not been able as yet to get particulars: One in Queen Street near Meeting; one at the corner of St. Michael's Alley and Church Street: one at the corner of Market and Anson streets; and one in State Street, between Queen and Chalmers. The first mate of the Royal Victoria is also sick on East Bay, and three of the crew on board of the vessel in the stream.

"The disease spreads so slowly as to induce strong hopes that we shall yet be spared the infliction of an epidemic.

"The foregoing sum up a total of forty-seven cases that have occurred on shipboard and in the city, out of which thirteen have died; twenty-eight recovered, and the balance under treatment."

Origin of Yellow Fever in New Orleans in 1856.—Case I.—July 27, 1856, James Hawkins, a native of Kentucky, but late a resident of Arkansas, entered ward 33, Charity Hospital. Patient is one of the "La Paz prisoners," and has recently returned to this country from his long captivity in Mexico. He reached Vera Cruz, from the city of Mexico, about the 10th of July, inst., remained there until the 20th, and took passage on the steamship Texas, for New Orleans. He reached New Orleans on the 25th of July, sick with fever, though able to walk a little. Had felt unwell on the 24th, and had a chill, followed by fever, on the 25th. On his arrival, he was taken to the Rainbow Hotel, corner of New Levee and Notre Dame Streets. Remained there until the 27th, when, being worse, he entered the hospital. When he entered the ward he had fever.

28th, morning. Skin hot and dry pulse 94; tongue coated white, with red edges; great thirst; pains in head and lumbar region; vomiting bile.

Evening. Fever still continues; still vomiting; skin moist and turning yellow.

29th, morning. Pulse 56; great nausea; vomiting clear fluid in small quantities; no pain; skin moist and cool.

2 P.M. Vomits dark matter; very restless: pulse 64, and undulating.

30th, morning. Pulse 62, and soft; tongue red, with a dark stripe down the centre; vomiting black matter without much effort.

3 P.M. Pulse quick and feeble; delirious; still vomits black matter; subsultus tendinum.

5½ P.M. Is dying.

The above is a history of Case No. 1, derived in part from notes taken by a very intelligent student of medicine, who marked the case down as yellow fever from the moment of first seeing him, and partly from a very clear and intelligent history given us by a comrade who came over on the Texas with Hawkins. We did not see the case until the morning of the 30th. At this time the man was yellow, delirious, and throwing up black vomit freely. Indeed we have never seen a "better" case of yellow fever.

An autopsy was performed in this case, and all the characteristics of yellow fever were present.

Case II.—Aug. 13, Eugene Claudel, native of France, aged 30 years, labourer, entered ward 13. Patient is from the city of Mexico, where he has resided for eighteen months past. Left that place on the 1st of August, on horseback. Arrived in Vera Cruz and spent two days and nights there, previous to his departure for New Orleans, on board the steamship Texas, on the 8th inst. Felt perfectly well when he left, but on the 10th, towards evening, felt some pain in the head, which was soon followed by a chill, and then a burning fever. Did nothing but drink water freely while on the boat. On his arrival at New Orleans, August 12, he was conveyed to a French boarding-house, but, being a stranger, he does not know the locality of the same. Was admitted into the hospital on the morning of 13th, died on the 14th.

We saw this patient, and he was a type case of yellow fever. A post-mortem was held, and confirmed the diagnosis.

Case III.—Lawrence Olsen, a native of Denmark, æt. 40 years. In New Orleans two years. Labourer. Entered ward 12, on the 14th of August. Died on same day.

This patient was delirious when he entered, and could give no account of himself, and unfortunately no further history than the above was elicited from those who brought him to the hospital. We have made every effort to trace him up, but in vain. He was undoubtedly a case of yellow fever.

Case IV.—Valentine Neu, a native of Prussia, æt. 23 years, shoemaker, six months in New Orleans, last from Pittsburg, entered ward 12, on 10th of August. Had fever, but yellow fever was not suspected. On the 16th, he became worse, threw up black vomit, and died. He was undoubtedly a case of yellow fever.

Since the death of this man we have used every exertion to trace up his place of residence, etc. We have succeeded in tracing him to the Rainbow Hotel, where Hawkins (Case No. 1) was sick after his arrival on the steamship Texas. The obliging proprietor of the Rainbow showed us his register, and there is the name of the patient. He had been boarding at this hotel since January last.

CASE V.—Edward Duffy, native of Lowell, Mass., though of Irish descent, æt. 21 years, entered ward 13, on 13th of August. Has been engaged running on towboats between the Balize and this city for three months past.

We saw this man on the morning of the 13th, when we went in to see Case II. He was lying on an adjoining bed, and had a high fever. We noted him more particularly as being one of seven men in the ward who had never had yellow fever, and we were anxious to see whether any such individuals would contract the disease from the Vera Cruz case. He died on the 16th, of genuine yellow fever, and the post-mortem revealed all the characteristics of this disease.

Such is a history of the five first cases occurring in the Charity Hospital this season. There were several other cases occurring simultaneously with these, one from Mexico, per steamship Texas, and one taken sick at the Rainbow Hotel; but as they were considered doubtful, or even more than doubtful by some medical gentlemen, we refrain from giving any account of them. We have shown that yellow fever has been introduced into the city from Vera Cruz, and in spite of quarantine; it remains to be seen whether it will spread—whether we are to have an epidemic.

Since writing the foregoing, there have been two or three other cases in the hospital, though they have certainly occurred since the introduction of the imported cases, and present comparatively little interest. We hear of two or three undoubted cases in private practice, though we have seen none ourselves. All are said to be among the labouring class of persons.

It will be perceived, by reference to the mortuary reports of the city, that seven deaths by yellow fever are reported for the four weeks ending August 23d. Five of these are the cases just cited in detail. Of the remaining two, only one is considered undoubted. This one was seen late in July by a physician in the lower part of the city, who reports the case to the Board of Health as yellow fever, but says he was called in only in time to see the man die. He learned that he had been taken from an American schooner just arrived at New Orleans, but could get no particulars.—*New Orleans Medical Times*, September, 1856.

Vaccina and Variola.—DR. MORLAND reported to the Boston Society for Medical improvement the following interesting case:—

"On the 13th of February last, he vaccinated a healthy male infant, six months old. On the 17th of the same month, a faint, but sufficiently distinct, eruption of measles was observed about the neck and shoulders. The usual symptoms of rubeola had declared themselves on the next morning after the vaccination, and the disease, consequently, must have commenced only a few hours previously to that operation, if four days be adopted as the period elapsing between the attack and the appearance of the eruption. The vaccine vesicle matured very slowly for several days, and the rubeolous eruption continued with varying distinctness, but always comparatively slight, until the 19th of February, when it disappeared. The vaccine vesicle then took a start, and went on rapidly to perfection. There seemed to be a retarding action reciprocally maintained for a time by the two affections, thus accidentally concurrent; vaccinia finally prevailing. The circumstantial record, made at the time, reads thus:—

"*February 17th.*—Vaccination apparently taking effect; measles appeared; will the vesicle be retarded?

"*18th.*—Vesicle advancing very slowly; measles retrograding; ordered a warm bath.

"*19th.*—Vesicle going on, but more slowly than is common; less redness around it; eruption of measles gone; will it recur?

"*20th.*—Vaccine vesicle much larger; child feverish; warm bath.

"*21st.*—At 7¼ o'clock in the morning, the child was seized with a severe general convulsion. He was seen by Dr. M. in about twenty minutes; a warm bath had been used. Wine of ipecac. and enemata, with cold lotions to the head, were at once resorted to, and, subsequently, three grains of calomel with five of rhubarb were given. Aspect of the little patient pale and confused. At 1¾ o'clock P. M., he had another convulsive attack, of rather greater severity. By previous direction, he was immediately placed in a warm bath, the body and limbs were well rubbed with the hand, and sinapisms were applied to the abdomen and to the feet; the face being dark-coloured and the scalp showing many turgid vessels, a large leech was applied to the left temple, and the wound was allowed to bleed for half an hour after the animal fell off. No more convulsions through the day. At 7½ o'clock P. M., mustard was applied to the back of the neck. The night of the 21st was passed by the patient in quiet sleep.

"*22d.*—Very bright and well, to all appearance, until 9½ o'clock A. M., when he had another very severe convulsion, lasting several minutes longer than the two previous ones. He was seen fifteen minutes after the access of the fit; was found stupid, with an occasional wild look of the eyes; had been placed again in the warm bath. Mustard-water frictions to the extremities were continued; the head being rather hot, cold applications were cautiously made to it; one drachm of castor oil was given; discontinued the breast milk. Dr. Storer saw the patient at this time, and recommended calomel and Dover's powder, one-eighth of a grain of the former to one-half a grain of the latter, every three hours. A continuance of the mustard-water frictions was also advised. Dr. S. believed that another leech might be needed. Dr. James Jackson, who had been sent for at Dr. M.'s request, visited the child shortly after, and gave a favourable prognosis. It was thought best by him to restrict the child's nursing to one minute's time every two hours; and, in the intervals, to allow sugar and water. Dr. J. thought that, although another leech might, possibly, be required, he should 'be slow to apply it.' The remainder of the management was concurred in. The powders above mentioned were commenced, and the other means continued. There seemed a degree of amendment in the afternoon of this day, and there had been some good sleep. The night of the 22d was quietly passed; there was only one dejection; a little colicky pain from flatulence; no convulsive action.

"*23d.*—Quite well, seemingly; pulse 118, rather sharp (yesterday, 128 to 130); skin moist; one powder was taken at bed-time last evening, and another this morning. The vesicle of vaccination has broken and partially dried into quite a large scab; it was full, yesterday. In the afternoon of this day the child seemed dull and stupid, possibly from fatigue; the lips and tongue somewhat swollen; suspended the regular use of the powders; renewed the mustard frictions, &c. He was now allowed to draw the breast during three minutes, not having nursed for three hours previously. Flatulence troublesome; relieved by mint-water.

"*24th.*—Night quiet; had one dejection; got one powder about midnight; the eyes somewhat red; no signs of returning rubeolous eruption; tongue white; occasional colic.

"*25th.*—Nearly as well as ever.

"*26th.*—Same record.

"*27th.*—A cervical gland, on the left side (that of the vaccination), much enlarged; otherwise very well and lively. Discontinued visits. From the last date to the present time, there has been no untoward occurrence, the child seeming better, even, than before his illness.

"The supervention of measles upon vaccination, by the doctrine of chances, must be rare; a purely accidental occurrence. The points of interest in this case are the evident mutually retarding influence of the two affections thus coexisting; the modification of the vaccine vesicle and of the eruption of rubeola by this action—not uncommonly witnessed under such, or similar, circumstances of complication—and, especially, the convulsions, as to their *cause*. Dr. M. was at first inclined to ascribe these to the retrocession of the measles; but it will be noted that they were manifested upon the eighth day after vaccination, when the vesicle should be perfect and the primary febrile action is usually observed—and consequently they may be more reasonably referred to the latter. This was Dr. Jackson's opinion. How much influence the conjunction of the two affections may have had, however, can hardly be determined. In his recently-published volume, Dr. Jackson gives an instance where convulsions took place in a child, on the eighth day after vaccination.

Some time previous to this, the patient had had pneumonia, which was ushered in by convulsions, and the same had occurred, also, during dentition. Dr. J. had apprehended they might take place after the vaccination, and had forewarned the mother on the subject. He refers to other cases in which convulsions were observed in children at the commencement of bronchitis and searlatina, but mentions only one after vaccination. In the case detailed above, there had not been any convulsions, previously, nor any threatening of them; there was, therefore, no reason to expect them.

"In this connection, the remark of Sydenham may appropriately be referred to, that 'an epileptic fit, in infants, is so sure a sign of smallpox, that if, after teething, they have one, you may predict variola—so much so, that a fit over night will be followed by the eruption next morning. This, however, will be generally mild, and in no wise confluent.' (*Works*, Syd. Soc. edit., vol. ii. p. 252.) Dr. Jackson also remarked that 'he believed convulsions are not rare in children, when the symptoms, so called, of smallpox first appear—corresponding to the eighth day of vaccination.' It would seem that the accident must be infrequent after simple vaccination."—*Boston Med. and Surg. Journ.*, June 19th, 1856.

Poisoning by Strychnia successfully treated by Camphor.—Prof. ROCHESTER communicated to the Buffalo Medical Association, February 11, 1856, the following example of this:—

"Feb. 2, 1856. I. De F., aged thirty-two years, was admitted about 5 P. M. He had taken strychnia with a view of self-destruction. It was swallowed at 4 P. M., and was said by him to have been four grains in amount. Supposing a fatal effect certain and speedy, he mentioned to an acquaintance what he had done. Large draughts of whiskey were poured down him immediately, and he was hurried to the hospital. In the absence of the house physician, Dr. B. H. Lemon, a messenger was dispatched for Dr. Rochester, who arrived at 7 P. M., and reports as follows:—

"'The patient, a robust and athletic man, was much excited; his eye was bright and wild; his countenance flushed, and his respiration hurried; he complained of great thirst, and of a burning sensation at the epigastrium. The pulse was slightly accelerated, but not increased in force. He had been vomiting very freely; the emesis being produced by copious draughts of warm milk administered by the Sisters of Charity. The iris responded readily to the tests of sensibility. I was informed that he had had several tetanic convulsions, the last of which had just taken place, and was unusually long and severe. I directed a large sinapism to be applied to the epigastrium, and gave him two grains of powdered camphor, with half a teaspoonful of the tr. of camphor, suspended in water. The sinapism had hardly been applied, and the camphor taken, when a spasm commenced, first manifesting itself in the cervical muscles, then in those of the arms and chest, the latter producing slight opisthotonos, and lastly, in those of the face, turning the eyes into their orbits, and setting the lower jaw firmly. The countenance became turgid, and the jugulars were enormously distended. The pulse numbered 88 per minute, and preserved its rhythm. Respiration seemed to be entirely suspended; no respiratory murmur was detected, but the heart's sounds were quite audible. The strong contraction of the pectoral muscles produced so much noise, that the pulmonary auscultation was incomplete. The nares were distended, and remained so. The paroxysm lasted about three minutes, and then ceased, with sudden muscular relaxation, and with a deep inspiration. The Sister of Charity in attendance told me that the preceding convulsion had been longer, and that it was cut short by the application to the nares of the vapour of strong aqua ammonia. The spasm over, the patient complained of slight headache and of intense thirst; his respiration was again hurried, and his wild manner returned. His aspect and condition were not unlike those of Myer, the hydrophobic patient whom I saw with Dr. Hawley, and other medical gentlemen, some two years ago.

"'I directed the sinapisms to be removed from the epigastrium, and placed over the cervical and dorsal vertebræ, and repeated the camphor as before, with the addition of half a grain of morphine. At 7.35 a spasm similar to the one described, occurred; confident in the antidote properties of the camphor, I directed it to be given every fifteen minutes, and left the patient in charge of Dr. J. D. Freeman, who kindly consented to remain with him until the arrival of Dr. Lemon. The latter returned to the hospital about 9 P. M., and reports: 'Respiration 55 per minute; pulse 80. A spasm at 9 o'clock and 10 minutes—duration two minutes. There was opisthotonos, with intense contraction of masseter, sterno-mastoid, pectoral, biceps, and gastrocnemii muscles. Spasms occurred at 9.25, 9.45, 10.15, and at 10.25. This proved to be the last, and was like a very severe chill; the one at 10.15 lasted five minutes, and was very severe. At 11.30 there had been no recurrence of either spasm or chill. I directed a little chicken broth and weak brandy and water, and left him with directions to be called if there should be any untoward symptoms. His respiration at this time had fallen to 40; pulse 88. He vomited several times on taking the camphor, but the dose was immediately repeated, and was not rejected on its second administration. To relieve the thirst and allay the vomiting, small pieces of ice were given.

" 'Feb. 3. Is much better this morning; has slept some; says he is hungry; is not thirsty, and has little or no pain at the epigastrium. Pulse 86; respiration 20; pupils natural; no headache.

" 'Directed light diet, and to remain in bed. The camphor, of which he took in all about ʒj, produced neither cerebral or gastric derangement.

" 'Feb. 4. Patient entirely recovered.'

"Dr. Rochester remarked that this was the second case reported by him to the society this year, where camphor had been successfully employed to counteract the effects of strychnia; he thought there was no doubt as to its properties as an antidote. Might it not possibly be successfully used in cases of traumatic and idiopathic tetanus?"—*Buffalo Medical Journal*, March, 1856.

Reduction of Dislocation into Axilla of Eighty Days' Standing; Rupture of Axillary Artery; Ligature of that Vessel; Death from Secondary Hemorrhage.—Dr. Geo. C. Blackman, in a letter to the editor of the *Western Lancet* (Aug. 1856), gives the following account of this case:—

"About the 10th of July, aided by yourself, I succeeded in reducing by manipulation, without the pulleys, a dislocation into the axilla, of eighty days' standing. The reduction was accomplished in a very few minutes, under the influence of chloroform and ether, and the next morning the patient left for the country, in a comfortable condition. Since that I have received no tidings from him. Encouraged by the result in this case, another patient, himself a physician, a tall, athletic man, and about fifty years of age, decided to submit to the same manipulation, although his arm had been dislocated for about sixteen weeks. The dislocation was downward and inward, and, about the tenth week, an unsuccessful attempt, by another surgeon, had been made with the pulleys, to which the force of six men was applied for two and a half hours. The patient being under the influence of chloroform and ether, aided by yourself, Drs. Fries, Cary, Graham, and Kaufman, I commenced my manipulations, adducting, rotating, abducting, and elevating the arm. These efforts had been made for about ten minutes, and the least possible violence employed, when a tumefaction appeared in the pectoral region, which in a few minutes attained considerable size. Supposing that the axillary artery was ruptured, as no pulse could be felt at the wrist, a ligature was immediately applied to the vessel at the upper part of its course. The operation was performed about 10 o'clock A. M., and compression of the pectoral region made by means of a sponge and broad roller. On removing this the next morning, the tumefaction had nearly disappeared. The patient continued comfortable, and, about nine days after the application of the ligature, I was compelled to leave the city on a professional visit to Indiana. I left on Friday afternoon, and returned on Monday morning, at which time I learned that my patient had died on Sunday morning, from hemorrhage at the seat of ligature. Two physicians, his most intimate friends, lodged in the same house with him, but before they reached his bedside, the quantity of blood lost was so great, that he sank exhausted in about two hours from the first and *only* attack of hemorrhage. Previous to my departure for

Indiana, I had suggested to the physicians in charge the importance of having compressed sponge at hand, to be used in any emergency of the kind, but this was not used by the attendant; instead of applying pressure instantaneously, he went in search of the physicians, who, at that early hour in the morning, were in bed. The time thus lost unquestionably led to the fatal catastrophe."

Removal of the Inverted Uterus.—Dr. C. G. PUTNAM, read before the Boston Society for Medical Improvement (Feb. 11, 1856), a history of three cases of removal of inverted uterus under the care of Dr. Channing and himself. The specimens were exhibited at a previous meeting.

It is now three years since the operations were done, and during this interval we have carefully watched the result. One of the patients was for some months subject to leucorrhœal discharges, and in another there had been an occasional approach to something like menstruation; but they are at present in excellent health and spirits, illustrating the observation of M. A. Petit, that the uterus belongs less to the individual than to the species, and proving that nature can support the loss without material disturbance in the harmony of her functions.

The first was that of a young woman, 20 years of age, with her second child. On application to Dr. Channing, she stated that "dreadful" pain attended the extraction of the placenta, and the "flowing" was excessive. She was able to nurse her child for three months, though flowing more or less all the time. Immediately upon the suspension of nursing, the hemorrhage became incessant; and when visited, twelve months after childbirth, she was bloodless, anasarcous, and hardly able to move about. He attempted, under the influence of ether, to re-invert the uterus; but failing in this, the ligature of cord was applied, and the ends brought through so that the pressure could be graduated by a screw. The ligature came off on the eleventh day. It was tightened more or less every day; but in this, as in the other two cases, whenever the pressure was carried beyond a certain point, there ensued vomiting, faintness, depression of pulse and other symptoms of strangulation, which made it necessary to relax it. Her recovery was perfect.

CASE II.—The result of this case was not so fortunate. The patient recovered from the effect of the operation, but died from the effects of ill-timed exertion, in the same manner as, after an exhausting hemorrhage, death sometimes follows the mere rising up in bed. A young woman, originally of healthy constitution, æt. 25. She had had two confinements within three years. The first time had twins, and was much enfeebled by nursing both. The third child she nursed nearly nine months, and was "pretty well," though frequently "flowing." When she ceased nursing, menstruation recurred at short intervals, and very copiously, and she began to suffer palpitation, throbbing in head, faintness, and dyspnœa on any exertion. It was evident that these symptoms were sympathetic with some uterine lesion, and upon further inquiry it appeared that at the time of delivery, though not aware of any extraordinary pain, hemorrhage, or faintness, yet she never "felt quite right" about the pelvis. During the first week sat up in bed and moved about the bed more freely than usual. On the eighth day, having got out of bed to evacuate the bowels, she felt something protruding from the external organs, considerably larger than an orange. She suffered much distress until it was replaced in the vagina; and though it never again appeared externally, she was occasionally obliged to press it upward in order to relieve a painful sense of pressure. The local uneasiness gradually diminished, and she continued to nurse her child till it died at the ninth month. Immediately upon weaning, she began to "flow" almost constantly, but was able to attend to her household duties for eight months, when she suffered so much from faintness that she was compelled to remain in bed.

The most prominent symptoms at this time, when I was consulted, were palpitation, throbbing in the head, dyspnœa on motion, urgent thirst. She was exceedingly pale; pulse 120, feeble; tongue white. On examination, a tumour was felt high up the vagina, apparently two inches in length, an inch and a half in thickness, and about two inches in breadth. The os uteri soft and distensible, and so nearly effaced that it might readily have been mistaken for a fold of the vagina encircling the upper part of the tumour. This sulcus, about two-thirds of an inch deep, could be traced all round the circle, and at no point could the finger or sound be passed further. The colour was a deep strawberry red.

She had just finished a menstrual period, and I decided to do the operation at once, so that it might be completed before the recurrence of another. The ligature was applied on the upper portion of the tumour (it could not be called a neck, for there was less narrowing than one would have expected), the ends being passed through a canula and made fast to a button moved by a screw.

The first constriction was followed in about four minutes by pain, failure of the pulse, which dropped from 120 to 90, coldness of the surface, vomiting, and other symptoms of strangulation. It was immediately relaxed, and the pain subdued by opiates and inhalation of ether. During the night, vomited twice. Slept at intervals. Opiate repeated. During the next day had copious serous discharge from vagina. The tumor tense, not tender to touch. Pulse 112. Skin soft. The ligature again tightened, causing very severe pain, which recurred in paroxysms. Opiates and ether repeated.

It will not be necessary to give the occurrences of each day, but I will merely say that the ligature was tightened every twenty-four hours as much as the patient could endure. The excretion of serum continued quite freely—at last attended with fetor. On the eighth day the tumour was less tense, but as it still seemed not to be entirely detached, no efforts were made to remove it.

Up to the 9th day, she was evidently improving in spirits, appetite, and strength. She had slept well the previous night, and in the morning, without asking leave, had her clothes changed and her bed made; and when visited, soon afterwards, she was very languid, unwilling to move, not faint but "terribly tired." From this state of depression, she never rose; her slight stock of strength had been entirely wasted by this unnecessary exertion, and she died in three days afterwards.

On examination after death, the tumour was found to be detached—hanging by a few shreds only. The pelvic organs were healthy, cicatrization perfect, the strangulation of the tumour having thus been effected without inducing peritonitis, and with comparatively slight constitutional irritation.

Case III.—A young woman, æt. 23. Second confinement. She stated to Dr. Channing that she had unusual pain and hemorrhage during the delivery of the placenta. Was unable to nurse the child on account of deficient nipples, and flowing continued for a year, almost without interval. The exhaustion became extreme, and she seemed to be failing rapidly.

In this, as in the other cases, an ineffectual attempt was made to re-invert the uterus before applying the ligature. She was unusually sensitive, and it was sometimes necessary to change the pressure of the ligature three or four times in the course of a day. The tumour was separated in about a fortnight.

From the symptoms which attended these three cases, it is probable that inversion occurred at the time of delivery. There is reason to believe, however, that it may take place gradually, and some evidence is offered to show that it may occur a considerable time after an apparently natural delivery.—*Boston Med. and Surg. Journ.*

Removal of the Entire Clavicle.—Dr. Geo. C. Blackman, Professor of Surgery in the Medical College of Ohio, states (*Western Lancet*, June, 1856) that on the first of May last, he saw, in consultation with Dr. Wm. Wood, a man aged 42, who had suffered from caries of the clavicle for more than a year. The first fistulous opening formed near the junction of the outer with the inner third of the bone, and just within this point it seemed excavated and expanded to a considerable extent. From its inferior margin there was a sharp and ragged bony projection which proved to be a true exostosis. About an inch external to the sterno-clavicular articulation, there was a second fistulous opening through which a considerable quantity of matter was daily discharged. The adjacent integuments were of an unhealthy aspect, presenting every indication of extensive disease at the articulation.

Assisted by Drs. Wood, Gray, and his pupil, Mr. Jones, Dr. B. proceeded at once to the removal of the bone. The patient having been brought under the influence of a mixture of chloroform and ether, he commenced his incision about the middle of the sternum, and carried it to the external fistulous opening. Great care was taken in isolating the bone from its important connections, and it was divided with a saw at the point above indicated, with the hope that the external third might be saved. On a more careful examination of the latter, however, it was found to be in an unsound condition, and was removed to its junction with the acromion. The interarticular cartilage at the sterno-clavicular articulation was softened, and a considerable portion of it had disappeared. The internal third of the bone was disorganized beyond the power of reparation or of removal, unassisted by art. The operation being completed, a little lint was introduced, the integuments brought together, and the whole neatly dressed by Dr. Wood, under whose skilful attention the patient was enabled in ten days to attend to his business. Three weeks have now elapsed since the operation, and not an unpleasant symptom has appeared; nor are there any indications of the extension of the malady to the sternum.

Fatal Hemorrhage from Tapping an Ovarian Tumour.—Dr. E. A. Peaslee presented to the New York Pathological Society (Feb. 13, 1856) an encysted ovarian tumour, weighing 45 pounds, removed from a lady aged 41, who first observed a tumour in the left iliac region between three and four years ago, which has gradually increased up to the present time (Feb., '56), with slight fluctuations in size. It had from the first been regarded as *ovarian.* The patient was first seen by Dr. P. in May, 1855, she wishing to obtain his opinion in regard to the propriety of an operation for its removal by the large abdominal section. On examination, he found the abdominal circumference to be 47 inches, the walls of the abdomen so tense that he could not decide whether the mass consisted of many or few distinct sacs. The general condition of the patient was so low, that he did not for a moment entertain the idea of an operation, and gave his opinion accordingly.

He did not again see her till the 25th of last month (Jan., '56) when he was again requested to remove the mass. To his surprise, her condition had much improved since May, '55 (though she had failed during the past summer); and, though the tumour had risen somewhat higher in the epigastrium, her circumference was but 48 inches. Appetite pretty good, respiration somewhat hurried, though, when sitting or lying quiet, there was no dyspnœa. Bowels regular; action of kidneys rather free. He did not, however, *advise* the operation of ovariotomy; though to her inquiry, whether she was apparently in as good a general condition as the two persons on whom he had operated successfully, he was obliged to reply in the affirmative; and, moreover, that it was impossible to ascertain whether the mass was adherent or not, without previously evacuating the sacs, by tapping, to such an extent as to admit a more exact examination, and that he could not express any opinion in favour of ovariotomy without previously tapping her; and if, in doing this, he found the mass extensively adherent, or could not decide that it was *not* adherent, in that event he would not entertain the idea of an operation. He did not advise the tapping even, since, though he regarded this operation as hardly dangerous in any degree, she was informed that the mass might be made up of very many small sacs, and without a single large one, and in that case she would be disappointed, and *he* should not arrive at any positive result as to the adhesion or non-adhesion of the tumour. The patient had a decided aversion to being tapped, unless she was assured that ovariotomy would follow, since a sister, who had been tapped a few years since, for the same disease, died a week after of peritonitis, and because she supposed, if once tapped, a repetition of the operation would be frequently necessary. After a deliberation of five days on the subject, the patient again sent for Dr. P., and informed him that she had decided to be tapped, as preliminary to the decision of the question whether he would perform ovariotomy or not. The operation was performed, in the usual way, on the 4th inst., assisted by Dr. Ranney, of Twenty-third Street. Her condition was good. Fluctuation indicated the existence of a distinct sac of considerable size, in and below the umbilical region, and another higher up. The former was at once reached by the trocar, and six pints of clear and highly gelatinous fluid (to the sense of touch) evacuated; and. on partially withdrawing the canula, two pints more of a milky fluid were withdrawn, evidently from another sac, which had been traversed by the instrument, while on its way to the larger one. On changing the direction of the canula to penetrate another sac, a few drops of venous blood flowed through the instrument. This he thought proceeded from a minute vessel on the interior of the sac, which had been punctured, as he had seen the same thing before. Several smaller sacs were then punctured, and, on withdrawing the canula as before, a few drops of venous blood again appeared. Fearing this might escape, through the puncture in the sac, into the cavity of the peritoneum, he waited until the dropping entirely ceased, and then withdrew the canula. With a curved trocar, other more distant sacs were evacuated. The mass now seemed to be composed of small cysts, and it seemed impossible to reduce the tumour much more. Further attempt was therefore discontinued. More blood now flowed through the canula; he waited till all oozing ceased, before finally withdrawing the instrument. Fifteen pounds of fluid had been withdrawn. The patient was fatigued by the prolonged operation, and depressed in mind from the fact that the operation must fail to demonstrate the adherence or non-adherence of the tumour; but, with the exception of some faintness and sickness of the stomach, nothing worthy of mention occurred. The tumour could be slightly moved below the umbilicus, but not at all at the upper part; the idea of the operation of ovariotomy was therefore abandoned. The next morning before 10 o'clock he was requested to visit the patient in haste, as she seemed to be sinking; before he arrived, she was dead. She had passed a tolerably comfortable night, with sickness of the stomach at times, but presented no grave symptoms till 8 o'clock, when her expression changed, and she became restless, and died before 10.

Post-mortem examination, 6½ hours after death.—Some bloody serum had escaped from the puncture through the abdominal walls. On cutting through the latter on the median line, a thick and very vascular membrane was found intervening between the parietal peritoneum and the ovarian mass; and a layer of bloody serum was seen between this and the mass, one or two inches deep. This membrane was found to cover over the whole tumour anteriorly and laterally, like an apron, it being also adherent to the tumour on both sides, as well as to the pelvis and the lower portion of the tumour. On further examination, the membrane just described was found to be the omentum major; and the hemorrhage had proceeded from a small vein, which had been punctured in penetrating it to reach the first sac. It had become so thick and firm, as well as vascular, by constant pressure and the motions of the tumour, that he had mistaken it for the wall of the sac first punctured, and the blood, which, during the operation, he supposed had flowed from the inner wall of the sac, had really flowed from the membrane just mentioned into the cavity, formed by the adhesions before specified, between itself and the diseased mass. But little bloody serum had escaped into the cavity of the peritoneum, and it was judged that not more than eight or ten ounces had been lost in all. The tumour (which was shown) was found extensively adherent to its upper and lateral portion, not so much so below the umbilicus. Its removal would not have been attempted during life, had it been exposed to view for that purpose, by any judicious surgeon. It was found to consist of an immense number of small sacs, as you perceive, and weighed forty-five pounds, making sixty pounds in all before the operation of paracentesis. It was chiefly developed from the left ovary, and both Fallopian tubes were closed up and distended with a putty-like substance, in which broken-up epithelial cells predominate.

It may be proper here to remark that, though a married lady for several years past, she had never been pregnant; menstruation had been regular till within the last year and a half. Dr. P. observed that the hemorrhage must be regarded as the "causa sine qua non" of death in this case. That is, had no hemorrhage occurred, death might not have taken place in any immediate connection with the operation. A quantity of blood between the omentum and the tumour, with a small amount also in the peritoneal cavity, must have in a few days led to a fatal result; but, in accounting for a death occurring within sixteen and a half hours after the operation, and where the amount of blood lost was so small, we should doubtless also take into consideration the exhaustion from the operation, and especially the mental shock produced by the knowledge that the operation had led to no positive result in diagnosis, and that therefore nothing further would be done.

The *source* of the *hemorrhage* was, as far as he knew, *peculiar*. Branches of the internal epigastric artery have sometimes been wounded; the bladder has been wounded; the uterus, happeuing to lie in front of the tumour, has also been punctured; and one of the Fallopian tubes, also, happening to be stretched over it in front, has been transfixed. But he has never heard of the greater omentum being injured by a puncture, at a point usually regarded as the safest, half way between the pubis and the umbilicus. Indeed, in all ordinary circumstances, where the abdomen is largely distended, it is impossible that the omentum should extend to this point. For it is not long enough, naturally, to extend even to the umbilicus in a case like this, even though it originally fall into the pelvis; and, moreover, it is uniformly, as far as he is aware, pushed up by the tumour during its development from below, and is generally found somewhat folded, and not reaching more than half the distance from the stomach to the umbilicus. In this case, the omentum was not less than two and a half feet long, as the specimen will show, since it completely covered the tumour anteriorly and laterally. And since, had it been free at its lower extremity at the time the tumour first began to grow, the latter would doubtless have merely lifted it up as is usual, Dr. P. inferred that the omentum had become adherent to some portion of the pelvic peritoneum before the tumour began to be developed. Thus the tumour grew upwards behind the omentum, which thus was expanded over the whole length of the tumour.

Finally, the whole extent of the omentum was equally vascular; and, had the puncture been made at any other point, there is no reason for believing that the hemorrhage would have been less than that which actually occurred.—*New York Medical Times*, May, 1856.

Bullet in Bronchial Tube, expelled after remaining there two weeks.—The following interesting case is related (*St. Louis Med. and Surg. Journ.*, Sept. 1856) by Dr. Samuel S. Emison, of Lafayette, Mo.:—

"On the 15th of May last, Emet Shannon, aged nine years, of good constitution, permitted a bullet, one-fourth of an inch in diameter, which he had in his mouth, to slip through the rima glottidis. He was instantly oppressed with violent dyspnœa and convulsive expiratory efforts, which continued ten or fifteen minutes, and were succeeded by prostration and pallor of face and lividity of lips.

"An hour after the accident, when I first saw him, he was cheerful and easy in all respects. There was no cough, dyspnœa, pain, nor was there any appreciable departure from the normal respiratory murmur. His whole appearance so little corresponded with what we supposed a foreign body, such as we have described, would produce, that we flattered his friends with the decided opinion, that it had passed into the œsophagus and that it would readily be expelled per viam naturalem. No change having taken place at the expiration of two hours, nothing was enjoined but quiet. Four hours after he was suddenly attacked with severe paroxysmal pain in the stomach and bowels. There being still no thoracic disturbance, the pains were ascribed to indigestible substances in the stomach, and an emetic given which brought up his unchanged breakfast, but no relief. A full dose of a mercurial and anodyne was given, and the anodyne repeated pro re nata, during the next twenty-four hours. During the afternoon of the 16th his pulse became frequent, face flushed and respiration accelerated: the pain in the stomach returned as soon as the effects of the anodyne abated. There were none of the physical signs indicative of congestion, or inflammation of the lungs. There was considerable indistinctness of the vesicular murmur in the subclavicular region, but no dulness on percussion of the left lung, anteriorly. Took hydr. submus. and comp. pul. opii et ipecac., every three hours. Afternoon of 17th—pulse 120; respiration very much accelerated; pain in the top of left shoulder; tenderness on percussion over the left subclavicular region; severe pain in the stomach and bowels, and tenderness and distension of both; complains now also of smothering sensations, and is disinclined to be raised up; there is now also an occasional hacking cough; no dulness, but almost entire want of vesicular murmur in the middle third of the left lung anteriorly. Could not examine posteriorly. Respiration in the right lung supplemental and great disparity in the movements of the two sides, the left being comparatively stationary. It was now clear that the ball had entered the left bronchus and was still occupying one of its branches. It was proposed to incline his head almost vertically downwards, with the hope, that while in that position, gravity aided by succussion would dislodge it, and that it would either be expelled, or if retained in the trachea might be removed by an operation. He would not consent to the experiment, and it was deemed hazardous to subject him to the use of chloroform for the purpose. A vein was opened, and after he had lost six or eight ounces of blood, his excitement from dread of the operation became so intense, that the vein was closed sooner than desirable; nevertheless the relief, so far as the thoracic distress was concerned, was immediate and decided. The pain in the stomach and bowels, which from the first was so severe as to mask other symptoms, was as severe as ever, except when he was fully under the influence of anodynes; and though its paroxysmal character and the absence of tenderness on pressure, for the first twenty-four hours, led to the conclusion that it was nervous and sympathetic, the tympanitic distension and tenderness now, the copious watery pea-green dejections which followed a dose of castor oil on the morning of the 18th, were thought to indicate a threatening of structural alteration. The mercurial and anodyne were continued till the 20th, when the general abatement of his distressing symptoms and the improved condition of alvine dejections induced a withdrawal of the mercurial.

"21*st.* Rests better; febrile excitement considerably abated; respiration very much less hurried, and the paroxysms of dyspnœa, or smothering as he called it, not troublesome; some dulness in the region where the vesicular murmur was noticed to have been obscured, and flatness and tubular respiration in the corresponding region behind, which could now be examined without giving him much pain.

"22*d.* Rests much better, and expresses for the first time some inclination for nourishment. Thoracic uneasiness not troublesome; physical signs same, no cough, but pain in the stomach and bowels still severe; febrile excitement confined principally to the early part of the night, followed by pretty free diaphoresis, not however colliquative. During the succeeding week his fever became less severe and of shorter duration each afternoon, his respiration during the remissions comparatively easy; little or no cough; dulness confined to the same region, neither increasing nor receding; appetite increasing, but the gastric and abdominal uneasiness persistent and alvine discharges were loaded with mucus. During this period he used comp. pulv. opii et ipecac., freely for his bowels, and assiduously warm fomentations. On the fourteenth day from the accident, he indulged his appetite quite freely, and had considerable fever with symptoms indicating an approaching extension of the pulmonary lesion. His bowels not having acted for several days, he was ordered three teaspoonfuls of castor oil, which operated harshly five or six times. He was excessively prostrated, and while being assisted to stool in this very relaxed condition, he had a very violent paroxysm of coughing, and the ball passed into his mouth, with inexpressible joy to those about him. For several hours after, he was on the verge of exhaustion, and took stimulants pretty freely.

"During the following night he expectorated considerable quantities of mucus and a small mammular sputum, resembling pus. His symptoms all gradually improved; the pain in the bowels, though troublesome, gradually disappeared. His appetite and strength improved slowly.

"*June* 10. Saw him to-day; dulness amounting to flatness over the region where it existed before, and tubular or blowing respiration in portions of the same district; no other sound audible. He is easily fatigued and respiration especially is hurried by exercise. His friends think he has had night-sweat for two nights past; no cough; pulse eighty; skin cold and relaxed; appetite good; walks about the room.

"*July* 20. His general appearance is as healthy as before the accident. Did not examine the chest, but suppose from his active and healthy appearance that his lung has resumed its normal state."

An Easy Mode of Constructing Bougies.—Dr. P. H. Cabell, of Selma, Ala., calls (*Virginia Med. Journ.*, April, 1856) attention to an easy and rapid mode of constructing bougies, which he thinks presents some advantages, both as to the qualities possessed, and the facility and cheapness with which they may be made. Reflecting upon the advantages the bougies made of elm bark possessed, from the ease with which they are introduced, and the expansion they undergo while in the urethra; and then thinking of the danger of breaking, the difficulty of treating deep-seated strictures, and the grave accidents which sometimes occur, Dr. C. determined to seek some substitute, which would possess its good qualities, and be free from all risk.

"The substance I finally selected was untanned cowhide; which may be obtained sometimes of great thickness. It is first to be well soaked in water, then cut into strips of suitable length and width, and tacked by the extremities over a block of wood of the proper curve. When wished straight, no form is necessary, they being merely stretched on a plane surface till dry. When dry, they are found very tough, unyielding, and of sufficient elasticity. They may be brought to the proper size by the knife, rasp, sandpaper, &c. and will be found to have a fine polish, which allows them to be introduced with ease; they are much more rigid than either the wax or gum instruments, but they are sufficiently yielding to be pefectly safe unless great violence is used, and even then I do not conceive that there could be much if any risk of making a false passage.

"There are two ways of preparing them for use—one by oiling as usual, and the other by dipping for a few moments in warm water. The point may be previously well softened by a longer immersion in water. It thus becomes almost jelly-like, and glides easily and painlessly along the urethra. If the surgeon does not wish to avail himself of their expansiveness in dilating the stricture, he may cover them with a solution of gutta percha, in chloroform, which will protect them from the action of the urethral mucus, and render them beautifully polished."

Vesico-Vaginal Fistula.—Dr. N. Bozeman, of Montgomery, Ala., has published (*Louisville Review*, May, 1856) some interesting "Remarks on Vesico-Vaginal Fistula, with an Account of a new mode of Suture, and seven Successful Operations."

Dr. B.'s new suture is, he observes, "only a modification of the twisted, as the clamp is a modification of the quill suture," p. 86. This suture Dr. B. calls the *Button Suture.*

"The essential parts of the apparatus consist of wire for the sutures, a metallic button or plate, and perforated shot to retain the latter in place. The wire should be made of pure silver, about the size usually marked No. 93, and properly annealed. A length of about eighteen inches should be allowed for each suture."

The button may be made of either lead or silver. "The former, hammered out to the thickness of 1-16th of an inch, answers the purpose tolerably well. The latter can be made still thinner, and does better on several accounts; it is lighter, less likely to yield under pressure, admits of a higher polish, and allows the wires to be drawn through the small holes without dragging.

"The object of the button is to cover the fistulous opening after the introduction of the sutures, and its size and shape will, therefore, vary somewhat according to circumstances. The shape of those that I usually employ is oval, but they may be made circular, semicircular, L or T shaped, to suit individual cases. The size will also necessarily vary, but it is seldom that one larger than 1 1-4 inches in length, and 5-8ths of an inch in breadth, is required. But, whatever the shape or size, it is a matter of great importance that the under surface should be slightly concave, and the edge turned up. Along the middle of the button are arranged perforations for the passage of the sutures, which should be sufficiently large to admit two thicknesses of the wire freely. The number of these openings will depend, of course, upon the number of the sutures, which are usually placed about 3·16ths of an inch apart."

Dr. B. claims for the button suture important advantages in the protection it affords to the denuded edges of the fistula. "It is a fact well known to surgeons," he observes, "that a simple incised wound will heal with much more rapidity when shielded from the atmosphere and all other extraneous influences, than, all other circumstances being equally favourable, when there is no such protection. Vesico-vaginal fistule, after the edges have been paired, being truly an incised wound, is subject, of course, to the same general laws. The button fulfils this indication of protection with positive certainty, if its application be properly attended to. It is true that in a deep cavity like the vagina, the opposite walls of which are nearly always in contact, the atmosphere can have little or no effect upon the affected parts. But there are other and far more obnoxious influences to shut out; and of these the urine, in cases of double fistule, is most hurtful, for, as it is not commonly the case that both openings are closed at the same operation, the one first operated on, without some protection, is continually bathed in this poisonous fluid. I say *poisonous*, for few will deny to urine such an influence upon raw surfaces, and the consequence is that failure, from this circumstance alone, oftentimes occurs. Leucorrhœal discharges are also more or less harmful, a fact of which Chelius was aware, but I do not know that any other author has made mention of it."

Dr. B. claims also for the button suture a superiority to the clamp suture of Dr. Sims in the following particulars:—

"1. It is simpler in its construction, and applicable to a greater number of cases.

"2. It affords complete protection and perfect rest to the approximated edges of the fistule.

"3. If two fistulous openings exist, one or both may be closed at the same sitting, according to the inclination of the operator or patient, without reference to the condition of the parts.

"4. The introduction of the sutures does not demand the same exactness in regard to the position of the points.

"5. The independent action of each suture renders parallelism unnecessary; and thus gives the operator the liberty of introducing them in whatever direction may best suit his purpose.

"6. If perfect coaptation be found wanting after the edges of the fistule have been brought together, it is not necessary to remove the sutures, but simply to loosen them in order to perfect the paring.

"7. The apparatus does not irritate, it matters not what the condition of the parts may be, provided they are not in a state of progressive ulceration or inflammation.

"8. The apparatus requires to remain in position seldom longer than ten days."

Experience must determine how far these claims can be sustained.

—

Kiesteine and the Urine of Pregnancy.—Dr. Geo. T. Elliott, Jr., Physician to Bellevue Hospital, New York, gives (*New York Journ. Med.*, Sept. 1856) a good résumé of the literature of this subject, and furnishes the results of numerous experiments made by himself, to determine whether there were any recognizable peculiarities in the urine of pregnancy.

He made a tabular record, he states, of over one hundred and fifty-three cases. "In order that we should be less exposed," he observes, "to the chances of deception or error, we obtained most of the urine from women who applied at my office for a ticket, which would enable them to be attended in their labour by the district physicians of the Asylum—though we did not adopt this plan until we had satisfied ourselves that the appearances did not appear to be affected by the time of day when the urine was passed; in other words, that the 'urina sanguinis' was not necessary to the experiment.

"The urine thus obtained was exposed at the proper temperature in shallow, wide-mouthed glass vessels, holding an ounce or more, and covered with a label referring to the number of the case in the record. A portion of each specimen was tested with heat and nitric acid—with litmus paper—often with acetic acid, as well as boiled with liquor potassæ, contained in bottles freed from lead.

"The daily changes were regularly noted until they could be almost foretold by us in many cases, and the microscope was brought to bear on every specimen many times.

"We thought, and still think, that these observatious should have been made more extensively on the urine of the earliest months of pregnancy, and on the urine of lower animals; but the drudgery of the task, and the result of our researches, have not stimulated us to continue further.

"It seemed to us desirable to notice whether the microscope could reveal any 'globular' or other bodies peculiar to pregnancy, and to this part of the examination Dr. Van Arsdale gave the most faithful and unwearied attention.

"Now, while the urine collected and thus exposed, furnished us with pellicles after various intervals of time, yet did these pellicles differ greatly from each other in appearance and modes of formation. While one-sixteenth of the whole number failed to present a pellicle, still their characteristics are readily referable to certain types.

"To begin with the changes which were the most satisfactory as coinciding with those on which the value of kiesteine as a test for pregnancy reposes.

"First day. Cloud-like deposit, like very thin blue milk dropped in the urine; or, like some fuzzy cotton carefully scraped.

"Second day. Shining specks in the urine, and commencing film on the surface.

"Third day. Film forming well, cheesy odour.

"Fourth day. Film very distinct, tenacious, about a line in thickness, concave on its upper surface, 'glistening like spermaceti,' lighter in colour than the rest of the urine, which has, however, assumed an opaline hue. The white specks which preceded the formation of the pellicle, are very distinct, and adherent to the sides of the glass. Brilliant crystalline specks on the surface. Cheesy odour very distinct.

"Seventh day. This state of things has continued, and the pellicle is now beginning to break up. It commences to crack and separate, showing a darker colour through its interstices.

"The microscope displays now, as it has done some days since, myriads of vibriones and monads, disporting themselves in a dark amorphous mass studded with opaque points, and having imbedded within it, very numerous and well-formed crystals of the triple phosphate, but no globular bodies whatsoever, either in the sediment, pellicle, or intermediate strata.

"Now could such appearances be found in the urine of pregnancy, and the urine of pregnancy alone, the need of the profession would be supplied; but the proportion of such classical specimens was small, and the cheesy odour rarely present, even in specimens equally well marked.

"We have seen a pellicle resembling the foregoing description in every single particular (saving the cheesy odour) form on the urine of a healthy woman, suckling a child four months old, and which required all the milk that the well-supplied breasts of its mother could furnish.

"A female servant in the asylum had been troubled with dysmenorrhœa. She would be faint, hysterical, very troublesome to deal with, and alarming herself, and all the women around her, when her turns came on. I examined the uterus at one menstrual period, drew off her urine with the catheter, and exposed it as usual.

"Hers passed through the changes described, and presented a well-marked, thick, tenacious, fatty scum on the surface, studded with cream-coloured spots, differing in no respect from numbers of our best marked specimens. The microscope displayed the appearances described above. I know that this woman had not been pregnant for two years, and she remained under my close observation for many months subsequently, and therefore these appearances occurred in the urine of pregnancy, in the urine of uninterrupted lactation, and in the urine of an unimpregnated female at a period of time amply remote from a previous pregnancy.

"Neither of these last two specimens gave the cheesy odour, but we soon learned that it was too infrequent to serve as a test of the urine of pregnancy.

"In three specimens from pregnant women presenting the same appearances, and undergoing similar changes, we might find the cheesy odour in one, the odour of putrescent beef in a second, and an unspeakable odour in the third.

"A very common variety of pellicle, and one that we acquired the habit of foretelling with great certainty, is apt to form on the urine of anæmic, anxious-looking women. It is generally of a pale colour, and contains a larger admixture of vaginal mucus. The changes occurring in this kind of urine are very much as follows: the specimen becomes rapidly opaline in colour, without the preceding whitish specks, twenty-four hours being, for the most part, more than sufficient for the transformation; and by that period of time the surface has assumed a glazed appearance from the presence of a film, which, as it does not differ in colour from the urine, might escape observation, unless a probe or sharp-pointed instrument were passed through it; when an even, regular, and slightly tenacious film would be detected. This would remain for variable periods, sometimes for more than a week, becoming thicker and better formed, and giving the best examples of the pellicle resembling the fatty scum of cooled mutton broth.

"Now, in this kind of urine we were able to foretell the appearance of vibriones and monads at an earlier period of time than in any other, they being visible before the crystals of the triple phosphate.

"In some of these specimens, while the change in colour just referred to, and the microsecpical appearances were the same, the pellicle would resemble a thin layer of collodion, adhering tightly to the centre, and sinking with the evaporation of the liquid.

"We have not observed the monads to appear at a later period than the vibriones, as a general rule.

"Again, some specimens of urine would give the cotton-like, cloudy deposit for the first day, and by the expiration of that time, the surface would be studded with brilliant crystals of the triple phosphate, as though diamond dust had been sprinkled there.

"This urine was generally alkaline from the beginning, and when we had recognized this appearance we no longer anticipated the opaline change in colour, nor any of the pellicles that have been described.

"These points would increase in number, become agglomerated, and form a pellicle, indeed; but one dry, irregular, and pointed, which broke up, and fell to the bottom as the others did.

"Another pellicle frequently met with, was one forming rapidly, dry and dark-looking, and rugous as though it had been blown with the breath and suddenly crisped. Under the microscope, vibriones and monads would first appear.

"A gentleman visiting my office, one day, passed some water at my instance, which was exposed under the same conditions as the others. To our amusement, a pellicle, precisely resembling the last described, formed and lasted some time.

"This variety, however, while presenting the cotton-like deposit, does not present the opaque spots and bright oblong points seen in others.

"Other specimens obtained from pregnant women would present a dense, turbid deposit. The urine would deepen in colour, and, after the usual time, from two to five days, an unadherent, clotted, dirty-looking pellicle would cover about two-thirds of the surface, presenting, as usual, the vibriones, monads, and triple phosphates.

"Indeed, so far as the appearances of the pellicles went, we found no type distinctive of the urine of pregnancy; for while the urine of women, whom we knew to be pregnant, furnished us with entirely different pellicles, under exposure to the same conditions of atmospheric temperature and light, we found, even among our limited number of specimens from the urine of unimpregnated females, and men, that pellicles would form similar to those on the urine of pregnant women.

"With regard to the microscopic appearances, we can say, that so uniform were the appearances of vibriones, monads, and triple phosphates, that we soon ceased to allude to them, otherwise, than by their initials.

"While the great proportions of our specimens were acid, we yet rarely met with crystals of uric acid. Urates of ammonia were not infrequent on the first day of exposure, and we have some cases recorded as presenting the urates of soda, and the oxalates of lime were often seen.

"We had hoped that Stark's views might bear the test of examination, and that it might be possible to observe with the microscope some appearance which should serve as a test for pregnancy.

"Nearly one hundred and sixty specimens of the urine of pregnant women have been thus examined, without the disclosure of anything peculiar to the urine of pregnancy.

"Torulæ were not unfrequently met with, and generally, without the stems, present in diabetic urine, and this led to our examination of the urine for sugar, which was done by boiling a portion with liquor potassæ, kept in bottles freed from lead.

"If this test should be considered at all reliable, the proportion of such cases was found to be large.

"While engaged in these examinations, a specimen of urine was brought by a student of medicine, Mr. Bedell, for examination. It was from a patient of his suspected of pregnancy.

"When I saw it (in the evening), it had already stood some days, and a thin, even, light-coloured pellicle had formed—lighter in colour than the subjacent urine, and commencing to crack. The urine was not albuminous, and the microscope disclosed numerous small globular bodies, perfectly circular; regular in size; whitish in colour; transparent in the centre, and opalescent on the edges; floating in the pellicle; sediment and intermediate strata; acetic, hydrochloric, sulphuric, and nitric acids did not affect them, nor were they changed by succussions with ammonia, ether, and chloroform.

"In a word, they answered so fairly to the description by Stark of his 'globular bodies,' that we suspected the woman of being pregnant by all the laws of 'Gravidine.' This patient remained under the care of Mr. Bedell, who knows that she was not pregnant during all the time that she continued under his observation. And as this was the only specimen that presented appearances resembling the globules described by Dr. Stark, we have not been able to confirm his observations.

"One of our specimens of urine from men presented appearances answering pretty closely to Dr. Stark's description, but by the seventh day they had commenced to germinate.

"In short, the result of our labours but enables us to say, that we have seen nothing conclusive as to recognizable peculiarities in the urine of pregnancy. We think that there is nothing positive in its indications, and that its appearances can scarcely even be called 'corroborative.'

"We reached this conclusion slowly, yet without regret; for we had no preconceived views to further, and only desired to marshal an array of facts which might speak to us for themselves.

"It may be interesting to add that one hundred and twelve specimens were tested with heat and nitric acid, in perfectly clean test tubes, for albumen, and but *two* presented that ingredient. They were both primiparæ, and had their feet and eyelids a little puffy, but without any symptom leading them to apply for advice. They were both kept on the use of gentle saline cathartics. In one the albumen disappeared before confinement. The urine of the other was not again examined, but both had natural labours."

INDEX.

CPSIA information can be obtained
at www.ICGtesting.com
Printed in the USA
BVHW081056211118
533723BV00011B/311/P

9 780483 398573